LINTON'S ANIMAL NUTRITION AND VETERINARY DIETETICS

LINTON'S ANIMAL NUTRITION AND VETERINARY DIETETICS

JOHN T. ABRAMS M.Sc., Ph.D.

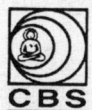

CBS Publishers & Distributors Pvt. Ltd.

New Delhi • Bengaluru • Chennai • Kochi • Kolkata • Mumbai
Hyderabad • Nagpur • Patna • Pune • Vijayawada

Linton's Animal Nutrition and Veterinary Dietetics

ISBN: 978-93-85915-89-5

First CBS Reprint: 2016

Published by:
Satish Kumar Jain for CBS Publishers & Distributors Pvt. Ltd.,
4819/XI Prahlad Street, 24 Ansari Road, Daryaganj, New Delhi - 110002
delhi@cbspd.com, cbspubs@airtelmail.in • www.cbspd.com
Ph.: 23289259, 23266861, 23266867 • Fax: 011-23243014

Corporate Office: 204 FIE, Industrial Area, Patparganj, Delhi - 110 092
Ph: 49344934 • Fax: 011-49344935
E-mail: publishing@cbspd.com • publicity@cbspd.com

Branches:
• *Bengaluru:* 2975, 17th Cross, K.R. Road, Bansankari 2nd Stage,
  Bengaluru - 70 • Ph: +91-80-26771678/79 • Fax: +91-80-26771680
  E-mail: cbsbng@gmail.com, bangalore@cbspd.com
• *Chennai:* No. 7, Subbaraya Street, Shenoy Nagar, Chennai - 600030
  Ph: +91-44-26681266, 26680620 • Fax: +91-44-42032115
  E-mail: chennai@cbspd.com
• *Kochi:* Ashana House, 39/1904, A.M. Thomas Road, Valanjambalam,
  Ernakulum, Kochi • Ph: +91-484-4059061-65
  Fax: +91-484-4059065 • E-mail: cochin@cbspd.com
• *Kolkata:* 6-B, Ground Floor, Rameshwar Shaw Road, Kolkata - 700014
  Ph: +91-33-22891126/7/8 • E-mail: kolkata@cbspd.com
• *Mumbai:* 83-C, Dr. E. Moses Road, Worli, Mumbai - 400018
  Ph: +91-9833017933, 022-24902340/41 • E-mail: mumbai@cbspd.com

Representatives:

• Hyderabad: 0-9885175004   • Nagpur: 0-9021734563
• Patna: 0-9334159340   • Pune: 0-9623451994
• Vijayawada: 0-9000660880

Printed at:
Neekunj Print Process, Delhi

Preface to the Third Edition

THE aims of the third edition of this book remain the same as for the first two, namely, to give a description of the fundamental bases of nutritional science and to provide an account of their application to the different species of animals. As before, Section I is concerned with the general properties of the main chemical constituents of feeding stuffs and with their metabolism in the animal body, thus providing a basis for Section II, in which the various foods are dealt with in turn. A new departure is Section III, wherein the basic needs of livestock for maintenance, growth, reproduction, lactation and work are considered from a general point of view. It is hoped that this section will provide a link between the preceding ones and Section IV, in which last section the practical feeding of the different animal species is dealt with.

Since the appearance of the second edition a great deal of nutritional research has been published; this has necessitated quite extensive re-writing of most of the book. Where there is so much material to choose from, and where, as in the case of nutrition, the field of study has so many related ones, the writer can only select topics to suit his own fancy and risk disagreement with other workers whose bias is slightly different. There are likely to be errors of omission and commission and I should be glad to have these brought to my notice.

So far as the student is concerned there has been no attempt to " write down " the subject. While the effort has been made to cover the field of study as completely and as coherently as possible, the difficulties of the subject and the gaps in our knowledge have not been hidden, for a course of study which leaves students incurious and believing that all the worth-while discoveries have already been made is a complete failure by any standards. Since a time-table which is so full of lectures and laboratory work that the student has no time to read widely for himself is also a failure, I have greatly increased the number of references to original papers, reviews and standard works. Some of the references are to classical papers of historical value, others are given for the sake of the experimental techniques they describe or for their surveys of particular

(iii)

topics, while a third group is included because it gives points of view on subjects still debatable. Although very many tables of data are included they are for the illustration of statements made in the text and not—though this pronouncement will not prevent one kind of student from trying—for memorisation. For "slide-rule nutrition" I have no respect; it is the condition of the animal which determines the course of mathematical calculations, not the converse.

New material for this edition includes chapters on the feeding of goats and on those laboratory animals which have produced the pilot work on which so many studies of the larger species have been based. Enough information is now available to enable a chapter to be devoted to the smaller carnivorous animals. The cat, used for so much physiological research, has received little serious nutritional study; fortunately there is now sufficient evidence relating to the carnivora for one to make reasonable assumptions as to its needs.

With the pressure of the rising world population behind it, nutritional research of the next few decades seems likely to be concerned more and more with efficiency. Problems of animal breeding and management are involved, quite apart from considerations of general agricultural practice, so that the services of many different groups of workers, including veterinarians, will be needed. It is clear that animal ill-health is a luxury the world will be increasingly less able to afford and that, for many veterinary surgeons, the emphasis on their work in the future must be on the prevention rather than the cure of disease. This may necessitate some changes of outlook in higher education since so many candidates for veterinary qualifications find the preservation of good health in livestock rather unattractive whereas the cure of disease seems fascinating. In the last chapter of this edition a very brief account of the efficiency factor in nutrition has been given. It is no more than a short exposition of the nature of the problem; the work has yet to be done.

For their help in preparing the third edition I wish to thank Prof. N. J. Scorgie, Prof. R. E. Glover, Drs. A. Z. Baker and M. Wright of Vitamins, Ltd., Dr. W. M. McKay and the Iodine Educational Bureau, Dr. W. S. Gordon, and Dr. John Hammond, F.R.S. To the Imperial Bureau of Animal Nutrition, the Cambridge University Press, the Nutrition Society and the authors quoted I am indebted for the use of plates 1–14.

My special thanks are due to my colleagues Margaret T. Williams, R. H. Marchant and G. A. Willis, who read through most of the manuscript for me and made valuable suggestions. I am grateful to Dr. H. E. Woodman and the Controller of His Majesty's Stationery Office for permission to use the tables of Appendix 1. Lastly I must acknowledge my indebtedness to the publishers, especially Dr. G. R. Thomson, and to the Eastern Press, Ltd., for their help and forbearance.

JOHN T. ABRAMS.

ROYAL VETERINARY COLLEGE, LONDON.

Preface to the First Edition

In the preparation of this book I have been fortunate in obtaining valuable aid from many friends. My colleague, Dr. R. Stewart MacDougall, contributed the botanical description of the Grasses, a reprint of a former publication in the Transactions of the Highland and Agricultural Society which should be of great assistance to students of agricultural botany; Miss H. Newbigin, of the Poultry Department of the Edinburgh and East of Scotland College of Agriculture, kindly consented to write the section dealing with the Feeding of Poultry; Mr. J. A. More, of the Agricultural Department of the University of Edinburgh, contributed the sections on Grassland and Calf Rearing; my colleague, Dr. Dryerre, wrote the article on Proteins; Dr. G. Scott Robertson, of the Chemical Research Division of the Ministry of Agriculture, Northern Ireland, wrote the section on The Minerals and their Functions; and my colleague, Mr. Wm. C. Miller, in addition to offering many valuable suggestions, wrote the section on Sheep Feeding. The Tables of the Composition and Nutritive Values of Foods given in the Appendix were compiled from many sources, and were prepared in collaboration with Dr. Scott Robertson.

I take this opportunity of expressing my gratitude to my collaborators, fully realising that the utility of the book and any success it may achieve will be due in no small measure to their co-operation.

To Messrs. Sutton & Sons, Reading, I am grateful for the loan of blocks illustrating some forage plants, while to the Publishers I am indebted for much stimulating help, and I thank the Printers for the care with which they have done their work.

R. G. LINTON

Edinburgh, February, 1927.

Contents

Section I

The chemical composition and metabolism of nutrients

Section II

The foods

Section III

Section IV

The feeding of animals

(ix)

Index to Plates

CHAPTER 1

WATER

1. Introduction.
2. The water content of foods.
3. The water requirements of livestock.

(1) Introduction

An animal can lose practically all its fat and over half its protein and yet live, but a loss of a tenth of its water results in death. Rubner's statement of fact emphasises the extreme importance of this element to all living tissue.

Animals can live for a long time without taking any solid food but very quickly suffer if there is a shortage in the water supply. Water dissolves food materials and helps to reduce them to a diffusible state so that the products may pass from the intestinal tract to the tissues. Without fluid the dry matter of food could neither be digested nor absorbed. As a constituent of blood and lymph, water conveys food material to those parts of the body requiring nourishment and removes, for excretion, waste materials which if allowed to accumulate in the body would cause auto-intoxication. The blood also carries ions, the normal concentration of which is a matter of great physiological importance. A sufficiency of fluid as affecting the concentration of the blood and lymph is necessary for satisfactory osmosis. In addition to these most important functions briefly mentioned above, water by acting as a cushion in and between the cells of the tissues provides that natural elasticity that is so essential for the life of the body.

Most of the water which an animal requires is consumed as drinking water or as an ingredient of the food though a small, but for some animals an important part is derived from the breakdown in the body of the carbohydrates, fats and proteins of the food. For example, the combined hydrogen in 1 g. of glucose, of an average protein, or of fat, will give rise to 0.6, 0.4 and 1.0 g., respectively, of water when those substances are oxidised. Thus a maintenance ration consumed by a bullock might produce 4 to 6 lbs. of what is called *metabolic water* per day. This is of little importance to the stock owner for he would be extremely unwise to restrict the supply of water to his stock so that such a small quantity would be of any significance, but is of interest in explaining how it is possible for certain animals to hibernate.

The total water needs of the body vary with (a) the animal itself, (b) its environment, and (c) the nature and quantity of food it consumes.

With regard to the first of these factors water requirements depend upon species, bodyweight, and whether the creature is producing new tissue—as in the case of a growing or fattening beast—or milk or eggs,

(1)

or is doing work. To balance the water used in the formation of tissue or other products and that lost via the lungs, skin, kidney and intestine, there is the water actually drunk, together with water present in the food consumed and that produced metabolically. Vaporisation losses of water depend on the coat covering: they are reduced by shearing.

Under exactly similar conditions the water requirement of the animal varies according to its species; the requirements of a camel are less than those of a horse and those of an old camel less than those of a young one, for in proportion to live weight water requirements vary with the stage of growth. At an early stage body tissues contain more water and require a bigger supply than they do at advanced age when a constant minimum requirement is attained. Shortage of water is thus much more serious in young animals than in old ones; even a moderate restriction may result in a decrease of growth sufficient to be economically important.

The environmental factors of importance include the temperature, relative humidity, and rate of movement of the surrounding air. A fall of temperature from about 22° C. to 15° C. approximately halves the water lost by evaporation from steers: further fall of temperature seems to produce much smaller changes[1]. Much more experimental evidence is needed on these points. It should be noted, too, that in dry regions the water content of the herbage may be little more than half of that of pasture in well-watered areas[2].

The nature of the food influences the amount of water required, for with increasing fibre, or protein, or minerals in the diet, more water is required. In the case of the protein the increase arises from the necessity to dilute the urea, the result of protein metabolism, in the body to an extent which renders it harmless and readily excreted. Thus mammals, especially when highly fed, require larger amounts for that purpose than do birds and reptiles whose waste from protein is excreted in the form of comparatively innocuous uric acid.

Common salt in the diet of an animal, when present in excess of its needs, requires additional water intake for its disposal. For that reason care must be taken when such foods as fish meal are being incorporated in the rations of livestock: the chlorine content of commercial compound foods for cattle, horses, pigs and poultry is governed by the Feeding Stuffs (Regulation of Manufacture) Order, 1947. (Appendix 2.)

For practical purposes it is doubtful if any healthy animal ever drinks too much water voluntarily, and the best results are obtained when all classes of farm stock have free, continual access to good, clean water. A deficiency, even for comparatively short periods, can have nothing but a detrimental effect. That is specially true in the case of high-producing dairy cows which may excrete gallons daily in their milk alone. Cattle, especially house-fed dairy cows when the supply of roots is short, are at times watered in a spasmodic and irrational manner and many veterinary surgeons of experience attribute the common intestinal and stomach complaints of these animals to an actual shortage of water. Other animals too are on occasions not allowed to meet their immediate needs. There is a common belief among horse owners and attendants that horses should not be given water while they are sweating. We know of no evidence in support of the custom, while there is much to be said against it. It is not suggested that horses, or any other animals for that matter, which have been deprived of water for long periods, should be allowed suddenly to consume large quantities of it, but it is true that a horse, provided that it is not to be immediately used at a fast pace, may with advantage be allowed to slake its thirst at any time. It was no doubt the frequent occurrence of colic in tired horses after they had returned from work to their stables that gave a foundation to the belief that they should not be watered immediately, but the virtual disappearance of that class of colic with the introduction of the law governing the length of man's working day showed where the fault in management lay.

The practice sometimes followed of giving fattening animals short supplies of water for a period just preceding sale for slaughter is not to be recommended. While there may be some slight reduction in " shrinkage " after slaughter, this should take second place to the humanitarian treatment of the living animal.

Although a healthy animal will not voluntarily drink too much water, there are occasions when it must consume more than it needs and more than is good for it. When pigs, for instance, are fed entirely on sloppy foods or when cows have an abundant succulent diet such as roots or grass supplemented by wet mashes, the food may thus be made so bulky that sufficient dry matter cannot be consumed. Moreover the moist food causes an undue dilution of the saliva which creates a tendency for the food to be swallowed without preliminary mastication and in a like manner the gastric juices are diluted to such a degree that their efficiency is greatly impaired.

(2) The water content of foods

All foods contain a certain percentage of water. It is found in greatest amount in roots, such as swedes, turnips and mangolds, and in wet brewer's grains, pasture grass, ensilage, etc., which contain 70 to 90 per cent. Any food that has been naturally air-dried retains a certain amount of moisture. The cereal grains such as wheat, oats and barley, contain on an average 11 per cent. of water, and the percentage of moisture is greater in newly threshed corn than in grain that has been stored. Grain that has ripened and matured in a hot, dry climate contains less moisture than that which has been grown in a moist climate and where the temperature is lower. An excessive amount of moisture in stored grain and other foods is undesirable as it favours the growth of moulds and encourages fermentation; the nutritive value of a food is thus decreased and in some cases toxic products may be formed.

The moisture content is important in relation to the keeping property of stored food, but the amount desired is not constant for all foods and conditions, and what may be regarded as a " safe " moisture content depends on several factors, e.g., the physical nature of the food and its chemical composition, the access of air, and the nature of bacterial or mould flora.

Moisture content is directly related to the relative humidity of the atmosphere in which the food is stored. In Great Britain the usual relative humidities of the open air are 60-70 per cent. in summer, and 80-95 per cent. in winter. With a food such as dried grass meal, these figures correspond to moisture contents of 10-12 per cent. in summer, and 18-30 per cent. in winter.' Unless storage rooms are kept closed to the external air, considerable absorption of atmospheric moisture is bound to occur.

The critical humidity for mould growth in dried grass meals is 67 per cent., corresponding to a moisture content of about 13 per cent. The rate of development of mould growth is a definite function of the relative humidity, provided there is free access of air. On very prolonged storage, mould growth may occur at relative humidities much lower than what is normally considered a safe level.

When individual food samples are considered, there are marked variations in moisture limits for mould growth, e.g., a sample of dried grass meal with 16.2 per cent. moisture has been stored for two years and not shown any mould growth, whereas another containing only 12.2 per cent. has shown considerable mouldiness. Much depends, of course, on the mould flora in the material.

Chemical composition affects storage of foods—e.g., high sugar or salt content inhibits bacterial or mould growth.

Hydrolytic rancidity, due to the lipase action of bacteria, moulds or yeasts, is largely dependent on the water content (as well as the temperature) of the food material. In dried whole milk, rancidity may occur if the moisture content is allowed to exceed 4 per cent.

Access of air is necessary for mould growth. If air is excluded it is often possible to store foods with very high moisture content for long periods. Thus silage with about 80 per cent. moisture may be kept without mould growth if well compacted to exclude air. Bacterial growth can occur until the concentration of acid produced is high enough to inhibit further multiplication of the organisms, when the rate of breakdown of the material is greatly arrested. Foods may also be compressed into cakes with a considerably higher moisture content than if stored as meals, but the cakes must be stored so that excessive moisture can evaporate.

Access of air needs to be encouraged in order to assist the drying out of damp foods—e.g., hay stacked at 20-25 per cent. moisture gradually dries out to 15-16 per cent. moisture, and at this figure such long material usually stores quite well. Hay may be baled at 30 per cent. moisture if not baled too tightly and space is left for the air to get in and for the moisture to evaporate.

The percentage of water naturally present in foods affords a convenient method of classifying them. Thus *succulent* foods are those which contain 70 per cent. or more of water, and *non-succulent* foods are those that contain less than 70 per cent.

(3) The water requirements of livestock

The recent review by Leitch and Thomson [4] shows how scanty is our knowledge of the water requirements of farm animals. The most desirable state of affairs is that where the animals have free access to water, but, since that is not always possible, some general relationship of water intake to food consumed needs to be described.

It appears to be desirable that the ratio of total water intake to dry matter content of the food should be about 3 : 1 by weight. For young stock the ratio is perhaps twice this figure, and if calves, for example, are not allowed to have free access to water in addition to receiving skimmed milk, hay and concentrates, they may fail to gain at the maximum rate.

Dairy cows (1,000 lb.) under average conditions in moderate climates, need some 8 gallons of water per day for maintenance alone and rather more than one gallon of water for each gallon of milk produced. If water is not freely available at all times, then it should be supplied not less than twice daily. The feeding of large amounts of succulent foods will diminish the need for drinking water.

Few experiments have been made concerning the needs of horses: it seems probable that the ratio quoted above holds good for them and that an average horse, doing moderately hard work under normal conditions, will need 8 to 10 gallons of water per day.

An adult suckling sow, eating 16 lb. of meal per day will require not less than 50 lb. of water. On the basis of his experiments Crowther [5] recommends a ratio of total water to dry matter of the feed of 3 : 1 at weaning, gradually falling to half of that value as the pig approaches bacon weight. As the moisture content of meal is usually low, these ratios can be interpreted as pounds of water needed per pound of meal fed.

The amount of drinking water required by sheep seems to depend on the pasturage they are grazing. In a temperate climate, with reasonable rainfall, the water content of the grass will be about 80 per cent., giving a water to dry matter ratio of 4 : 1. With high temperatures and low rainfall the ratio may only be 1 : 1, so that sheep may then need about 1 gallon of drinking water per day. The needs for water are also greater during pregnancy [4] and during lactation.

Among other factors the water requirements of poultry depend upon egg production, and the few experiments which have been reported suggest that a hen in full lay should receive not less than 0.05 gallon per day.

The necessity to bring large quantities of cold water up to body temperature causes a heat loss which can well be afforded by any properly

nourished animal which drinks the water. Where an animal is being fed
so sparingly that it is deemed advisable to heat the water in order to
avoid such a loss, a false economy is being practised. The creature should
be fed better, for it is not likely to be suffering from an energy deficiency
alone.

REFERENCES

1. Mitchell, H. H., and T. S. Hamilton, (1936). J. Agric. Res., 52, 837.
2. Cashmore, A. B., (1934). Counc. Sci. Indust. Res., Australia, Bull. No. 81.
3. Wright, N. C., (1941). J. Agric. Sci., 31, 194.
4. Leitch, I., and J. S. Thomson, (1944). Nutrition Abs. Rev., 14, 197.
5. Crowther, C., (1931). J. Roy. Agric. Soc. England, 92, 1.

THE CARBOHYDRATES

(1) Introduction

The carbohydrate group includes a great many substances of different composition, ranging from the monosaccharides, or simple sugars, to the much more complex polysaccharides. Carbohydrates all contain the elements carbon, hydrogen and oxygen, and in most cases the two latter are present in the molecule in the same proportions as they are in water: hence the name carbohydrate. In addition the carbohydrates are either simple sugars alone, or are largely or entirely condensation products of sugars.

The carbohydrates form the greatest proportion of plants used for food. Foods containing a high percentage of them are called carbonaceous foods: examples of these are maize, potatoes and molasses. Calculated on 100 per cent. dry matter basis, maize contains 79 per cent. of carbohydrate (exclusive of crude fibre), molasses 88 and potatoes 84 per cent. Foods of animal origin contain very little; thus greaves (or cracklings) may have 3 per cent. or less and fish meal very little or none at all.

The most important carbohydrates occurring in foods may be classified as shown in the following analysis: —

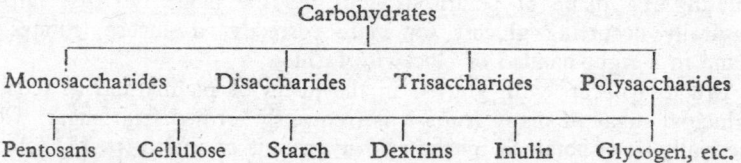

Lignin and hemicellulose† are less well defined substances than the above, but because of their occurrence in close association with those

† See also p. 13.

materials, they are usually considered with them, as are the pectins, gums and mucilages.

(2) The saccharides

(a) Monosaccharides.

The monosaccharides or simple sugars are the simplest of the carbohydrates and, except rhamnose, have the general formula CnH_nOn. They are further classified according to the number of carbon atoms the molecules contain. The most commonly occurring monosaccharides are the pentoses and hexoses (C_5 and C_6 respectively) and these are of importance in animal nutrition; they are soluble in water and diffusible through semi-permeable membranes and can thus be absorbed from the intestinal tract into the blood stream of animals.

The important pentoses ($C_5H_{10}O_5$) in plants usually occur as constituents of the complex carbohydrates pentosans, which frequently serve an important purpose in the structure of plants. Thus xylose occurs as xylans in the xylem of woody stems in most plants and in the hulls of oats, straw, etc. Arabinose occurs as arabans in many gums, and rhamnose (a methyl pentose) occurs in many glucosides and saponins. Ribose is a constituent of plant nucleo-proteins and also occurs in certain animal nucleotides.

The principal hexoses ($C_6H_{12}O_6$) which need to be considered are glucose (dextrose or grape sugar), fructose (lævulose or fruit sugar), galactose and mannose. All the simple sugars possess the property of reducing alkaline copper solutions (e.g., Fehling's solution) and in glucose, mannose and galactose, which may be called aldose sugars, the reducing power is due to the presence of an aldehyde grouping. Fructose, however, owes its reducing power to a ketonic group and so may be termed a ketose sugar.

Glucose occurs in plant seeds, roots, and in various juices (e.g., sugar cane). Of the animal foods it occurs chiefly in root crops, such as swedes and turnips. It circulates in the blood of animals (p. 14) and is formed in the mammalian intestine during the digestion of starch, sucrose and lactose. Commercial glucose is made by boiling starch with dilute sulphuric acid and is often called "brewers' sugar". All the simple sugars have asymmetric carbon atoms and, as a result, are capable of rotating the plane of polarised light. As the name dextrose implies, naturally occurring glucose (or more correctly, d-glucose) rotates the plane in a right-handed or clockwise fashion.

Fructose occurs with glucose in the juices of plants, and as it is the principal sugar of many fruits it is frequently termed fruit sugar. Commercially, it is obtained by the acid hydrolysis of inulin (p. 13). As the name lævulose indicates, naturally occurring fructose rotates the plane of polarised light in a left-handed or anti-clockwise manner.

Galactose does not occur naturally, except in combined form, as in the disaccharide, lactose, in the trisaccharide, raffinose, and in brain and nerve tissue.

Mannose also occurs chiefly in the combined form as one of the more complex carbohydrates.

(b) Disaccharides.

The disaccharides of common occurrence all have the formula $C_{12}H_{22}O_{11}$ and may be regarded as formed from the condensation of two hexose molecules with the elimination of a molecule of water, thus:—

$$C_6H_{12}O_6 + C_6H_{12}O_6 = C_{12}H_{22}O_{11} + H_2O.$$

Similarly, on hydrolysis such a disaccharide molecule will unite with water to produce two hexose molecules: —

$$C_{12}H_{22}O_{11} + H_2O == C_6H_{12}O_6 + C_6H_{12}O_6.$$

The most important disaccharides are sucrose (cane sugar), lactose (milk sugar) and maltose (malt sugar).

Sucrose is the granulated sugar of domestic use and is present in the juices of many plants, such as carrots, beets, and sweet fruits; it is particularly abundant in sugar cane and sugar beet. Digestive enzymes in the mammalian intestine convert sucrose to glucose and fructose : sucrose itself is not found in the animal body. Sucrose is dextro-rotatory but on hydrolysis yields both dextro-rotatory glucose and lævo-rotatory fructose; the influence of the latter sugar is the greater, so that the hydrolysis mixture is lævo-rotatory. Thus when sucrose is hydrolysed an *inversion* of the rotation occurs, so the process is frequently referred to as *the inversion of cane sugar*. Sucrose does not reduce alkaline copper solutions.

Lactose does not occur naturally except in milk, the secretion of the mammary gland, and, occasionally, in the blood and urine of females in whom that gland is very active. This carbohydrate is indeed the only one available to sucklings, in whose intestines, apart from its being hydrolysed there to glucose and galactose, it produces such conditions of acidity and of growth of particular micro-organisms as to assist in the absorption of other constituents of the food, for example calcium and phosphorus. Its presence in skim milk and in whey thus makes these by-products very useful for the nourishment of young animals which are not receiving whole milk. Lactose is a reducing sugar, is dextro-rotatory, and is neither so soluble nor so sweet as sucrose. (See also p. 222)

Maltose is produced by the hydrolysis of starch by the enzyme diastase and therefore occurs in large amounts in germinating seeds, when the reserve carbohydrate (starch) is being mobilised for use by the growing plant. During the hydrolysis of starch, dextrins are first formed and these are then further hydrolysed to maltose. The enzyme maltase, present in the intestinal secretions, can still further hydrolyse maltose to two molecules of glucose, in which form the sugar can be absorbed by the animal. Acid hydrolysis of starch usually gives complete conversion to glucose, so that maltose cannot be prepared by this means. Maltose is the chief constituent of malt extract, accounting for about 50 per cent. of the solid matter. It is not so sweet as sucrose, is íextrorotatory, and reduces alkaline copper solutions, though not so readily as glucose.

(c) Trisaccharides.

The trisaccharides are formed from the simple sugars by the combination of three hexose molecules, with the elimination of water, and may be hydrolysed by an exact reversal of the process.

$$C_6H_{12}O_6 + C_6H_{12}O_6 + C_6H_{12}O_6 = C_{18}H_{32}O_{16} + 2H_2O.$$

Trisaccharides and tetrasaccharides (produced from four simple sugar molecules) are sometimes included in the group polysaccharides, but the latter name is usually reserved for the more complex carbohydrates with very large molecules.

Raffinose is a trisaccharide occurring commonly in plant foods, especially in sugar beet, wheat, barley and cotton seed. Complete hydrolysis of raffinose produces glucose, fructose and galactose.

(d) Polysaccharides.

The polysaccharides may be regarded as built up from a large number of monosaccharide molecules with the elimination of water. They differ from one another (a) in the nature of the simple sugars from which they are derived, (b) in the way in which the sugar residues are linked together, and (c) in the number of sugar molecules condensed together to give the polysaccharide molecule, i.e., in molecular weight. Those which are derived solely from the hexoses may be represented by the general formula $(C_6H_{10}O_5)_x(H_2O)_y$. The pentosans are derived from the pentoses, while the combination of pentoses and hexoses may give rise to perhaps another group of polysaccharides.

Such substances as lignin, pectin, and hemicellulose, which contain substantial amounts of non-sugar residues combined with sugars in the macro-molecule, will not be dealt with in this section.

Starch is the most important carbohydrate, as it constitutes the main food store in most seeds and tubers. In the plant cells it forms characteristic granules, the size and shape of which vary with the botanical species and so give a valuable means of identifying flours and ground foods. Starch grains contain at least two separate carbohydrates, amylose and amylopectin. The latter has a greater molecular weight than amylose, which forms the major part of the starch grain, is soluble in cold water and has no gelatinising power; amylose is also called "soluble starch." Amylopectin, however, swells considerably in hot water, producing the typically mucilaginous starch paste. The starch molecule is a condensation product of glucose. Acids and digestive enzymes gradually convert starch to glucose, but, except at the final stages, the reaction mixture contains an ill-defined assortment of substances, usually described as dextrins, of varying molecular complexity. Those dextrins which are first produced and which have the highest average molecular weight, give a blue colour with iodine: they are called amylodextrin. As hydrolysis proceeds and the mean molecular weight of the products falls, the colour given with iodine changes gradually to red (erythrodextrins) and then to colourless (achroodextrins). Further hydrolysis of the material yields maltose and finally dextrose.

Glycogen, or " animal starch ", which is also derived from glucose, differs from plant starch in molecular structure. Though substances of rather similar type have been found in plant materials, glycogen is regarded as a typical product of animal origin. As isolated from various sources its mean molecular weight ranges from about one to thirteen millions, a very high value for a · substance which is water soluble. Glycogen gives a red or violet colour with iodine. It is most abundant in muscular tissue and in liver, especially in the latter: its function is that of a reserve of energy. It is not attacked by strong alkali.[1]

Inulin, which replaces starch as a food reserve in the tubers of the dahlia and artichoke, is a polysaccharide which yields fructose on hydrolysis. It gives no colour reaction with iodine.

Cellulose is also a condensation product of glucose, but the manner of condensation of the glucose units is different from that in starch, with the result that the two materials differ in some important respects. Both can be hydrolysed to glucose by mineral acids, but cellulose needs much more drastic conditions than starch, and, while starch is easily broken down by the enzymes of the digestive tract, cellulose appears to be quite unaffected. As in the case of starch—and probably most of the more complex polysaccharides—cellulose is a mixture of molecules, all of high but varying molecular weight, rather than a single substance. An important property of cellulose which has been used in modern methods of analysis is its solubility in cold 72% sulphuric acid: when the solution is afterwards diluted and boiled under controlled conditions, the cellulose is fully hydrolysed.

(3) General analytical methods for foods

(a) Limits to the value of analyses.

The chief object of the chemical analysis of foodstuffs is to obtain information as to their probable nutritive value, without having to resort ro time-consuming and relatively expensive animal feeding trials. Such analyses can never be more than rough guides to the livestock owner, and, in order that he may obtain the maximum benefit from such information, he should have some appreciation of the general principles of the analysis of foods.

Plant foods vary in composition from year to year, from season to season, from one district to another, from one plant to another, and from one part of the plant to another: foodstuffs of animal origin are likewise subject to variations in chemical composition. It is important, therefore, that the sample examined by the analyst should be representative of the whole of the material available.

(b) Moisture, ether extract, ash and protein estimations.

A weighed portion of the sample is dried in an oven, under standard conditions of temperature and pressure: the loss of weight gives the water content of the sample, while the residual substance represents the total dry matter. There are various alternative methods for this determination.

Next an aliquot portion of the dry substance is extracted exhaustively with ether for about 16 hrs., the residue then being freed from solvent by drying in an oven. Its loss in weight gives the amount of ether soluble extract present in the food. In some cases the extractable fatty substance (glycerides, sterols, phosphatides, etc.) is weighed directly.

For the determination of the ash content of the sample, a small, weighed portion is heated carefully until all water, fat, protein, carbohydrate, etc., have been completely removed.

It is extremely difficult to isolate and weigh directly the protein of foodstuffs. Usually the nitrogen content of the material is determined by Kjeldahl's method, the nitrogen percentage of the sample then being multiplied by 6.25 to give the protein percentage of the food. The value of 6.25 is only an average one, but the error likely to be introduced by using it, instead of the correct one for the food concerned, is usually small.

(c) Crude fibre determinations.

A weighed portion of the dry,† fat-free substance is then boiled successively, under precisely specified conditions, with 1.25% sulphuric acid and 1.25% sodium hydroxide solution. The insoluble residue is filtered off, washed in turn with water, alcohol and ether, and then dried and weighed. By subtracting from the weight of dry insoluble substance the amount of ash it yields on ignition, the crude fibre content of the food may be calculated. The method here described is the Weende method.

The percentages of moisture, ether soluble material, ash, protein and crude fibre, when subtracted from 100, give the soluble carbohydrate or nitrogen-free extractive content of the food. This last figure, therefore, being a difference figure is affected by all the errors inherent in the other determinations.

(d) Crude fibre content in relation to type of food.

When foodstuffs are thus analysed, a study of the data leads to the following conclusions : —

(i) Fibre is a typical product of plant, not of animal, cells: nitrogen-free extract occurs in traces only in most animal tissues.

(ii) Comparing the foods on a dry matter basis, there are differences between plants. The fibre content of oat grains, for example, is about 10%, that of maize grains 2%. This difference is used as the basis for the further classification of foods, for those containing 15% or more of fibre, based on dry matter, are called coarse foods, the remainder being described as concentrated foods. Thus, although silage contains 5 to

---

† Care must be taken in drying the sample.

13% of fibre, as it stands, it is designated a coarse food, since this is equivalent to 25 to 30% on dry matter.

(iii) As plants become mature, their fibre content increases.

(iv) The fibre in a given plant occurs largely in the stem and the outer parts of the seed coat; that is, it is present in those parts of the plant where mechanical strength is needed. Fibre thus stiffens the stems of plants and gives hard, protective coats to the seeds.

If the analytical data referred to above are compared with the nutritive values of the various plant foodstuffs, when used as the sole item of the diet for a given species of animal, it is found to be generally true that the higher the fibre content of the food the lower is its feeding value: hence the sub-division of foods into coarse or concentrated classes, the latter class yielding the more nutriment.

On the basis of the known behaviour of the simple sugars, the di- and trisaccharides, dextrin, starch, glycogen and inulin, it would be expected that they would appear as monosaccharides in the nitrogen free extract of the Weende process. Cellulose, on the other hand, would be expected to be found in the fibre fraction, which has long been known to contain two other types of material, the hemicelluloses and lignin, which must now be described.

The hemicelluloses are an ill-defined group of substances derived from the pentoses, hexoses and uronic acids, the last named substances being compounds closely related to the sugars and from which they get such names as glucuronic acid, etc. The hemicelluloses have been classified on the basis of their insolubility in water, wherein they differ from starch, and their solubility in dilute alkali, in which they differ from cellulose. Dilute mineral acid converts them to their simple molecular constituents.

When the cellulose and hemicellulose is removed from fibre by the action of cold, 60 to 70% sulphuric acid, there remains a yellow or dark brown residue which consists of lignin, together with some entrained mineral matter. Although lignin contains carbon, hydrogen and oxygen, those elements are not present in the proportions in which they are found in the usual carbohydrates: furthermore lignin contains large amounts of non-sugar residues condensed in the molecule. It is relatively inert and insoluble, and, even more perhaps than the polysaccharides, probably consists of a group of closely related compounds of high molecular weight rather than a single substance.

Lignin, cellulose and hemicellulose are the major constituents of the walls of plant cells, whereas starch and the simpler carbohydrates are present in the cell contents. As plants become mature there is an increased deposition of lignin, and, because of its insolubility, not only is the quantity of lignin in plant tissues important but the manner of its distribution is also of significance. As an outer coating for cellulose and hemicellulose it will protect them to some extent during the Weende digestions with acid and alkali.

(4) The metabolism of nitrogen-free extractive

A big disadvantage of the Weende fibre determination is that the fibre obtained is defined solely in terms of the method of analysis, there being no requirement that it shall be of fixed composition, and, in actual fact, it has long been known that crude fibre is of variable composition. Before discussing the limitations of the Weende method, however, some attention must be paid to what is known of the digestion and metabolism of both fibre and nitrogen-free extractive.

Of the substances which make up the nitrogen-free extract the monosaccharides, present as such in foods or produced by the action of the digestive enzymes on di- or trisaccharides, dextrins or starch, are absorbed from the intestine of the non-ruminant. After absorption such simple sugars may be oxidised to supply the heat and energy for the normal physiological processes of the body; or they may be stored as glycogen; or, as first shown by Lawes and Gilbert, they may be converted to fat, which is then stored.[2] Although the glycogen reserve is readily converted into glucose when required by the body, and although the glycogen⇌glucose transformation occurring in the liver is very important, the actual storage capacity of that organ for glycogen is very limited: it is easily depleted of its glycogen by a few days fasting. To prevent the damage to the body which is produced by an excessively high blood glucose level (hyperglycæmia) storage of glucose as glycogen occurs after a normal carbohydrate meal, while, during later periods, the reverse change is used to prevent harmfully low blood sugar levels. Glycogen may be formed in the body from several sources, including several monosaccharides, but, on hydrolysis it gives glucose only.

In adult ruminants starch and the simple sugars meet a large bacterial population in the rumen, where an unknown and perhaps variable proportion of them is broken down by bacteria and converted into other substances. Starch, dextrin, etc., which reaches the intestine, is absorbed as in non-ruminants.

Information concerning the digestion of hemicellulose is incomplete. Air dried vegetables may contain hemicelluloses so labile as to be broken down by digestion at pH 8,[3] but different species of animal vary so much in their capacity for such digestion that hemicellulose breakdown is best dealt with simultaneously with fibre (p. 17).

Soluble carbohydrate is the main source of energy and is the chief source of body fat; except for carnivora it forms the major portion of the diet of livestock. Fat which is derived from carbohydrate tends to be of the hard, saturated type (p. 24). A dietary deficiency of carbohydrate could be met by increased fat and protein intake, but it is unwise to feed livestock in such a way. Soluble carbohydrates are easily digested and there is nothing to gain and much to lose by underfeeding with them: excessive body-fat formation is to be avoided, however, under any feeding regime, except in the case of livestock being deliberately fattened for slaughter.

(5) The metabolism of crude fibre

The percentage of *digestible* fibre in a food depends on (a) the species and age of the animal consuming it, (b) the nature of the food itself, and (c) the nature of the rest of the ration. .

The young of all species are unable to digest fibre. Just before weaning, under normal conditions, herbivora acquire some capacity for fibre digestion, but even adult omnivora and carnivora fail to deal with more than a small fraction of the fibre of foods. Adult ruminants have the greatest capacity for fibre digestion, an ability which they owe largely to the microbial fermentation which proceeds in the rumen before the commencement of gastric and intestinal digestion. Other herbivora, by reason of similar processes which occur in the cæcum and colon *after* digestion in the stomach and small intestine, come next on the list. Pigs, dogs, and poultry have limited ability to digest fibre.

On the average ruminants digest 55 to 60% of the crude fibre of hay, but the range of values may extend from 20 to 80% depending upon the nature and maturity of the crop.[4][5][6] The corresponding range for the horse is 13 to 33%. Of mixed feeds sheep have been reported to digest 35% of their fibre,[7] corresponding values for pea and bean haulms being 55 and 61% respectively. Pigs have been found to digest 2 to 36% of rye-meal fibre, but it would be unwise to credit that species with greater capacity for fibre digestion than 5 to 10%. The reported data for dogs also vary,[8] and the same general low standards can probably be applied to pigs, dogs and poultry. Present views on the abilities of livestock to deal with food fibre are reflected in the following requirements for compound foods (Feeding Stuffs [Regulation of Manufacture] Order, 1947).

TABLE 1

Species	Maximum permitted fibre content of food, %.
Dairy cows	10.0
Cattle, young stock	8.5
Horses	10.0
Pigs	8.5 – 9.0
Poultry	8.5 – 9.0
Poultry, baby chick	6.0

Although cattle can deal with more than 10% of fibre in their rations, high milk production in cows and good work performance in horses are not compatible with rations high in fibre.

Most of the data which have been recorded for fibre digestibility relate to cattle, and reference to tables (p 469) shows the variation of digestibility of different foods by a given species. The fibres of dried sugar beet pulp, of cotton seed cake, barley grains, wheat bran, and beans are 80, 20, 50, 25, and 60% digested respectively. In general the fibre of woody stems, straws, and seed coats is least digestible: the fibre of young growing plants is more easily digested than that of mature plants. Thus, though the fibre content of young dried grass may be as high as 20%, it is highly digestible and such food must be considered to be a concentrated one. Further points of this kind are made in discussing modern work on the digestibility of cellulose and lignin.

Enzymes capable of attacking fibre are not secreted from the digestive tracts of livestock, and fibre breakdown is the result of bacterial action in the alimentary canal. The balance of nutrients in a diet is important, for it probably affects the relative numbers of organisms in the digestive tract of the animal consuming the food: fibre is less well digested in rations which are high in starch.

The principle products of the digestion of fibre are glucose, the waste gases hydrogen, carbon dioxide and methane, and the lower fatty acids, acetic, propionic and butyric. Though it is not yet known what precise metabolic paths the fatty acids take after their absorption from the rumen, recticulum, omasum and large intestine, they are produced in significant amounts, " in sufficient quantity to supply at least 40% of the fasting energy requirements " of cattle and sheep.[9]

As it is isodynamic with other digestible carbohydrate, digestible fibre is a source of heat and energy for physiological purposes, and it is important in assisting the digestion of compact concentrated foods by opening them up and increasing the surface area of food exposed to the digestive juices. There has, however, been much unscientific speculation as to the part fibre plays in nutrition. Calves have been reared on fibre-free rations and Mead and Goss[10] kept heifers for six years on a concentrate ration low in fibre and found digestion to be normal, though bloating tended to occur if the concentrate were not fed in small portions. On the other hand 5 to 15% of cellulose added to a purified fibre-free diet has been shown to improve the growth of chicks.[11] From the practical point of animal feeding, a fibre-free ration is likely to be deficient in several factors: on those grounds, except in the case of carnivores, it is not to be recommended.

Too much fibre in the ration is undesirable for all very young stock, for pigs, poultry, hardworking horses, and high-yielding dairy cows, as well as for carnivora. Some of the very coarse foods, for example wheat straw, require so much energy expenditure for their digestion that, even in the case of ruminants, the animal consuming them may derive no positive energy gain. Not only is fibre poorly digested in many cases, but its presence may diminish the digestion of the accompanying fat and protein. Barton Mann has attributed increased incidence of coccidiosis in poultry to too high a fibre content of the diet.[12]

Since samples of particular foodstuffs, especially those of plant origin, may vary widely in chemical composition, tables of analyses of foods give only general guidance as to the make-up of a given food. Furthermore, when the chemical composition of the food is known, such factors as the species, age and sex of the animal consuming it, have to be considered in assessing its nutritional value.

From the nutritional standpoint the analysis of foods should be rapid in execution, the chemical fractions isolated and estimated should be constant in composition, and there should be a reliable body of evidence to correlate chemical composition with feeding value.

The Weende method of fibre determination is rapid, but the fibre isolated is of varying composition, and Norman [13] has said that " it would be an important advance if . . . its use in expressing composition were abandoned as inadequate, unreal and misleading ". Numerous attempts have been made during the last two decades to devise better schemes for the analysis of the carbohydrates in foods and it seems likely that the Weende method is approaching the end of its usefulness.

In a sample of foodstuff which has been freed of fat, protein, sugars and starch by enzymic digestion and has then been subjected to the controlled action of sulphuric acid, lignin remains behind as an insoluble residue, cellulose is converted to glucose, and hemicellulose is hydrolysed to a mixture of glucose and pentoses. By combined copper-reduction and fermentation methods attempts have been made to assess the cellulose and hemicellulose contents of the food from the above hydrolysis products.[7] The "total indigestible residue", which is the sum of the three fractions, is appreciably higher than the fibre content: for example the respective fibre contents of clover hay, wheat straw and oat hulls were given at 21, 36 and 30 per cent. whereas the totals of lignin, hemicellulose and cellulose were 33, 57 and 61.

As the accuracy of distribution of the three components within the total indigestible residue is not beyond question in the above method, some attention has been concentrated on the accurate separate determinations of the lignin and cellulose contents of foods. As defined by modern methods of estimation, lignin is virtually indigestible, even by ruminants. Ellis, Matrone, and Maynard found it to be undigested by the cow, sheep and rabbit,[14] Forbes and collaborators found its coefficient of digestibility to be 1% when clover-timothy hay was fed to sheep,[6] and Gray, from a total of 4862 g. in the fodder of animals of the same species recovered 4803 g. from the fæces.[15] Hale, Duncan and Huffman, in their studies of rumen digestion, found 3% digestion of lignin during the twelve hours of active rumen fermentation.[16]

Improved methods of cellulose determination showed little correlation between the fibre and cellulose contents of grass and legume hays: in the growing crops it was found that the rates of increase of fibre and cellulose were about equal in the legumes, whereas the cellulose increased at a greater rate than the fibre in the grasses. There was a steady increase in lignin content as the plants matured. Digestion trials with sheep showed that cellulose content was a better index of digestibility than fibre percentage, so far as those foods were concerned.[17]

Woodman and Evans [18] observed fodder cellulose, obtained by alkali treatment of wheat straw, to be equally well digested (82%) by sheep and pigs when it constituted some 30% of the ration although it had adverse effects on the digestibility of the protein of the rest of the ration.

The results of a number of workers suggest that the cellulose of hay is about 60% digested by sheep.[4][6][7][15]

Although it seems probable that better methods of analysis will lead to improved understanding of the importance of hemicellulose, cellulose and lignin in the fodder of livestock, it must be remembered that the presence and mode of distribution of other insoluble material in plant foods plays a part in the digestion of such foods. Cutinised plant material is highly resistant to digestion,[19] and silica is another substance which appears to have protective properties.

Associated with the fibre of a ration, and sometimes confused with it, is its bulk. The term is used here not to denote the weight associated with a standard volume of food, but with its capacity to form a bulky mass in the intestine. Used in this sense bulk is more concerned with power to take up, and to hold, water from the digestive tract than with fibre content,[20] but far too little is known about the physiological processes which are involved for any standards to be set for the bulk of a foodstuff.

REFERENCES

1. Bell, D. J., (1948). Biol. Rev., *23*, 256.
2. Lawes, J., & J. Gilbert, (1859). Trans. Roy. Soc., 2, 493.
3. Williams, R. D., & W. H. Olmsted, (1935). J. Biol. Chem., *108*, 635.
4. Rutledge, W. A., & R. H. Common, (1947). J. Agric. Sci., *37*, 60.
5. Schneider, B. H., (1947). "Feeds of the world; their digestibility and composition."
6. Forbes, E. B., R. F. Elliot, R. W. Swift, W. H. James, & V. F. Smith, (1946). J. Animal Sci., *5*, 298.
7. Heller, V. G., & R. Wall, (1940). J. Nutrition, *19*, 143.
8. Lössl, H., quoted by E. Mangold, (1934). Nutrition Abs. Rev., *3*, 647.
9. Phillipson, A. T., (1947). Nutrition Abs. Rev., *17*, 12.
10. Mead, S. W., & H. Goss, (1935). J. Dairy Sci., *18*, 163.
11. Davis, F., & G. M. Briggs, (1947). J. Nutrition, *34*, 295.
12. Barton Mann, T., (1947). J. Agric. Sci., *37*, 145.
13. Norman, A., (1939). J. Amer. Soc. Agronomy, *31*, 751.
14. Ellis, G. H., G. Matrone, & L. A. Maynard, (1946). J. Animal Sci., *5*, 285.
15. Gray, F. V., (1947). J. Exp. Biol., *24*, 1 & 15.
16. Hale, E. B., & C. W. Duncan, (1947). J. Nutrition, *34*, 747.
17. Matrone, G., G. H. Ellis, & L. A. Maynard, (1946). J. Animal Sci., *5*, 306.
18. Woodman, H. E., & R. E. Evans, (1947). J. Agric. Sci., *37*, 202.
19. Baker, F., & S. T. Harriss, (1947). Nutrition Abs. Rev., *17*, 3.
20. Procter, F., & N. C. Wright, (1927). J. Agric. Sci., *17*, 392.

THE FATS

1. **The substances found in the ether extract of foods.**
    (a) Glycerides.
    (b) Waxes and sterols.
    (c) Phosphatides.
    (d) Other substances.
2. **The fatty acids and glycerides.**
    (a) Chemical properties.
    (b) Absorption from the intestine.
    (c) The utilization of absorbed fat.
    (d) The nature of milk fat.
    (e) Fatty acid synthesis and degradation.

(1) The substances found in the ether extracts of foods

When a food is subjected to the action of a solvent such as ether or light petroleum, the fatty substances are dissolved out. In addition to the true fats, various other substances, such as waxes and certain pigments, are also dissolved so that the total material removed by solvent extraction cannot truly be called " fat ", but is more correctly described by the terms " ether extractives " or " crude fat ".

(a) Glycerides.

True fats or *glycerides* are esters of the trihydric alcohol, glycerol—

$$CH_2OH$$
$$|$$
$$CHOH$$
$$|$$
$$CH_2OH$$

With a fatty acid RCOOH, where R represents an alkyl† group with the general formula C_nH_{2n+1}, this alcohol can yield esters of three different types, according to whether one, two or three of the hydroxyl groups are replaced by fatty acid radicles, as shown below : —

(1) Monoglyceride, e.g.,

$$CH_2OOCR \qquad\qquad CH_2OH$$
$$| \qquad\qquad\qquad\qquad |$$
$$CHOH \quad and \quad CHOOCR$$
$$| \qquad\qquad\qquad\qquad |$$
$$CH_2OH \qquad\qquad CH_2OH$$

(2) Diglyceride, e.g.,

$$CH_2OOCR \qquad\qquad CH_2OOCR$$
$$| \qquad\qquad\qquad\qquad |$$
$$CHOOCR \quad and \quad CHOH$$
$$| \qquad\qquad\qquad\qquad |$$
$$CH_2OH \qquad\qquad CH_2OOCR$$

(3) Triglyceride, e.g.,

$$CH_2OOCR$$
$$|$$
$$CHOOCR$$
$$|$$
$$CH_2OOCR$$

† or unsaturated olefinic groups.

(19)

Naturally occurring monoglycerides and diglycerides are rare except in fats which have undergone some decomposition, so that the true fats occurring in natural foods may be regarded as consisting entirely of triglycerides. A triglyceride may be further classified as a *simple* or *mixed* triglyceride according to whether it contains one or more than one particular fatty acid in its structure. Thus a mixed triglyceride may be given the general formula

$$\begin{array}{l} CH_2OOCR^1 \\ | \\ CHOOCR^2 \\ | \\ CH_2OOCR^3 \end{array}$$

where R^1, R^2 and R^3 represent different alkyl † groups. Natural fats are, in general, mixtures of mixed triglycerides, for a simple triglyceride derived from a given fatty acid tends to be formed only when that particular fatty acid constitutes 70% or more of the total fatty acids in the fat.[1] It is unusual for fats to contain as high a proportion of one fatty acid as this, though ground-nut oil is one such example.

Since three different fatty acid molecules can be combined with a single glycerol molecule in three different ways, and thereby produce three structurally different glycerides of slightly different physical and chemical properties, the physical and chemical characteristics of natural fats do not depend on their fatty acid compositions alone. Cacao butter and mutton tallow, for example, have very similar fatty acid compositions, but the distributions of the acids within the glycerides are quite different, and the physical properties of the fats differ quite appreciably.

(b) Waxes and sterols.

Waxes do not contain any combined glycerol, but are esters of other alcohols, mostly the monohydric aliphatic alcohols of high molecular weight as, e.g., cetyl (hexadecyl) alcohol, $C_{16}H_{33}OH$ which occurs in spermaceti, and myricyl (triacontanyl) alcohol, $C_{30}H_{61}OH$, occurring in beeswax. Waxes are usually hydrolysed with greater difficulty than glycerides. They are not known to have any feeding value for the common species of livestock.

Sterol esters of fatty acids are sometimes included with the waxes. The sterols, however, are complex alcohols very different from those of the paraffinoid series which give rise to the typical hard, non-greasy waxes, and the sterol esters should be differentiated from the aliphatic wax esters. In most crude fats the proportion of sterol compounds is very small, but there are relatively large amounts in wool fat and in some liver oils. The sterols have been subdivided into two main groups, those characteristic of all animal fats being termed zoosterols or cholesterols and those limited to the vegetable kingdom being called phytosterols. Of the zoosterols the most common is cholesterol, $C_{27}H_{45}OH$, which is abundant in wool fat and to a lesser extent in liver oils, and in still smaller amounts in other parts of the animal body. Cholesteryl

† or unsaturated olefinic groups.

esters (C_2H_5OOCR) occur in blood and other similarly complex lipoids are found in the brain. Many different phytosterols occur in plants, sitosterol, $C_{29}H_{49}OH$, being most common. It has been found in the oils from many cereals, as well as maize, cottonseed, peas, beans and numerous other seeds.

(c) Phosphatides.

The phosphatides, like the glycerides, are fatty acid derivatives. They are soluble in ether, but differ from the glycerides in their solubilities in other organic solvents.

As a group they may be further divided into the lecithins, cephalins and sphingomyelins, the first two classes being quite closely related to the glycerides, for they can be regarded as being derived from glycerides in which one fatty acid radicle in the molecule is replaced by phosphoric acid. In turn the phosphoglyceride molecule is combined with aminoethyl alcohol in the cephalins and with the related alcohol, choline, in the lecithins. It will be seen from the constitutional formulæ of these compounds that there will be different lecithins and cephalins depending on (a) the particular fatty acids which are combined with glycerol, and (b) whether the phosphate linkage is on the middle or on one of the two end carbon atoms of the glycerol molecule. There is evidence to show that one of the two combined fatty acids is an unsaturated one always.

The lecithins and cephalins are important constituents of living cells. Cephalin is concerned in the clotting of blood, but, although the phosphatides have been said to be associated with fat synthesis and transport, their precise functions are not yet determined.

Sphingomyelins are substances which on hydrolysis give rise to fatty acids, phosphoric acid, choline and another base, sphingosine.

(d) Other substances.

In addition to the glycerides and phosphatides, crude fat may contain small amounts of free fatty acids, and there are other substances, such as the glucolipoids, which may be found, though their amount is likely to be small unless the material from which the crude fat was derived contained large amounts of nerve tissue. The glucolipoids are derivatives of fatty acids, the base, sphingosine, and a sugar, usually galactose.

Volatile or essential oils occur in plant foods, but only in small amounts. They may be present in crude fats, but they are usually members of the terpene family, and are in no way related to glycerides or phosphatides. Apart from their power to flavour food, they appear to have no nutritional value, though they may affect the taste of the flesh of animals which consume foods containing them.

Reference is frequently made in the scientific journals to the unsaponifiable matter of fats. This is the fraction of natural fats which can be extracted with solvents such as ether and benzene after the fats have been boiled with an alcoholic solution of potassium hydroxide and the resultant solution has been cooled and well diluted with water: in the unsaponifiable matter occur such substances as the sterols, carotene and vitamin A. During this process the fatty acids, usually present largely in combined form in the fats, are converted into water-soluble soaps. The procedure is often used to separate the vitamin-containing fraction of fats from the rest of the material prior to the quantitative determination of the vitamin potency of the fat.

(2) The fatty acids and glycerides

(a) Chemical properties.

With one single, unimportant exception, the acids which are found in natural glycerides are all straight chain fatty acids, saturated or un-saturated, and containing an even number of carbon atoms in the molecule.

Of the saturated fatty acids, palmitic acid, $C_{15}H_{31}$. COOH, is the most characteristic, with myristic acid, $C_{13}H_{27}$. COOH, and stearic acid, $C_{17}H_{35}$. COOH, perhaps next in abundance, though both are much less common than palmitic acid. Milk fat is unique in showing a complete range of saturated fatty acids, from C_4 to C_{20}.

Of the unsaturated fatty acids, oleic acid, $C_{17}H_{33}$. COOH, is by far the most common, for " in very many fats it forms more than half of the total fatty acids, in relatively few does it form less than 10% of the total fatty acids, and up to the present it has been found absent from no natural fat or phosphatide ".[1] Oleic acid differs from its saturated counterpart, stearic acid, in having a double bond in the $\triangle^9$ position, i.e. between the ninth and tenth carbon atoms, counting that of the carboxyl group as the first;

$$CH_3.(CH_2)_7.CH = CH.(CH_2)_7.COOH$$

while linoleic acid has two such bonds in the $\triangle^9$ and $\triangle^{12}$ positions. Linoleic acid is also widely distributed in natural fats. Of the unsaturated fatty acids which contain three double bonds in the molecule, linolenic acid is found in many vegetable fats: fish oils contain even more highly unsaturated fatty acids.

A glyceride which is derived from a saturated fatty acid has a higher melting point than those derived from the corresponding unsaturated fatty acids with one or more double bonds in their carbon chains. Largely because of this, fats which contain a high proportion of un-saturated fatty acids tend to have low melting points: fish, and many vegetable, fats are thus fluid at normal atmospheric temperatures, while the body fats of land animals tend to be solid or semi-solid under such conditions.

By virtue of their double bonds the unsaturated fatty acids are more reactive than the saturated ones, their most important characteristic in this respect, from the nutritional point of view, being their power to combine with atmospheric oxygen, the change which thus ensues being called " oxidative rancidity ". In general there are two characteristics of the fats themselves which help to determine the rate at which oxidation proceeds. Broadly speaking, the more highly unsaturated the fat, the more rapidly will it tend to become oxidised: linseed oil oxidises quite rapidly to give a tough oxidation product and is thus called a drying oil. The oxidation process is deliberately hastened in the paint trade, so that boiled linseed oil, which has been treated with lead or manganese for such purposes, is not suitable for feeding to livestock. Olive oil is an example of a non-drying oil, and cottonseed oil, less reactive than linseed oil but more so than olive, is a semi-drying oil. Apart from unsaturated fatty acids, the second factor which affects the rates of oxidation of natural fats is their respective contents of anti-oxidants, such as the tocopherols. These protective substances may be largely destroyed during the production of highly refined fats, which then oxidise far more rapidly than the untreated ones. The actual chemical changes which occur during such oxidation processes are complex, there being usually an induction period during which oxidation goes on slowly, followed by a phase of greatly accelerated change. It is not necessary for the change to have proceeded very far before an unpleasant rancid taste is acquired by the fat. What makes oxidative rancidity even more undesirable is the con-comitant destruction of carotene and vitamin A.

A second unwanted type of change which may occur in natural fats is hydrolytic rancidity, when free fatty acid is liberated as the result of the presence of moisture (which retards oxidative rancidity) and lipase. Hydrolytic rancidity is probably less common than the oxidative type, though it is likely to occur where foods have been stored in a damp condition.

(b) Absorption from the intestine.

It was formerly believed that the glycerides are absorbed from the intestine only after they have been converted into free glycerol and the sodium salts of the fatty acids, the reverse change occurring as soon as the absorbed material has passed into the cells of the body: it was necessary to postulate this second reverse reaction since much the greater part of the blood fat is present as triglyceride and not as free fatty acid or sodium soap.

The intestinal contents are seldom so alkaline, however, as to permit the existence there of such sodium salts, and more recent research has yielded two theories of fat absorption. In both instances the bile salts are given an important part to play in emulsifying the fat ingested and in rendering fatty acids diffusible in aqueous media in which the normal long chain fatty acids are normally insoluble.

Verzar [2] believes that the whole of the ingested fat is hydrolysed, that the fatty acids enter the body in the form of bile-salt complexes which are water soluble, and that the phosphatides then play a big part in the conversion of the fatty acids to triglycerides. The triglycerides enter the systemic circulation via the lymphatic system.

Frazer, however, thinks that only a fraction of the fatty acids in the ingested glycerides is hydrolysed, the liberated fatty acids, with bile salts and mono- and diglycerides, then forming a powerful emulsifying system, which rapidly reduces the rest of the food fat to a fine emulsion. When the fat particles have once been reduced to a given particle size they may then be absorbed from the intestine as glyceride, reaching the blood via the lymphatic system and traversing many of the organs of the body before they pass to the liver. The liberated fatty acids, however, are said to pass straight to the liver, thus following a different path from the triglycerides and perhaps undergoing very different fates.'

The problem is a very complex one, with many details as yet unsettled, but Frazer's partition theory has perhaps better experimental support than Verzar's lipolytic hypothesis.

(c) The utilization of absorbed fat.

In the normal case the rise in the blood fat content which follows the absorption of dietary fat disappears within a few hours, either because the fat has been laid down in the tissues, or because, after suitable modification, it has been secreted as milk fat by the lactating female, or because it has been completely oxidised to provide energy for the body.

In well nourished animals masses of fatty tissue tend to accumulate in certain well defined sites, the so-called fat depots. Such sites include the omentum, the subcutaneous tissues and the region around the kidneys. Fat which is stored in this way constitutes a reserve supply of food: it may also function as a thermal insulator and as a barrier against mechanical shock. Much of this reserve fat can be used up with no apparent harm to the animal concerned, though it will lose weight, and, by losing its subcutaneous fat, may forfeit the sleekness of the well nourished animal.

Although the size of the fat depots may not vary much during long periods of time, this does not signify the existence of a static condition, but simply that the flow of fat into those regions is balanced by the outward flow. When food is taken temporarily in excess of the needs of the animal the rate of inward movement of fat to the depots is increased, but the outward transport does not stop, though it will now be smaller than the inward flow, so that the size of the fat depots is increased. During periods of food scarcity the rate of outward flow becomes greater than the rate of deposition and the amount of depot fat diminishes.

Apart from those glycerides which may be carried via the bloodstream from one fat depot to another, the fat which flows into the depots arises from two dietary sources, namely the food fat, and the carbohydrate and protein of the food. Both carbohydrate and protein can be converted into body fat, as was proved long ago, in the case of the former, by Lawes and Gilbert, but, from the quantitative aspect, dietary protein is a minor source of body fat.

When carbohydrates are converted into glycerides in the animal body they yield a rather characteristic firm type of fat, rich in oleic, palmitic and, though to a lesser extent, stearic acids. The absorbed *dietary fat,* however, may vary widely in composition, and, as it is possible to consume quite considerable amounts of fat in the diet, it may be wondered what effect such variation has upon the nature of the depot fats.

The absorbed fat first passes to the fat depots, but the dynamic process to which reference has already been made enables the body to obtain some measure of control of the nature of the depot fat. If, for example, food fat containing a large proportion of one of the shorter chain saturated fatty acids, such as lauric acid, $C_{11}H_{23}.COOH$, is consumed, it may be deposited immediately in the fat depots, but, during the subsequent mobilization of such fat, the lauric acid seems to be preferentially metabolized and does not return to the fat depots. To maintain a reasonable level of such a fatty acid—as glyceride, of course—in the fat depots, there must be steady consumption of dietary fats containing that acid in large amounts. Short chain fatty acids particularly are eliminated by this kind of selection: ingested butyric acid, for example, remains in the tissues for very few hours.[4]

Apart from this the tissues can introduce double bonds into certain positions in the carbon chains of fatty acids molecules so as to give more highly unsaturated fatty acids, or they can reverse the process. In this connection it should be noted that linoleic acid, one of the " essential " fatty acids necessary for the maintenance of life, cannot be made by the body from the closely related oleic acid, and therefore it must be supplied preformed in the diet, albeit only in quite small amounts. The body can also build up (p. 28) fatty acids of higher, from those of lower, molecular weight: this process too is reversible.

However, the ability of the animal body to regulate the nature of its body fat is not unlimited, a fact which is of commercial importance. If, for example, pigs are fed on foods rich in fats containing large amounts of the highly unsaturated fatty acids, then glycerides containing such acids will tend to accumulate in the body fat. Because of the low melting points of the glycerides of this kind, the value of the animal after slaughter may be seriously diminished on account of its liquid or semi-solid carcase fat, and because fats containing large proportions of the highly unsaturated fatty acids tend to become rancid rather quickly.

It has been stated already (p. 14) that a diet consisting predominantly of carbohydrate gives rise to a characteristic type of body fat—at least in the case of land animals. In all cases palmitic acid accounts for about one-third of the total fatty acids, the remaining two-thirds consisting of oleic and stearic acids. The proportions of oleic and stearic acids vary in a manner which is fairly typical of the species, though the amount of oleic acid is seldom less than 40% nor more than 50%. Mutton fat for example usually contains more stearic and less oleic acid than beef fat, which accounts for the differences in hardness and melting point between the two fats. Hilditch has suggested that the experimental evidence implies that the glycerides which are formed in the animal body from carbohydrates consist of palmitodioleins or their hydrogenated derivatives, namely oleopalmitostearin and palmitodistearin. (Note that isomeric forms of these are possible. See p. 19).

CH₂O.P	CH₂O.P	CH₂O.P
CH.O.R	CH.O.R	CH.O.S
CH₂O.R	CH₂O.S	CH₂O.S
Palmitodiolein	Oleopalmitostearin	Palmitodistearin

$$P = \text{Pamityl,} \qquad C_{15}H_{31}.CO—$$
$$R = \text{Oleyl,} \qquad C_{17}H_{33}.CO—$$
$$S = \text{Stearyl,} \qquad C_{17}H_{35}.CO—$$

For a given species there are also differences between the kinds of fat which are laid down in different parts of the body. Fat which is nearer the body surface, for example subcutaneous fat, usually has a lower melting point and contains more oleic and less stearic acid than deeper seated fat. This phenomenon is believed to be associated with the need for fat to be fluid at body temperatures and with the slightly lower temperatures of those parts of the animal body which are near the external surfaces.

In connection with the above relationship attempts have been made to explain species differences in the composition of body fats on the basis of differences of mean body temperatures. Since marine animals have body temperatures about 100°F. and yet their body fat is highly unsaturated and is fluid at normal atmospheric temperatures, it is clear, as Hilditch has pointed out,[1] that the part played by body temperature is not well defined, though, as the preceding paragraph shows, temperature is not without some influence on the nature of the depot fats. It should be remembered that the carbohydrates of foods suffer different fates in different species. In the adult ruminant a significant fraction is converted in the rumen into fatty acids: in the non-ruminant herbivore a similar conversion, though perhaps on a smaller scale, occurs in the caecum: it is only in the omnivorous and carnivorous animals that most of the digestible carbohydrate of the food is absorbed in the form of simple sugars.

High or low planes of nutrition will affect the nature of the depot fats in accordance with the principles already outlined. A high plane of nutrition enables more body fat to be laid down, but the kind of fat which is thus deposited will depend on the nature of the dietary fat and on the proportion of it which is present in the ration. On low planes of nutrition large amounts of dietary fat of low melting point are to be avoided in the case of animals bred for slaughter: for most livestock the fat content of the diet should not be above 3-4%.

The colour of body fat and the manner in which it is deposited have long been used as indications of quality in meat carcases. When animals go back in condition the pigment which colours the fat becomes concentrated and the yellow colour is thus intensified. Old cows which have had many periods of alternating gain and loss of body fat, have a fat which is much deeper coloured than that of young animals which have been gaining throughout their life. Colour of the fat is not an infallible guide to quality, however, as it is also influenced by the nature of the diet and by the breed of animal. Thus grass-fed bullocks, receiving ample supplies of carotene, will yield excellent beef even though the fat is relatively highly coloured. Cattle of the Channel Island breeds, which are noted for their dairying rather than beef qualities, have a much deeper-coloured body fat than other cattle, but amongst the other breeds there may be considerable variations in fat colour which are not always consistently related to poor beef quality. The manner of deposition of fat in a meat carcase has a very important influence on tenderness as it affects the size of the muscle bundles. Meat from young or small animals is tender, having small muscle bundles of what is often termed a fine " grain ". In older or larger animals the grain is coarse, i.e., the muscle bundles are large, and the meat is correspondingly tough. In a well-fattened animal the lean meat is " marbled " by an infiltration of fat between the muscle fibres; this breaks up the bundles and makes the meat more tender.

The fat depots of land animals consist very largely of glycerides, whereas their organs contain, in relation to their glyceride contents, substantial proportions of phosphatides. As a rule the fatty acids in liver phosphatides are, as a group, more unsaturated than the liver or depot glycerides. This appears to be due to the presence in the phosphatide fatty acids of rather less oleic acid, but substantially greater amounts (ca. 20%) of highly unsaturated C_{20} and C_{22} acids than is present in the glycerides. It has been suggested that liver phosphatides play a part in the intermediary stages of glyceride re-synthesis.

Diets which are rich in fat and low in protein or choline tend to produce excessive deposition of fat in the liver: an increase in the choline content of the ration causes a reduction in the liver fat. A number of other dietary constituents have a lipotropic action of this type, but the explanation of the phenomena is far from clear.

(d) The nature of milk fat.

It has been mentioned that ingested fat may also be used to form milk fat. Although the composition of milk and of milk fat seems to be a species characteristic, it is generally true that the milk fats of land animals differ from their depot fats in containing the lower members of the saturated fatty acid series. In carnivorous and omnivorous animals the amounts of butyric and caproic acids present in milk fat are small, but appreciable quantities are found in the milk glycerides of herbivorous animals. Another common feature of milk fats is the presence of lower members of the unsaturated fatty acid series with their double bonds in the same, i.e., $\triangle^9$ position with respect to the carboxyl group as in oleic acid. In the case of the milk fats of the cow, goat and sow palmitic acid constitutes about 25-30% of the total acids.

Milk glycerides are derived from blood fat, not from blood sugar. The precise mechanism is not fully established, but it is believed that such oleo-glycerides as go normally to form the body fat of the cow, for example, are converted into glycerides of the short chain saturated fatty acids by the step-wise alteration of the original unsaturated acids, chiefly oleic acid. The way in which this change might occur is dealt with in the following section.

Since milk fat is derived from blood fat it would seem that the nature of the dietary fat of a lactating animal would influence the kind of milk fat produced, subject to any compensatory mechanisms the mammary gland might possess for stabilizing the chemical composition of that fat. It is important to note that while dairy cows can metabolize linoleic and linolenic acids, present as glycerides in oil seeds or in oil seed cakes, in such a manner as to leave the composition of their milk fat largely unchanged, they are not able to do so with the highly unsaturated C_{20} and C_{22} acids of cod-liver oil. As a result, dairy cows which are given more than slight amounts of cod-liver oil in their rations produce a milk fat which contains appreciable amounts of such long chain fatty acids, whereas the quantities of the lower saturated fatty acids are well below normal. It is undesirable from the point of view of taste and keeping quality of butter fat for such an event to occur, especially when it is associated, as it usually is, with diminished milk yield. The disturbance ceases, however, when the amount of cod-liver oil given to the cattle is reduced to about 2 oz. a day.

Fasting, besides producing a diminished milk yield in lactating cows, also results in the production of milk fat containing much more oleic acid than normal and only about a half of the amount of lower saturated fatty acids: there is also a significant rise in the content of unsaturated C_{20} acids. Recent work has shown that ketosis in dairy cattle brings about somewhat similar, though smaller, changes in the composition of the milk fat. With rapid recovery from the ketosis—following glucose therapy—there was a return to normal composition of the milk glycerides.

(e) Fatty acid synthesis and degradation.

The manner in which fatty acids are built up and broken down in the animal body has long occupied the attention of biochemists, but in this section only those points which have some significance in nutrition may very briefly be considered.

By feeding to animals such types of fatty acid as it is possible to recognize when they appear in the tissues, fæces or urine, several groups of workers during the past forty years have shown that when fatty acids are degraded, the point of disruption is the β-carbon atom, i.e., that which is next but one to the carboxyl group. From a given fatty acid the next lower member of the series, plus either acetic acid or a derivative of acetic acid, e.g., acetyl phosphate, are produced. The new fatty acid may then be broken down in just the same way. This breakdown of fatty acids by two carbon atoms at a time, recalls the fact that the natural fatty acids contain even numbers of carbon atoms in the molecule; it suggests that the synthesis of fatty acids may take place by a reversal of the process and, in truth, some evidence to support this hypothesis has been obtained.[5]

Recent research has also suggested that the two-carbon fragments are disposed of by their becoming involved in the later stages of carbohydrate breakdown (the " citric acid cycle "). Where there is little carbohydrate metabolism, as in starvation, this method of disposal is blocked and it has been postulated that the acetic acid, or acetyl phosphate, produced by fatty acid breakdown then forms the acetoacetic acid which is found in relatively large amounts in the blood and urine of animals in such a condition.

Apart from β-oxidation it is also known that the terminal CH_2-group of the longer chain fatty acids may be oxidized to -COOH. Fatty acid breakdown in the β-position to this new carboxyl group may then occur.

In these kinds of changes there would seem to be the beginnings of an explanation for the existence of the characteristic types of fatty acid which are found in body fats and in milk.

REFERENCES

1. Hilditch, T. P., (1947). " The chemical constitution of natural fats."
2. Verzár, F., and L. Jeker, (1936). Arch. ges. Physiol., 237, 14.
3. Frazer, A. C., (1946). Physiol. Rev., 26, 103.
4. Schoenheimer, R., (1942). " The dynamic state of body constituents."
5. Baldwin, E., (1947). " Dynamic aspects of biochemistry."

THE PROTEINS

(1) The Chemistry of Proteins and Related Compounds

(a) Introduction.

The nitrogenous substances of natural, unprocessed foodstuffs are of two kinds, firstly, the proteins, peptides and amino-acids, and secondly, such compounds as lecithin, choline, etc., which are not chemically related to the first group and which are usually minor constituents from the quantitative point of view.

The direct quantitative isolation and weighing of food proteins is so difficult and tedious an operation that it is seldom attempted. Instead the nitrogen content of the sample is found by Kjeldahl's method and the nitrogen percentage is multiplied by 100/16 to give the " crude protein " percentage. The factor 100/16 is used simply because the average nitrogen content of different proteins is 16%.

The term " crude protein " is employed since non-protein nitrogen is not differentiated from protein nitrogen by this method of analysis. Sometimes the expression " amides " is used to cover all of the material that cannot be classified as " true protein " †, and a distinction is made between the nutritive values of the true protein and the " amides " of a food. Though there may at times be some justification for this (p. 58), the system of nomenclature used and the arbitrary assessment of nutritive values on so casual a method of analysis leave much to be desired.

Knowledge both of the chemical properties and the nutritive values of proteins, peptides and amino-acids has been accumulated with much difficulty during the last hundred years, and the treatment given to them in this chapter is not in the chronological order of development of the subject.

(b) The amino-acids.

(i) Formulæ.

Some twenty * different amino-acids are related to the proteins and peptides in a manner which somewhat resembles the relationship of the simple sugars to the polysaccharides, though the problems of protein structure are much more complex than those of the carbohydrate family.

The names, structural formulæ and other details of the amino-acids concerned are given in the accompanying table, from which it will be seen that all of them contain the elements carbon, hydrogen, oxygen and nitrogen, two of them having sulphur in addition. Each amino-acid contains the characteristic grouping

$$\text{R} \qquad\qquad \text{R}$$
$$\text{HOOC.}\overset{.}{\text{C}}\text{.NH}_2 \quad \text{or} \quad \text{HOOC.}\overset{.}{\text{C}}\text{.NH-}$$
$$\overset{.}{\text{H}} \qquad\qquad \overset{.}{\text{H}}$$

that is, they all have a nitrogen atom linked directly to the carbon atom, the latter being the first carbon atom attached directly to the carboxyl group. In most cases the nitrogen atom carries two hydrogen atoms, the exceptions being those amino-acids, namely proline and hydroxy-proline, where it is linked both to the α - and to another carbon atom, and to one hydrogen atom only.

According to whether the molecule contains equal numbers of –COOH and –NH₂ groups, a preponderance of carboxyl groups, or an excess of amino-groups the natural amino-acids are divided into three main classes, namely the neutral, acid, and basic amino-acids. This classification is a convenient one because the members of a given group, for example the basic amino-acids, usually have some chemical properties in common, which serve to differentiate them from the other groups and which assist in their separation from mixtures of amino-acids.

Within the chief subdivisions there are further sections. The neutral amino-acids, for example, may be divided into the aliphatic, sulphur-containing, aromatic and heterocyclic classes, depending upon whether

† i.e., protein which is insoluble in the presence of copper hydroxide.
* The exact number is not quite certain.

TABLE 2

Class and common name	Structural formula	Mol.formula	Mol.Wt.	N%
1. *Neutral Amino-acids.*				
(a) Aliphatic:				
Glycine	$CH_2(NH_2).COOH$	$C_2H_5O_2N$	75	18.7
Alanine	$CH_3.CH(NH_2).COOH$	$C_3H_7O_2N$	89	15.7
Serine	$HO.CH_2.CH(NH_2).COOH$	$C_3H_7O_3N$	105	13.3
Threonine	$CH_3.CH(OH).CH(NH_2).COOH$	$C_4H_9O_3N$	119	11.8
Valine	$(CH_3)_2:CH.CH(NH_2).COOH$	$C_5H_{11}O_2N$	117	12.0
Leucine	$(CH_3)_2:CH.CH_2.CH(NH_2).COOH$	$C_6H_{13}O_2N$	131	10.7
Isoleucine	$(CH_3)(C_2H_5):CH.CH(NH_2).COOH$	$C_6H_{13}O_2N$	131	10.7
(b) Aromatic:				
Phenylalanine	$C_6H_5.CH_2.CH(NH_2).COOH$	$C_9H_{11}O_2N$	165	8.5
Tyrosine	$p\text{-}HO.C_6H_4.CH_2.CH(NH_2).COOH$	$C_9H_{11}O_3N$	181	7.7
(c) Sulphur containing:				
Cystine	$S.CH_2.CH(NH_2).COOH$	$C_6H_{12}O_4N_2S_2$	240	11.7
Methionine	$CH_3.S.CH_2.CH_2.CH(NH_2).COOH$	$C_5H_{11}O_2NS$	149	9.4
(d) Heterocyclic:				
Tryptophane		$C_{11}H_{12}O_2N_2$	204	13.7

Proline	CH$_2$—CH$_2$ CH$_2$ CH.COOH NH	C$_5$H$_9$O$_2$N	115	12.2
Hydroxyproline	HO.CH—CH$_2$ CH$_2$ CH.COOH NH	C$_5$H$_9$O$_3$N	131	10.7
2. Acidic Amino-acids				
Aspartic acid	HOOC.CH$_2$.CH(NH$_2$).COOH	C$_4$H$_7$O$_4$N	133	10.5
Glutamic acid	HOOC.CH$_2$.CH$_2$.CH(NH$_2$).COOH	C$_5$H$_9$O$_4$N	147	9.5
3. Basic Amino-acids				
Lysine	NH$_2$.(CH$_2$)$_4$.CH(NH$_2$).COOH	C$_6$H$_{14}$O$_2$N$_2$	146	19.2
Arginine	NH$_2$.C(:NH).NH.(CH$_2$)$_3$.CH(NH$_2$).COOH	C$_6$H$_{14}$O$_2$N$_4$	174	32.2
Citrulline	NH$_2$.CO.NH.(CH$_2$)$_3$.CH(NH$_2$).COOH	C$_6$H$_{13}$O$_3$N$_3$	175	24.0
Histidine	CH=C.CH$_2$.CH(NH$_2$).COOH NH—N CH	C$_6$H$_9$O$_2$N$_3$	155	27.1

the group "R" is alkyl, contains sulphur, or contains a benzene or heterocyclic nucleus.

All of the natural α–amino-acids except glycine are optically active by virtue of the asymmetric α-carbon atom: furthermore, although they do not all rotate the plane of polarisation of light in the same way, they are all configurationally related, the hydrogen atom, amino group, carboxyl group, and radical "R" all occupying the same relative positions in three dimensions with respect to the α–carbon atom.

$$COOH$$
$$|$$
$$H—C—NH_2$$
$$|$$
$$R$$

This phenomenon is of biological significance, for, in a number of cases, the animal body appears to be unable to metabolize that geometrical form of certain amino-acids which does not occur naturally.

(ii) *Physical and chemical properties.*

Except for cystine and tyrosine, the amino-acids are quite readily soluble in water. Though glycine has a sweet taste, from which it derives its name, the amino-acids as a class have no characteristic taste.

Apart from that general reactivity of amino and carboxyl groups which is typical of them in whatever compounds they occur, as for example the tendency towards solution of the compound in dilute alkali which the COOH group confers, the chemical reactions of the amino-acids are of interest from two points of view. First there is the diversity of chemical reactions which follows the different natures of the radicals shown as "R" in the above formula, and secondly there is the ability of the carboxyl group of one amino-acid to unite with the amino group of the second, water being eliminated in the process and a "dipeptide" being formed. In this reaction the grouping –CO–NH– is formed, which is typical of proteins and is called the "peptide linkage".

(c) The Proteins.

(i) *Peptides.*

(1) $CH_2(NH_2)COOH + H_2NCH_2COOH$
      Glycine   Glycine
                    $= CH_2(NH_2)CONHCH_2COOH + H_2O$
                                        Glycyl-glycine

(2) $CH_3CH(NH_2)COOH + H_2NCH_2COOH$
      Alanine   Glycine
                    $= CH_3CH(NH_2)CONHCH_2COOH + H_2O$
                                        Alanyl-glycine

(3) $CH_2(NH_2)COOH + CH_3CH(NH_2)COOH$
      Glycine   Alanine
                    $= CH_2(NH_2)CONHCH(CH_3)COOH' + H_2O$
                                        Glycyl-alanine

In the first example of peptide formation shown in the above equation only one "dipeptide", glycyl-glycine, so called because of its origin from two molecules of glycine, is possible. With two different amino-acids, however, as in the second and third examples, two different dipeptides, depending upon which of the amino-acids retains its free carboxyl group, may be formed.

The dipeptides formed in this way still possess both free NH₂ and free COOH groups, and may thus condense with yet a third molecule of an amino-acid to give tripeptides. From three molecules of glycine only the tripeptide glycyl-glycyl-glycine may be obtained, but three different amino-acids reacting together may give rise to six tripeptides. For example, glycine, lysine and alanine will form

1. Glycyl-lysyl-alanine   4. Alanyl-glycyl-lysine
2. Lysyl-glycyl-alanine   5. Lysyl-alanyl-glycine
3. Glycyl-alanyl-lysine   6. Alanyl-lysyl-glycine

and it will be clear that peptides which may be derived from as few as four or five different amino-acids, in this manner, will be very numerous. In this respect the proteins show a type of complexity which is not found in polysaccharides such as cellulose and starch.

(ii) *The structure of proteins.*

By stepwise condensation under carefully controlled conditions, poly-peptides containing between ten and twenty amino-acid residues in the molecule have been synthesised in the laboratory. With increasing molecular weight the physico-chemical properties of such polypeptides, e.g., solubility in water, tend toward those of the simpler natural pro-teins. The essential feature of the protein molecule is, therefore, the repetition of the grouping –C.CO.NH– in long chain, with radicals " R ", which are characteristic of the different amino-acids, disposed to the sides, thus :

$$
\begin{array}{cccccc}
\text{H} & \text{H} & \text{H} & & \text{H} & \text{H} \\
\text{NH}_2\text{CCONHCCONHCCONH} & \cdots\cdots\cdots\cdots & \text{COONHOOOOH} \\
\text{R} & \text{R} & \text{R} & & \text{R} & \text{R}
\end{array}
$$

Where there is a glycine residue in the molecule, " R " will represent a hydrogen atom; where there is a tyrosine residue " R " stands for the group HO.C₆H₄.CH₂, and so on.

Earlier evidence as to the nature of proteins was obtained by studying their hydrolysis to mixtures of amino-acids by acids, alkalis and enzymes. Studies of peptide synthesis, and of the physico-chemical and biological properties of proteins, all of which have contributed to the elucidation of protein structure, followed later.

Plant and animal tissues contain mixtures of proteins rather than single pure proteins. The latter may differ from one another in one or more of the following ways (a) in amino-acid composition, (b) in molecular weight, (c) in the order in which the amino-acids are joined up in the peptide chain, (d) in the geometrical shape of the whole molecule, and (e) the manner and extent of attachment to non-protein moieties, such as carbohydrates. Differences of these types are respon-sible for the very diverse physical, chemical and biological properties of proteins from different sources.

TABLE 3

PLANT PROTEINS

	Arginine	Histidine	Lysine	Tyrosine	Tryptophane	Phenylalanine	Cystine	Methionine	Threonine	Leucine	Isoleucine	Valine	Glutamic Acid	Aspartic Acid	Glycine	Alanine	Proline	Hydroxyproline	Serine
1. Cereal.																			
Wheat	4.2	2.1	2.7	4.4	1.2	5.7	1.8	2.5	3.3	6.8	3.6	4.5							
Maize	4.8	2.2	2.0	5.5	0.8	5.0	1.5	3.1	3.7	22.0	4.0	5.0							
Oats	6.0	2.2	3.3	4.6	1.2	6.6	1.8	2.4	3.5	8.3	5.6	6.3							
Rye	4.3	1.7	4.2		1.3	5.6		3.0	6.2	4.0	5.0								
Rice	7.2	1.5	3.2	5.6	1.3	6.7	1.4	3.4	4.1	9.0	5.3	6.3	24.1		10.3				
2. Cereal by-products.																			
Maize germ	8.1	2.9	5.8	6.7	1.3	5.5	1.8	1.6	4.7	13.0	4.0	6.0							
Wheat germ	6.0	2.5	5.5	3.8	1.0	4.2	0.8		3.8	6.7									
Maize gluten	3.1	1.6	0.8	6.7	0.7	6.4	1.1	2.5	4.1	24.0	5.0	5.0	24.5		4.3				
3. Green crops																			
Vegetables	7.0	2.1	5.7	5.4	1.9	4.5	2.0	2.3	4.1				13.1	5.3			2.5		
Lucerne	4.3	2.1	4.9	5.7	1.6	4.5	1.6	2.3	3.3	6.6	3.6	4.4							
4. Yeast (Av.)	4.3	2.8	7.5	3.6	1.3	4.1	1.0	1.9	5.5	7.4	5.9	5.0							
5. Leguminous and oil seeds.																			
Peas	8.9	1.2	5.0		0.7	4.8	1.2	1.0	3.9	6.4	4.1	4.0							
Soyabean	7.1	2.3	5.8	4.1	1.2	5.7	1.9	2.0	4.0	6.6	4.7	4.2	21.0		17.4	8.8			
Linseed	8.4	1.5	2.5	5.1	1.5	5.6	1.9	2.3	5.1	7.0	4.0	7.0							
Groundnut	9.9	2.1	3.0	4.4	1.0	5.6	1.6	1.2	1.5	7.0	3.0	8.0							
Cottonseed	7.4	2.6	2.7	3.2	1.3	6.8	2.0	2.1	3.0	5.0	3.4	3.7			5.6				
Sunflower	8.2	1.7	3.8	2.6	1.3	5.4	1.3	3.4	4.0	6.2	5.2	5.2			5.3				

ANIMAL PROTEINS

6. Milk, cow																			
Whole	4.3	2.6	7.5	5.3	1.6	5.7	1.0	3.4	4.5	11.3	8.5	8.4	24.2	6.3	0.6	2.8	8.0	0.0	77.5
Casein	4.2	3.0	7.9	6.9	1.2	5.6	0.3	3.5	4.1	9.9	6.5	6.7	13.4	9.7	0.0				4.9
Lactalbumin	3.9	2.1	9.6	4.4	2.5	5.4	4.1	2.7	5.4	10.4	6.4	6.4							
7. Egg.																			
Whole	6.4	2.1	7.2	4.5	1.5	6.3	2.4	4.1	4.9	9.2	8.0	7.3	16.3		2.2		4.3		
Albumin	5.7	2.4	5.0	4.2	1.4	6.4	2.9	5.5	3.8	9.4	7.1	7.3	8.2		3.3				7.6
8. Meat and fish.																			
Beef, musc.	7.7	2.9	8.1	3.4	1.3	4.9	1.3	3.3	4.6	7.7	6.3	5.8	15.4	6.0	5.0	4.0	6.0		5.4
Beef heart	7.4	2.7	7.4	4.4	1.4	5.1	1.2	3.2	4.7	8.4	5.2	6.3	13.3	6.9					5.9
Liver	6.6	3.1	6.7	4.6	1.4	6.1	1.4	3.2	4.8	8.4	5.6	6.2	12.2	6.9	8.5				7.3
Meat scraps	7.0	2.0	7.0	3.2	0.7	4.5	1.0	2.0	4.0	8.0	6.3	5.8							
Meat meal	5.9	2.7	7.2	2.9	0.7	5.1			3.0	7.7	2.7	5.4							
Blood meal	3.7	4.9	8.8	3.7	1.3	7.3	1.8	1.5	6.5	12.2	1.1	7.7	10.3	5.9	23.6	9.2	15.3	13.0	3.3
Gelatine	8.7	0.9	5.8	0.7	0.0	2.1	0.1	0.8	2.0	3.1	1.7	2.8							
Keratin	10.7	1.0	3.2	5.1	1.4	3.7	14.0	1.0	7.2	10.0	5.0	6.0							
Sardine meal	7.4	2.4	7.8	4.4	1.3	4.5	1.2	3.5	4.5	7.1	6.0	5.8							4.9
Wool	10.5	0.7	2.9	5.5	1.5	4.2	13.6	0.6		11.2		5.3							

In Table 3 [1,2] are shown the quantities of the different amino-acids which are to be found in those weights of various proteins which contain equal amounts (16 gm.) of nitrogen. Not all of the data are equally accurate, nor have full amino-acid analyses for all of the proteins been determined, but the values given are sufficient for some interesting comparisons to be made. As a group the plant proteins contain less lysine, histidine, and cystine and methionine than do the animal proteins, but there are big differences within each group. Among the vegetable proteins the cereals are rather poor in lysine, whereas the leguminous seeds tend to contain relatively little cystine and methionine: of the animal proteins gelatine contains almost no cystine, very little trypto-phane and small proportions of methionine, histidine, leucine and isoleucine, while wool protein and the keratins of horn and hoof are rich in cystine. Again there are differences to be observed between the proteins of whole grains and those of by-products such as maize germ. Differences of this kind have profound influences upon the physical, chemical and biological properties of the different proteins.

The molecular weights of the proteins range from about 15,000 to several millions, so that the numbers of amino-acids condensed may be as great as several hundreds of thousands in one protein molecule.

One phenomenon which depends upon the order in which the con-stituent amino-acids are linked together in a peptide chain is that of digestion, for Bergmann [3] has shown that the digestive enzymes are specific in the nature of the peptide linkages which they can hydrolyse. Pepsin, for example, cannot attack all linkages between the amino-acids in the molecule. A linkage between an aromatic and an acid amino-acid is broken by pepsin, under appropriate conditions, only if the second –COOH group of the latter amino-acid is uncombined and there are no nearby free –NH₂ groups to neutralise its effect. Protein digestion thus appears to be an orderly attack upon the protein molecule by a group of digestive enzymes, each of which can perform certain specific functions.

It has been suggested that two peptide chains may become cross-linked, to give a net-like structure, by interaction between reactive atoms or groups of atoms at adjacent points in the peptides.[4] For example, by oxidation of two HS– groups from two simple polypeptides, the grouping –S.S.– bridging the two molecules, might be formed. Though the geometrical form of the protein molecule may have a marked effect on the chemical changes which follow the heating of proteins, or on the resistance of proteins to attack by digestive enzymes, very little is yet known which is of practical application to nutritional problems.

The most important of the proteins which have a non-protein portion attached to them are those enzymes which are built up from proteins, phosphoric acid and members of the vitamin B– complex, and which are vitally concerned in the metabolism of fats, carbohydrates and proteins.

The preceding paragraphs will suffice to show that it is difficult to classify the proteins in a simple manner, and the system usually adopted, though of great value in other fields, as yet has little practical application to problems of animal nutrition.

(d) Non-protein Nitrogenous Constituents of Foods.

In foodstuffs non-protein substances containing nitrogen are found. They consist of a very diverse group of compounds, which includes ammonium salts, nitrates, alkaloids, creatine, and phosphatides. Apart from their being classed as " protein ", unless a more elaborate analytical technique than the simple Kjeldahl nitrogen estimation is carried out, they have some significance in animal feeding. For example, the nitrate content of mangolds which have not been matured by storage, has been blamed for causing scouring in cattle, and there are cyanogenetic glucosides in linseed which, under certain conditions, give rise to hydrogen cyanide to whose effects the deaths of calves have been attributed.

(2) The Digestibility of Proteins
(a) Introduction.

Animals which are given diets free from proteins nevertheless continue to excrete nitrogen in their fæces and urine and fairly soon die in an emaciated condition. Proteins are thus essential constituents of foodstuffs, but research during the past thirty years has shown that the nutritive value of proteins seemingly depends upon their breakdown into *amino-acids* in the alimentary tract and upon the ability of the amino-acids, thus liberated and then absorbed, to meet the qualitative and quantitative needs of the animal concerned. There is no evidence to show that intact proteins or even peptides are absorbed from the intestine under normal conditions, except perhaps during the first day or two of post-natal life.

(b) Protein digestibility.

(i) *Definition.*

The digestibility, that is, the proportion of a given protein which is broken down to amino-acids by the successive action of the gastric and intestinal secretions, depends upon a number of factors, which include (a) the nature of the protein itself, (b) the quantity of protein which has been fed during a given period, (c) any heat treatment or other processing to which the protein has been subjected, (d) the nature of the rest of the ration and (e) biological factors, such as the species and age of the animal concerned.

Because of experimental difficulties (p. 12) digestibility trials do not involve measurements of protein intake and fæcal output as such, but are based upon determinations of the food nitrogen and fæcal nitrogen by Kjeldahl's method.

(ii) *Digestibility of different food proteins.*

The digestion of pure proteins separated from the other components of foodstuffs is not of much practical importance and needs little consideration here. Animal and fish foods perhaps approximate most closely to this ideal, and in their case it is possible to say that tissues which have a protective function in the animal, akin to that of fibre in plants, tend to be least digestible. The proteins of tendon, skin, hair, feathers, and hoof are relatively indigestible, especially the last three, although recent work has shown that even these may be partly digested, provided that they are sufficiently finely divided.[5] The digestion of plant proteins cannot be satisfactorily considered separately from the fibre content of plants.

(iii) *Influence of level of dietary protein.*

Data, collected from the literature, on the apparent digestibility by sheep of the protein of roughages were as shown below[6]:

TABLE 4

Average Protein content of food (on dry basis)	3	5	7	9	11	13	15	17	19	21	23
App. Dig.% ...	21	35	51	55	61	68	72	72	75	78	79

These results with sheep suggest that there is little chance of any appreciable fall in digestibility as the amount of a given protein is increased in a ration up to about 30% of the dry matter, a limit which is normally high enough to satisfy those animals which have the greatest need of dietary protein, namely the very young. Experiments carried out with other species than sheep and with proteins from other sources than those mentioned above have produced substantially the same results.

(iv) *Influence of fibre.*

The relationship between the percentages of protein in roughages and the digestibility of the protein is partly a reflection of the tendency for the fibre and protein contents of hay, straw and other coarse foods to vary reciprocally. In Table 5 data are presented to illustrate this point. The percentage digestibilities refer to cattle, and it is important to remember that, among the plant foods, *wide* variations of fibre content and protein digestibility are found within each group of foodstuffs; the data presented are average ones only. With rising fibre content protein digestibility tends to fall.

TABLE 5

Foodstuff	Crude Protein Dig.%	Fibre Content of Food (dry matter basis)
Straw	40 or less	>30
Hay	60	25–40
Green fodder, fresh ...	70	20–30
Cereal grains	80	2–10
Leguminous seeds	85	4–10
Meat (muscle), fish ...	>80	Nil
Egg, milk	95	Nil

The digestibilities given are called " apparent " because the fæcal " protein ", which is excreted by test animals fed on the foods listed, is assumed to be derived entirely from the food ingested, whereas some of it actually comes from digestive juices poured out into the alimentary tract during digestion. The " true percentage digestibility ", which takes into account such losses, is always higher than the corresponding apparent digestibility. In Table 6 are given averaged data for protein digestibility percentages (true) for different dietary proteins, with sheep as the experimental animals.[6]

TABLE 6

Food			True Dig.%	Food			True Dig.%
Grass Hay	...	...	79	Lucerne Hay	...	...	88
Grass, Pasture	...	...	93	Cereal Straws	...	...	67
Root Crops	...	...	91	Silages	...	...	80
Oil-seed cakes and meals			91				

(v) *The effects of heat treatment.*

There are at least three factors which determine the effect of heat on the digestibilities of food proteins; these factors are, firstly, whether moist or dry heat is used; secondly, the duration of the time of heating; and thirdly the temperature attained. These considerations are relevant to the feeding values of such foodstuffs as hay, silage, dried grass, oil-seed cakes and dried blood-meal, and to the cooking of swill and similar products.

Usually, but not invariably, moist heat treatment of a protein is less destructive than dry heat, other factors being equal. A slightly different but important case is the protection against the effects of high temperatures which the water of foodstuffs exerts: for example, provided that sufficient water remains in the material to prevent its temperature rising much above 100°C., grass may be dried in air currents at temperatures as high as 800°C. without the digestibility of the protein being adversely affected.[7]

With prolonged times of heating, at fixed temperatures, protein digestibility tends to diminish. In the case of some leguminous seeds, *short* periods of heat treatment cause the digestibility to rise, but increasing time then leads to a gradual fall; raw soya-bean, with a protein digestibility for chicks of 77%, is improved by being heated to 130°C./30 min., when the digestibility rises to 88%,[8] an increase sufficient for it to be economically important. Another important example is that of dried grass, which begins to deteriorate progressively, when it is left in the drier after all of the initial mosture has been removed.[9]

High temperatures tend to produce diminished protein digestibility. There is evidence to suggest that solvent-extracted coconut meal, which is processed at relatively low temperatures, contains protein of higher digestibility than samples produced by other methods at higher temperatures,[10] and blood meal is another food which benefits by more gentle treatment. There are a few foods, however, in which an improvement is brought about by moderate heat treatment: soya-bean meal is improved by being heated to 140°C. for about 2 min., although it shows deterioration if the temperature is raised much above that figure for an equal interval of time.

A great deal of work remains to be done on this important subject.

(vi) *Species differences with respect to protein digestibility.*

Relatively few experiments have been made to study the abilities of different species of animals to digest the protein of the same food. Where the fibre content of a food is low, e.g., 10% or less on a dry matter basis, there are few indications of species differences, but the advantage lies increasingly with the adult ruminant as the fibre content of a ration increases. In the case of such foods as maize, oats, decorticated groundnut cake, processed swill and wheatfeed, all foods of low fibre content, the protein is as well digested by pigs as by cattle, but the digestibility of the protein of palm kernel cake meal (fibre 16%) is about 90% for cattle and only 60% for pigs, while comparable values for dried sugar beet pulp (fibre 18%) are 60% and 35% respectively. Pigs are less successful with pasture grass, too. Differences of this kind are also to be expected when one is comparing protein digestibilities in very young and in mature stock.

(3) The Biological Values of Proteins

(a) Introduction.

The proteins of the body-fluids and tissues of animals have to be built up *within* the animal body from amino-acids, and, in the normal case, the only materials available for synthetic purposes are the amino-acids, or substances derived from them, which are absorbed from the intestine following protein digestion. Such dietary sources, which include the proteins produced by micro-organisms in the rumen of ruminants and subsequently digested by the host, must conform to requirements with respect to quantity, digestibility, and amino-acid composition.

(i) *Functions of dietary proteins.*

Dietary protein is needed by the young animal for the increase of tissue it has still to produce, by the pregnant one for the growth of the foetus and the development of the maternal organs of reproduction and lactation, by the lactating female for the milk protein she secretes, and by birds to satisfy the needs for egg production. Even livestock which have simply to maintain their bodyweights must receive protein to offset the otherwise steady loss of body protein due to the continual need for the elaboration of enzymes, hormones, etc., while the convalescent beast has to make good the wastage due to sickness or injury.

Previous mention has been made of the variation of digestibility and of amino-acid composition of food proteins. Since the different organs and tissues of the animal body do not necessarily develop at equal rates, and since the amino-acid compositions of such substances differ from one another even in animals of the same species, the requirements of the body for amino-acids will vary, qualitatively and quantitatively, from time to time. It is not to be expected that the needs for amino-acids for maintenance, growth, pregnancy and lactation respectively will be identical, or even that they will remain constant during any one of these phases. It is clear, therefore, that the problem is complex and that the dietary protein needs of livestock can only be expressed in the most general terms, unless more precise information is available about the food protein concerned and the animal consuming it.

(ii) *Nutritive importance of amino-acids.*

It was proved many years ago by Hopkins [11] that zein, the protein of maize, would only support the growth of mice if it were supplemented with tryptophane, while Osborne and Mendel showed that one of the proteins of wheat, gliadin, which contains little lysine, was not quite adequate for the maintenance of the body weight of rats, and would not support growth unless lysine were added to it. Hopkins later showed that there were big differences between the powers of a mixture of cystine, tyrosine, lysine, tryptophane and histidine and one of leucine, valine, alanine, glycine and glutamic acid to sustain life in rats. In 1912 Abderhalden almost succeeded in satisfying the needs of dogs by feeding a mixture of sixteen amino-acids as the sole source of " protein ".[12]

It was Rose and his collaborators who finally solved the problem.[13] Finding that a mixture of amino-acids, of the kinds and in the amounts which were then believed to exist in casein (which was known to be a satisfactory protein for growth), would not support the growth of young rats, he began a search for missing amino-acids and eventually found a new one, threonine, which was an effective supplement for his hitherto inadequate mixture. Having now a satisfactory growth-promoting mixture of amino-acids at his disposal, Rose then began a painstaking series of researches, in which he studied the effects on the growths of young rats of omitting each of the different amino-acids in turn. Although all of the amino-acids are physiologically essential, i.e., they are an integral part of body protein, not all of them are nutritionally essential and hence need to be supplied preformed in the diet. In Table 7 are shown the essential and non-essential amino-acids for the rat, as given by Rose, in his final paper [14] on the subject.

TABLE 7

Dietary amino-acids for rat growth	
Essential	Non-essential
Lysine	Glycine
Tryptophane	Alanine
Histidine	Serine
Phenylalanine	Cystine
Leucine	Tyrosine
Isoleucine	Aspartic acid
Threonine	Glutamic acid
Methionine	Proline
Valine	Hydroxyproline
Arginine	Citrulline

Subject to certain conditions the growing rat can synthesize the nutritionally non-essential amino-acids when they are not provided in the diet; it cannot synthesize the essential ones except arginine, in whose case synthesis by the body is sufficient for some, though not optimum, growth. In the absence of sufficient quantities of the essential amino-acids (in the form of digestible protein, under normal conditions of animal management), either failure to grow or sub-optimal growth results.

The word " essential " needs explanation. Given a suitable source of amino-groups, $-NH_2$, the body is apparently able to produce at an adequate rate a suitable keto-acid to serve for the synthesis of the non-essential amino-acids. Pyruvic acid, a product of carbohydrate metabolism, can thus give rise to alanine;

$$CH_3COCOOH \quad . \quad . \quad . \quad CH_3CH(NH_2)COOH$$

Although ammonium salts are able to furnish amino-groups in this way, the paramount sources are those amino-acids which are absorbed from the gut in excess of the body's present need for them.

It is known that the young chick needs dietary supplies of glycine, which is not an essential amino-acid for the rat. Again, whereas the maintenance of nitrogen equilibrium (p. 47) in the dog and in adult man requires the presence of lysine, the sexually mature adult rat does not need it [15] even when it has been depleted of body protein.[16] It seems to be clearly established that there are definite differences between the methionine requirements of the rat, dog and man [17][18][19][20] under comparable conditions. Relatively little of the necessary research, especially on the needs of farm livestock, has yet been carried out, but present evidence suggests that roughly the same group of nutritionally essential amino-acids is concerned in the case of each of the different species.

Little is known of the specific amino-acid requirements for pregnancy and lactation, but a body of evidence is now available for comparing the needs of essential amino-acids for growth, simple maintenance, and protein repletion (after being depleted on low protein diets) in the rat.[16][20] Arginine is needed for growth, but apart from that, the same nine essential amino-acids appear to be involved in each case.[21] Here again the subject is in its infancy, however.

The developed ruminant requires special consideration, for, quite early in life, a large, and not necessarily invariable [22] bacterial population becomes established in the rumen. From both the protein and non-protein fractions of the ingested food, amino-acids are synthesized by micro-organisms, and though comparatively little information is available as to the nature of the amino-acids so produced, there is no reason to suppose that those which are essential for the host are lacking. Factors which tend to alter the nature of the bacterial population may thus influence the nature of the amino-acids synthesized and hence affect protein production in the ruminant.* The young ruminant, before the rumen has developed and symbiosis has been established, depends almost entirely on its ingested food material for its supply of essential amino-acids.

Certain relationships within sub-groups of the amino-acids require comment; for example, though phenylalanine and tyrosine are very similar in chemical constitution

Phenylalanine $C_6H_5.CH_2.CH(NH_2).COOH$

Tyrosine $p\text{-}HO.C_6H_4.CH_2.CH(NH_2).COOH$

they are not interchangeable in the diet of the growing rat. The former needs to be supplied in adequate amount in the diet, but, though the animal requires tyrosine, it seems not to matter whether that amino-acid is supplied as such or whether additional phenylalanine is supplied from which the animal can make its own. On the other hand phenyl-alanine formation from ingested tyrosine does not occur: dietary phenyl-alanine is essential.

Methionine is also indispensible for rat growth, but about one sixth of it can be replaced by the other sulphur-containing amino-acid, cystine; since the latter compound cannot alone support growth, clearly cystine may be formed in the tissues from methionine whereas the reverse reaction is not possible.

Glutamic acid or proline may serve as substitutes for arginine in the diet of the growing rat, but they are very inefficient ones.

As in the case of the glycerides and fatty acids (p. 24), a dynamic equilibrium exists in the tissues with respect to proteins and amino-acids. If, for example, muscle protein appears in a particular animal to be constant in amount this is not due to the chemical inertness of this protein but to protein synthesis and degradation proceeding at equal rates.

Any amino-acids which enter the body, following the digestion and absorption of dietary protein, become a part of this dynamic system. If, to take an extreme example, glycine were to be the only amino-acid absorbed after such a meal, there would be an exchange of tissue glycine for blood glycine, and, for a short period of time there might exist in the blood an increase in its glycine content corresponding to the amount absorbed, but because of the dynamical nature of the body processes, such an increase would be derived partly from the food and partly from the tissues.

The animal body cannot synthesize protein from a single kind of amino-acid, however, nor have experiments shown that it has any ability to store, even for a few hours, amino-acid mixtures which are unbalanced for protein production. The amount of protein which may be synthe-sized is limited by the amino-acid present in least proportion. Any surplus of a single amino-acid, such as glycine in the example quoted, or of a mixture of such substances, is rapidly degraded in the liver, where removal of the amino-groups goes on. There is evidence that, for a matter of a few hours, some of this *nitrogenous* portion of the amino-acid molecule may be stored, but failing fresh opportunities for protein synthesis, it is excreted (as urea or uric acid) in the urine within 24 hours. These facts have a very important bearing upon the way in which proteins should be fed to livestock.

(b) Measurements of biological values of proteins.

The argument of previous paragraphs (p. 42) shows that the value of a dietary protein may well depend upon the purpose for which it is needed; for example, a protein which may maintain the bodyweight of a mature animal may be unable to produce a satisfactory level of growth in a young one. Attempts have been made in the past, however, to compare the nutritive values of proteins and therefore some account must now be given of the older and newer methods of approach.

(i) *Use of protein efficiency ratio.*

One method which has been much used because of its apparent simplicity is that in which the nutritive value of a protein is measured by its ability to promote growth in young animals. The original method was that of feeding to a number of groups of animals of the same age and condition a series of diets containing gradually increasing percentages of the protein to be examined. At very low levels of protein intake too little protein would be furnished for optimum growth; at very high levels the protein needs of the animals would be more than satisfied, so that some protein would be broken down and used for other purposes than tissue formation. There would thus be some level of protein in the diet for which the ratio of weight gained to protein consumed (the " protein efficiency ") would be a maximum. Proteins from different sources might therefore be compared on such a basis.[23]

Many workers, however, have found this method too tedious and have simply compared the respective weight gains of suitable groups of animals when given different dietary proteins at some quite arbitrary level in the diet, usually about 10%. A favourite reference protein for this purpose is whole egg protein, which is of very high biological value.

Gains in weight give no indication of the kind of body substance laid down, and the increases might be due largely to bone or fat formation. This point is important from the standpoint of practical feeding, for it is far more economic to produce body fat from dietary fat and carbohydrate than from protein. By selection of animals of suitable age and by careful attention to the adequacy of the non-protein fraction of the diet, such difficulties may be avoided when protein efficiency ratios are being measured.

Using this method in its simple form it is not possible to separate the *two* factors which are concerned in the gains in weight, namely, the digestibility of the protein and the nutritive value of the absorbed fraction. Nor is it easy, though attempts have been made, to say how much of the protein consumed is used for maintenance and how much for the formation of new tissue. Boas-Fixen[24] has reviewed the early work in this field.

A survey of the results obtained with rats, using this method, leads to the conclusions that " protein efficiency is a function of gain in weight rather than a characteristic of the protein fed " and that " proteins are classified relative to each other, and with equal accuracy, by either gain in weight alone or protein efficiency ".[25] There is thus little point in measuring the protein intake of growing animals in this way when they are fed *ad libitum*.

For comparative purposes it may be said for the growing rat, that meat, egg and milk proteins have efficiency ratios of 2.6 to 3.8, barley, wheat and oat proteins give values of 1.5 to 2.2, and peas, beans, and coconut and cottonseed meals about 1.0 to 1.5. It seems probable that this is approximately the order of efficiency for other non-ruminant species.

(ii) *Nitrogen balance methods.*

The second method of comparing the nutritive values of proteins, a method which has a number of variations, avoids the difficulty of trying to trace entire proteins or even amino-acids through their various metabolic paths in the body by concentrating solely on the nitrogenous portion of the molecule. Kjeldahl nitrogen determinations are made on ingested food, on the corresponding fæces, and on the urine which is voided, and it is assumed that the amounts of consumed, undigested, and catabolized protein are proportional to the quantities of nitrogen so determined.

This is the " nitrogen balance " method. An animal which, during a given period, is excreting in its fæces and urine just as much nitrogen as it consumes in its food, is said to be in nitrogenous equilibrium. Where the amount consumed is less than that lost in urine and fæces, the creature is said to be in negative nitrogen balance: in such a case the stores of body protein are obviously being drawn upon. A positive nitrogen balance indicates the laying down of tissue protein, with a nitrogen intake in excess of fæcal and urinary losses.

The limitations of the method in its simplest form are fairly clear. No differentiation is made between the nitrogen, which is derived from true protein or amino-acids in food and fæces and that which is non-protein in nature. Furthermore, it is not possible to trace the paths of particular amino-acids in this way.

Technically the method is comparatively simple, which is one of its greatest advantages, but the theoretical interpretation of the results has caused much discussion. As in the previous method, the determination of nutritive values by nitrogen balances necessitates a careful consideration of the purpose which the dietary protein is expected to serve, i.e., whether it is for maintenance, growth, lactation, etc. The different ways in which nitrogen balance experiments have been used for measuring the nutritive values of proteins are given below.

Method of Thomas.[26]

Thomas determined the amounts of nitrogen lost in fæces and urine by subjects who were receiving a diet which was almost protein free: this loss was assumed to represent the effects of " wear and tear " Milk

or other dietary protein was then added to the diet in known amounts
and the fæcal and urinary excretions were again determined. The subjects were still in negative balance, but the loss was smaller than in the
first experiment. The amount of body protein thus spared by the
absorption of 100 g. of the test protein was taken as its "biological
value". Such values are not constant for a given protein but depend
upon the amount of it included in the diet: different proteins had to
be compared one with another at fixed percentages of the diet. Thomas's
method is concerned with the *maintenance* needs of the body.

Method of Mitchell.[27]

Mitchell attempted to adapt the nitrogen balance principle to the
measurement of the biological values of proteins for growing animals,
namely young rats. He accepted the findings of Folin that after such
animals have been placed on nitrogen-free diets for a certain period of
time (upwards of about four days), the urinary and fæcal nitrogen
excretions attain fairly constant values, the amount of nitrogen found in
the urine representing the constant *endogenous* metabolism, which is
assumed to be independent of the catabolism of dietary protein. In
such experiments the protein content of the diet must not be at too
high a level, or else more than enough may be supplied to meet the
requirements of the body (p. 57): usually the level is fixed at about 10%.

In Mitchell's method a group of animals is put on a nitrogen-free
diet: after the lapse of a few days it may be assumed that the fæcal
and urinary excretions have reached constant and minimal values.
Fæces and urine are then collected over a period of four to seven days
and their amounts of contained nitrogen are measured. Next the animals
are transferred to the test diet and allowed to remain on it for a few
days. The animal body having become adapted to the new conditions,
fæces and urine are collected and analysed as before, the nitrogen of
the food intake corresponding also being measured. There are various
precautions to be adopted.[10] [28]

If, during equal periods of time, "N" represents the nitrogen intake,
"F" the fæcal nitrogen excretion on the test diet, "f" that on the
nitrogen-free diet, "U" the urinary loss on the protein-containing diet,
and "u" the endogenous urinary loss of nitrogen, then the following
relationships are true. ("Protein" and "nitrogen" are here used inter-
changeably.)

Apparent digestibility of protein $\dfrac{(N - F) \times 100}{N}$ % ....(1)

True digestibility $\dfrac{N - (F - f) \times 100}{N}$ % ....(2)

True amount of *dietary* protein absorbed $N - (F - f)$ ....(3)

True amount of absorbed dietary protein
catabolized $\quad\quad\quad\quad\quad$ U – u $\quad\quad\quad\quad$ ....(4)

Amount of dietary protein converted
into body protein (3) minus (4) = N – (F – f) – (U – u) $\quad$ ....(5)

The biological value of the protein for growth, which is the percentage
of absorbed dietary protein laid down as tissue protein, is

$$\frac{N - (F - f) - (U - u) \times 100}{N - (F - f)} \quad\quad\quad ....(6)$$

Numerous researches have been made using this method of determining the nutritive values of proteins. Highest on the list for the growing
rat comes whole egg protein, while meat muscle, milk and isolated egg
proteins give figures which range from 70 to 90 (Av. 80). Rolled oats,
barley and whole wheat give values of 66, 64 and 67 respectively, but
peas and beans are much lower at 48 and 38. Vegetable proteins of
fairly high efficiency include wheat bran, 74, heated soya bean, 75,
maize germ, 78, and cottonseed and coconut meals, 80 and 70 respectively.

Such data as are available for the *adult* human tend to be slightly
higher than the above values, whereas corresponding figures for the
young chick are generally 10-20% lower. It should be noted that the
data given are true when the proteins in question are the sole ones in
the diet: mixtures of dietary proteins present a more complex problem
(p. 53).

Recent discoveries concerning the dynamic nature of the body constituents make it difficult to differentiate between food nitrogen and body
nitrogen, so that this method of assessing the nutritive values of proteins
has been criticized,[29] though Mitchell has pointed out that not all of
Folin's postulates have been proved invalid.[1] It is now known, however,
that the feeding of *single* amino-acids to animals which are on nitrogen-
free diets may actually lead to a diminution in loss of urinary nitrogen,[30]
despite the fact that one amino-acid by itself cannot form body protein.
Recently Bosshardt and Barnes[31] have shown that when a protein is fed
at different dietary levels to a group of animals (mice) and faecal
nitrogen/100 gm. food consumed is plotted against nitrogen intake/100
gm. food, a straight line is obtained. When the line is extrapolated back
to zero nitrogen intake, the value for faecal nitrogen thus obtained is
not identical with that experimentally observed in animals which are
given nitrogen-free diets. Titus,[32] in experiments on cattle, had earlier
obtained results which suggest that faecal nitrogen excretion on a
nitrogen-free diet is not a safe index of the amount of the metabolic
excretion on diets containing protein. Such evidence as this certainly
puts in doubt the distinction between dietary and endogenous nitrogen
metabolism.

Possibly the sparing of body nitrogen by a single amino-acid, as
described, may be due to the fact that the body is constantly forming
certain proteins, e.g., enzymes, from others of quite different amino-acid

composition, and hence the provision of single amino-acids enables some use to be made of the residue from such operations which otherwise would be wasted.

It is scarcely to be viewed with surprise that such an empirical concept as that of the biological value of proteins should fail to describe fully phenomena which are certainly very complex. The more recent studies take greater account of the complexities of the problem than the earlier ones had the chance of doing, however.

Method of Sumner, Pierce and Murlin.[33]

One of the difficulties of Mitchell's original method is the un-palatability of protein-free diets, the subjects losing appetite, so that the amount of food consumed tends to fall below that which is eaten on a protein-containing diet. In such cases there is a doubt whether the allowance made for " wear and tear " is correct.

Sumner, Pierce and Murlin, using the nitrogen balance technique for adult subjects, took as their basal diet one which contained *small* amounts of whole egg protein, instead of being nitrogen free. Appetite is improved by the presence of the protein. Rather like Thomas, these workers then compared the powers of various proteins to prevent the loss of body nitrogen with that of whole egg protein. The test proteins and the reference protein (whole egg) were added to the basal diet at the usual fairly low levels.

Method of Melnick and Cowgill.[34]

Several observers, e.g., Martin and Robison,[35] have noted that for nitrogenous intakes which are about sufficient to produce nitrogenous equilibrium, a graph of the nitrogen gained or lost by the body against nitrogen intake is a straight line. Melnick and Cowgill proved that this was true for dogs even when the proteins being fed were of widely different nutritive values.

Bricker, Mitchell and Kinsman,[35] showed that the curves relating nitrogen intake to nitrogen balance—both expressed in mg. of nitrogen per basal calorie—were linear in the case of adult human beings, for nitrogen intakes ranging from 0 to 4 mg./Cal. The curves could be expressed in the form

$$Y = aX - b \qquad\qquad \dots\dots\dots\dots (7)$$

where " Y " is the nitrogen balance corresponding to nitrogen intake, " X ". For nitrogen equilibrium, where " Y " is zero, the amounts of nitrogen intake were 2.76, 4.76, 2.88, 3.38 and 3.12 mg. for the proteins of milk, white flour, soya-flour, white flour and soya-flour mixed, and mixed foods respectively. These values thus indicate the relative values of the various proteins for maintenance purposes.

The points where the curves cut the " Y " axis give the total loss, faecal and urinary, on a nitrogen-free diet. It is also possible to show that " a " represents the product of the true digestibility of the protein tested and its conventional " biological value " (Section b above).

This method, with the variation of plotting nitrogen absorption instead of nitrogen intake, has been applied to normal adult dogs.[37] The curves are linear only over the range from negative to slight positive nitrogen balances.

In this instance the equation for the curve is

$$Y = kA - m \qquad \ldots\ldots\ldots\ldots (8)$$

where "Y" represents the nitrogen balance, "A" is the nitrogen absorbed and "m" is the total loss of nitrogen on a protein-free diet. If one makes the conventional assumptions as to endogenous nitrogen loss, then, using the symbols previously employed,

$$Y = N - F - U \qquad \ldots\ldots\ldots\ldots (9)$$
$$A = N - (F - f) \qquad \ldots\ldots\ldots\ldots (10)$$
$$\text{and} \qquad m = f + u \qquad \ldots\ldots\ldots\ldots (11)$$
$$\text{whence} \qquad k = \frac{N - (F - f) - (U - u)}{N - (F - f)} \qquad \ldots\ldots\ldots\ldots (12)$$

Thus "k", if expressed as a percentage, has then the same form as the conventional biological value of Thomas and Mitchell, and should not exceed unity, since biological value is defined as the percentage of absorbed protein laid down as tissue protein. Since values of "k" greater than unity have been observed, it is clear that assumptions regarding endogenous losses are open to doubt.[18]

The term "nitrogen balance index" has therefore been suggested for "k": it is the rate of change of nitrogen balance with respect to nitrogen absorbed. Values of "k" for different dietary proteins have been measured to compare their abilities to regenerate plasma protein in protein-depleted dogs.

A more recent method which has been suggested for the assessment of the biological value of dietary proteins, is to feed the protein at a low level of the diet and then determine the ratio of creatinine nitrogen to total nitrogen in the urine: a linear relationship between biological value and this ratio may hold good, but further work will have to be carried out to test the method more exhaustively.[38]

It is of practical importance that experimental evidence has been obtained of a reduction of total calorie intake increasing the amount of body nitrogen utilised, though it does not affect the utilisation of dietary nitrogen. The importance for protein metabolism of having diets which are adequate with respect to total calorie intake has been stressed several times.[39][40]

(iii) *Values based upon amino-acid composition*

The third tentative method of assessing the nutritive values of proteins is that which is based upon considerations of amino-acid composition. It is not yet possible, except in the most general of terms and with the utmost reserve, to express the needs of an animal of a given species and in a particular state of development, for the various amino-acids, so that Block and Mitchell[1] have taken the protein of whole egg, which has a very high biological value for growing rats and whose amino-acid composition is known with fair accuracy, as a standard.

When they wish to compare whole maize protein with their standard, these authors use, not equal weights of the two proteins, but such weights as contain equal amounts of nitrogen. The amount of each of the essential amino-acids, plus the related tyrosine and cystine, in the maize protein, is then expressed as a percentage of that found in the equivalent quantity of whole egg. The percentages for whole maize worked out in this way are: arginine 75, histidine 95, lysine 28, tyrosine 122, tryptophane 53, phenylalanine 79, cystine 63, methionine 76, cystine and methionine together 71, threonine 76, leucine 239, isoleucine 50, and valine 68. Lysine, the most deficient of the maize amino-acids compared with the whole egg, is called the " limiting amino-acid ", and 28 is said to be the " chemical score " for maize protein.

(iv) *Comparison of biological values obtained by different methods*

When these authors compiled a list of dietary proteins in order of descending chemical score (despite the fact that lysine was the limiting amino-acid in some cases only, methionine, cystine plus methionine, etc., being other examples), they found that to a fair approximation it was also a list of diminishing protein efficiency ratios and of biological values for rats.

The correlation was not at all satisfactory, however, when the results were considered in the case of growing chicks. The reason for the discrepancy is not known, though it may be related to the fact that glycine, an essential amino-acid for the growing chick, was not considered. It should be noted that dried whole egg has not the high biological value for the chick which it has for the rat. There are other possible explanations, however, which are best considered separately, after this introduction to the various methods used for the assessment of nutritive vaiues.

(v) *Whole proteins, hydrolysed proteins and amino-acid mixtures*

A question which is of theoretical and practical importance, is whether the respective nutritive values of a whole protein, of an equal weight of the hydrolysed protein, and of its exact chemical equivalent in pure amino-acids, are *strictly* the same.

Unless mild methods of hydrolysis are employed there is always the chance of destroying some of the chemically more unstable amino-acids; differences of nutritive value might arise from such a cause, but over and above this, there is the problem of whether some additional factor is present in whole proteins which is destroyed by hydrolysis. Woolley [41] has claimed that a substance (" streptogenin ") occurs in proteins which is a mouse growth stimulant when added to hydrolysed proteins. Such effects might be due to the presence in streptogenin of a new amino-acid, or of a peptide, which in some unknown way is of value to the organism. In this latter connection it has been pointed out that evidence for a 100% conversion of protein to amino-acids in the intestine has never been presented;[42] it is not the kind of phenomenon which could be proved very easily in any case.

The ultimate cause of the effects reported by Woolley have still to be explained, but in the meantime comparisons of the nutritive values of whole proteins with the equivalent mixtures of amino-acids may be considered. It has been claimed for man that mixtures of the essential amino-acids, in proportions such as are found in whole egg, yeast, cotton-seed meal, etc., and with as much nitrogen, have as great a biological value as the intact protein.[43] This is subject to the reservation that the amino-acids must be of the natural form (p. 34): in actual fact some racemic amino-acids, containing an equal amount of the unnatural form, were fed, and it was only when allowance was made for this fact that the amino-acid mixtures were as good as the intact proteins. For the weight recovery of protein-depleted rats, a mixture of sixteen amino-acids produced as good results as an amount of casein containing the same quantity of nitrogen.[26]

In a review of the needs of the growing chick for amino-acids and protein, however, Almquist[44] says that better growth is obtained with whole proteins than with mixtures of amino-acids.

It seems, therefore, that there is a little doubt still, concerning the adequacy of amino-acid mixtures. This is not solely a theoretical point, although it affects Mitchell's " chemical score " method of assessing nutritive values. Almquist has given a list of the factors which might lead to differences between the nutritive values of amino-acids and those of the corresponding whole proteins. These are, (a) decreased appetite and food consumption of animals on amino-acid mixtures, (b) increased rates of destruction of the more rapidly absorbed amino-acids in the mixture, (c) increased loss of such amino-acids in the urine, (d) increased destruction by intestinal bacteria of amino-acid mixtures, (e) the passage into the body of " ready-made " and biologically important peptides from the digestion products of whole proteins, or (f) the presence in such proteins of new growth factors.

Almquist's first four suggestions have as their basis the idea that an amino-acid mixture may temporarily overload the capacity of the body for absorbing amino-acids and for synthesizing protein from the absorbed material. His fifth suggestion might imply, either that the absorbed peptides could be built up into body protein without further degradation, or that being peptides they would not be so susceptible to abnormally high losses as a correspondingly rapid intake of amino-acids. Almquist doubts whether the sixth postulate is of any great probability. It would seem that the processes of protein digestion and absorption need re-examination.

(c) Supplementary values of dietary proteins.

Related to the last subject are the practically important matters of the supplementary values of proteins and of the effect of processing upon the nutritive values of these food constituents.

It has long been known that some, but not all, mixtures of food proteins, give better growth of young animals and are of higher biological value than the component proteins when the latter are fed *singly* upon a comparable basis. Until Mitchell viewed this phenomenon from the point of view of limiting amino-acids, there was very little chance of predicting the biological value of a certain mixture of dietary proteins from a knowledge of that of each of its constituents. Mitchell suggests that a mixture of two or more proteins will be of higher biological value than its constituents, if its chemical score is higher than theirs, or, in other words, if the proportions of the amino-acids (essential amino-acids plus related ones) in the mixture approximate more closely to the " ideal " whole egg protein, than do those of the individual dietary proteins. The following data are taken from Mitchell's review:

TABLE 8

(Adapted from the data of Block and Mitchell [1])

Dietary Protein (nitrogen)			Chemical score	Protein eff. ratio	Biological value	Limiting Amino-acid
Cow's	milk	100%	68	3.4	84	cystine-methionine
Cow's White	milk flour	50% 50%	60	3.4	—	cystine-methionine
Cow's White	milk flour	33% 67%	53	2.9	71	lysine
Cow's White	milk flour	20% 80%	40	—	50	lysine
White	flour	100%	28	1.1	52	lysine
Cow's	milk	100%	68	3.4	84	cystine-methionine
Cow's Oats	milk	43% 57%	66	—	93	cystine-methionine
Rolled	oats	100%	46	—	66	lysine
Beef (musc.)		100%	71	3.1	—	cystine-methionine
Beef White flour		50% 50%	59	3.0	—	methionine
White	flour	100%	28	1.1	52	lysine
Beef (musc.)		100%	71	3.1	—	cystine-methionine
Beef Maize meal		50% 50%	64	3.2	—	Isoleucine
Maize	meal	100%	28	1.2	—	lysine

It is especially noteworthy that where admixture of dietary proteins gives a chemical score higher than the single components, then, within reasonable limits of experimental error, the protein efficiency or biological value of the mixture is higher also.

The results quoted by these authors apply to rat growth; it is pertinent therefore to enquire whether the method can be applied to other species, or to other physiological conditions than growth.

The adult ruminant is unique, in that it can draw upon bacterial protein in addition to that in its fodder. It might be thought, therefore, that food proteins of different biological values for the rat would differ much less when tested on such species. Trials with sheep have supported this contention,[45] but it has also been suggested, and received experimental support, that lysine is a critical amino-acid for milk production in cattle, since many vegetable proteins are deficient in this amino-acid as compared with milk protein; beans and peas, being relatively good sources of lysine, supplement the relatively deficient cereal grains. Almquist and Grau [46] have applied the method successfully to rations for chicks, using the protein from sesame seed or soya-bean alone, or from mixtures of various proportions of the two; they found that the best ratio was that which they had calculated beforehand on the basis of the methionine contents of the two proteins.

Mitchell's method of approach is thus useful, provided it is realized that a protein may be very deficient in more than one amino-acid and that one cannot expect too great a precision, in the prediction of relative nutritive values of proteins and protein mixtures based solely upon amino-acid composition, no matter how accurately the latter may have been determined. Recent work has shown that the amino-acids of food proteins are not all released at the same rates during the process of digestion. For rats the essential amino-acids of beef were completely available, but only 65% of the lysine in cottonseed flour was absorbed.[47] Similar phenomena are doubtless characteristic of other species and other foods (the influence of dietary fibre on protein digestibility should be remembered).

There are numerous other examples of the supplementary values of proteins which have more of an empirical basis than a theoretical one as yet. Maize and meat meal together are more effective for the growth of pigs than either is alone; the cereal grains, in fact, fit in very well with meat, fish and milk proteins in this way. For rats dried yeast has proved an efficient supplement for whole wheat and whole maize respectively.[48] For poultry soya-bean meal provides a better supplement for mixtures of maize and maize gluten, and of maize and wheat middlings, than the animal proteins derived from fishmeal and meat scrap respectively;[49] a ration containing wheat, wheat middlings and fishmeal was less successful than one which contained only the vegetable proteins. With cows as the experimental animals Morris and Wright made interesting use of the nitrogen balance method to study the biological values for milk production of a number of dietary proteins, these last being given with oats as supplement to maintenance rations. Under these conditions the values for blood meal, pea meal, bean meal, meat meal, and decorticated groundnut cake, plus flaked maize were 73, 64, 59, 55 and 52 respectively. The groundnut alone gave a value of 50, and linseed one of 46.[50] In this research the possible importance of the amino-acids lysine and tryptophane for milk production was suggested. Spring grass, whether fresh, dried or ensiled, also has a biological value of 75-80, but autumn grass gives values 10-15 units lower. The high figures for peas, beans and grass are noteworthy.

No mention has yet been made of the time factor in these supplementary relationships. It is, however, a very important one, for the animal body cannot store surplus amino-acids for any appreciable period of time. For example, although tryptophane, methionine and lysine are each effective supplements for certain protein preparations when they are fed together with them, they have no such virtue if they are given several hours afterwards.[51] In terms of animal management, and especially in the case of non-ruminants, this means that rations should be so compounded that full use is made of the amino-acid composition and availability of each of the constituents, the various ingredients being fed *together*. Quite apart from any supplementary values of the proteins it should be noted that, on numerous occasions, a very rapid loss of appetite has been reported in animals which are given food deficient in an essential amino-acid; it is quite possible that partial deficiencies may lead to some loss of appetite. Almquist[41] has observed that even though all the rest be present in full amount, the omission of a single essential amino-acid has the same effect on chicks as a complete lack of protein.

(d) Effect of processing upon biological values.

The processing and cooking of food proteins can have marked effects on their nutritive values, either by direct effect on digestibility, as described previously, or by chemical changes in the actual amino-acids. Casein loses some of its nutritive value when it is heated to 140°C.,[52] such loss being made good when lysine is added to the heat-treated protein. From this it might appear that lysine is chemically changed and made unavailable to the animal organism by the heat treatment, but recent work suggests that rather than the complete destruction of lysine, such heat may result in the second amino-group in lysine forming new types of peptide linkages which are resistant to digestion.[53] Lysine, though the most sensitive to the influence of heat, is probably not the only amino-acid to be affected; information is lacking on this point, the practical importance of which may be gauged by the change of a protein efficiency ratio from 3.3 to 0-0.8 as a result of drying a food and then baking it at 130°C. for forty to sixty minutes.

The grinding of proteins has also been found to have a deleterious effect upon them,[5] although it is probably negligible for ordinary foods. It has also been shown, that the bleaching of flour by the use of nitrogen trichloride—a former commercial operation—produces changes in the protein, such that the subsequent feeding of the product in adequate amounts to dogs can lead to a form of canine hysteria.[54]

(e) Net utilization of proteins.

The biological value of a protein, though a useful index of the nutritive value of the latter, is only one of three equally important factors from the point of view of economic efficiency.

The product of biological value and corresponding true digestibility, is an index of the " net utilization " of a protein:[1] it is the percentage of food protein *ingested* which is converted into body protein.

If one wishes to compare two foods as suppliers of body protein, this may be done by multiplying their respective protein contents by the net utilization. The figure obtained gives, as a percentage, the fraction of the *food* which is convertible to body protein. The following example illustrates this point.

TABLE 9

1 Food	2 Protein %	3 Biol. Value (rat)	4 True % dig.	5 Net utilization	2 x 5
Wheat Germ	.20	75	95	71	14.2
Pea Meal	22	48	92	44	9.6
Linseed Cake	30	78	94	73	21.9

Calculations of this kind should only be made, bearing in mind that digestibility data and biological values should be selected for the species of animal to be fed and for the particular purpose envisaged.

(f) Importance of suitable levels of dietary protein in animal feeding.

Protein is not stored in the normal adult animal except to a very limited degree (the building up of body tissue during pregnancy is a special case). A beast which has been undernourished during a lengthy period may have used up some of its own body protein during that time and a loss of such a kind will be gradually made good when it is again fed on a higher nutritional plane. Apart from cases of this type, however, the feeding of rations containing high proportions of protein is uneconomic and perhaps physiologically undesirable, if only for the reason that a diet containing disproportionately large amounts of one food constituent is likely to be equally deficient in some others. Above certain limits of protein intake, it has been shown that neither the growth rate nor the leanness of the carcase of pigs, nor the yield or composition of the milk of cows is improved by high protein feeding.

Though this subject is dealt with in detail elsewhere, it may be said that a *rough* guide to the amounts of average dietary protein to be fed to livestock in different conditions, is as follows:

Growth, early stages	25%	of total digestible energy of diet from protein
Maintenance	5-10%	„ „ „ „ „ „ „ „
Pregnancy, last third of	15%	„ „ „ „ „ „ „ „
Poor lactation	12%	„ „ „ „ „ „ „ „
Heavy lactation	16%	„ „ „ „ „ „ „ „
Work	5- 7%	„ „ „ „ „ „ „ „

(g) Non-protein nitrogen compounds as substitutes for dietary protein.

A great deal of work has been done in recent years to determine how efficiently, and in what quantity, the micro-organisms of the digestive tracts of ruminants can synthesise protein from non-protein nitrogen, such synthetic protein being digested subsequently by the host.

McNaught and Smith[55] have recently reviewed this important subject. They re-emphasize the bacterial degradation of protein which, in addition to protein synthesis, is brought about by the bacteria of the rumen, and point out the logical conclusion, that determinations of the biological values of proteins for non-ruminants have little application to the growth and maintenance needs of ruminants. They state that the efficiency of utilization of dietary nitrogen will depend on the balance between the amount of protein synthesised by the bacteria and the quantity of simple nitrogenous material in the diet, whether the latter consists of non-protein substances, such as urea, or of easily degraded soluble protein. In turn the rate of synthesis of bacterial protein depends upon the starch supply. Simple nitrogenous substances not used for protein synthesis are lost to the body.

As a result of these considerations, the above authors conclude that the use of urea and similar simple nitrogen compounds will only be successful when the diet is rich in starch and poor in protein, and when, moreover, that protein is sparingly soluble in rumen fluid. They also conclude that it may be wise to continue to regard the non-protein, or amide, nitrogen of foodstuffs as having only half the nutritive value of true protein for ruminants.

Experiments, not only with urea but also with ammonium compounds, which have been made to test the efficiency of non-protein nitrogen as a source of protein for cattle and sheep, tend to show that there is maximum efficiency of utilization of these materials, when they constitute about 40% of the total dietary nitrogen. From the aspect of toxicity that level should not be exceeded.

The problem of using urea for the production of milk protein by ruminants is more complex than that of making provision solely for maintenance and growth. In the case of high yielding cows the required rate of production of milk protein is so high as to cause doubt concerning the capacity of the rumen bacteria to produce it from simple nitrogen compounds.

Experiments made with non-ruminants have failed to show that urea has any value for protein synthesis.

REFERENCES.

1. Block, R. J., & H. H. Mitchell, (1946-47). Nutrition Abs. Rev., 16, 249.
2. Block, R. J., (1945). " Advances in Protein Chemistry, II ", 119.
3. Bergmann, M., (1942). " Advances in Enzymology ", 2, 49.
4. Chibnall, A. C., (1942). Proc. Roy. Soc. (B)., 131, 136.
5. Newell, G. W., & C. A. Elvehjem, (1947). J. Nutrition, 33, 673.
6. Blaxter, K. L., & H. H. Mitchell, (1948). J. Animal Sci. 7, 351.
7. Watson, S. J., (1934). Third International Grassland Congress, 1.
8. Evans, R. J., J. McGinnis & J. L. St. John, (1947). J. Nutrition, 33, 661.
9. Watson, S. J., (1935). J. Roy. Agr. Soc. England, 95, 1.
10. Mitchell, H. H.; T. S. Hamilton, & J. R. Beadles, (1945). J. Nutrition, 29, 13.
11. Hopkins, F. G., & E. G. Willcock, (1906-7). J. Physiol., 35, 88.
12. Abderhalden, E., (1912). Z., Physiol. Chem., 77, 22.
13. Rose, W. C., (1938). Physiol. Rev., 18, 109.

14. Rose, W. C., M. J. Oesterling & M. Womack, (1948). J. Biol. Chem., *176*, 753.
15. Mitchell, H. H., (1947). Arch. Biochem., *12*, 293.
16. Frazier, L. E., R. W. Wissler, C. H. Steffee, R. L. Woolridge & P. R. Cannon, (1947). J. Nutrition, *33*, 65.
17. Cox, W. M., A. J. Mueller, R. Elman, A. A. Albanese, K. S. Kemmerer, R. W. Barton & L. E. Holt, Jr., (1947). J. Nutrition, *33*, 437.
18. Allison, J. B., J. A. Anderson & R. D. Seeley, (1947). J. Nutrition, *33*, 361.
19. Johnson, R. M., H. H. Deuel, Jr., M. G. Morehouse & J. W. Mehl, (1947). J. Nutrition, *33*, 371.
20. Brush, M., W. Willman & P. P. Swanson, (1947). J. Nutrition, *33*, 389.
21. Wissler, R. W., C. H. Steffee, L. E. Frazier, R. L. Woolridge, & E. P. Benditt, (1948). J. Nutrition, *36*, 245.
22. Baker, F., & S. T. Harriss, (1947-8). Nutrition Abs. Rev., *17*, 3.
23. Osborne, T. B., L. B. Mendel & E. L. Ferry, (1919). J. Biol. Chem. *37*, 223.
24. Boas-Fixen, M. A., (1934-5). Nutrition Abs. Rev., *4*, 447.
25. Hegsted, D. M. & J. Worcester, (1947). J. Nutrition, *33*, 685.
26. Thomas, K., (1909). Arch. Anat. Physiol., 219.
27. Mitchell, H. H., (1924). J. Biol. Chem., *58*, 873.
28. Graves, H. C. H., (1945). Chem. and Indust., 146.
29. Schoenheimer, R., (1942). "Dynamic State of the Body Constituents."
30. Miller, L. W., (1944). J. Biol. Chem., *152*, 603.
31. Bosshardt, D. K., & H. R. Barnes, (1946). J. Nutrition, *31*, 13.
32. Titus, H. W., (1927). J. Agric. Res., *34*, 49.
33. Sumner, E. E., H. B. Pierce, & J. R. Murlin, (1938). J. Nutrition, *16*, 37.
34. Melnick, D. R., & G. R. Cowgill, (1937). J. Nutrition, *13*, 401.
35. Martin, C. J. & R. Robison, (1922). Biochem. J., *16*, 407.
36. Bricker, M., H. H. Mitchell & G. M. Kinsman, (1945). J. Nutrition, *30*, 269.
37. Allison, J. B., & J. R. Anderson, (1945). J. Nutrition, *29*, 413.
38. Murlin, J. R., L. A. Szymanski, & E. C. Nasset, (1948). J. Nutrition, *36*, 171.
39. Cuthbertson, D. P., & H. N. Munro, (1937). Biochem. J., *31*, 694.
40. Cuthbertson, D. P., & H. N. Munro, (1939). Biochem. J., *33*, 128.
41. Woolley, D. W., (1945). J. Biol. Chem., *159*, 753.
42. Van Slyke, D., (1942). Science, *95*, 259.
43. Murlin, J. R., L. E. Edwards, S. Fried, & T. A. Szymanski, (1946). J. Nutrition, *31*, 715.
44. Almquist, H. J., (1947). J. Nutrition, *34*, 543.
45. Maynard, L. A., (1947). "Animal Nutrition," 351.
46. Almquist, H. J. & C. R. Grau, (1944). Poultry Sci., *23*, 341.
47. Kuiken, K. A., & C. M. Lyman, (1948). J. Nutrition, *36*, 359.
48. Sure, B., (1948). J. Nutrition, *36*, 59.
49. Van Landingham, A. H., T. B. Clark, & B. H. Schneider, (1945). Poultry Sci., *24*, 105.
50. Morris, S., & N. C. Wright, (1933-4). J. Dairy Sci., *5*, 1.
51. Geiger, E., (1947). J. Nutrition, *34*, 93.
52. Greaves, E., A. F. Morgan & M. K. Loveen, (1938). J. Nutrition, *16*, 115.
53. Block, R. J., P. R. Cannon, R. W. Wissler, C. H. Steffee, R. L. Staube, L. E. Frazier & R. L. Woolridge, (1946). Arch. Biochem., *10*, 295.
54. Mellanby, E., (1946). Brit. Med. J., *2*, 885.
55. McNaught, M. L. & J. A. B. Smith, (1947). Nutrition Abs. Rev., *17*, 18.

THE INORGANIC ELEMENTS

(1) Occurrence in biological materials

(a) Introduction.

Careful examination of plant and animal tissues has revealed the presence therein of many inorganic elements, quite apart from the hydrogen, oxygen and nitrogen which are associated with the major organic components of living cells. The list includes sodium, potassium, magnesium, calcium, iron, copper, manganese and cobalt among the metals, and chlorine, iodine, sulphur, silicon, and phosphorus of the non-metals. This does not exhaust the list but it includes the major components and most of the elements whose functions are known or suspected.

A close relationship exists between (a) the nature and composition of the soil of a given region, (b) the mineral elements in the plants of that area and (c) the inorganic elements in the bodies of the animals which graze the herbage. In some cases the balance may be such that both plant and animal thrive; in other cases the soil may be deficient in certain elements, with the result that only certain species of plant will grow and the beasts grazing the herbage may become unthrifty due to lack of an essential element; in yet other instances the soil contains some

† The terms " inorganic elements " and " mineral elements " are both in common use.

toxic material which finds its way into the plants growing thereon with the unhappy result that the grazing beasts are poisoned.

(b) Plant products.

As might be expected from the above paragraphs, there are rather marked differences between the amounts of the various inorganic elements which are found in different plant species. When land is cultivated, the mineral fraction of the herbage which grows upon it often shows the results of such cultivation. The following table, for example, gives some idea of the variations which may be found in the contents of the major mineral elements of pasture.[1]

TABLE 10

	No. of Samples	Silica-free Ash	CaO	P_2O_5	Na_2O	K_2O	Cl
		%	%	%	%	%	%
Cultivated Pasture	24	6.64	1.00	0.74	0.25	3.18	0.95
Natural Pasture " all grazed "	22	5.85	0.65	0.67	0.37	2.66	0.64
Poor Hill Pasture " partly grazed "	35	5.49	0.56	0.60	0.41	2.60	0.60
Island of Lewis ...	1	—	0.29	0.24	0.38	0.68	0.12
Falkland Islands ...	55	4.65	0.29	0.54	0.31	2.20	0.70

Leguminous plants flourish on soils which are rich in lime, for which reason the clovers are very useful feeding stuffs for many species of livestock, since these plants are substantially richer in calcium than the grasses.

These facts are extremely important for, in certain natural grazing areas, conditions of mineral deficiency in the soil, often aggravated by climatic variables, give rise to serious deficiency diseases in the grazing stock. Tremendous losses to the livestock industry of South Africa have resulted from the very low phosphorus content of some of the pastures: more recently deficiencies of copper, cobalt and other elements have been associated with disease conditions in grazing animals. Calcium deficiency in herbage seems to be less pronounced though there is no doubt that the calcium content is frequently far below the optimum level, especially when the pasture is grazed by milking cows or growing animals. Legume pasture or hay generally contains enough calcium to meet the animal's needs, as these crops quite commonly fail to grow normally when calcium is deficient, but grasses are much less affected by soil acidity and lime status so that a satisfactory growth is no proof of the plant's adequate calcium content.

Grass and fresh green foods generally contain some 2-4% of mineral ash, but the exact amount varies with the seasonal conditions, with the stage of maturity of the plants and with respect to the different parts of the same plant. As plants mature the proportion of insoluble siliceous matter increases. The amount of phosphorus is usually much greater in plant seeds than in the leaves and still greater than that in the stems; on the other hand the leaves are much richer in calcium than are the seeds, a fact which is of considerable nutritional importance. The outer coat of seeds contains more inorganic matter than the inner portion : in the case of the legume seeds the husk tends to contain a high proportion of calcium to phosphorus, but with the cereal grains the outer part is rich in phosphorus and low in calcium. For both of these groups of food-stuffs, the kernel is relatively rich in phosphorus and poor in calcium, though the leguminous seeds are better than the cereal grains in this respect.

The mineral variations in the cereal products may be quite consider-able, as is evident from the figures for phosphorus given by Snook,[2] who reports an average total phosphorus (P) content of 0.24 per cent. for Western Australian wheat, as compared with 0.47 per cent. for standard British wheat and figures of 0.20 and 0.23 per cent. for Australian oats as compared with 0.39 per cent. for standard British oats.

(c) Animal tissues.

About 3 per cent. of the weight of the animal body consists of the elements already listed. Two-thirds of this are accounted for by calcium and phosphorus, chiefly in the form of bone, although calcium is present in soluble form in the body fluids and phosphorus is one of the most widely distributed elements in the organism both with regard to place and function. Potassium, sulphur, chlorine and magnesium, in that order, account for a further 0.6-0.7 per cent. Iron and the rest of the inorganic elements contribute the remaining half per cent. or so.[3] It is not easy to say to what extent the total amount varies from one species to another, but there is no reason to believe either that the range is large or that the proportions of the different elements are very different from the figures quoted above. Almost the whole of the iron of the body is to be found in the blood, liver and spleen, much of the copper occurs in the liver and the greater part of the iodine is located in the thyroid gland.

The above facts are reflected in the composition of foods of animal origin. Rich sources of calcium and phosphorus, for example, are meals, such as meat-and-bone meal, which contain a large proportion of bone. Dried milk is fairly rich in mineral matter (7 per cent. of ash), some two-thirds of which is derived from calcium and phosphorus : it is low in iron and copper, however. Fish meal, which usually includes the ground bones, yields about 20 per cent. of ash, mainly as calcium phosphate.

(2) Functions of the inorganic elements

There are some inorganic elements which are found in the animal body, usually in mere traces, whose function is not known : aluminium is one example of this kind. In other cases it can be shown experimentally that the element in question plays some part in metabolism, although the extent of the knowledge we possess about this varies greatly from one element to another. To do justice to the subject would need a monograph, so that the following account is a summary of the main functions of the inorganic elements, further details with regard to the different elements being given in the appropriate sections.

(a) Protective.

Under this heading may be included the part played by calcium in helping blood-clot formation and the functions of calcium, phosphorus and perhaps fluorine in forming the hard enamel of the teeth.

(b) Structural.

Sulphur, in the sulphur-containing amino-acids, is an important constituent of such materials as hair, horn and hoof: calcium, phosphorus and magnesium are vitally concerned in the formation of bone. This last function is a most important one, since satisfactory bodily size and proportions, with their secondary effects on such physiological phenomena as reproduction, are involved.

(c) Regulatory.

Iodine is taken up into organically combined form by the thyroid gland and is thus concerned in the general regulation of the metabolic rate of the body; sodium and chloride ions, principally, are concerned in the maintenance of the osmotic pressure of the body fluids, while the ions of sodium, potassium, calcium, magnesium and chlorine play a part in the maintenance of the blood at a slightly alkaline level (pH 7.4). In the preservation of the normal rhythm of heart muscle, sodium, potassium and calcium ions are involved.

(d) General metabolic.

In this subsection may be included varied examples of the activities of the inorganic elements in the metabolism of the animal body. Iron, combined with an appropriate protein, is essential for oxygen transport to the tissues; it is also an important constituent of enzymic oxidising systems. The magnesium ion is an activator for a number of enzyme reactions involving phosphates; manganese is the activator for certain digestive enzymes. In the processes of digestion chloride and sodium ions are essential. Apart from its activities in a number of enzymic oxidation systems, copper is necessary for the satisfactory formation of haemoglobin, while cobalt is present in combined form in vitamin B_{12} and is therefore intimately concerned with the prevention of nutritional anaemia, apart from its being needed by the micro-organisms of the digestive tract of the ruminant. In addition to the part it plays in phospho-proteins and in phosphatides, phosphorus is an essential factor in the synthesis and breakdown of the carbohydrates and probably of fats and proteins also.

These brief summaries of the various functions of the inorganic elements in the animal body show that though the elements may be minor constituents in the quantitative sense, they are in fact indispensable. From the nutritional point of view some are more important than others only in so far as they are more likely to be deficient in animal rations. Even that statement must be made with reserve, however, since the variety of reactions which is governed by this group of elements is only now becoming apparent.

(3) The availability of mineral elements to livestock

Under this heading will be briefly outlined the various factors which have an influence upon the amounts of the different inorganic elements that pass into the body through the wall of the digestive tract and are derived from ingested food.

The quantities of such elements absorbed from the gut will depend first of all upon their concentration in the food consumed. There is the complicating factor of solubility to be considered, however, for it may be assumed with a good degree of confidence that solids insoluble in the digestive fluids do not pass in any quantity across the walls of the stomach or intestine. This point may be illustrated with reference to the compound " salt licks " which are sometimes given to livestock. As a source of iron, where it is thought necessary to provide additional amounts of this element, either a soluble or an insoluble compound may be chosen. Very often ignited ferric oxide, as a finely divided powder, is included. This substance is so insoluble that very little of it can be absorbed from the gut and certainly no more than would be afforded by the use of a more soluble iron salt in much smaller proportion in the ration. The problem of solubility will also be concerned where, for example, ground limestone is being used as a dietary source of calcium; fine grinding of the substance can be depended upon as being one factor which will tend to facilitate solution and absorption.

Another related variable to be considered is the acidity or alkalinity of the contents of the digestive tract. The common salts of the metals which are at present under discussion are soluble in acid solution but, except for sodium and potassium, give rise to a number of insoluble compounds in neutral or alkaline ones. In the stomach of the mammal compounds of such metals will thus tend to dissolve: in the small intestine, however, the addition of alkaline digestive secretions gradually makes the food mass alkaline, although it seems to be true that a pH of greater than 7 is not reached for some way along the small intestine. Lactose is believed to facilitate the absorption of calcium from the gut[5] because of the acidic type of fermentation it undergoes in the small intestine; it is thus an important sugar in the nutrition of young stock. The acidity of the food itself is important, as for example in the feeding of silage. Though the absorption of calcium may be facilitated, this is not necessarily an advantage to the body, for reasons which are given later (p. 66).

Once the various elements have been brought into solution, in ionic form, it seems that the simple laws of chemical equilibrium operate, although there are many factors, such as the presence of the semi-permeable wall of the gut, which help to complicate the overall picture. In a reaction between calcium and phosphate ions, one would expect an increasingly large proportion of calcium (or phosphate) to be converted into the sparingly soluble calcium phosphate, $Ca_3P_2O_8$, as the concentration of phosphate (or calcium) is increased, and it is certainly true that a great disparity between the amounts of calcium and phosphate in a ration is more likely to produce nutritional disorders than one which is better balanced. On the same basis the poorer absorption of iron and magnesium in presence of too large proportions of phosphate may be accounted for. The phytic acid of cereals, an acid derived from inositol and phosphoric acid, presents a more complex problem (p. 68), although it certainly seems to hinder the absorption of calcium, magnesium and phosphorus from the diet. Oxalic acid, in certain vegetable foods, may diminish calcium absorption, probably because of the formation of the insoluble calcium oxalate.

(4) The loss of inorganic elements from the body

In the previous section the availability of the inorganic elements to the animal body was treated from a physical and chemical point of view, with few or no references to the powers of the animal organism to interfere in the process. Its powers of this kind are very considerable, however, and have a great influence on the proportions of ingested inorganic elements which escape from the body, although the fine details of the various regulatory mechanisms are still being investigated.

Mineral elements are lost in fæces, urine, sweat and, in the case of the lactating female, in milk. In sweat the main inorganic constituents are sodium and chlorine. In milk the chief losses are, roughly in order of their magnitude, potassium, calcium, sodium and magnesium of the metals and chlorine and phosphorus of the non-metals. Since potassium is a major mineral constituent of plant foods, efficient feeding, during the lactation of the common species of livestock, is mainly concerned with seeing that the other elements are present in sufficient quantity in the ration.

So far as the kidneys and intestine are concerned the inorganic elements may be lost to the body, (a) by secretion in the urine, (b) by their not being absorbed from the intestine, or (c) by their being absorbed at one time but excreted into the intestine somewhat later. Some elements, for example sodium, are eliminated chiefly by the first route, whereas others, such as calcium, are lost to the body mainly by routes (b) and (c). There is little advantage in discussing here the details of the phenomena which occur: it is sufficient to say that the animal body probably has the capacity to vary somewhat the paths of elimination to suit particular conditions at different ages.

As with many other nutrients, there seems to be most efficient retention of the inorganic elements when they are present in rather small amounts in the diet. Secondly, the animal body is selective in its behaviour and does not necessarily excrete two or more elements in the same proportions as they are provided in its food. In the third place the power of selection for an animal of a given species will vary with its age and condition, so that a young animal may retain a greater proportion of its dietary calcium than would an older one. Other factors of the diet, acting through the animal and not in a simple physicochemical way, can produce differences of retention. As an example of this type of mechanism there is the increase in the amount of calcium absorbed from the gut as a result of the administration of vitamin D. Previously (p. 64) it was stated that increased acidity of the contents of the gut would facilitate calcium absorption. In the case of the consumption of silage made by the use of mineral acid the acid taken in from the intestine would require neutralisation by the bases in the blood, as a result of which the loss of certain bases via the urine might well exceed their increased intestinal absorption. For this reason, among others, such silage should be brought near to neutrality, using chalk for the purpose, before it is fed to livestock. Although the body thus seems to have the power to regulate its intake of minerals to suit its purposes, its capacity is by no means unlimited. Thus with high yielding dairy cows cases have been recorded where more than 90 per cent. of the total mineral intake was excreted in the faeces and urine, although the 10 per cent. left was inadequate to supply the minerals contained in the milk and the animals had to draw on their skeletal reserves. Similarly it seems that laying hens are never able to provide sufficient mineral matter for egg shell formation without drawing on their body reserves, at least temporarily, as their maximum daily absorption of mineral matter is less than that contained in a single egg shell.

(5) Mineral deficiencies in practice

The opinion is sometimes expressed that mineral deficiencies in practice are limited to sodium, chlorine, calcium and phosphorus. Such statements presuppose complete knowledge not only of the precise composition of all foods, natural and processed, but also of the functions of all the inorganic elements, singly and in combination; they are completely unwarranted.

The growth of young stock requires adequate amounts of calcium and phosphorus for bone formation, while the production of milk necessitates further a satisfactory level of salt intake. Extreme deficiencies of these substances from the ration are soon manifest, but suboptimal levels may result solely in a slightly diminished growth rate or somewhat lower milk yield and these are symptoms not so easily observed. The same kind of principle applies to the other elements.

Quite apart from calcium and phosphorus deficiencies, the second of which is very widespread, there are known to be regional iodine, cobalt and copper deficiencies. The adjective ".regional" must not be taken in too narrow a sense, for it may mean areas of many hundreds or, on the other hand, of very few square miles. Livestock which are living more or less completely on the local produce may thus be more liable to show such deficiencies than animals whose food comes from several different areas.

The undesirable result of an imbalance of calcium and phosphorus in foods has already been stressed. This is not the only case of its kind and here the point must be made that an element which is benevolent in its action at one level of intake in the diet may prove toxic at a much higher one: copper is an example of this type. When it is said, therefore, that the toxicity of molybdenum is reduced by an increased copper intake,[6] that of selenium by arsenic[7] and that of zinc—an essential element *in traces*—by iron, copper and cobalt together,[8] it should be clear that the phenomenon is probably one of wide application, many details of which remain to be explored.

Where the mineral needs of livestock cannot be met by the inorganic elements in the food supplied they may be met by the provision of a salt lick or by the inclusion of a suitable mineral mixture in the ration. The chief minerals used for this purpose are common salt, chalk or ground limestone, steamed bone flour and calcium phosphate, together with small amounts of potassium iodide. A salt lick, which enables the individual beast to take just as much as it requires, has some advantage over the actual mixture of the minerals with the ration, in which method there is no opportunity for the independent selection of the bulk of the inorganic fraction apart from the chief organic constituents of the diet. Moreover, finely dispersed iron and copper compounds are very effective catalysts for the oxidation of many unsaturated organic compounds, including fatty acids and carotenoid substances. From the substance of this paragraph and the preceding one, the need for clear thought and judgment with respect to the nature and amounts of the mineral elements with which a ration is to be supplemented will be apparent.

(6) Consideration of the individual elements

(a) Calcium and phosphorus.

The utilizations of calcium and phosphorus are here considered together as these two minerals are often very closely associated in their metabolism by the animal body, which requires a sufficient supply of each element, with—for most species—a suitable source of vitamin D. Where vitamin D is deficient or where the level of either calcium or phosphorus in the diet diminishes towards the minimum amount needed for satisfactory bodily function the ratio between the calcium and phosphorus in the ration may have an important influence on the physiological condition which develops.

Recently Mitchell[9] has reviewed the information available on the mineral needs of livestock. Data on calcium and phosphorus, taken from his tables, have been adapted to give the abbreviated version in Table 11 below, requirements being expressed in terms of the dry matter of the ration.

TABLE 11

Calf, Holstein Wt. Ca. Ca/P			Colt, Percheron Wt. Ca. Ca/P			Sow or barrow Wt. Ca. Ca/P			Lamb, male. Wt. Ca. Ca/P		
lb.	%		lb.	%		lb.	%		lb.	%	
200	0.8	1.6	440	0.7	1.6	75	0.6	1.8	20	0.24	1.5
400	0.4	1.5	660	0.5	1.6	150	0.5	1.7	50	0.18	1.4
1200	0.2	1.4	880	0.4	1.4	250	0.4	1.5	90	0.17	1.2
—	—	—	1320	0.2	1.3	350	0.2	1.1	120	0.15	1.2

In each case there is a fall in the required calcium content of the food and also a fall in the Ca/P ratio as the early stages of growth are passed. For growing chickens 0.6% calcium is needed for a body-weight of 0.5 lb.; this level is maintained up to weights of 3 to 4 lb., but the Ca/P ratio remains at about 2.0. In the case of the pregnant animal the general trend of the above values is reversed, the percentage of calcium in the ration and the Ca/P ratio beginning low and then increasing. The above theoretical requirements should be increased in practice by a suitable safety margin: for ordinary rations of natural foods such a margin might be about 50%, provided that adequate supplies of vitamin D are available. Where coarsely ground minerals are being used a rather higher margin may be needed, but some discretion should be exercised since too high a level of calcium in a ration seems to interfere with the proper assimilation of iron, iodine and manganese, as well as phosphorus. Considerable variation may occur in the Ca/P ratio, however, without any untoward effects unless the supplies of vitamin D, and available calcium or phosphorus are inadequate.

Absorption of both calcium and phosphorus from the intestinal tract is favoured by the feeding of substances such as lactose, which produce a high acidity in the digestive tract. On the other hand, large intakes of iron, aluminium or magnesium by forming insoluble phosphates, reduce the absorption of phosphorus. Fatty acids may form insoluble calcium soaps and so restrict calcium absorption, and a similar effect may be noticeable in the case of natural foods containing oxalic acid, which forms insoluble calcium oxalate.

In many of the cereal grains, and especially in the bran derived from them, much of the phosphorus is present as phytin. This last substance consists of the salts—chiefly of magnesium and calcium—of phytic acid, the acid hexaphosphoric ester of inositol. Phytic acid forms insoluble calcium salts, like phosphoric acid,[10] and the availability to the animal organism of the calcium and phosphorus of rations containing cereal foods, has been the subject of much investigation. The exact position is still not too clear, but there is evidence to show that the phosphorus and calcium of such foods require adequate amounts of vitamin D in the ration for their full utilization.

In contrast to the effects of phytic acid, it has been found that calcium and magnesium carbonates and phosphates, which are insoluble at the normal pH of the intestine, tend to form soluble co-ordination compounds with amino-acids. The presence of protein in the ration thus facilitates the absorption of these elements: it provides another example of the importance of rations being " well balanced " for the function they are intended to serve.

Only about a quarter of the average calcium excretion is via the urine: phosphorus excretion varies with the different species of animal; in herbivora it is principally via the fæces, but in carnivora mainly in the urine.

Calcium and phosphorus are deposited together in the formation of bone, cartilage being first converted to ossein and then calcified. In the young animal a deficiency of calcium or phosphorus or, in some species, of vitamin D, leads to imperfect calcification, so that mechanical stresses exerted on the bones cause them to bend or their ends to become enlarged, with the production of swollen, knobbly joints. This condition is called rickets; severe cases are becoming more rare but the more difficultly observed mild cases still exist. Apart from " permanent " structural bone, reserve calcium and phosphorus are deposited in the trabeculæ for mobilisation whenever required. These reserves are of very considerable importance and may be used during heavy milk secretion or for the building of structural bone during periods of rapid growth. Because of these reserves a normal animal can resist the adverse effects of calcium or phosphorus deficiency for a considerable time without showing any symptoms of either rickets or tetany. Thus the skeleton acts as a buffer in calcium and phosphorus metabolism, depleting itself when the need is urgent, as during lactation or when the diet is deficient, and replenishing itself when the needs are easily covered by the diet. Even an old animal can store calcium and phosphorus in its skeleton when supplied with adequate amounts. This depletion of the trabeculæ during deficiency normally involves no physiological harm, since the reserves are readily built up again during periods when the body needs are less, but, under conditions of prolonged deficiency, the condition known as osteomalacia may result in adult animals. In this disease not only have the reserves in the trabeculæ been exhausted but some of the calcium and phosphorus of the structural bone have been mobilized in the blood, leaving the residual bone weak, brittle and easily fractured. Cases have been recorded of fractures of the pelvis in lactating cows. Apart from these troubles the condition is characterised by low calcium and phosphorus levels of the blood, negative balances of these elements and a lowered productivity. In phosphorus deficiency, which is common, there may be depraved appetite (pica), the animals consuming earth and the dead bones of other animals, etc., apparently in an attempt to make good their lack. Lowered fertility is another accompaniment of low phosphorus intakes, while the function of phosphorus as an intermediary in protein synthesis[4] seems to be reflected in the lowered biological values of dietary proteins for sheep when there is a deficiency of that element in the ration." In the case of diets which are phosphorus deficient, the animal organism may be forced to draw upon its skeletal reserves to an appreciable extent. Phosphorus deficiencies of pastures are accentuated by drought, which reduces the phosphorus content of the herbage.

It should be borne in mind that the skeleton cannot liberate one of the elements, calcium or phosphorus, without liberating an equivalent amount of the other. As both calcium and phosphorus are withdrawn from the skeleton simultaneously, fragile bones may result from aphosphorosis or from calcium deficiency or from both. Poultry would appear to present an exception to the above statement regarding the simultaneous withdrawal of calcium and phosphorus from the skeleton. Thus Tyler [12] has shown that the laying fowl, even when receiving adequate amounts of calcium carbonate, removes calcium intermittently from the skeleton for shell formation without removing phosphate in significant amounts; this worker has suggested [13] that whereas calcium from the gut is carried as a calcium-phosphorus complex, that liberated from the bone in laying hens may be carried as calcium proteinate. The composition of bone in laying hens is by no means constant, varying according to the diet and the calcium balance.

Although the antirachitic factor, vitamin D, apparently regulates the absorption of calcium and phosphorus from the intestine and the deposition of these minerals in osseous tissue to form bone, no amount of vitamin D will compensate for an absolute deficiency of either element. Within reasonable limits the greater the imbalance of calcium and phosphorus, or the nearer the amounts of these elements approach to the animal's minimum required daily intake, the more vitamin D is needed to ensure their efficient utilisation. The precise action of vitamin D is far from being fully understood, however, and it should be remembered that there are species differences with respect to the magnitude of the response to a given dose of the vitamin, or to different forms of the vitamin.

Sheep and horses seem to be less susceptible to phosphorus deficiency than cattle. When drought accentuates the deficiency, there is usually a fall in both the protein and carotene contents of pasture, so that the livestock tend to be subjected to simultaneous lack of water, protein, phosphorus and carotene.

(b) Magnesium.

Absorption of dietary magnesium from the intestinal tract does not appear to depend on the presence of either an acidic or a basic reaction and it seems that the conditions governing its absorption are quite different from those of calcium, although, like calcium, excretion of magnesium is chiefly via the faeces. More than 70 per cent. of the body magnesium occurs in the skeleton but the remaining portion is widely distributed and the amount in the soft tissues exceeds that of calcium. Apart from its structural functions magnesium is concerned in the activation of the phosphatase enzyme and is thus involved in the metabolism of carbohydrates. The percentage of magnesium in bone ash decreases with increasing age, probably as a result of the decrease in the organic matrix of bone, as calcification proceeds.

A beneficial effect on calcium metabolism has sometimes been claimed to result from the addition of magnesium to the diet, but as little is known of magnesium requirements, the observed effect may not be a direct one but may be a result of increased growth or an alteration in the amounts of calcium and phosphorus absorbed, or other similar factors.

Where both calcium and phosphorus are adequate in amount, the ingestion of a moderate excess of magnesium will not markedly diminish calcium retention, although it may increase the requirement for calcium and phosphorus. Dolomitic limestone, containing magnesium carbonate as well as calcium carbonate, is quite a satisfactory source of calcium in rations containing liberal amounts of phosphate.

Under conditions of disease where there are large losses of calcium from the body and where calcium absorption may be negligible, magnesium metabolism does not appear to be affected, and for this reason it would appear that the metabolism of magnesium may be very different from that of calcium. Moreover, the distribution of magnesium in the soft tissues of the body is more closely related to the distribution of the phosphorus than to that of calcium, and the magnesium level in the blood tends to vary with the phosphorus content. Very little is known about the effects of vitamins on magnesium metabolism.

Magnesium deficiency results in a cessation of growth, a lowered magnesium level in the blood and bones, but an increase in the bone calcium. There appears to be a fundamental disturbance of normal calcium metabolism resulting in a pathological precipitation of calcium salts in soft tissues and possibly an interference with normal calcification in bone tissues. Lactation tetany or grass tetany is associated with low levels of blood magnesium and calcium, whereas the normal tetany of magnesium deficiency is associated with low magnesium but a normal serum calcium. It seems probable that tetany can be produced in more than one way, and a study of blood changes may be inadequate to indicate the causes. The formation of renal calculi may be associated with both magnesium deficiency and magnesium excess. In acute magnesium deficiency calcium is deposited in large amounts in the kidney, but the addition of phosphate to the ration, probably by precipitating and so preventing the absorption of calcium, has a preventive action. Excess of magnesium may also produce calculi in rats and Eveleth and Millen [14] have reported a high incidence of renal calculi in sheep kept on diets high in magnesium and relatively low in calcium.

Recent work on the magnesium requirements of dairy cattle suggests that 30-40 g. of magnesium are needed per day to prevent the onset of tetany or nervous symptoms in cows. [15] Experimental tetany, apparently identical with " grass tetany ", was produced in cows on diets containing only about 10 g. of magnesium in the daily ration. In every case of tetany it was found that appreciably lowered serum magnesium values were observed *before* the onset of acute symptoms. It was not found possible, however, to show an exact correlation between the quantity of the magnesium in the ration and the subsequent degree of hypomagnesaemia in the animals. Some factor involving utilization may perhaps be involved. Calves reared exclusively on milk may also suffer from magnesium deficiency and show evidence of pathological calcium deposition.

(c) Sodium, potassium and chlorine.

These three elements occur almost entirely in the soft tissues and body fluids, and there is usually more potassium than sodium. Meat diets contain equal quantities of sodium and potassium but vegetable foods usually contain only a small proportion of sodium relative to the potassium content. Carnivorous animals thus obtain a sufficiency of both sodium and potassium from their meat diet, whereas herbivorous animals require much more sodium than they get in their natural food and it is necessary to add common salt to the rations of these animals unless they have access to salt licks. Chlorine occurs mostly as chlorides, which contribute very largely to the anions in blood and play an important part in the acid-base equilibrium.

The soluble sodium and potassium chlorides are readily absorbed and circulate throughout the body. Excretion of sodium and potassium is largely in the form of chlorides or phosphates and mostly occurs through the kidneys, although perspiration may account for quite a considerable proportion of the excretion under certain circumstances. Although a certain storage of chlorine may occur in the skin and subcutaneous tissues, sodium and potassium are not stored appreciably, any excess over the body needs being immediately excreted. Whereas the skeleton of the body provides valuable reserves of calcium and phosphorus, there are no large reserves against deficiencies of sodium, potassium and chlorine. All foods are relatively rich in potassium so that there is rarely a deficiency of this element, but many foods are relatively deficient in both sodium and chlorine. A shortage of common salt is probably the most frequent cause of mineral deficiency in farm stock.

Sodium deficiency results in retarded growth, reduced fertility and impaired ability to utilise digested protein and carbohydrate material. In laying hens there is frequently an outbreak of cannibalism as well as loss of weight and lowered production. Chloride is an essential constituent of the gastric secretion, as well as forming about two-thirds of the anions of the blood. Its deficiency is rarely distinguished from sodium deficiency as the two elements usually occur together in the form of common salt. When the amount of common salt in the ration is low, urinary sodium and chlorine excretion falls, but when large amounts are fed there is a large excretion and a considerable increase in water requirement. Owing to the ability of the animal to control to some degree its excretion of sodium chloride, when the food is deficient in salt relatively little wastage of the body supplies occurs and it frequently takes some time for ill effects to be noticeable. Salt deficiency symptoms usually appear first in the more productive animals, for example, there may be a fall in the milk yield of a dairy cow. Excessive intakes of salt, on the other hand, result in a considerable retention of water in the body, causing œdema. Mitchell is of the opinion that there is no need to have more than 0.5 per cent. of common salt added to the grain ration of cattle and sheep. Salt poisoning in poultry is relatively common and the condition may also occur in pigs fed with kitchen waste as this frequently contains an unusually large amount of salt. There are now legal limits to the amounts of chlorine (as sodium chloride) which may occur in "National" foods for livestock; in no case is the permitted amount greater than 1 per cent. (Appendix 2.) Other animals do not often suffer from excess of salt although cases have been recorded of death ensuing from an over-consumption of salt by farm animals given free access to it after a long period of deficiency.

(d) Iron.

Although only small amounts of iron are present in the animal body, it is an essential constituent of hæmoglobin and is thus of fundamental importance. Green foods are rich in iron which appears to be completely available, and, with the exception of milk, most natural, unprocessed foods seem to contain enough iron for the needs of the animal body. Iron compounds can be absorbed if they are are soluble and ionisable and ferrous salts are probably more easily utilised than ferric. Inorganic iron has often been considered to be the only form of any use to the animal, as highly complex organic compounds which are not completely broken down in the digestive tract are not likely to provide any available iron; recent evidence, however, suggests that some organic iron compounds may serve as quite useful sources of this metal. An excess of iron has a detrimental effect on phosphorus assimilation as it forms an insoluble phosphate. The principal excretion of iron is in the fæces.

Absorbed iron is utilised for hæmoglobin formation and as the red blood corpuscles only have a life of four to six weeks before being replaced, iron metabolism must be constantly very active. For hæmoglobin synthesis a small amount of copper, together with a number of other factors, is necessary, though copper is not present in hæmoglobin itself. Although iron in the body occurs largely as hæmoglobin, there are small amounts present in other parts of the body and storage may occur in the liver, spleen and kidneys.

During breakdown of the red blood cells hæmatin is liberated and further broken down to a simpler iron compound together with various pigments which pass to the liver and are secreted in the bile. Iron released in erythrocyte breakdown is normally used again for hæmoglobin synthesis so that the constant regeneration of the blood which takes place in the body does not necessitate any great loss of iron. Under certain conditions of disease, however, there is an accelerated destruction of blood cells and iron may be converted to a form in which it cannot be used and so is excreted and lost. Very active multiplication in the number of red blood cells is necessary in young growing animals and if this does not occur, or if in adult animals destruction exceeds regeneration, *anæmia* results, characterised by a low level of blood hæmoglobin. Nutritional anæmia results from a shortage of iron or from lack of the copper, cobalt, or other factors essential to hæmoglobin synthesis. It may occur at any time in life when the mineral supply is inadequate for normal hæmoglobin formation; it is particularly common in suckling animals, especially pigs. Milk being deficient in iron, young animals, if they are of such a species that milk is their sole food for the early part of life, are usually born with relatively large iron reserves. The hæmoglobin content of the blood of new-born pigs is very much greater than at weaning and the percentage of iron in the total ash of the body is also relatively high at birth. Anæmia in suckling pigs may be prevented by dosing with ferrous sulphate to which a trace of copper salt is added. In the absence of copper, storage of iron in the liver may take place without resulting in hæmoglobin synthesis. As most farm foods contain adequate amounts of iron, nutritional anæmia, due simply to lack of this element, does not often occur in weaned animals.

(e) Sulphur.

The animal can obtain all the sulphur it requires from proteins containing this element and thus inorganic sulphur is not necessary in the food supply. In the animal body sulphur occurs in the amino acids cystine and methionine as well as in various amino-acid derivatives; small amounts of sulphates and thiocyanates are also present.

The sulphur-containing proteins are broken down and absorbed from the digestive tract in the same manner as other food proteins but the various metabolic changes which occur after absorption are not fully understood. Numerous enzyme reactions are involved in the formation of compounds such as sulphates and taurocholic acid and in the conversion of methionine to cystine. Excretion of sulphur occurs in both fæces and urine and largely results from protein catabolism. Urinary sulphur is chiefly in the inorganic form but there are also present many organic compounds representing various stages in the breakdown of the sulphur amino-acids.

Much of the sulphur retained by the body is deposited as keratin, the name given to a group of proteins, characterised by hardness, insolubility and resistance to enzyme digestion, which occur in the skin, nervous system, hair, claws, feathers and wool. Although the amount of cystine stored in wool may be practically equal to the dietary intake, attempts to improve wool growth by feeding additional cystine have not been successful, from which it would seem that cystine can be synthesised either by the intestinal flora or by the animal itself from other sources of dietary sulphur.

Sulphur deficiency cannot occur without involving a deficiency of essential amino-acids so that the symptoms specifically indicative of sulphur shortage are not known unless these are taken to be identical with the symptoms of essential amino-acid deficiency. Excess of sulphur in the form of amino acids or sulphates has no nutritional value and excess of elemental sulphur has a toxic action.

(f) Iodine.

Iodine is one of the trace elements essential for normal nutrition. Although only very small amounts (about 0.00005 per cent.) of iodine are to be found in the mammalian body, most of it in the thyroid gland, this element is extremely important. Through its conversion into the iodine-containing amino-acid, thyroxine, iodine is concerned in the regulation of the metabolic rate of the organism. In the absence of sufficient of the hormone, the basal metabolic rate is diminished, and the animal becomes physically and mentally retarded. An excess of iodine can cause the reverse of this condition.

Iodides are readily absorbed from the digestive tract and excretion of iodine occurs through the kidneys largely in the form of iodide: considerable storage in the thyroid gland may take place.

Due to lack of sufficient iodine an enlargement of the thyroid gland, known as goitre, occurs, while pregnant animals receiving inadequate amounts of iodine may produce dead or very weak offspring showing marked evidence of goitre. Goitre is associated with certain areas of the world where the water, soil and crops are relatively deficient in iodine, and in these areas the administration of iodine is found to be an effective preventative. It may also occur through the inability of the animals to use iodine adequately or as a result of the presence of goitrogenic substances, such as have been reported in cabbages and in soyabeans, which interfere with iodine metabolism. The occurrence of goitre in certain areas where the soil iodine is relatively high indicates that there are factors other than simple iodine deficiency contributing to this condition: among these may be included a high calcium content of the water supply.

The administration of small amounts of iodine in the food of domestic animals is very beneficial where there are symptoms of a deficiency. There is increasing evidence which suggests that such deficiencies may be geographically very localised. Moreover, although the clinical symptoms of extreme deficiency are so very visible, the results of suboptimal intakes are not so easily seen. On the other hand, the feeding of iodine supplements should be carried out with care, since too high a proportion of this element in the ration can have very undesirable results on the health of livestock. The general consensus of opinion on this matter is that 0.05% of iodine, based on the sodium chloride included in a mineral mixture, is quite sufficient.

In view of the conversion of absorbed iodide into thyroxine and the enhancement of the metabolic rate by this hormone, attempts have been made within recent years to iodinate dietary proteins by treating them, under suitable conditions, with iodine; the iodinated proteins have then been fed to different species of livestock in an attempt to stimulate production. A very extensive attempt to increase the production of milk by dairy cows has been reported by Blaxter.[16] The daily intake of iodinated protein was 20 gm./cow, which led to a mean increase in daily milk yield of 22% for an increase in feeding of 12% above the standards. However, 20% of the cows lost weight and there were some other undesirable effects. Such feeding practices require further investigation; present indications are that they may ultimately prove of use, but that very careful control is essential. Similar experiments have been carried out on the feeding of thyroprotein to pigs to determine its effects on their growth rates; the results were generally unsatisfactory.[17] Blaxter has also reported the influence of iodinated casein on sheep,[18] the basal metabolic rate of which was capable of being increased some 80% thereby. Whether iodocasein has any beneficial effects on laying hens seems to be a matter of doubt.[19]

(g) Copper.

In experiments on hæmoglobin regeneration in nutritional anæmia, copper was shown to be unnecessary for iron assimilation but to be essential for the conversion of absorbed iron into hæmoglobin. Although iron appears to be the primary deficiency in the anæmia of very young animals, better curative results are sometimes obtained when both iron and copper are administered. Copper, although only present in very small proportions in the animal body, is widely distributed in the tissues and is present in the blood (although not in the hæmoglobin) and in relatively large amounts in the liver. Milk is deficient in both iron and copper. There is now ample evidence that deficiencies of copper in the pasturage of many countries leads to much ill health in the livestock which consume the herbage. Although there are a number of complicating factors to be considered, copper deficiency is, at least in part, associated with " salt sick" in Florida,[20] " coast disease " and " falling disease " in different parts of Australia, " scouring disease " and " licking disease " in continental Europe and " swayback " in lambs in Britain. In some cases there seems to be a simple pasture deficiency, but in other instances the availability of the copper of the herbage is involved. A high Ca/P ratio, or high lead, or zinc content of the pastures has been suggested as being responsible for the copper of the herbage failing to perform its normal functions;[21] the use of copper as a curative agent for scouring due to excess molybdenum is another example in this class which has already been mentioned.

Anæmia has been described as the typical symptom of copper deficiency, the liver and spleen of affected animals showing excessive deposition of iron. In " falling disease " the deficiency produces sudden death in cattle; there is usually poor condition and evidence of anæmia, but scouring does not seem to be so common. " Swayback " is a nervous disorder of new-born and young lambs, muscular inco-ordination being the characteristic feature;[22] the lambs become stiff in gait, unthrifty, and retarded in growth; Dunlop and Wells [23] in Britain showed that feeding salt licks containing 0.3% of copper to pregnant ewes in districts where swayback was endemic reduced the incidence of disease in the lambs, while similar results were obtained in Australia.[24]

Another characteristic feature of copper deficiency seems to be loss of wool or deterioration of its quality in sheep [25] or loss of hair or poor pigmentation in other species.[26]

(h) Cobalt.

Although " wasting diseases " had been observed in grazing livestock in different parts of the world, the first evidence of the cause of the trouble, in which sheep and cattle would graze the herbage for several months, then lose appetite, waste away and finally die though surrounded by ample food, came from Australia. In most cases the animals were anæmic. Curiously enough, horses appeared to be unaffected. Eventually, after it had been found that the curative powers of various (impure) iron compounds did not parallel their iron contents, the beneficial agent was found to be cobalt,[27] which was one of the impurities. Treatment of the animals themselves, or of the pastures, with *small* amounts of cobalt is curative; high dosage is undesirable.

" Bush sickness " in New Zealand, " Grand Traverse Disease " in areas of the United States, " Pine " in Britain, " Nakuruitis " in Kenya and " Enzootic Marasmus " in Australia are examples of the different names given to wasting diseases affecting ruminants in widely separated parts of the world: in each case cobalt is both a preventative and curative agent.

Non-ruminants seem to need very little cobalt in their diets, but it has been shown that rumen organisms take up cobalt from the surrounding medium.[28] Moreover, sheep which were given cobalt orally, after having been rendered cobalt deficient, gained weight, had restored appetites and increased hæmoglobin values while comparable control, undosed animals and those given cobalt by injection, continued to decline. It was also shown that there were changes in the types of rumen organisms, and a marked reduction in their numbers, in sheep on a cobalt deficient diet and in those given cobalt by injection.[29] In some way, therefore, the bacterial population of ruminants is involved in cobalt deficiency disease.

The problem is more interesting on account of the fact that vitamin B_{12} which is active in cases of human pernicious anæmia, has been found to contain about 4% of cobalt.[30]

In experiments on copper and cobalt deficiency in sheep, Marston [31] has described the clinical symptoms of sheep suffering from lack of cobalt. They are lethargic and listless, with dull and rheumy eyes; their buccal and conjunctival mucosæ become pale and their skins change to a dull greenish colour as well as becoming fragile enough to break when the wool is parted.

In some parts of the world, deficiencies of both cobalt and copper occur in the herbage. The " Coast Disease " of Australia is due to such causes.

(i) Manganese.

Small amounts of manganese are essential for normal reproduction and as an activator for various enzymes, such as arginase.[32] Manganese is stored chiefly in the liver, and is excreted via the fæces; the amount present in the body can be appreciably increased by suitable feeding. A deficiency in rats results in testicular degeneration and imperfect development of the fœtus after conception; growth may also be retarded. In poultry a deficiency results in perosis or " slipped tendon ", a gross enlargement and malformation of the tibio-metatarsal joint with displacement of the gastrocnemius.[33] This condition is most frequent in battery-fed birds and is aggravated by large amounts of calcium and phosphorus, which possibly prevent manganese absorption. Hens on a manganese-deficient diet produce eggs of low percentage hatchability, with a large proportion of chondrodystrophic embryos having short thick legs and wings and globular heads.

Manganese is widely distributed in the plant kingdom and although it may be deficient in milk, the amounts present in the usual animal foods are adequate for normal nutrition except, perhaps, for poultry.

(j) Zinc.

Although no instance of zinc deficiency in farm animals kept under natural conditions has been reported, zinc is an essential element for the nutrition of rats and presumably for other animals, since it is an activator for carbonic anhydrase, the enzyme responsible for the reversible formation of carbonic acid from water and carbon dioxide. Rats deprived of zinc exhibit retarded growth and a deterioration in the fur. The element is widely distributed in very minute amounts in the body and by feeding zinc these amounts can be considerably increased, although they are not permanently retained. Excretion is via the fæces. Milk contains more zinc than copper or manganese and other foods contain more than enough for nutritional requirements. A dietary excess of zinc seems to have little influence on laboratory animals, but Godden [34] has stated that there is some evidence that it may have harmful results with pigs.

(k) Other minerals of unknown function.

In addition to the mineral elements already discussed, which have been proved to be essential for animal nutrition, many other inorganic elements have been shown to occur in the animal body. Although these are not known to be necessary and are generally considered as being merely contaminants arising from their accidental occurrence in the food supply, refinements in analytical technique may eventually show some of them to be essential in extremely minute amounts.

Bromine is invariably found in animal blood and this element is a normal constituent of plants. Occasionally considerably more bromine than iodine is to be found in the blood and tissues, and this is attributed to a high intake and a slow rate of excretion.

Nickel is very closely related to cobalt and although there is no conclusive evidence of any physiological role for nickel there have been indications that this element might increase the effect of cobalt in the treatment of enzootic marasmus, when suboptimal levels of cobalt are fed.

Aluminium is present in all plants and animals but only traces can be absorbed from the intestine, so that relatively large amounts have been fed experimentally without producing any harmful results. Godden[34] reports that pigs may consume considerable amounts of alum for long periods without any harmful results. Aluminium may, however, interfere with the absorption of phosphorus and large intakes of aluminium salts, in excess of the total phosphorus, will produce rickets. Normal foods contain such a small amount of aluminium that there is little or no effect on phosphorus absorption.

Silicon is present in all soils and occurs in all plant and animal tissues. Herbivorous animals normally consume large amounts of silicon and they have the capacity to metabolise and store appreciable quantities. Although various animals have been successfully reared on silicon-deficient rations and no essential function has been claimed for this element, the very high percentage occurring in feathers suggests that it may be important in maintaining their rigidity.

Barium and *strontium* occur occasionally in animals; barium has always been found in the eyes, and a relationship to pigmentation has been suggested.

(1) Toxic elements.

Several minerals which have no useful nutritional function sometimes occur in the food or water supply in amounts which render them of significance for their toxic effects.

As *lead arsenate* is now a very commonly used insecticide, there arises the possibility of lead or arsenic poisoning resulting from the feeding of crops treated with this chemical. The amount of readily soluble lead in soil, however, is found to be very small and the uptake of lead by growing plants is chiefly confined to the roots. Owing to the ability of soil to fix most of the lead reaching it, lead poisoning arising from the use of sprays containing lead would seem to be unlikely. Lead poisoning has more frequently been reported amongst stock grazing on shooting ranges or around disused lead mines, although it has been found that sheep are very resistant to lead poisoning.[35] While the primary effect of soil arsenic is to reduce plant growth, there is an increased arsenic content of the crop which may have a harmful influence on the animal consuming it. Although arsenic normally occurs in the body, anything other than very minute traces is dangerous. Arsenic poisoning from natural sources has been reported from an area in New Zealand where the soil and water contained relatively large quantities of the poisonous element. It has recently been suggested that arsenic may be of value in preventing selenium intoxication.[7]

Fluorine occurs regularly in teeth and bones but when ingested in too large amounts it has a toxic effect characterised by mottled enamel of the teeth: as a result of the rapid wearing down of the teeth the animals are unable to eat. Bone and teeth injuries are the usual signs of fluorine toxicity but an excessive or prolonged intake also affects food consumption and consequently productivity. Fluorine occurs in many foods and in certain areas the amounts in the drinking water are dangerously high. In affected areas in various parts of the world chemical investigations have shown the soil, vegetation and animal bones to contain ten times as much fluorine as similar materials from healthy districts. Apart from these special areas, however, the most important cause of fluorine poisoning in farm animals is the use of calcium phosphate supplements containing fluorine. Many natural rock phosphates contain up to 3.5 per cent. of fluorine and their use as mineral supplements has resulted in harmful effects. Acid phosphate and dicalcium phosphate made from such rock phosphate for feeding purposes also contain harmful amounts of fluorine unless special precautions are taken, and as mineral phosphate fertilisers frequently contain 3 or 4 per cent. of fluorine and considerably increase the fluorine content of the drainage waters, their use may result in a dangerously increased fluorine content of the water supply. Bone meals and dicalcium phosphate made from bones normally contain only very small amounts of fluorine and can be considered as safe mineral supplements. It has been stated that mineral phosphate supplements for feeding purposes should not contain more than 0.1 per cent. of fluorine—and probably less if it is given over long periods to breeding stock and dairy cattle—although the form in which the fluorine occurs seems to be important. American workers[36] carried out feeding experiments with pigs, chickens and rats and found that fluorine in calcium fluoride was not nearly so toxic as in sodium fluoride; rock phosphate limestone and triple superphosphate containing fluorine were intermediate in their harmful effects. Even though the toxic effects of fluorine are cumulative, rock phosphates containing 3.5 per cent. of fluorine were fed as 0.5 per cent. of a pig ration for 20 to 25 weeks without harm. Although chickens are also prone to fluorine poisoning they may stand higher levels and excrete fluorine faster than mammals; up to 2 per cent. of the fluorine-containing rock phosphate was safely included in chick rations.

Selenium in quite small concentrations can have very injurious effects and whilst it is of little importance in this country, selenium toxicosis is common in certain areas in America. The so-called " alkali disease " of cattle in the Great Plains of America, characterised by a loss of vitality and appetite, emaciation and loss of hair, is now known to be a selenium poisoning. Any soil containing 0.5 parts per million of selenium is potentially dangerous but there is considerable variation in the selenium contents of the various plants, some apparently benefiting from this element and showing enhanced growth and yield. There is no satisfactory means of preventing selenium poisoning, although it has been found that the addition of sodium arsenite to the drinking water combats the toxicity of both organic and inorganic selenium, as also does increasing the protein content of the diet. In practice the only satisfactory treatment so far has been to transfer the animals to unaffected areas and to avoid selenised foods.

Molybdenum is toxic to animals and is responsible for the "teartness" of pastures in certain areas of England. The characteristic symptom is a violent form of scouring, which is usually treated by removing the animals from the affected pasture and feeding roughage foods. The administration of copper sulphate will cure the diarrhœa.[36] Teartness occurs on soils derived from the lower lias formations, which are relatively rich in molybdenum, and the absorption of molybdenum by the herbage is increased by the use of lime or manures containing lime. Clovers and Yorkshire fog absorb molybdenum most readily and so are not desirable on teart land, and the molybdenum in young leafy growth generally is the most harmful, hay crops grown on teart land usually being safe to feed. Recent work[37] has indicated that the use of manures containing cobalt may have the harmful effect of increasing the molybdenum content of the herbage to an undesirable extent.

Nitrite and *nitrate* poisoning have been reported from several sources. Cases of "oat hay poisoning" in America, causing trembling, staggering and rapid perspiration have been ascribed to the presence in the oat hay of potassium nitrate.[38] The condition is most common in ruminants. Post-mortem examinations show that hæmoglobin is converted to methæmoglobin, and since this is a change associated with nitrites it is probable that a conversion of nitrate to nitrite occurs in the digestive tract. Olson and Moxon[39] have examined the possibility of the conversion of nitrate to nitrite in the plant food before ingestion, and have found that when the material is wet, reduction of nitrates by bacterial action may occur over a wide temperature range.

Plants other than oats, *e.g.*, other cereals and certain weeds, may sometimes contain enough nitrate to produce the characteristic symptoms, and there is evidence that the trouble may occur repeatedly in certain areas. There is a possibility that nitrate fertilisation may produce crops which are toxic, and Crawford[40] has reported a case of 16 cattle dying after grazing an area dressed with sodium nitrate, although in this case it appears that dry weather had prevented the solution of the manure which had itself been licked up by the stock.

(7) Mineral requirements of domestic animals

In determining the mineral requirements of domestic animals and the necessity or otherwise for supplementing the food supply with a mineral mixture, consideration must be given to the stage of maturity of the animals, their production—of growth, fat, fœtus, milk or eggs—and the mineral composition of the foods usually given. The addition of mineral supplements cannot raise production above certain levels, but is only effective in remedying any deficiencies in the diet. Although there are a considerable number of mineral elements essential for adequate nutrition the majority of them are *usually* present in sufficient quantity in most foods.

In an attempt to summarise the needs of livestock for the inorganic elements, Mitchell [9] has given the following table.

TABLE 12

Element			Rat	Pig	Chicken	Calf	Lamb	Horse
Calcium	...	...	0.36	0.40	0.66	0.27	0.18	0.23
Phosphorus	...	...	0.22	0.30	0.40	0.19	0.15	0.21
Magnesium	...	...	0.005	—	0.04	0.07	—	—
Potassium	...	...	0.17	0.15	0.17	—	—	—
Manganese	...	...	—	—	0.004	—	—	—
Cobalt ...	...	...				0.07	0.07	
Copper	...	...	3	8		3	5	
Iodine ...	...	...			1	0.09	0.11	
Iron	...	...	...	60					

The above average requirements are given as percentages of the dry matter of the ration for the first five elements, and as parts per million for the last four.

The values refer to the growing animal, but they will not be quite sufficient for the very young animal. Moreover, though the calcium figure will not need to be increased very much for a pregnant beast, that of phosphorus is at least 40% higher for the ewe. During heavy lactation, but not perhaps otherwise, additional calcium is likely to be necessary; the amount of phosphorus will need to be increased 33-50%, however. For the laying hen, of course, the calcium requirements can rise to as much as 3% of the ration. There is no evidence of an added need for calcium and phosphorus for muscular work, though extra potassium may be necessary.

Mitchell concludes that from the practical point of view it would be difficult to make a ration, well balanced with respect to its major organic constituents, which would be deficient in potassium or magnesium, or, save in certain regions, in copper, cobalt, iodine or iron. Poultry rations may lack sufficient manganese, however. There is a definite chance of calcium being present in insufficient quantities in rations containing large amounts of cereals, cereal by-products and vegetable-protein concentrates. If the ration is adequate in protein, however, Mitchell believes that it will also be adequate with respect to phosphorus, provided that a good combination of foods is used to furnish the protein. Only in the very young chick or pig may there be a need for mineral supplements to supply phosphorus. As there is no body storage of salt, deficiency of this mineral can very easily occur.

Among the many reviews which have appeared concerning mineral deficiencies in livestock, that of Miss Russell [41] is especially useful, since it surveys the whole field and gives many references to original work.

REFERENCES

1. Orr, J. B., (1929). " Minerals in Pasture in Relation to Animal Health."
2. Snook, L. C., (1938). Empire J. Exp. Agric., 6.
3. Hogan, A. G. & J. L. Nierman, (1927), quoted by Maynard " Animal Nutrition ", 1947.
4. Rittenberg, D. & D. Shemin, (1946). Annual Rev. Biochem., 15, 247.
5. Robinson, C. S., C. F. Huffman & M. F. Mason, (1929). J. Biol. Chem., 84, 257.
6. Ferguson, W. S., A. H. Lewis & S. J. Watson, (1943). J. Agric. Sci., 33, 44.
7. Moxon, A. L. & M. Rhian, (1943). Physiol. Rev. 23, 305.
8. Smith, S. E. & E. J. Larson, (1946). J. Biol. Chem., 163, 29.
9. Mitchell, H. H., (1947). J. Animal Sci., 6, 365.
10. Bruce, H. M. & R. K. Callow, (1934). Biochem. J., 28, 517.
11. Morris, S. & S. C. Ray, (1939). Biochem. J., 33, 1209.
12. Tyler, C., (1940). Biochem. J., 34, 202.
13. Tyler, C., (1942). J. Agric. Sci., 32, 43.
14. Eveleth, D. F. & T. W. Millen, (1939). Vet. Med., 34, 106.
15. Ender, F., K. Halse, & P. Slagsvold, (1949). Proc. 14th Int. Vet. Congress, London.
16. Blaxter, K. L., (1946). J. Agric. Sci., 36, 117.
17. Braude, R., (1947). J. Agric. Sci., 37, 45.
18. Blaxter, K. L., (1948). J. Agric. Sci., 38, 207.
19. Hutt, F. B. & R. S. Gowe, (1948). Poultry Sci., 27, 286.
20. Neal, W. M., R. B. Becker & A. L. Shealy, (1931). Science, 74, 418.
21. Shearer, G. D., J. Innes & E. McDougall, (1940). Vet. J., 96, 309.
22. Stewart, W. L., (1932). Vet. J., 88, 133.
23. Dunlop, G. & H. Wells, (1938). Vet. Rec., 50, 1175.
24. Bennetts, H. W. & F. Chapman, (1937). Austral. Vet. J., 13, 138.
25. Marston, H. R. & H. J. Lee, (1948). J. Agric. Sci., 38, 229.
26. Smith, S. E., M. Medlicott & G. Ellis, (1944). Amer. J. Physiol., 142, 179.
27. Underwood, E. & J. Filmer, (1935). Austral. Vet. J., 11, 84.
28. Tosic, J. & R. L. Mitchell, (1948). Nature, 162, 502.
29. Gall, L., S. E. Smith, D. Becker, C. Stark & J. Loosli, (1949). Science, 109, 468.
30. Lester Smith, E., (1948). Nature, 162, 144.
31. Marston, H. R., H. J. Lee & I. W. McDonald, (1948). J. Agric. Sci., 38, 216.
32. Folley, S. J. & A. L. Greenbaum, (1948). Biochem. J., 43, 537.
33. Wilgus, H. S., Jr., L. C. Norris & G. F. Heuser, (1937). J. Nutrition, 14, 155.
34. Godden, W., (1939). Chem. and Indust., 58, 791.
35. Shearer, G. D., J. R. M. Innes & E. I. McDougall, (1940). Vet. J., 96, 309.
36. Kick, C. H., (1935). Ohio Agric. Exp. Sta. Bull., 558.
37. Mitchell, R. L., R. O. Scott, A. B. Stewart & J. Stewart, (1941). Nature, 148, 725.
38. Bradley, W. B., H. F. Eppson & O. A. Beach, (1940). Wyoming Agr. Exp. Sta. Bull., 241.
39. Olson, O. E. & A. L. Moxon, (1942). J. Amer. Vet. Med. Assoc., 100, 403.
40. Crawford, M., (1941). Vet. Rec., 53, 650
41. Russell, F. C., (1944). " Minerals in Pasture Deficiencies and Excesses in Relation to Animal Health ", 69.

VITAMINS

1. Introduction.
2. General chemistry of the vitamins.
3. Some physiological properties of the vitamins.
4. Requirements for the different vitamins.
   (a) Species differences.
   (b) Differences due to microbial agents of the digestive tract.
   (c) Differences due to physiological condition.
5. The occurrence and stability of the vitamins in foods.
6. The individual vitamins.
   (a) Vitamin A.
   (b) Vitamin D.
   (c) Vitamin E.
   (d) Vitamin K.
   (e) Vitamin B_1, aneurin or thiamine.
   (f) Riboflavin, vitamin B_2.
   (g) Nicotinic acid (niacin) and nicotinamide.
   (h) Pyridoxine, pyridoxal, pyridoxamine, vitamin B_6.
   (i) Pantothenic acid.
   (j) Biotin.
   (k) Inositol.
   (l) Choline.
   (m) Folic acid.
   (n) Other factors included in the vitamin B-complex.
   (o) Ascorbic acid, vitamin C.
   (p) Vitamin P.

(1) Introduction

The vitamins are a group of organic compounds, differing from the fats, proteins and carbohydrates in chemical structure, whose presence in minute amounts in foodstuffs is generally necessary for the well-being of mammalian and avian species. Although vague knowledge of the functions of some of them has been available for many, even hundreds of years, their scientific study goes back only to the end of the nineteenth century, while their actual isolation in pure form has been a problem, still continuing, of the last few decades.

Some of the vitamins can be synthesised from simpler materials by micro-organisms, so that modern research is revealing more and more the importance of these lower forms of life in the maintenance of the health of many species of livestock, especially, but not solely, the adult ruminants.

There is a great deal of diversity of chemical constitution and of function among the vitamins as a class. Moreover, in a number of instances, as for example vitamin D, a single name is given to a group of substances of related though not identical structure, which have common physiological functions. In a few cases, the position is made more complicated by the different members of such a group having different nutritional values for different species. Again the members of the vitamin D group may be quoted as an example.

(2) General chemistry of the vitamins

Full details of the chemistry of the vitamins must be sought in text-books and monographs,[1][2] attention here being directed to such aspects of their properties as are of nutritional significance.

It was discovered in 1913 that the substances needed for life and health, over and above protein, fats, carbohydrates and mineral elements, must consist of at least two types, one kind being soluble in fats and the other in aqueous solutions. To the present time, the grouping of the vitamins into " fat-soluble " and " water-soluble " classes is preserved, even though riboflavin, a member of the second class, is sparingly soluble in water, though more soluble than it is in lipoid solvents.

The fat-soluble vitamins A, D, E and K—the letters are more indicative of the order in which they were discovered than anything else, but are retained because of their simplicity—are organic compounds of complex structure, differing in the numbers and kinds of carbon-rings in their molecules and in the attached side chains. Oxygen is present in some of the vitamins of this group, but none of them contains elements other than carbon, hydrogen and oxygen.

Vitamin A is decomposed by exposure to oxygen (air) and by light; vitamin D is destroyed by ultra-violet radiation; vitamin E is sensitive to the presence of oxygen but exerts a protective action on any vitamin A which accompanies it; it is broken down by ultra-violet light; vitamin K is prone to decomposition by light, heat and oxygen. Since the four vitamins, in their various forms, often occur in the same foods, the above properties underline the necessity for storing such foods in cool, dark rooms without too much access of air.

The water-soluble vitamins include a group which is sometimes described as the " vitamin B-complex ", the individual members of which, in very many cases, have now been named and their chemical structures determined as well as their physiological functions studied. Two other water-soluble vitamins, C and P, respectively, are usually present in different classes of foodstuffs from those in which the others occur in substantial proportions.

The vitamin B family now includes aneurin, riboflavin, niacin, pyridoxine, pantothenic acid, folic acid, biotin, p-aminobenzoic acid, choline, inositol and the cobalt-containing B_{12}, quite apart from another group of impure substances whose functions are suspected but whose chemical constitutions are not yet settled. Chemically they are a very diverse group of compounds, but many foodstuffs which are rich in one member of the family are often potent sources of the others, too. Some noteworthy points about the members of the vitamin B-complex are the instability of riboflavin, pyridoxine and folic acid to light, and that of aneurin and riboflavin to alkali. Aneurin is relatively easily decomposed by heat. These matters are relevant to the processing of foods containing members of the vitamin B-complex.

(3) Some physiological properties of the vitamins

In many cases full details of the physiological functions of the vitamins are lacking; the following list is intended merely to give some idea of the general importance of this group of compounds. Species differences in requirements are considered later.

Vitamin A is concerned with vision and with the maintenance of the epithelial tissues of the body; in some as yet unknown way it is involved in protein synthesis. Vitamin D, on the other hand, operates in the metabolism of calcium and phosphorus and thus plays a part in bone formation. Over the exact functions of vitamin E there has been much discussion; it is concerned in the maintenance of normal reproduction in some species and in keeping muscular tissues in healthy condition, while vitamin K assists in the preservation of the clotting power of the blood, thereby preventing hæmorrhages.

During the last decade or so, several members of the vitamin B-complex, including aneurin, riboflavin, niacin, pyridoxine and pantothenic acid, have been proved to be important constituents of enzyme systems which are concerned with the metabolism of carbohydrates and proteins in the body. Usually the vitamins are linked to phosphoric acid and act in conjunction with specific proteins.. They are thus very necessary for the well-being of the organism.

Of the other members of the B-complex, folic acid and vitamin B_{12} are factors in the prevention of certain types of anæmia, choline is an agent for the transference of methyl groups from one compound to another within the organism, and the rest are, as yet, too little understood to have had definite reactions assigned to them. It may ultimately prove to be the case that some of the less well identified substances are compounds of previously known function; mistakes of that kind are difficult to avoid when one suspects the existence of an unknown factor as a dietary essential for some species and, with this vague knowledge as the only guide for the early experiments, has to produce an experimental diet complete in every other essential save the one doubtful entity.

Vitamin C helps to maintain in health the intercellular substances of the body. On the precise nature and exact functions of vitamin P there is yet no general agreement, but the vitamin, or group of compounds, is said to prevent the development of capillary fragility.

(4) Requirements for the different vitamins

The reactions in which many of the vitamins are known to participate are so fundamental in the life of the organism, that it may be assumed that they are essential for the well-being of all the mammalian and avian species. In this book, however, the main theme is not that of the basal reactions of living tissues but of the nutrients which must be provided in the diet of livestock. For this reason it is essential to consider briefly the general factors which influence the required dietary intakes of the various vitamins under different conditions.

(a) Species differences.

There are marked differences between livestock of the various species for dietary supplies of vitamins. Vitamin A, in one or other of its different forms, is needed by animals of all species, at all ages and in all conditions. On the other hand vitamin C must always find a place in the diet of man, the primates, the guinea-pig, but only in certain conditions for some other species. Normal healthy adult ruminants are seemingly independent of dietary supplies of members of the vitamin B-complex, but only because the rumen bacteria synthesise the vitamins in sufficient amounts from other constituents of the ration. The horse, which seems to make rather less efficient use of micro-organisms than the developed ruminant does, takes a place somewhere between such creatures as the pig or fowl and the sheep or cow, the former of which are completely dependent upon dietary sources of riboflavin, for example, while the latter are normally independent of it.

Differences between the needs of the different species for supplies of vitamins in the ration, apart from varying degrees of enlistment of the aid of micro-organisms of the digestive tract, may also reflect varying capacities of the animal tissues for synthesis of the vitamins. Too little is yet known of this interesting subject.

(b) Differences due to microbial agents of the digestive tract.

These differences are due to increasingly complex symbiotic relationships between host and micro-organisms of the digestive tract. The young of all species have a general dietary need for vitamin A and for members of the B-complex. As growth proceeds the normal herbivore, and especially the growing ruminant, obtains more and more of its requirements for vitamin B from bacteria, whereas the omnivorous and carnivorous species remain almost entirely dependent on ingested food. All of them continue to need vitamin A.

This has a bearing on the practical feeding of young livestock which are taken from the dam at an early age and are given milk substitutes; the foods provided should be efficient sources of the required vitamins, bearing in mind the age and species of the animals.

(c) Differences due to physiological condition.

The different physiological conditions which it is desirable to cover under this heading are respectively, the maintenance of the adult beast in health, the growth of young stock, and work, reproduction and lactation in mature animals.

When new body-substance, or milk, or eggs, is being produced, there are additional needs for vitamins over and above those required for the maintenance of normal health and weight. This means that special attention must be paid to growing, pregnant and lactating animals; too low an intake, as for example, of vitamin A will lead to less than optimal growth, or diminished fertility, or the production of feeble or stillborn young. Two or three times as high an intake of vitamin A may be needed for satisfactory reproduction as for keeping the animal in what appears to be excellent health. This last point is a very important practical one, for it means that one cannot judge the reproductive capacity of a beast by its general appearance and, since to find that conception has not occurred or that the young are feeble at birth is to be wise after the event, steps must be taken to see that the diet of breeding stock always contains all the vitamins which will be needed and in optimal amounts.

Although it has been stated that the normal, healthy, developed ruminant is more or less independent of dietary sources of vitamin B, because of the effects of the rumen bacteria, the full implication of the symbiotic relationship between animal and micro-organisms must be remembered. Different types of micro-organism synthesise the various vitamins of the B-complex in different relative proportions and, since the numbers and kinds of rumen bacteria are influenced by the nature of the ration given to cattle, sheep and goats, there is in fact a relationship between the food ingested by those species and the amounts of vitamin-B which are made available to them. Synthesis by the animal itself and by rumen bacteria may well be sufficient for the moderate or low producing dairy cow, but whether that is true for the high producer is not so sure: the matter should not be left solely to chance.

Hard work, involving as it does the metabolism of large quantities of carbohydrates, probably requires the vitamins involved in oxidative processes in amounts proportional to the energy metabolism concerned. Since the horse is known to have limited powers for the synthesis of riboflavin, for example, it follows that attention should be paid to the intake of riboflavin when horses are doing hard work.

The breeding performance of cattle and horses is improved by the inclusion of vitamin C in the ration, although for normal maintenance little or none seems to be required.

If a surplus of the fat soluble vitamins is given to livestock, a considerable proportion of the excess may be stored in the liver and in other parts of the body, to be used when there is a temporary dietary deficiency. On the other hand there is little or no capacity for the storage of the water soluble vitamins in the animal body, so that their supply becomes a day-to-day problem. Scouring, in all species, may bring about insufficient absorption of such factors; the administration of some of the sulphonamide type of drugs, by reducing substantially the numbers of micro-organisms in the gut, may also produce temporary deficiencies.

(5) The occurrence and stability of the vitamins in foods

Details of the precise contents of the different vitamins in various foods are not a matter of very great practical interest; the following table is intended to give a general picture of the relative potencies of the different foodstuffs commonly given to livestock.

TABLE 13

	Vitamin.	Rich sources.	Poor sources.
Fat-soluble	A — As carotene or pro-vitamin A.	Good pasture and fresh green crops; good dried grass; good green silage; carrots; yellow maize.	Poor hay; oil seeds; most cereals and cereal by-products; roots except carrots; bleached, dried crops.
	As vitamin A itself.	Fish liver oils; milk and livers of animals on good pasture, or on good animal sources.	Lean or fat-extracted meats.
	D	Fish liver oils; synthetic vitamin D.	Almost all other foods.
	E	Fresh green crops; cereal grains, especially germ; germ-oils; some vegetable oils.	Foodstuffs low in fat content.
	K	Fresh green crops; soya-bean.	Most seeds and roots.
Water soluble	B-complex, as a whole.	Fresh green crops; oil seeds and cakes; legume seeds; liver; dried yeast; bran; (fresh milk is a moderate source).	Highly extracted flour; starches; fats; low-protein foods.
	C	Fresh green crops; roots; fresh milk.	Fats; cereal grains; most foods of animal origin.
	P	Green leaves.	Most other foods.

The list is noteworthy for the way in which fresh green foods are shown to be rich sources of most of the vitamins, both fat and water soluble kinds. Other foods which are good all-round sources of the vitamins are fresh liver and, bearing in mind its high water content, fresh milk. As potent sources of the B-complex, bran, wheat germ, liver and dried yeast may be indicated. The poverty of most foods in vitamin D is discussed in the section dealing with this vitamin.

Sufficient has been said of the general chemistry of the vitamins to give some idea of their stability in foodstuffs. A number of them are decomposed by heat treatment, so that the cooking of foods is of no advantage from the point of view of vitamin content, but so far as animal foodstuffs are concerned, most harm probably results from exposure to air and light, either in the field after harvesting or after the foods have been ground. Losses of potency of vitamins A, E, and C and of riboflavin can easily amount to some 50 per cent., when foods are ground and left exposed to light and air for a day.

(6) The individual vitamins
(a) Vitamin A.

The expression vitamin A is often loosely used to denote either pro-vitamin A or the true vitamin: actually the pro-vitamins are the products of plants, from which the animal organism can produce the actual vitamin.

(i) *Pro-vitamin A.*

A group of closely related compounds, the α-, β-, and γ-carotenes, all of them having the molecular formula $C_{40}H_{56}$, occurs in the unsaponifiable fraction of the ether extract of green leaves and of carrots. A vast amount of chemical research has been carried out on these substances, which have been shown to be highly unsaturated compounds containing some chemical structures in common in their molecules. It is due to the fact that they have common structures that they each possess what may briefly be described as " vitamin-A-like activity " when they are included in the diets of livestock. Because the three molecules are not absolutely identical, however, the three different carotenes are not equal in physiological activity. From all points of view, β-carotene is the most important; it constitutes some 85 per cent. of the total carotenes of plants. A fourth compound, cryptoxanthine, a hydroxy derivative of the carotenes, occurs in yellow maize and is also of biological importance.

The pure carotenes are deeply coloured substances, which give yellow solutions in fats, though the colour is usually masked by the chlorophyll of plant leaves. Oxygen quickly decomposes them, with the formation of physiologically inactive derivatives; light also has a destructive action on them. So far as green foods are concerned, the depth and vividness of the green is usually an indication of the amount of carotene present both with regard to the fresh crops and the conserved materials made from them (except silage); this is by no means an infallible guide but is a useful general one, where no accurate method is available.

A detailed study of the chemical constitution of the carotenes in relation to their physiological properties is much beyond the scope of this book; it is sufficient to indicate here that each of the carotenes may exist in several isomeric forms, due to the many double bonds in the molecule, with corresponding changes in biological value.[3]

Carotene is much better absorbed from the digestive tract when some suitable solvent is present; normally this is the rest of the ether extract of plant materials. Moore[4] first showed that the feeding of carotene to rats which had been depleted of their reserves of vitamin A led to the deposition of vitamin A in the liver; in other words the animal body can convert carotene into actual vitamin A. At first it was thought that the liver was the chief site of the conversion, but more recent work[5][6] has shown that the intestinal mucosa is also involved. It does not follow, however, that all of the absorbed carotene will be converted into vitamin A at once; some may be stored in the body-fat, for example. There are marked differences between the different species of livestock regarding their powers of absorption of carotene from rations and the proportions of the absorbed material which they store as carotene: birds differ from mammals in that they store little carotene, either in the body or in the yolk of their eggs. The colour of egg yolk is due to related but apparently biologically inactive pigments: egg yolks which are very pale may yet be rich in vitamin A, but the deeply coloured yolks are not necessarily rich in the vitamin.

(ii) *Vitamin A.*

There are at least two substances, both of them highly unsaturated alcohols and of very similar constitutions, which have the formula, $C_{20}H_{30}O$. One of them is found in the fat of animals which have received carotene, and in the liver and gut of salt-water fish, the other being found in fresh-water fish. Unlike carotene, the common form of the vitamin, designated A_1, is a very pale yellow, which is almost colourless in dilute solutions. The colour of a fat such as butter is thus no guide to its vitamin A potency.

When a solution of antimony trichloride in dry chloroform is added to a sample of vitamin A, a deep blue colour, the depth of which is proportional to the amount of the vitamin present, quickly develops, although the colour relatively soon fades. This reaction, discovered by Carr and Price, has been much used for the estimation of the amounts of the vitamin in fats and in the fatty extracts of foods, the potency of the material being expressed in "Blue Units". Attempts have been made to overcome the difficulties of the transient colour.[1] Carotene under similar conditions gives a much weaker blue-green colour. Other methods of estimation are either biological or spectrographic.

The chemical formula for vitamin A, together with its general reactions, would suggest that its molecule might be derived from half a molecule of carotene. It has indeed been suggested that the molecule of β-carotene may be broken down into two molecules of vitamin A in the animal body, whereas the other carotenes, less physiologically potent than the β-compound, can only form one because of their slightly different chemical constitutions. After the publication of much conflicting evidence, this does now seem to be the case.[2] Vitamin A_2 is less potent for mammals than the more abundant A_1.

In its sensitivity to light and other destructive agents, the true vitamin resembles the carotenes.

(iii) *The physiological properties of pro-vitamin A and vitamin A.*

In the absence of sufficient dietary amounts of vitamin A or of the carotenes, or in conditions which prevent their absorption from the gut, (a) the growth of young animals slows down or ceases entirely, death eventually ensuing if the deficiency is absolute and is continued, (b) hyper-keratinization of the epithelial tissues occurs, as the result of which there may be reduced resistance to disease, so far as the eyes, respiratory and alimentary tracts are concerned, or reduced fertility, due to imperfect functioning of the membranes of the reproductive organs, (c) "night blindness ", being an ability to see properly in dim light, is produced or (d) there may be some muscular inco-ordination, resulting in a stiff gait, or even convulsions may occur.

Though many of the ways in which vitamin A functions in the organism are not understood, it is known that the vitamin combines with a protein to form the retinal pigment, rhodopsin or visual purple, which, by the action of light on the retina, is converted into visual yellow. The last named is a protein-vitamin-A-aldehyde complex.[9] It is this sequence of changes which is responsible for vision in subdued light, so that a deficiency of vitamin A in the blood results in there being too little visual purple for such conditions. There is thus " night blindness ", often the first symptom to be noticed in mature stock.

Mellanby[10] showed that animals may be born blind, or may become blind at an early age for another reason connected with vitamin A deficiency, namely, malformation of the bones of the skull and compression of the optic nerve.

In some way vitamin A is concerned with the synthesis of the body protein,[11] so that the failure of young stock to grow fully may partly be due to this factor. Whether the diminished capacity for protein synthesis produces a desire for less food, or whether the poor appetite which accompanies vitamin A deficiency operates quite independently is not clear : both factors would hinder the increase of bodyweight. The more rapidly the young animal grows under optimal conditions, the more serious is a lack of vitamin A in the ration; birds are particularly affected, the turkey more than the fowl.

In domestic animals an unsteady gait, due to nerve degeneration, is a common symptom of vitamin A deficiency, while a swollen condition (generalised œdema or anasarca) is found in cattle quite often.

The hyper-keratinization of the epithelial tissues which follows upon a lack of vitamin A in the diet affects the appearance of the animal. Its coat is usually roughened and dry. Apart from the eye troubles already mentioned, the changes in the epithelial tissues and perhaps alterations in the composition of the fluid bathing the eyes, usually produces pronounced " watering ", or, in the case of the fowl, the secretion of a viscous fluid which may cause the lids to adhere to one another. Inflammation of the eyes, probably due to secondary infections, may or may not occur. A related phenomenon is the tendency for deposits to accumulate in the kidneys and ureters due to the degenerate epithelial tissues impairing the function of the kidney tubules. Cornification of the uterine and vaginal membranes results in diminished fertility.

(iv) *The units of carotene and vitamin A.*

The interest of the livestock breeder with respect to the amounts of vitamin A or carotene in foods relates to the physiological effects the rations are likely to produce. Two problems follow directly from this, (a) whether it is possible to measure accurately the quantities of the different pro-vitamins and vitamins in the food and (b) knowing the amounts which are present in the ration, whether it is possible to predict with accuracy their physiological action.

So far as the first point is concerned, the active factors are present in such small amounts that their separation and estimation is a matter of difficulty; some compromise is almost inevitable if the analyst is to give his data with sufficient speed. The second problem is even more serious. The precise physiological effects produced by a given amount of a given pure vitamin are conditioned by the amount of it which is absorbed from the gut, and by the species, sex, age, etc., of the animal concerned. So far as the diet is involved, then the amount and nature of its fat are important factors, while there is evidence that the presence of vitamin E in the ration prevents the destruction of some vitamin A in the gut.[11][13]

In the early days of vitamin A research, the chemical nature of the factor was not known with real precision. Consequently the amounts of the vitamin present in foods had to be measured by comparing the growth-promoting power for rats of the unknown food as compared with a standard oil, known to be active. Later on when fairly pure carotene became available, the International Unit of vitamin A potency was defined as the biological power (growth-promoting power under standard conditions) of one millionth of a gramme (one microgramme, or μg.) of this supposedly pure carotene. A few years later the multiple nature of carotene was realised, and the old standard solution of mixed carotenes was replaced by one of " pure " β-carotene. In order to cause as little confusion as possible, the amount of biological activity for the International Unit was kept the same as before, but, because the β-compound is the most active of the carotenes, the International Unit of vitamin A activity is that of only 0.6 microgramme of β-carotene.* Because of the complexities of the problem the position even now is very unsatisfactory, as Gridgeman has shown in his monograph [14] and it is probable that in future the regular estimation of the " vitamin A " content of foods will be by purely physical and chemical methods. The exact effect of a given amount of carotene or vitamin A, as indicated above, depends on the nature of the ration, but there is a sufficient body of evidence available to suggest reasonable limits for the amounts of these vitamins which are needed for specific purposes. When the vitamin A requirements of live-stock are being considered, International Units may be used, but the above limitations must be kept in mind.

From the practical feeding point of view the relationship of carotene to vitamin A is most important, for there seems to be no doubt that it is the latter substance which is the important one for the organism, carotene being of use only in so far as it can be converted into the true vitamin.

So far as rats are concerned it has been shown that if the basal diets of vitamin A depleted animals are satisfactory, especially with respect to vitamin E content, and if the doses given are relatively small, then the two substances (vitamin A and β-carotene) have equal potencies on a weight for weight basis.[8] This is of fundamental interest in showing that

* This has more recently been replaced by 0.34 microgramme of pure vitamin A acetate, equivalent to 0.3 microgramme of the pure vitamin.

when the molecule of β-carotene is broken down in the animal body it does give rise to two molecules of vitamin A.

It is not necessarily of much practical consequence, however, for these reasons: (a) it does not follow that the two substances are equally well absorbed from the gut of other species, (b) it cannot always be assumed that the rest of the ration will be satisfactory in all respects, (c) it does not follow that all species and breeds are equally efficient in converting carotene into vitamin A, even though the mechanism be the same, and (d) it is unsatisfactory to give either substance to livestock at very low levels, with no safety margin. Lastly, one should not assume that criteria which are suitable for growth are satisfactory for other physiological conditions. In a review of the needs of farm mammals, Hart[15] concludes that the minimal requirements of cattle, sheep, swine and horses are about 5 microgrammes of vitamin A, or about 20 International Units, or 20-30 microgrammes or 40-50 International Units of β-carotene per kilogramme of bodyweight; birds need even more. For practical purposes Hart recommends feeding *at least* 5-10 times these minimal levels. The needs for good reproduction are several times the levels which will keep the normal adult beast in a healthy condition, while evidence has been produced that in rats relatively high levels of intake (probably 400-600 I.U./Kg. bodyweight) led to better growth, longer life, longer reproductive life with more and better young, than at lower (and perhaps higher) levels.[16]

High levels of intake allow greater storage of vitamin in the liver and thus provide a safeguard against temporary shortages, but it is not possible to increase the levels in milk above very moderate values (400 I.U. per gramme of milk fat) even when very large doses of vitamin A are fed to cattle. The efficiency of transfer of vitamin A from food to milk is only of the order of 2-3 per cent.,[17] when such high doses are given. There is some evidence that the vitamin A reserves in the livers of newly born animals may be materially increased when the dam is given high levels of vitamin A during the last third of pregnancy; this has been shown to be true of the pig and goat[18] and perhaps of the cow. Evidence is also beginning to accumulate that there is an antagonistic relationship between the thyroid glands and vitamin A at very high dosage levels of the latter, but this does not materially affect normal feeding.

(v) *The significance of vitamin A in animal feeding.*

Cattle.—Since the precursor of vitamin A, carotene, is present in abundance in all fresh green leafy plants, grazing animals normally get sufficient not only for their immediate needs but for the storage of reserves to be used in periods of shortage or extra demand. However, the supply may be insufficient during prolonged periods of drought, when the grazing of fresh green grass is reduced and winter feeding conditions lengthened. Moreover, an abnormally dry summer and short grazing period usually mean a reduced supply of good class hay for winter use. These conditions are most pronounced in countries like America and India where summer droughts are liable to be very severe and of particularly long duration. Avitaminosis A, i.e., deficiency of vitamin A in the body, occurs in the United States under such conditions, the most common manifestations being premature expulsion of the fœtus, or death at full term, severe diarrhœa in weak, new-born calves and ophthalmia in young growing animals; in the latter instance complete blindness may result. Night blindness is the first clinical symptom, but this can only be detected when the condition is suspected and the vision of the animals is tested at twilight, for example by placing obstacles in their way in the yard as they are moved about.[18]

The time taken for symptoms of vitamin A deficiency to appear when there is neither carotene nor vitamin A in the food, depends principally upon the reserves built up during the period of abundance. Guilbert and Hart,[19] using cattle which had previously consumed an abundance of carotene, detected symptoms of deficiency after 230 days of continuous feeding with vitamin-deficient food; the total reserves were exhausted after 282 days. A daily withdrawal of reserves of 9-11 microgrammes per kg. live weight was suggested.

In parts of Britain, particularly on high-lying land, store cattle are wintered in either closed or open courts from September to March or April. During this time of 200 days or longer the diet is generally deficient in carotene, consisting largely of oat straw or inferior weathered hay. Before spring grass is available, therefore, animal reserves of vitamin A may quite commonly reach a low level. To feed these cattle merely on low quality hay to tide them over to the spring is therefore an unsound practice.

While definite evidence of avitaminosis A has not been proved, there are districts where catarrhal conditions and calculi in the urinary tract are common among young cattle. It must, however, be stressed that the absence of definite symptoms which are usually attributed to a deficiency of vitamin A does not necessarily imply that the animal has a sufficiency for normal health and growth. In fact, a hypovitaminosis may occur without definite symptoms. Hart[16] has drawn attention to the difficulty of diagnosis of the milder forms of avitaminosis A and to the fact that the state of maturity, lactation, gestation, development, production and rate of growth all influence the onset of symptoms.

Stewart and Macallum[20] showed that the vitamin A content of the colostrum of cows may be materially affected by the length of the non-lactating period between successive calvings. This is a discovery of real practical importance, for while it has long been known that cows should have a rest between milking and calving (a dry period), its full significance was not hitherto recognised.

Stewart and Macallum[21] have also found that calves born of mothers whose colostrum had a low vitamin A content, were more liable to infections such as white scour, navel ill and joint ill than were calves from mothers whose colostrum was rich in vitamin A.

Linton (1935) determined the vitamin A content in the livers of 58 calves, of which 34 were known to be diseased and 24 were apparently healthy calves slaughtered for food, the ages ranging from birth to 3 months; a higher percentage of cases with little or no liver reserves was found in the diseased calves than in the healthy animals. Similar results have been reported by Barron,[22] while a group of American workers[23] showed that dairy calves which had received less than about 20 microgrammes of carotene/Kg. bodyweight/day suffered from enteritis, together with some degeneration of kidney, liver and testis. The observations of the last named workers were generally confirmed and extended by others[24] who stated that yearlings may need intakes of about 100 μg. carotene/Kg./day.

The importance of satisfactory intakes of vitamin A for bulls has also been stressed.[25] About 50μg. or more of crude carotene/Kg./day is needed for satisfactory semen production. Two bulls which had been efficient in this respect, were then put on carotene deficient rations and " semen samples collected as the depletion progressed showed marked increases in percentage of abnormal spermatozoa and cellular debris, with progressive decline in motility ". Furthermore " histological evidence of previous testicular injury due presumably to vitamin A deficiency was evident after as long as 20 months of carotene feeding ".

Horses.—In the horse faulty hoof formation, e.g., brittleness,[26] general debility and loss of condition,[27] partial blindness,[28] little or no store of vitamin A in the liver,[29] and low fertility,[30] which have been reported in various parts of the world, all tend to show the inability of many of the conventional rations, such as oats and hard hay, to provide adequate vitamin A for this species, which must be among the worst fed of domestic animals.

When horses do not get access to grazing, the vitamin A must be supplied by giving soiling crops when available, and by the addition of cod liver oil, or dried grass, during the winter months.

Sheep.—Under normal conditions of husbandry sheep are not known to be liable to vitamin deficiency; indeed, sheep's liver usually carries a substantial reserve of vitamin A. Linton[29] found six ewes that had had no other food than that supplied by lowland grazing and which were slaughtered during May at intervals from shortly before full term to three weeks after parturition, to be fairly rich in vitamin A. The same worker provided evidence to suggest that the liver of the newly born lamb is very low in vitamin A content under normal conditions. Similar results have been described by Barron.[22]

While such high reserves may generally be present in the livers of grass-fed sheep, this is not necessarily the case with sheep, such as tup lambs, which have been artificially nourished by box feeding for the purpose of forcing an early maturity. For such animals cod liver oil should be added to the artificial food.

Although the frequency with which urinary calculi occur in sheep which have been folded on roots may seem significant in view of the poverty of most roots in carotene, there is no definite evidence to prove or disprove such a hypothesis as to the cause of the trouble.

Pigs.—Pathological conditions due to deficiency of vitamin A in the diet were at one time very common among sty-fed pigs, and for long were attributed to rheumatism and " cramps ". The pig is peculiarly susceptible to dietary deficiencies due to the demands created by the production of two litters of 10 or 12 piglings in the course of 12 months. In general, the cereals and their by-products as fed to pigs are deficient in carotene, and swill, while in itself a most valuable addition to the cereals, has by an order of the Ministry of Agriculture to be thoroughly boiled, as the result of which its vitamin content is greatly reduced, if not destroyed. It is not surprising, therefore, that unless the diet is fortified by the addition of vitamin A, hypovitaminosis A is common.

In the pig, in contrast to other domestic animals, nervous symptoms are primary, affected animals showing inco-ordination of movement, stiffness and spasms. There may be hemeralopia and also dryness and itchiness of the skin. Diarrhœa may also be present. Abortion may occur, or if the young are born at full term, they may be weakly and prone to catarrhal conditions, and to pneumonia.

Foot and Kon[31] found that they could not bring to marketable condition pigs which were receiving vitamin A deficient rations. Loss of appetite, poor growth, diarrhœa, awkwardness of gait, poor vision and fits were observed in the animals; a drooping ear and staring eye were characteristic symptoms.

Cure by the administration of vitamin A could be achieved in the milder cases, while weanling pigs, given a massive dose of the vitamin, were then able to manage without further supply right up to slaughtering. A constant level of 0.5 per cent. of cod liver oil in the ration, or 1 per cent. during the first three or four months only, so as to lessen the risk of spoiling the carcase fat by later feeding of the oil, have been suggested. Green food will provide some carotene for such animals, of course, but its intake is usually rather small.

Poultry.—According to Downham,[32] poultry, both young and mature, have a very high requirement of vitamin A. If the egg has been well supplied with the vitamin the young chick will probably have a reserve sufficient for two or three weeks, but not longer. Downham found that with chickens and turkey poults fed experimentally on a vitamin A deficient diet the mortality was 100 per cent. by the 45th day with the turkeys, and by the 60th day with the chicks. The greater requirements of young turkeys for vitamin A, as compared with young chicks, are in keeping with the more rapid growth of the former birds: the example is one of fairly general application to other constituents of the diet.

The symptoms of a deficiency in the diet are inco-ordination of movement, staggering and crouching on the hocks. Soreness and pastiness of the eyelids are pronounced. Colds are common and bronchial affections are usually the ultimate cause of mortality. " Nutritional roup " is the name given to a group of symptoms commonly seen in fowls fed on a diet deficient in vitamin A. Nutritional roup is therefore not a specific disease. The first symptoms usually noticeable are swelling of the infra-orbital sac, sero-mucous or muco-purulent rhinites with occlusion of the nasal passages and consequent difficulty in breathing. Concomitantly there is xerophthalmia and later keratomalacia. There are well marked lesions— membranous exudations and cheesy pinhead nodules—of the mouth and œsophagus.[33] Heavy deposits of urates in the kidneys and ureters, so that the organs take on a white, rather swollen appearance, is another symptom of vitamin A deficiency.

Dogs.—Although many of the diseases of dogs are suggestive of a deficiency of vitamin A in the diet, astonishingly little has been done towards clarification by assaying the liver reserves of vitamin A after death. Deafness in dogs (Mellanby), ulceration of the cornea, imperfect dental development, gastro-intestinal and kidney disturbances, skin affections and general systemic derangements are suggestive of hypovitaminosis A.

Some of the diets supplied to dogs, e.g., a preponderance of wheaten flour biscuits, are definitely deficient in either vitamin A or carotene, and it would be surprising therefore if a deficiency of vitamin A were not in part responsible for many canine ailments.

Linton and Brownlee[34] determined the liver reserves in 100 apparently healthy dogs and found great variation, many dogs having but low reserves. It is advisable to guard against a possible deficiency, particularly in the case of breeding dogs and young puppies, by the provision of cod liver, or higher potency oils, e.g., halibut oil.

Foxes.—The minimum vitamin A requirements of fox pups to prevent the onset of the first symptoms of vitamin A deficiency are between 15 and 25 I.U./Kg. bodyweight/day, but no storage in the liver was observed until 50 to 100 I.U. were fed.[35] The first and characteristic symptoms of deficiency are nervous, namely, " trembling and ' cocking ' of the head, periods of whirling and in some cases coma ". Abortions were also observed in deficient animals: no specific effect on the quality of the fur was noticed.

It will be noted that the dosage needed is of the same order as for herbivorous species (p. 94) and the likelihood is that the fairly constant ratio of dosage to bodyweight is a characteristic of growth in most species of mammal.

(b) Vitamin D.

(i) Introduction.

In the early years of this century there were two separate schools of thought with regard to the problem of rickets: in the one case it was held that rickets could be cured by dietary agencies, while the alternative belief was that sunlight was a curative agent. Mellanby[36] showed that a fat-soluble substance was concerned in satisfactory bone growth in puppies. Huldschinsky, on the other hand, believed that ultra-violet light was the responsible factor.[37]

In 1922 McCollum, using air and heat to destroy what we now know to be carotene and vitamin A, showed that the butter fat he had used still had calcifying power for the bones of young rats.[38] This was the first proof of the existence of two fat soluble vitamins and is an interesting reflection on the comparative stabilities of vitamins A and D.

Within a short time, American observers reconciled the two opposing schools of thought by showing that the irradiation of certain foods with ultra-violet light could convert inactive material into substances which had a curative action on rickets.[39 40]

It was not long before the activity was traced to the unsaponifiable portion of fats and in particular to certain sterols. Workers in England and Germany, investigating irradiated ergosterol prepared under carefully controlled conditions, finally isolated a pure substance, also a member of the sterol family, which was extremely active and which, to signify its action, was called calciferol.[41 42].

The progress of research in this field and the comparison of the synthetic vitamin with the naturally occurring one led to the discovery that there were marked species differences with respect to the relative activities. It was thus suggested that at least two substances were probably concerned and eventually the isolation of the pure natural vitamin D (a) from fish liver oil and (b) from the irradiation products of a sterol slightly *different* from the precursor of the first crystalline vitamin D, was achieved. Calciferol is also known as " vitamin D_2 " and the second active substance as " vitamin D_3 ". In all, something like a dozen related compounds are now known to have some degree of anti-rachitic activity. In the physical, chemical, physiological and clinical fields the investigation of vitamin D has provided one of the most difficult and fascinating of nutritional problems.

(ii) *Chemistry of Vitamin D.*

The active compounds are all white, crystalline members of the sterol class, containing carbon, hydrogen and oxygen in the molecule. In addition to a hydroxyl group and to side chains which differ from one compound to another, they have—or are closely related to—certain cyclic systems. Apart from the general properties characteristic of the hydroxyl group and the double bonds in the molecule, they show few reactions which are distinctive enough to be used for their estimation in foods. Assays are therefore carried out by biological methods, although a useful colour reaction, which may have some application, has been reported recently.[43] Although there are several anti-rachitic substances, the most common and most important members are D_2 and D_3.

By contrast with vitamin A, vitamin D is fairly stable to heat and oxygen. It is converted into less active substances by the action of ultra-violet radiation and is much less stable than was once thought when it is in intimate contact with alkaline materials for long periods. Because of this and because also of the catalytic powers for oxidation possessed by traces of iron and copper, it is not advisable to incorporate vitamin concentrates into rations until relatively soon before they are to be used.

(iii) *Physiological properties of vitamin D.*

Despite all the work which has been done on the physiological properties of the vitamins of this group, very little is known of their mode of action. They appear to facilitate the absorption of calcium and phosphorus from the gut and perhaps to prevent their excretion: apart from assisting the formation of bone by an increase in the serum calcium level in this way, they may actually influence the manner of deposition of these elements in bone. In the absence of sufficient intakes of calcium and phosphorus, of course, no amount of vitamin D can remedy the position and, from the practical feeding point of view, it is best to remember that the vitamin facilitates the absorption and use of calcium and phosphorus from foods and to ensure that the ration contains suitable levels of the three components.

Where insufficient vitamin D is provided in the ration, there may be thickening or swelling in the metatarsal and metacarpal regions, bending of the long bones, swollen and stiff joints, stiffness of "gait" and retarded growth in young cattle, pigs, sheep, horses and dogs. In growing birds, with relatively higher needs than mammals, similar symptoms, including a softened beak and bending or depression of the sternum, may be found. Loss of appetite often occurs, but is not symptomatic of avitaminosis D only.

In older animals increased liability of the bones to fracture, or dead, weak or deformed offspring may result. Among laying birds, the production of thin-shelled eggs, or diminished egg production and lowered hatchability, occurs.

Though much work still remains to be done, it is already clear that there are marked differences between the potencies of vitamins D_2 and D_3 with respect to bone formation in birds and mammals. For the rat—and perhaps for most mammals—vitamin D_3 is about 30 per cent. more active, weight for weight, than calciferol[4] but for the chick the ratio of the potency of D_3 to that of calciferol is about one hundred to one. When, therefore, chicks are being given a dose of a given number of International Units of vitamin D, they should receive it in the form of vitamin D_3.

Quite apart from differences between the various species of livestock with regard to their relative abilities to use the different forms of the vitamin, the nature of the rest of the diet is of importance, as described previously with reference to calcium and phosphorus in rations (p. 67). On a "normal" diet the rat seems to need little if any vitamin D, so that, to make animals rachitic for assay purposes, the ration includes some 3 per cent. of chalk, to give a high Ca/P ratio.

(iv) *The occurrence of vitamin D in foods and its bioassay.*

Vitamin D is the least widely distributed of the known vitamins. It occurs, principally as D_3, in fish-liver oils and in the bodies of animals which have been exposed to plenty of sunlight: it may appear in the products, e.g., milk, or eggs, or livers, of stock which have obtained vitamin D in this way. Calciferol, on the other hand, is produced by the action of ultra-violet light on sterols of vegetable origin: it occurs in hay, which has been well cured but not weathered and bleached, and it is produced by the irradiation of yeast. Both vitamins are now available as pure synthetic compounds, or in the form of potent solutions of these.

For the measurement of the amounts of vitamin D in foods, the effects of the vitamin on bone development on young animals are measured, rats and chicks being the usual test animals. Either the creatures are made rachitic by the use of vitamin D deficient and imbalanced diets, following which the curative value of the food is studied (therapeutic method) or the food is mixed with a known deficient (control) diet and its ability to prevent the onset of rickets, when it constitutes different percentages of the ration, is observed (prophylactic method).

As with all bioassays large numbers of animals are needed and strict precautions, with statistical checks, have to be taken.[45][46] Observation of the effects on bone formation can be made in three ways, using for the purpose animals which have received known amounts of the food and of the standard solution of vitamin D respectively and comparing (a) the percentages of ash in the dry, fat-free bones, e.g., femurs, or (b) taking X-ray photographs of a suitable joint, and measuring the uncalcified gap between the adjoining bones, e.g., tarso-metatarsal distances in chicks, or (c) killing the animals, removing a suitable bone, e.g., radius and ulna of rats, and measuring the blackened " areas of healing " rendered visible by putting longitudinally cut sections of bone in silver nitrate and then exposing them to light. Much skill, time, and care are needed. The International Standard of vitamin D_2 is a solution of calciferol in a suitable vitamin-free oil; one International Unit is the activity of 0.001 g. of the solution. Provisional standards of vitamin D_3 are in use [45] for the standardisation of products to be used for birds.

Cod liver oil of known and declared minimal potency may be purchased, its standardisation having been carried out by the manufacturer. The potency of the oil as obtained from the fish varies seasonally, its average value being about 100 I.U./g. Halibut liver oil is several times more active. The potencies of cow's milk, and of ox and pig livers depend on the intake of the beasts or their degree of exposure to sunlight, but they are seldom more than 1 I.U./g.

Pure calciferol has an activity of 36 I.U. (rat) per microgramme, the corresponding value for D_3 being 47 [45]; for work with fowls, a provisional standard has been introduced, the activity of which is defined as 40 units (chick) per microgramme. Natural products, fortified by the addition of synthetic vitamin D, are now available for use with livestock; where they are to be used for chicks the purchaser should see that the more suitable vitamin D_3 is being bought, otherwise it will only have a fraction of its nominal potency.

(v) *The significance of vitamin D in animal feeding.*

It will be realised that the required intake of vitamin D is dependent on the species and condition of the animal concerned and on the nature of the rest of the diet, particularly the Ca/P ratio. For this reason, and because some of the vitamin will be formed in the body as the result of the action of sunlight on the skin, only a very general rule can be framed as to the amount which is needed in the diet. Some 6-10 I.U./Kg./day may be taken as representing average requirements for mammals and more for birds, but it is a figure to be modified according to conditions. The importance of calcium, phosphorus and vitamin D in the rations of livestock cannot be too strongly stressed, for failure to supply the requisite amounts at the right time can result in diminished growth, through lack of skeletal development, to bone malformations which may make their presence felt only during the reproductive phase in the life of the female, or to difficulties during lactation.

In some cases massive doses of vitamin D have been given in order to avoid the trouble of daily administration; 500-1,000 times the normal daily dose has been given once or twice per year. Despite the fact that large doses of ten to one hundred times the average daily dose may be given without harm, the practice requires careful control, since too high a dose can produce harmful effects, including calcification of the soft tissues and death. Very high doses do not lead to correspondingly high levels in the milk of the lactating animal.

In Britain, at least, there are strong arguments in favour of ensuring the presence of the appropriate form of the vitamin in the rations of all livestock, particularly young growing stock and pregnant and lactating animals. Cod liver oil is normally quite effective in cattle and pigs at levels of intake which should not disturb milk fat production nor adversely affect the quality of the body fat, but for those who prefer it, more potent preparations, free from such risks, are available.

(c) Vitamin E.

Vitamin E is a fat-soluble vitamin, known chemically as *tocopherol*, of which there are α, β and γ forms. Wheat germ oil, the principal concentrated source of vitamin E, contains both α and β-tocopherols. The three compounds contain ring systems (chromane) in the molecule; there is a hydroxyl-group attached to the nucleus and also a long side chain. α-tocopherol has the molecular formula $C_{29}H_{50}O_2$. The α-compound is about twice as active as the β-compound [47] and ten times as potent as the γ-isomer; the natural products are optically active. Various homologues of the tocopherols have been synthesised and it is evident that biological activity may be exhibited by many related compounds.

Vitamin E is reasonably stable to heat, especially *in vacuo*, but is slowly decomposed by ultra-violet light. It is fairly resistant to oxidation, but is decomposed by oxygen in the presence of suitable catalysts, e.g., iron salts, and is also destroyed by fats which have developed oxidative rancidity. For this last reason, while it remains fairly stable in the germ of uncrushed wheat, vitamin E begins to deteriorate, unless special precautions are taken, when once the wheat has been crushed or the oil expelled.

The effects of vitamin E deficiency on male and female rats have been thoroughly studied; in the female, the œstrous cycle and ovulation and fertilisation are normal, but pathological changes in the embryo result in resorption at about the second week; in the male, testicular degeneration results in permanent sterility. Disturbances in the anterior pituitary also occur in the female subjected for a long period to a deficiency of vitamin E. Symptoms of prolonged deficiency in the rat and rabbit also include muscular dystrophy, degeneration of muscle fibres leading to discolouration of the uterus and seminal vesicles, and a characteristic degeneration of the convoluted tubules of the kidney. The necessity for prolonged deficiency before some of these symptoms develop results from the fact that, as in the case of vitamin A, reserves of vitamin E can be stored in the animal body for a considerable time.

" Stiff-lamb disease " has been attributed to a deficiency of vitamin E in the milk of lactating ewes, when the latter have been fed rations of red kidney beans and lucerne, mixed or grass hay during the winter period [48]; the condition was cured by giving the vitamin in the form of wheat germ oil, either to the lambs or the ewes. About 10 ml. of cold pressed oil per lamb per day, equivalent to 30 mg. of mixed tocopherols, was effective. A similar condition has been observed in calves. While the physiological action of the vitamin is far from being understood and the hopes that were once raised with respect to the use of vitamin E in correcting infertility in farm livestock have not been realised, increasing evidence has accumulated of other useful properties which this group of compounds possesses. It has a protective action on vitamin A, while recent studies, though by no means complete so far as explanations of the observed effects are concerned, seem to show that feeding 1 g. of natural mixed tocopherols to cattle fed on cereals, maize silage and hay led to an increase in the fat content of the milk and, when the yields were compared on a standard 4 per cent. fat basis, to slightly increased yields (5–15 per cent.).[49] Other workers have presented evidence which suggests that vitamin E may be concerned in protein utilisation.[50] Quite clearly much more research needs to be carried out in this field to confirm and extend such observations.

Vitamin E is present, in varying degree, in all green leafy foods and in hay. Cereals are well supplied, the germ being a particularly rich source. The oil extracted from the germ, especially from wheat, is very potent when extracted at low temperature and *in vacuo*. Rice oil (obtained from rice polishings), cotton seed oil, maize oil and palm oil also contain considerable amounts. Active preparations have been made from the fatty material of lettuce leaves. The international unit of vitamin E is the activity of 1 mg. synthetic racemic α-tocopherol acetate in solution in 0.1 g. olive oil.

How much vitamin E the livestock of a farm receive in their rations is clearly conditioned by the system of feeding used. If the food is well chosen, so as to provide other nutrients in good supply, then vitamin E will probably be present in adequate amounts, but rations which contain large proportions of roots, straw, dried beet pulp, poor hay, etc., may well be unsatisfactory.

Several workers have investigated the effect of vitamin E on the fertility and hatchability of hen's eggs, and although a gross deficiency leads to infertility, the results do not point to the need for additional vitamin E in ordinary hen foods. Vitamin E deficiency has been noted [51] in the puppies from dogs kept on a diet of commercially evaporated milk; there was progressive muscular paralysis, which began in the pups on about the 20th day after birth; there was also hypersensitivity to pain and loss of hair of the head and limbs. In the dams there was marked loss of weight, while sores developed on the teats: cure was effected by administration of synthetic α-tocopherol. A bitch needs about 1 mg./Kg. bodyweight/day.[52] Clinical evidence claiming beneficial results accruing from the administration of vitamin E which is unsupported by controlled experimental evidence, should be accepted with caution.

(d) Vitamin K.

Vitamin K is another case of a fat-soluble vitamin which occurs naturally in several slightly different forms, derivatives of naphthoquinone. In vitamin K_1, the side chain is a phytyl group, $C_{20}H_{39}$, and there is also a methyl group in the quinone nucleus. Several synthetic naphthoquinones, simpler than the natural substance and, in some cases even more potent, have been prepared; for ease of administration water-soluble, physiologically active compounds have been synthesised. The vitamin is sensitive to light and, as it contains a quinone group, to alkalies also.

Dam [53] noticed that chicks which were put on to fat free diets eventually died of multiple intramuscular and subcutaneous hæmorrhages. Ten years passed, however, before the nature of the pure vitamin was elucidated: in the meantime it was shown that vitamin K exerted its effects by maintaining the prothrombin level of blood, so that, in normal birds, clotting soon followed small lesions whereas the bleeding continued in the deficient ones.

Suitable sources of the natural vitamin are fresh green foods, soya beans and good quality fish meal (not solvent extracted meal); cereals, seeds and roots are poor sources. The vitamin needs to be provided in the diet of chickens and other birds and, among mammals, rats, rabbits, and dogs. In farm mammals it seems to be synthesized in sufficient amount in the digestive tract for normal purposes, but is being found useful in the treatment of " sweet clover disease ", which cattle acquire through consuming the spoiled crop. The active toxic agent is a phenol, dicoumarol, the effect of which is to lower the prothrombin level of the blood and hence produce continued hæmorrhages.[54]

In the bioassay of the vitamin, day old chicks are placed on vitamin K free diets: at the end of about a fortnight the blood clotting time may then be as much as an hour. Using different levels of the material to be tested and of a standard preparation of pure vitamin K, the blood clotting times of the chicks in the different groups are again measured several hours after the two preparations have been fed. One unit of the vitamin is the activity of one microgramme of pure vitamin K_1. Chemical methods of estimation, which depend on the reactions of the quinone grouping in the molecule, are also available.

(e) Vitamin B_1, aneurin or thiamine.

(i) *Introduction.*

Although the work of Eijkman, in the closing years of the last century, had shown that nervous symptoms followed in birds which were given a diet of unpolished rice,[55] it was not until many years later that the water soluble factor which seemed to be involved in the metabolic disturbances produced by such a diet, was seen to be of a dual nature. The symptoms which followed the complete omission of the water-soluble vitamins of the B-complex from the ration and which could be cured by the administration of suitable aqueous extracts, were only partially alleviated if the extract were heated at a sufficiently high temperature for a sufficiently long time. Eventually the heat-sensitive vitamin was isolated in crystalline form and its chemical structure settled.[56 57]

(ii) *Chemistry of aneurin.*

Aneurin is usually obtained in the form of its white, crystalline hydrochloride, readily soluble in water. Its aqueous solution has a faint smell and a bitter taste both of which are reminiscent of yeast. Aneurin hydrochloride has the molecular formula $C_{12}H_{18}ON_4SCl$ and contains two ring systems in the molecule, the pyrimidine and thiazole rings.

It will withstand being heated in aqueous solution at 100° C. for an hour with comparatively little decomposition, provided the solution is neutral or acid, but at higher temperatures the rate of decomposition is increased. Losses in normal cooking are very largely due to the rejection of aqueous liquors in which the food is cooked and in which the vitamin has dissolved. In alkaline solutions the vitamin is fairly rapidly destroyed.

With mild oxidising agents in alkaline solution, aneurin gives a pigment with a blue fluorescence: this is the base of one of the chemical methods of estimation.

(iii) *Physiological properties of aneurin.*

In the form of its pyrophosphate, aneurin takes part in some of the essential steps in the metabolism of carbohydrates: the pyrophosphate, also known as diphosphothiamine, is the coenzyme which is responsible for the breakdown of pyruvic acid in the metabolism of carbohydrate by nervous tissue.[58] In the absence of sufficient vitamin B_1, there is incomplete oxidation of carbohydrates, pyruvic acid accumulates in the blood, and loss of muscular co-ordination, retraction of the head, and paralysis follow. These last named were some of the symptoms which the early workers had observed in their work.

One of the very earliest symptoms of aneurin deficiency is loss of appetite. This, with the other symptoms, rapidly vanishes (within a day or two) when the vitamin is included in the ration.

The body has little storage capacity for aneurin and a deficiency in the diet is made worse by increased intake of carbohydrate. The needs of the organism more or less parallel the amount of carbohydrate absorbed from the diet; this is a point to be remembered when diets rich in starch are being fed.

In addition to the purely chemical methods of assay of aneurin, two biological procedures are used which are specific, (a) that involving changes in the rate of uptake of oxygen by slices of brain of aneurin depleted birds in response to dosing with the vitamin and (b) the more convenient one depending upon the slowing of the heart rate (brady-cardia) of rats, due to aneurin lack, and its alleviation when the vitamin is added to the ration in controlled amounts.[59] The International Unit of aneurin is the activity corresponding to 3 microgrammes of the pure hydrochloride.

(iv) Sources of aneurin.

Whole grain, legume seeds, green foods, bran, dried yeast and liver are very good sources of the vitamin: dried yeast is ten to twenty times as potent as the rest of the foods in the list and is very useful. Doubtful sources are foods which have been cooked for long periods or those produced from refined flour. Hinton[60] has shown that, in wheat, rye, maize and barley, some 60 per cent. of the total aneurin of the grain may be found in the scutellum, which constitutes only about 1.5 per cent. of the weight.

(v) Aneurin in the feeding of livestock.

Adult herbivorous animals, on natural diets, are normally independent of dietary sources of aneurin, for the vitamin is produced in sufficient amounts by the micro-organisms of the digestive tract. The young of this group of livestock depend upon the milk supply they receive until a sufficiently abundant microbial population is established in the gut: where young stock, for example calves, are being taken off milk at a relatively early age, care should be taken during weaning period to make sure that the foods given during the transition are satisfactory. Apart from this contingency and the case of the animal of any age which is receiving drugs of the sulphonamide class, there seems to be little evidence that the herbivorous species, except the horse,[61] need dietary aneurin. The hard-working horse, on the conventional hay and oats regime, may well get insufficient of this vitamin: bran will supply the deficiency and is best included in the ration each day and not once a week. An alternative very useful source is 1 - 3 per cent. of good dried yeast.

Pigs and poultry with free range do not suffer from aneurin deficiency, nor will they if good grain and bran are freely available, but diets for either species which include rather large proportions of cooked potatoes, household waste and, in the case of pigs, processed swill, will benefit from the inclusion of 2 - 3 per cent. of dried yeast in the ration. Dogs and other carnivorous species which get fair amounts of good raw meat should also be in little need of supplementary aneurin: where, as is often the case, the meat is of such a kind that it must be cooked, or where a fair part of the ration consists of biscuits, which may consist largely of well-cooked cereal products, aneurin-rich food may be needed. It is of note that the offal—skin, skeleton, head and viscera, but not muscle—of some *raw* fish, when constituting 10 per cent. or more of the ration of foxes, causes paralysis ("Chastek paralysis"). This effect is one of aneurin deficiency, caused by an enzyme which destroys the vitamin: cooking the fish inactivates the enzyme and the food may then be safely incorporated in a ration. Other species to whom raw fish is given may perhaps be affected in some degree, when the fish is mixed with the rest of the ration and left for a time at room temperatures.

(f) Riboflavin or vitamin B_2.

(i) *Introduction.*

The presence of the compound now known as riboflavin in whey, to which it gives the characteristic greenish yellow colour, has long been known.[62] Much later, when the vitamins of the B-complex were being studied, the growth promoting power of milk came to be associated with that same compound.[63] Other groups of workers, investigating not vitamins but the nature of the enzymic oxidising systems in living cells, found that they were dealing with riboflavin also,[64] and it was not long before the nature of the molecule had been investigated and its synthesis accomplished.[65]

(ii) *Chemistry of riboflavin.*

Riboflavin, $C_{17}H_{20}O_6N_4$, is a deep orange-yellow powder, whose aqueous solutions, despite the rather low solubility of the vitamin (0.01 per cent. at room temperatures), are markedly coloured and show a greenish fluorescence. It shows stability to heat in acid and neutral solutions but not in the alkaline ones in which it is much more soluble. Light, both visible and ultra-violet, destroys the vitamin quite rapidly, e.g., the riboflavin potency of bottled milk may be halved by a few hours' exposure to sunlight.

The riboflavin molecule consists of three fused ring systems (isoalloxazine system) to which is attached a side chain closely related to the sugar, ribose.

(iii) *Physiological properties.*

In the form of its phosphoric ester, and allied to specific proteins, riboflavin is an essential component of several enzyme systems which are concerned in oxidations in living cells.

Its omission from the diet may cause inhibition of the growth of young animals, diarrhœa, dermatitis, nerve degeneration and lesions of the mouth and lips; in some instances eye disorders, which may lead to blindness, follow.

(iv) *Sources of riboflavin.*

Although the vitamin is fairly widely distributed in foods, the cereals are rather poor sources of it: good supplies may be found in fresh green foods, milk, wheat germ and dried yeast, the last named being twice as potent a source as dried whole milk and six or seven times as rich as kale, one of the most important of the vegetable sources. Liver, though not often available for animal feeding, except as dried whale liver, is about two-thirds as potent as dried yeast.

(v) *Riboflavin in the feeding of livestock.*

The normal, healthy adult ruminant is apparently independent of dietary supplies of riboflavin but it should not be forgotten that its independence is related to the microbial population of the rumen and, since the types and numbers of bacteria in the digestive tract may be influenced markedly by the nature of the ration, it by no means follows that cattle fed in any careless or supposedly cheap fashion will get all the riboflavin they need. In the horse the disease known as "equine periodic ophthalmia" has been associated by Jones with riboflavin deficiency [65] and on the basis of the urinary excretion of riboflavin in relation to the dietary intake by horses, other workers have come to the conclusion that some of the vitamin should be present in the ration. Pigs need riboflavin in their rations and so do the carnivorous mammals. Lack of sufficient riboflavin in the diet of the laying hen leads to the production of eggs of low hatchability, the embryos that fail to hatch being dwarfed and with a characteristically defective development of the down: needs for hatchability, i.e., for breeding, are much higher than for the simple maintenance of health or for ordinary egg production.

Young growing stock of all species need dietary supplies of riboflavin in the early stages of growth. Normally there is enough present in the milk of mammals to meet the needs of the young, while young ruminants soon become independent of dietary supplies of the vitamin because of rumen development. Grazing animals are not likely to suffer from riboflavin deficiency, but lack of this vitamin in the diet of the growing pig or dog or bird soon results in a diminished growth rate. In the chick "curled-toe paralysis", in which the birds sink down on the hock with the toes turned under in a characteristic manner, is produced by lack of sufficient riboflavin in the diet.[66] Deficiency symptoms in pigs include stiffened limbs, poor hair growth with skin eruptions, and eye (corneal) lesions. Diarrhœa is commonly met with in many species on deficient diets.

(g) Nicotinic acid (niacin) and nicotinamide.

(i) *Introduction.*

Nicotinic acid was the first vitamin to be isolated from foods in a pure crystalline state,[67] but at that time (1913) knowledge of the multiple nature of the vitamins was so limited that the new compound could not be related to any clear symptoms of nutritional deficiency. Two or three years later Goldberger in the United States came to the conclusion that human pellagra was, the result of faulty diet. In 1929 evidence was forthcoming that canine " black-tongue " disease was cured by the same foods as was pellagra [68] and, after Knight had shown that nicotinic acid was essential for the growth of certain micro-organisms [69] the curative value of this agent both for pellagra and black-tongue was demonstrated.[70]

(ii) *Chemical properties of niacin.*

Both the free nicotinic acid, $C_5H_4N.COOH$, and the corresponding amide, are white, crystalline solids, readily soluble in water. Furthermore, they are both unaffected by light, and, save for the conversion of the amide to the free acid or its salts, are quite stable in neutral, acid or alkaline solutions. From the point of view of chemical structure, they are the simplest of the vitamins, their molecules consisting simply of the pyridine ring with the attached carboxyl or amide group.

(iii) *Physiological properties of niacin.*

Despite the amount of work which has been done on these compounds their precise clinical properties are still uncertain. Linked to phosphoric acid, ribose and adenine, niacin forms coenzyme I, which is an essential enzyme for many tissue oxidations, especially those of carbohydrates, so that a deficiency of niacin in the organism can be expected to produce rather extensive changes in metabolism. Loss of appetite, loss of weight, diarrhœa and dermatitis are some of the symptoms which have been described in niacin-deficient livestock. In human beings pellagra, with its mental derangement, responds rapidly to administration of the vitamin, while black-tongue in dogs meets with an equally rapid cure, but it now seems to be clear that some of the older diets which produced such diseases were probably faulty in other respects. While the omission of the vitamin from the diet of the pig, dog, fowl, and man soon leads to disease, the nature of the syndrome characteristic of simple niacin deficiency needs further investigation.[71]

There is an interesting relationship between proteins and nicotinamide, for it has been found that in some animal species a deficiency of niacin may find partial compensation when the protein content of the ration is increased. The amino-acid, tryptophane, seems to be the one from which niacin may be synthesized, so that, as proteins differ from one another in tryptophane content, so they vary in their powers of compensation for deficiency of the vitamin. Intestinal micro-organisms seem, in part at least, to be concerned in this phenomenon.[72]

There are some slight differences between the physiological properties of the free acid and its amide, but from the nutritional aspect they are unimportant. In the animal body both compounds are converted into methyl derivatives, the CH_3- group being attached to the nuclear nitrogen atom.

(iv) *The occurrence of niacin in foods.*

Meat, especially liver, fish, legume seeds, groundnut cake and the cereal grains—except maize—are quite good sources of the vitamin. In green foods and in maize it is present in moderate amounts only, but maize compares poorly with the green foods because of its high ratio of carbohydrate to protein. Much the most potent source is dried yeast, about twice as good as liver and groundnut cake and six or seven times as potent as fresh meat.

(v) *Niacin in the feeding of livestock.*

The amount of niacin needed daily by animals depends on such factors as their species, weight, the protein content of the ration and the amount and nature of the carbohydrate metabolized. Ruminants, both young and mature beasts, are normally independent of dietary sources,[73] while, of the non-ruminant herbivores, the horse seems to need little or none in its ration.[74] In pigs niacin deficiency leads to diarrhœa, to failure to grow or to loss of weight,[75] and to ataxia and anæmia.[76] In dogs and birds mouth symptoms (black-tongue in dogs) follow on the supply of insufficient amounts of the vitamin in the diet, the birds showing poor growth and general unthriftiness. It is impossible to give fixed requirements for niacin, but they are of the order of 300 microgrammes/Kg. bodyweight/day for such species as need dietary supplies.

Both chemical and microbiological methods of estimation are available.

(h) Pyridoxine, pyridoxal, pyridoxamine, vitamin B₆.

(i) *Introduction.*

First evidence of the existence of another vitamin of the B-complex followed soon after the observations of Goldberger and Lillie in 1926, that rats, which were put on diets believed to be deficient in the " pellagra preventing " factor, developed acrodynia, a characteristic dermatitis involving the head and paws of the experimental animals. György[77] obtained evidence that the diet was actually deficient in more than one vitamin and suggested the name vitamin B₆ for the unknown substance which produced the acrodynia in rats: within four years the vitamin had been isolated by several different groups of workers, including György.[78] A year later the vitamin, to which the name pyridoxine was given, had been synthesized.

Subsequent work showed that some three closely related compounds, of slightly different physiological properties, were concerned; the other two were named pyridoxal and pyridoxamine.

(ii) *Chemistry of vitamin B₆.*

The three vitamins of this group have in common in their molecules, (a) the pyridine ring, and (b) a methyl, a hydroxyl, and a $-CH_2OH$ group attached to corresponding carbon atoms in the pyridine nucleus. Where they differ is that, attached to the carbon atom in the 4-position to the nitrogen of the pyridine ring, pyridoxine itself has the group $-CH_2OH$, pyridoxal the group $-CHO$ and pyridoxamine the group $-CH_2NH_2$. Their molecular structures thus bear some resemblance to nicotinic acid.

Pyridoxine is a white crystalline solid, readily soluble in water, its solution having a definitely bitter taste. All three substances are destroyed by exposure to light, especially by ultra-violet light under neutral or alkaline conditions. Pyridoxal, on account of the presence of the –CHO group is unstable to hot aqueous alkali, but with this exception the three compounds are stable in solution at 100°C.

(iii) *Physiological properties of vitamin B.*

All three compounds are found in living tissues, a large proportion of them in combined form. The animal body converts pyridoxine into pyridoxal and pyridoxamine, which appear to be the actual agents concerned in protein metabolism. In the form of its phosphate, pyridoxal is concerned in two types of enzyme systems whose functions are vital for living cells. Firstly it acts as coenzyme for transaminations, in which process an amino-group is transferred from one amino-acid to a keto-acid to produce a second amino-acid;[79] the substance is thus of great importance in protein metabolism. Secondly pyridoxal phosphate is a coenzyme for the decarboxylation of amino-acids such as glutamic acid, tyrosine and arginine.[80] Pyridoxine is also connected with the metabolism of tryptophane in the animal body. The functions of pyridoxamine phosphate are less clearly defined.[81] As pyridoxine is concerned in such fundamentally important reactions, the need for its inclusion in the ration where the animal concerned has no powers of synthesis or the bacteria of the digestive tract are unable to produce it in sufficient amount, requires no stressing.

(iv) *The occurrence of pyridoxine in foods.*

Vitamin B₆ occurs in foods chiefly in association with proteins. Seeds and cereals, especially the germ in the latter case, are good sources and so is bran. Dried yeast is rich in the vitamin, while liver and milk are good animal sources.

(v) *The significance of vitamin B₆ in animal feeding.*

Although all species of livestock are said to require dietary supplies of Vitamin B₆, deficiency symptoms in cattle and sheep under conditions of normal husbandry have not been reported. On account of the association of the vitamin with the protein fraction of foods a simple deficiency is rather unlikely. Cattle on suitably restricted rations show loss of appetite, poor growth and unthriftiness.[82] On deficient diets the young of all species exhibit impaired growth, with nerve degeneration which ultimately leads to convulsive seizures both in mammals and birds. Dermatitis is apparently specific to rats, while pigs and dogs develop severe microcytic, hypochromic anæmia.

Chemical methods of assay are available for vitamin B₆, while microbiological assays, using different strains of organisms which react differently to the three forms, have also been much used. In addition a biological method has been developed in which the curative value of foods for the specific rat dermatitis is examined.

(i) Pantothenic acid.

(i) *Introduction.*

The search for a growth stimulant for yeast, " bios ", was begun by Wildiers [53] at the beginning of the century. Later the existence of other growth factors, required by bacteria and by rats and chicks, was revealed. Eventually the different lines of approach converged until, in 1933, a crystalline compound was isolated, which was effective in the several different circumstances.[54] The structure of the compound was elucidated and the substance itself was called pantothenic acid, to denote both its nature and its very wide distribution.

(ii) *Chemistry of pantothenic acid.*

Pantothenic acid is a pale yellow oil, which gives white crystalline salts, the calcium salt being the one most commonly available. It is unstable towards heat both when it is dry and when it is present in acid or alkaline solution.

Pantothenic acid is derived from β-alanine (an unusual example of a natural β-amino-acid) and the dihydroxy-acid of the following structure, $HOCH_2C(CH_3)_2CH(OH)COOH$, so that the molecule contains a peptide linkage.

(iii) *Physiological properties of pantothenic acid.*

In view of the fact that some species of bacteria and yeasts, as well as mammals and birds, require a supply of pantothenic acid, the vitamin would appear to be involved in one or more of the fundamental reactions of living cells. In association with proteins pantothenic acid is concerned with the oxidation of pyruvic acid and with the acetylation of various substances in the animal body, as for example, the formation of acetylcholine from choline. One of the coenzymes has been examined in some detail and has been found to contain 11 per cent. of combined pantothenic acid.[55] It is quite probable that the vitamin may have other functions in fat and protein synthesis.

(iv) *The occurrence of pantothenic acid in foods.*

Although pantothenic acid occurs widely in foods, there are rather marked variations in the quantities present in different materials. A study of a variety of foods of animal and vegetable origin,[56] showed that fish meals of 40 - 70 per cent. protein content contained between 5 and 23 microgrammes of the vitamin per gramme of food, ordinary meat-scrap, 6 - 26 μg., dried liver, 82 μg., and dried milk or whey, 20 - 55 μg. Plant concentrates which were examined provided the following data; groundnut cake or meal, 30 - 50 μg., sesame, linseed and coconut meals, 6 - 8 μg., sunflower-seed, cotton-seed and soya-bean meal, 10 - 16 μg. The grains proved to be poor sources, yielding only 4 - 8 μg./g., except rice meal which showed five or six times as much; wheat bran contained about 23 μg. Lucerne meal, 20 - 40 μg., and dried baker's yeast, 50 μg., showed themselves to be good sources of the vitamin. On a dry matter basis lucerne was found to contain 44 μg./g. in the early stages of growth but only two-thirds of that amount when in full bloom, while corresponding data for clover showed a fall from about 20 μg./g. down to half that value.

In a report on the recommended nutrient allowances for swine " it has been pointed out that conventional (American) rations derived from maize, soya-bean meal, barley, linseed meal and a small amount of lucerne meal or meat meal, provide a good margin of safety for aneurin and niacin, a much smaller one for riboflavin and none at all for pantothenic acid.

(v) *The significance of pantothenic acid in animal feeding.*

Adult ruminants appear to require no dietary source of the vitamin, microbial synthesis producing what is needed; there is little information available as to the needs of calves. There is evidence, however, that horses may need dietary supplies of about 40 μg./Kg. of bodyweight, the corresponding figures for the dog and pig being some 100 and 200 μg. respectively. The requirements of birds are also high.

The symptoms of deficiency vary a good deal. In young mammals and birds failure to grow is often the first sign of deficiency; in dogs and pigs there may be diarrhœa. Chicks, at a later stage, show a typical dermatitis. Lesions of the spinal cord in chicks and nervous disorders, ending in convulsions, may occur in dogs. In pigs there is a characteristic " goose-stepping " walk. Disturbances involving the thymus gland are found in several species. Failure of normal hair pigmentation in the dog and fox has led to the vitamin being given the name the " anti-graying " factor, but the effect is not a specific one nor does it apply to all species of livestock.

Laying hens put on to rations deficient in pantothenic acid may continue in lay for a long period, but the hatchability of the eggs soon falls to a very low percentage. Good condition in the birds may be maintained on intakes of 150 μg./100 g. of ration, whereas the hatch-ability of the eggs produced falls to zero in ten weeks; for good hatch-ability, four to five times this level of vitamin intake is necessary, which is also about the level needed for satisfactory growth.[88]

(j) Biotin.

The earliest evidence for the existence of the vitamin now known as biotin was provided by Boas,[89] who showed that dermatitis and loss of muscular control in rats followed their being given large amounts of raw, dried egg-white. Later it was shown that the same factor was needed for the stimulation of yeast growth and eventually the substance was isolated and synthesised.[90]

Biotin is a white, crystalline solid, soluble in water, whose molecular formula is $C_{12}H_{16}O_3N_2S$; its molecular structure is complex. It is present so universally in foods and is synthesised so readily by the intestinal flora that difficulty is experienced in producing a deficiency in livestock, whose requirements are very small in any case. Evidence has been obtained that biotin, in association with proteins, may be concerned in decarboxylation and deamination mechanisms in the animal body.[91]

(k) Inositol.

Inositol is a sweet-tasting, white crystalline solid, $C_6H_{12}O_6$, a hexahydroxy derivative of cyclohexane, which has long been known to exist in animal and plant tissues (combined as " phytin " in the latter). It is present in good quantity in natural foods so that deficiencies are not likely to occur on ordinary rations.

Recent work suggests that, apart from inositol being a constituent of some of the lipoids in the body, it may play a part in the activity of pancreatic amylase.[92] The substance is already known to be concerned in the prevention of " fatty liver " under certain conditions.

(l) Choline.

Choline, $(CH_3)_3N(OH)CH_2CH_2OH$, which has long been known, is a colourless base, fairly stable in dilute aqueous solution and especially in the presence of acids. It is found in combination in phosphatides in plant and animal tissues alike; foods which contain little or no ethersoluble matter are unlikely to contain much of the base.

In the form of phosphatides choline plays a vital part in the life of living cells. Its conversion to acetylcholine in the animal body produces a powerful physiological agent concerned in nerve function; it is also one of a small group of substances which act as methylating agents in living tissues.[93] Often by virtue of the last named characteristic, choline is concerned in the prevention of liver and kidney damage, especially on diets high in fat, and of perosis in chicks and poults. For normal growth and function it appears to be required for dogs, chicks, poults and young pigs [94] at levels of about 0.15 to 0.3 per cent. of the diet. Ruminants are not known to require dietary supplies. Choline is likely to be present in sufficient amount in all normal rations, unless they have had their fatty matter extracted.

(m) Folic acid.

Folic acid is the name now given to a group of closely related chemical compounds, the individuals of which were sought by groups of workers in different fields during a period of two decades or more.

In the case of each substance there are combined in the molecule (a) a pteridyl group, (b) p-aminobenzoic acid and (c) one or more molecules of glutamic acid. Pteridine is a benzenoid type of compound with four nitrogen atoms in its two fused rings. Substances with one combined aminobenzoyl residue (pteroylglutamic acid), with three (recognised in bacterial metabolism as " L. casei factor ") and with seven (known as vitamin B_c) are all known.

Pteroylglutamic acid is a yellow, sparingly-soluble solid, although its sodium salt is reasonably soluble in water; its solutions are unstable to light.

For bacteria the different forms of the vitamin have rather different properties, but for the higher animals their effects seem to be very similar. In man, the monkey, dog, pig, chicken, turkey and rat—and doubtless in many other species—folic acid is one of the factors concerned in the prevention of a macrocytic type of anaemia, of nutritional origin. Despite the large amount of work being done in the field, the position is still not clear.[25][96] Potent dietary sources of the vitamin are liver and liver extracts, yeast and yeast extracts, and green leaves.

(n) Other factors included in the B-complex.

A cobalt-containing vitamin B_{12} in the form of a red crystalline solid, has been isolated by two groups of workers.[97][98] Beyond the fact that it seems to be concerned in the cure of pernicious anaemia in man and that it contains about 4 per cent. of cobalt, relatively little is yet known about the substance. One interesting point is that though the substance is active for man, all of the evidence at present suggests that cobalt is not an essential element for him, only ruminants apparently requiring it. Although the substance is present in liver and is active in very minute doses, little is known about the distribution of the compound in foods.

(o) Ascorbic acid, vitamin C.

(i) *Introduction.*

Of all the vitamins, ascorbic acid has perhaps the longest history as a distinct entity; the known association of scurvy in man with dietary faults and the prevention of the disease by the use of citrus fruits go back two or three centuries. The definite need for some dietary factor to prevent symptoms of scurvy appearing in guinea pigs was shown in 1907 by Holst and Frölich,[99] but twenty-five years elapsed before the isolation [100] and synthesis [101] of the vitamin was accomplished.

(ii) *Chemistry of ascorbic acid.*

Ascorbic acid is a white, crystalline, water-soluble acid, $C_6H_8O_6$ (the molecular formula is that of the internal ester or lactone), which is closely related to the hexoses. In aqueous solution the vitamin is relatively unstable; at a pH of about 5 or less, ascorbic acid is converted reversibly by mild oxidising agents, e.g., air, into dehydro-ascorbic acid which is still biologically active. At a pH of more than 5, however, an irreversible oxidation occurs and biological potency is lost. Ultra-violet light increases the rate of destruction of the vitamin.

(iii) *Physiological properties of vitamin C.*

Ascorbic acid is concerned in the maintenance and formation of the inter-cellular substances of the animal body. In this way the vitamin is involved in the production of good bone as well as soft tissues. Where there is severe deficiency, bone lesions, especially at the joints, bleeding of the gums and loosening of the teeth (the historic symptoms of scurvy in man), haemorrhage internally or externally from slight mechanical causes which normally would produce no damage, anaemia, and finally death result. Reproductive performance may be affected. There is evidence that the requirements for vitamin C may be higher than normal in certain diseases.

Capacity for storage of vitamin C is limited, as in the case of other water-soluble vitamins. Where large doses are ingested, any excess above the immediate needs and limited storage of the body is excreted in the urine.

(iv) *The occurrence of vitamin C in foods and its assay.*

Good sources of ascorbic acid are fresh green leafy vegetables, especially kale and turnip tops, potatoes and turnips, and the citrus fruits. Fresh liver and fresh milk are the only animal foods which contain appreciable amounts, and the latter food has only about 1 per cent. of the potency of kale.

Two assay methods have been used for vitamin C assay. In the chemical method the quantitative oxidation of ascorbic acid under controlled conditions, using the dye, 2 : 6-dichlorophenolindophenol, for the oxidation, is used. The dye serves as its own indicator, its pink colour (in acid solution) changing to colourless as oxidation proceeds. For the biological method of assay young guinea pigs are put on a vitamin C-deficient diet, and the power of the material to be assayed to prevent the onset of scorbutic symptoms or to cure them once they have become established is compared with that of pure ascorbic acid.[102]

(v) *The s'_,nificance of ascorbic acid in animal feeding.*

Under normal maintenance conditions a dietary source of ascorbic acid seems to be needed by man, the other primates and the guinea pig only, other species having a metabolic need for the vitamin but being able to synthesise it at a rate sufficient for their needs.

It is largely during the last decade that knowledge of the higher levels of nutrients, which are needed for productive purposes than for simple maintenance, has been slowly growing. Although the evidence is still controversial, there are indications that the very young animal may need dietary sources of ascorbic acid[103] and that mature animals, especially where there is a sub-optimal intake of vitamin A, may also require vitamin C in their rations.[104][105] To what extent these findings may be substantiated by later research is not very important in livestock feeding provided that some care is taken to provide a balanced ration. Where, for the sake of the many other factors present in it, fresh green food is included regularly in the diet, there seems to be small chance of vitamin C deficiency.

(p) Vitamin P.

Vitamin P is the name given to a group of compounds, rather than a single pure substance, which it has been said are necessary for the maintenance of normal capillary permeability. These compounds occur in green leaves and citrus fruits. There is much confusion about their real function and no evidence that they are of significance in practical livestock feeding. There are a number of recent reviews concerning vitamin P,[106][107] which give accounts of the complexities of the problem.

REFERENCES

1. Bicknell, F., and F. Prescott, (1942). " The vitamins in medicine."
2. Heilbron, I., W. E. Jones, and A. L. Baccarach, (1944). Vitamins and Hormones, 2, 155.
3. Deuel, H. J., C. Hendrick, E. Straub, A. Sandoval, J. Pinckard and L. Zechmeister, (1947). Arch. Biochem., 14, 97.
4. Moore, T., (1929). Biochem. J., 23, 803.
5. Mattson, F. H., J. W. Mehl, H. J. Deuel, and C. E. Wiese, (1947). Arch. Biochem., 15, 65 and 75.
6. Glover, J., T. W. Goodwin and R. A. Morton, (1947). Biochem. J., 41, xlv.
7. Gibson, G. P., and R. J. Taylor, (1945). Analyst, 70, 449.
8. Koehn, C. J., (1948).. Arch. Biochem., 17, 337.
9. Morton, R. A., M. K. Salah, and A. L. Stubbs, (1946). ·Biochem. J., 40, lix.
10. Mellanby, E., (1938). J. Physiol., 93, 42.
11. Brown, E. F., and A. F. Morgan, (1948). J. Nutrition, 35, 425.
12. Moore, T., (1940). Biochem. J., 34, 1321.
13. Hickman, K. C. D., M. W. Kaley, and P. L. Harris, (1944). J. Biol. Chem., 152, 321.
14. Gridgeman, N. T., (1945). " The Estimation of Vitamin A." (Unilever Ltd.)
15. Hart, G. H., (1941). Nutrition Abs. Rev., 10, 261.
16. Sherman, H. C., and H. Y. Trupp, (1949). J. Nutrition, 37, 467.
17. Blaxter, K. L., S. K. Kon, and S. Y. Thompson, (1946). J. Dairy Res., 14, 225.
18. Thomas, J. W., J. K. Loosli, and J. P. William, (1947). J. Animal Sci., 6, 141.
19. Guilbert, H. R., and G. H. Hart, (1934 and 1935). J. Nutrition, 8, 25 and 10, 409.
20. Stewart, J., and J. Macallum, (1938). J. Agric. Sci., 8, 428.
21. Stewart, J., and J. Macallum, (1938). J. Comp. Path. and Therap., 51, 290.
22. Barron, N. S., (1942). Vet. Rec., 54, 29.
23. Thorp, W., H. A. Keener, S. I. Bechdel, and N. B. Guerrant, (1942). Amer. J. Vet. Res., 3, 27.
24. Boyer, P., P. Phillips, N. Lundquist, C. Jensen and I. Ruppel, (1942). J. Dairy Sci., 25, 433.
25. Madsen, L., O. Eaton, L. Heemstra, R. Davis, C. Cabell and B. Knapp, (1948). J. Animal Sci., 7, 60.
26. Klemola, V., (1933). Biedermanns Zentralbl., (B) Tierenährung, 5, 657.
27. Chatelain, M. P., (1933). Bull. Acad. Vet. France, 6, 452.
28. Meadows, D., (1919). Vet. J., 26, 140.
29. Linton, R. G., (1943). " Animal Nutrition," 2nd Edn.
30. Marshall, F. H. A., and J. Hammond, (1947). " Fertility and Animal-Breeding." Min. Agr. Fisheries Bull. No. 39.
31. Foot, A. S., and S. K. Kon, (1938). Agriculture, J. Min. Agric. Engl., 45, 913.
32. Downham, K., (1938). Vet. Rec., 50, 785.
33. Edwards, J. T., (1937). J. Army Vet. Corps., 9, 6.
34. Linton, R. G., and A. Brownlee, (1939). Nature, 144, 978.
35. Smith, S. E., (1942). J. Nutrition, 24, 97.
36. Mellanby, E., (1918). J. Physiol., 52, xl.
37. Huldschinsky, K., (1919). Deut. med. Wochenschr., 45, 712.
38. McCollum, E. V., N. Simmonds, P. G. Shipley, and E. A. Parks, (1922). J. Biol. Chem., 51, 41.
39. Steenbock, H., and M. T. Nelson, (1924). J. Biol. Chem., 61, 405.
40. Hess, A. F., and M. Weinstock, (1924). J. Biol. Chem., 62, 301.

41. Askew, F. A., R. B. Bourdillon, H. M. Bruce, R. K. Callow, J. St. L. Philpot, and T. A. Webster, (1932). Proc. Roy. Soc. (London), *109B*, 488.
42. Windaus, A., O. Linsert, A. Lüttringhaus, and G. Weidlich (1932). Ann., *492*, 226.
43. Palasi, V. V., (1947). Nature, *160*, 88.
44. Gridgeman, N. T., (1945). Quart. J. Pharm. Pharmacol., *18*, 24.
45. " Biological Assay of Vitamin-D3 by the Chick Method " (1940). British Standards Inst. Bull. No. 911.
46. Morgan, R. S., (1934). Biochem. J., *26*, 1144.
47. Harris, P. L., J. L. Jensen, M. Joffe, and K. E. Mason, (1944). J. Biol. Chem., *156*, 491.
48. Whiting, F., J. P. Willman, and J. K. Loosli, (1949). J. Animal Sci., *8*, 234.
49. Harris, P. L., W. J. Swanson, and K. C. D. Hickman, (1947). J. Nutrition, *33*, 411.
50. Harris, P. L., and E. L. Hove, (1947). J. Nutrition, *34*, 571.
51. Anderson, H. D., C. A. Elvehjem, and J. E. Gonce, (1939). Proc. Soc. Exp. Biol. Med., *42*, 750.
52. Michaud, L., and C. A. Elvehjem, (1943). Nutrition Abs. Rev., *13*, 323.
53. Dam, H., (1935). Biochem. J., *29*, 1273.
54. Overman, R. S., J. B. Field, C. A. Baumann, and K. P. Link, (1942). J. Nutrition, *23*, 589.
55. Eijkman, C., (1897). Virch. Arch. path. Anat., *149*, 187 and 523.
56. Williams, R. R., (1936). J. Amer. Chem. Soc., *58*, 1063.
57. Todd, A. R., and F. Bergel, (1937). J. Chem. Soc., 364.
58. Peters, R. A., (1940). Chem. and Ind., 373.
59. Harris, L. J., and P. C. Leong (1936). Lancet, *1*, 886.
60. Hinton, J. J., (1944). Biochem. J., *38*, 214.
61. Carroll, F. D., H. Goss, and C. E. Howell, (1949). J. Animal Sci., *8*, 286.
62. Blyth, A. W., (1879). J. Chem. Soc., *35*, 530.
63. Kuhn, R., P. György, and T. Wagner-Jauregg, (1933). Berichte., *66*, 317 and 576.
64. Warburg, O., and W. Christian, (1932). Biochem. Z., *254*, 438.
65. Jones, T. C., (1949). J. Amer. Vet. Med. Ass., *114*, 326.
66. Bethke, R. M., and P. R. Record, (1942). Poultry Sci., *21*, 147.
67. Funk, C., (1913). J. Physiol., *46*, 173.
68. Goldberger, J., C. H. Waring, and D. G. Willets, (1915). U.S. Pub. Health Rep., *30*, 3117.
69. Aykroyd, W. R., and M. H. Roscoe, (1929). Biochem. J., *23*, 483.
70. Knight, B. C. J. G., (1937). Biochem. J., *31*, 731.
71. Krehl, W. A., N. Torbet, J. de la Huerga, and C. A. Elvehjem, (1946). Arch. Biochem., *11*, 363.
72. Ellinger, P., and M. M. Abdel Kader, (1947). Nature, *160*, 675.
73. Johnson, B. C., A. C. Wiese, H. H. Mitchell, and W. B. Nevens, (1947). J. Biol. Chem., *167*, 729.
74. Pearson, P. B., and R. W. Luecke, (1945). Arch. Biochem., *6*, 1945.
75. Chick, H., T. F. Macrae, A. J. P. Martin, and C. J. Martin, (1938). Biochem. J., *32*, 10, and 844.
76. Cartwright, G. E., B. Tatting, and M. M. Wintrobe, (1948). Arch. Biochem., *19*, 109.
77. György, P., (1934). Nature, *133*, 498.
78. György, P., (1938). J. Amer. Chem. Soc., *60*, 983.
79. Lichstein, H. C., I. Gunsalus, and W. W. Umbreit, (1945). J. Biol. Chem., *161*, 311.
80. Gale, E. F., (1946). " Recent Advances in Enzymology," 6, 1.
81. Umbreit, W. W., D. J. O'Kane, and I. C. Gunsalus, (1948). J. Biol. Chem., *176*, 629.
82. Anon., (1947). Nutrition Reviews, *5*, 98.
83. Wildiers, E., (1901). La Cellule, *18*, 313.
84. Woolley, D. W., H. A. Waisman, and C. A. Elvehjem, (1939). J. Amer. Chem. Soc., *61*, 977.
85. Lipmann, F., N. O. Kaplan, and G. D. Novelli, (1947). Federation Proc., *6*, 272.
86. Bondi, A., R. Etinger, and H. Meyer, (1949). J. Agric. Sci., *39*, 104.

87. Hughes, E. H., E. W. Crampton, N. R. Ellis, and W. J. Loeffel, (1944). Recommended nutrient allowances for domestic animals, No. 2, N.R. Council, U.S.A.
88. Gillis, M. B., G. F. Heuser, and L. C. Norris, (1948). J. Nutrition, *35*, 351.
89. Boas, M., (1927). Biochem. J., *21*, 712.
90. Harris, S. A., D. E. Wolf, R. Mozingo, and K. Folkers, (1943). Science, *97*, 447.
91. Lichstein, H. C., and W. W. Umbreit, (1947). J. Biol. Chem., 170, 329 and 423.
92. Lane, R. L., and R. J. Williams, (1948). Arch. Biochem., *19*, 329.
93. Anon., (1947). Nutrition Rev., *5*, 131.
94. Neumann, A. L., J. L. Krider, M. F. James, and B. C. Johnson, (1949). J. Nutrition, *38*, 195.
95. Spies, T. D., (1948). Ann. Rev. Biochem., *17*, 455.
96. Anon. (1948). Nutrition Rev., *6*, 131.
97. Ricke, E. L., Science, *107*, 396.
98. Smith, E. L., (1948). Nature, *161*, 638.
99. Holst, A., and T. Frölich, (1907). J. Hyg., *7*, 634.
100. King, C. G., and W. A. Waugh, (1932). Science, *75*, 357.
101. Ault, R. G., et alia. (1933). J. Chem. Soc., 1419.
102. Coward, K., and 'E. W. Kassner, (1936). Biochem. J., *30*, 1719.
103. Lundquist, N. S., and P. H. Phillips, (1943). J. Dairy Sci., *26*, 1023.
104. Braude, R., S. K. Kon, and J. W. G. Porter, (1948). Biochem J., Proc.
105. Bassett, C. F., J. K. Loosli, and F. Wilke, (1948). J. Nutrition, *35*, 629.
106. Scarborough, H., (1945). Biochem. J., *39*, 271.
107. Oser, B. L., (1948). Ann. Rev. Biochem., *17*, 405.

CEREAL GRAINS

(1) Introduction

The cereal grains constitute a particularly important class of food-stuffs, of world-wide distribution and significance. They are all concentrated foods, containing about 10% of protein, 60-70% of soluble carbohydrate, up to 4% of oil and up to 10% of fibre. They tend to be low in mineral matter and to have too low an available-calcium content so that, by themselves, they are rachitogenic.

The cereal grains are essentially carbohydrate concentrates and useful counterparts to the protein-rich foods for the production of rations for livestock. Their protein is of moderate biological value, tending to be lacking in lysine; with milk protein there is usually satisfactory supplementation.

Within the group there are, however, differences sufficiently great to affect their respective values as animal foodstuffs. Oats, rice (unpolished) and millet are rather high in fibre, barley occupies an intermediate position and the rest of the class contain only about 2% of fibre. Oats, maize, dari and millet are relatively rich in oil, while maize is the most deficient in mineral matter. If these differences are kept in mind and compensation is made for them, then it may be said that in a large measure, the cereal grains are interchangeable, one for another, in many rations.

(The following table is included to show the nature of the cereal grains; more comprehensive data are given in the tables at the end of the book.)

TABLE 14

Grain	Dry matter	Crude protein	Oil	Soluble carbohydrate	Crude fibre	Ash	N.R.	Starch equiv.†
	%	%	%	%	%	%		%
Oats ...	87	10	5	58	10	3	7	60
Wheat ...	87	12	2	69	2	2	7	72
Barley ...	85	10	2	66	5	3	9	71
Maize ...	87	10	4	69	2	1	9	78
Rice ...	89	8	2	65	9	5	—	—
Rice (polished)	87	7	—	78	1	1	13	82
Dari seed	89	10	4	71	2	2	9	74
Millet ...	88	11	4	61	8	4	7	59
Rye ...	87	12	2	70	2	2	7	72

Excluding unpolished rice, dari seed and millet, the following digestibilities apply to the cereal grains:

Protein: approximately 80 per cent. for cattle, sheep, pigs and horses.

Soluble carbohydrate: 80-90 per cent. for the same species.

Oil: about 80 per cent. for herbivorous species, rather less for pigs.

Fibre: 30-40 per cent. for cattle and sheep, about 40 per cent. for such of the grains as are commonly fed to horses and about 20 per cent. for pigs.

The digestibilities of the other three foods seem to be rather lower than the figures quoted above. In many cases there are few reliable data upon which conclusions may be based and it must be remembered, too, that the nature of the rest of a ration may affect the foodstuffs which are now being discussed.

(2) Oats (*Avena Sp.*)

(a) Varieties and their characteristics.

The following are often recognised as distinct species of the genus *Avena*, though it is certain that some of them are descendants from a common stock or are closely related: *Avena sativa*, the common or European-cultivated oat; *Avena orientalis*, the Tartarian oat; *Avena nuda*, the China oat; *A. fatua*, the wild oat; *A. strigosa*, the bristle-pointed oat; *A. sterilis*, the "animated or fly oat"; *A. barbata*, a Mediterranean oat; and *A. brevis*, the short oat. Of these there are many varieties.

Avena fatua, the wild oat sometimes found growing among other cereals, usually has a husk of a brown or yellow colour and a seed which can be readily distinguished from the cultivated oat by the presence of the characteristic hairs at the base of the grain. The outer palea (husk) carries a bent and prominent awn and the ear is sparse.

† For definition see p. 286.

Avena strigosa, or the bristle-pointed oat, is grown as a cereal crop in Wales and the northern and western islands of Scotland. Of *A. orientalis* there are several varieties, such as white tartarian, black tartarian, etc. *A. nuda*, the naked oat of China, falls away from the husk when ripe, hence its name.

There are many varieties of oats, but there is very little difference between them as far as their composition or nutritive value is concerned. *The potato oat* is a variety which for over a century has been extensively cultivated in Scotland.

Winter Oats.—The two varieties of these autumn sown oats most commonly grown are winter grey, or dun oat, and black winter oat. The black variety possesses somewhat stronger straw than the grey, but winter straw is not so palatable as that of the finer spring varieties.

New Oats.—Oats are cut before they are fully mature. As they become older they lose moisture and become more mature and harder; new oats, which are those less than about five months old, may cause indigestion unless introduced gradually into the ration.

Foreign oats are variable in quality, samples from some countries, e.g., New Zealand, Canada and Australia, being very good, whereas oats from other sources may be poor, dirty and contaminated with weed seeds. It is possible, by an examination of the weed seeds, to determine from what country a sample of oats has come, or if foreign oats have been mixed with those that are home grown.

The oat plant is characterised by its large, open and spreading panicle. When threshed the "seed" comes away enclosed within the inner and outer paleæ, the *husk*, and leaves on the straw the glumes or *chaff*. Most of the modern cultivated varieties are awnless. The grains should be of uniform size; where there is much variation in size and appearance it usually indicates that the oats are of varied origin. Good oats should weigh at least 40 lb. per bushel * (500 g./litre). The weight per bushel gives an indication of the proportion of husk to kernel; the greater the proportion of husk to kernel the less the weight per bushel. Of the total weight of the grain, 20-35 per cent. is husk. The average proportion of grain to straw in winter oats is 30-35 per cent. and in spring oats 40-50 per cent. Due to uneven ripening the proportion of husk to kernel varies considerably even in oats of the same variety. A superior sample has a plump, evenly-filled appearance. The colour of the kernel should vary very little, even though the enclosing husk may be white, dark yellow or black; it should be white and firm with a clean, fresh appearance, have a pleasant taste and not be tainted or musty.

Clipped Oats are oats which have had the ends of their husks clipped

---

* In measuring the weight per bushel of any grain, the bushel measure is filled rapidly, the grain being poured in without tapping or shaking the measure. When the measure is full the "strike" is applied (a board is pulled over the measure) to ensure a level top. The contents are then weighed.

off by machinery so as to increase the weight per bushel, or to improve the sample for show purposes.

Canadian Feed Oats.—When wheat, especially foreign wheat, is screened prior to milling there is obtained, in addition to the screenings of broken grain and weed seeds, a quantity of oats which have grown up with the wheat. These are usually poor in quality and light in weight, and are known as *Canadian feed oats,* and sometimes as *sport oats.*

Kiln Dried Oats.—New oats contain a high proportion of moisture, and if they are stored in this condition fermentation is liable to occur with a resulting deterioration in value. In order to give the, oats a better keeping quality they are sometimes dried in the kiln, particularly before shipment. Sometimes weathered and musty oats are treated in this way to prevent further fermentative action, but kiln drying does not convert damaged grain into good oats.

Bleached Oats.—Poor quality oats, such as those which have become dull, discoloured, or mouldy, by weathering in the field, are sometimes bleached with sulphur dioxide in order to give them a better colour. (Such samples may give a sulphurous smell if warmed gently.) The nutritive value of the sample is not improved by this process.

Musty Oats.—When oats are stored damp they undergo fermentation and acquire a musty smell, and a dull, unpleasing appearance. The term *foxy* is often given to oats that have heated when they have been stacked or shipped while containing too much natural moisture. The kernel loses its pleasant flavour and becomes bitter and sometimes of a reddish colour. Musty or foxy oats are dangerous to feed, especially to horses, and cause indigestion, polyuria and rapid wasting.

(b) Oat by-products.

(1) Oat chaff consists of the glumes which are separated from the straw during the threshing. It is a coarse food, about as good as oat straw, which it may be used to replace.

(2) Oat clippings, obtained in the preparation of clipped oats, resemble oat husks (see below) in nutritive value.

(3) Oat screenings, consisting of broken grain, weed seeds and particles of straw chaff, are used for poultry food, and are sometimes ground up and incorporated in compound foods.

(4) The products given in the table below are all fibrous food obtained as by-products during oat milling;

TABLE 15

	Water	Protein	Percentage composition Ether Ext.	N. Free Ext.	Fibre	Ash
Oat husks	16	3	1	53	33	4
Scree dust	7	9	6	50	20	5
Oat dust	7	10	11	56	14	4
Meal seeds	9	5	2	51	30	3
Oat mill feed ...	8	5.5	1.7	50	28	6.4

The last named is a mixture of the other offals which is sold in the U.S.A. The digestibility of its organic matter has been found to be [1]: cattle 33.8, horses 35.2, sheep 37.9, pigs 22.4 per cent.

The fibre contents of these foods limits their usefulness. Young cattle can utilise oat husks, whose feeding value, when added to a ration of molassed beet pulp plus protein and mineral supplements, was about two-thirds that of hay.[2]

Scree dust, oat dust and meal seeds are useful pig foods, especially when they are added to rations which are very low in fibre. They are thus useful adjuncts to maize meal. As might be expected such by-products tend to be rather variable in quality; they may contain undesirable amounts of dirt and sand.

(c) Oatmeal.

This is the ground kernel of the grain after it has been cleaned and the husk and hairs removed. It is rich in protein (16 per cent.), in ether-soluble extract (9 per cent.) and contains little fibre (2 per cent.). Except for calf-rearing and for sick horses and for pigs being fattened for shows, its use is not general for animals owing to its high cost.

Oat Flour is made from oatmeal which is ground and sifted through silk bolting to remove the coarser particles. Oat flour is suitable for dogs and cats suffering from intestinal complaints.

Rolled Oats are obtained by passing scoured oats, after they have been steamed to soften them, between rollers in order to flatten them. After being rolled they are dried.

Sussex Ground Oats are whole oats ground to a fine meal. They are a popular food for poultry but, unfortunately, are sometimes adulterated by the addition of ground oat husks.

(d) Crushed Oats.

Since the husks of oats are fibrous and relatively indigestible, experiments have been carried out to determine whether oats gain in digestibility and nutritive value by being crushed.

For those species, such as pigs and poultry, which are not well adapted to the digestion of fibre, it is advantageous to crush the grain, or even to grind it to a meal. Very young pigs benefit by having the husks removed altogether.

For animals which are in high production or which are being fattened, such as dairy cows, fattening cattle, or pigs, where rapid results are desired, crushed or ground oats may again be given with profit.

Young stock, such as colts and calves, also gain advantage from having crushed, instead of whole oats. Crushed oats, together with skim, separated or buttermilk to provide calcium and additional protein, are a good food for calves from the age of three or four weeks.

Except in the case of tired, sick, emaciated or old animals, there appears to be little advantage, other than that mentioned in the preceding paragraphs, in feeding crushed oats. So far as horses are concerned the gain, if any,[3] is only about 5 per cent. It is not desirable to grind oats before they are fed to horses; light crushing is sufficient.

Crushed oats should be made from good grain, and in batches sufficient for a few days only; long storage is apt to lead to considerable deterioration.

(e) Nutritive value of oats for different species of livestock.

Oats are a good concentrated food for horses, the ratio of digestible protein to the digestible non-protein constituents being suitable, and the proportion of fat not too high; moreover, the fibre content of oats also seems to be about right for these animals. Like all cereals, however, oats are calcium deficient, so that calcium should be provided in ample amount by careful attention to the rest of the ration. Unless this provision is made abnormal bone formation is likely to occur, especially in young stock.[4] It is a mistake to imagine that oats are essential for horses. This is not the case, and a properly balanced mixture of other grains and concentrates may replace oats very largely, if not entirely, in the ration of horses. The quantity of oats given to horses depends of course upon the work that the animals are called upon to perform, and also upon the rest of the diet; for hard-working horses an ordinary allowance is from 10 to 20 lb. per day. For young colts the allowance may be from 1 to 3 lb. per day, increasing up to 4 or 5 lb. when two years old and from 6 to 10 lb. per day when from two to four years of age.

Oats are an excellent food for dairy cows and unless too expensive may always form part of the ration. Mixed with other concentrates they are helpful in starting the fattening of cattle and sheep.

Reference has already been made to the use of Sussex ground oats for poultry feeding; crushed or ground they are also a good food for pigs. For horses it is only necessary to crush lightly or bruise the grain, grinding to a meal is not desirable. When oats are bruised there is an increase of about 50 per cent. in their bulk.

(3) Wheat (*Triticum sativum*)

(a) General characteristics.

The wheat flowering head consists of a compact arrangement of spikelets around a central stalk. On threshing, the grain comes away naked from the husk, in which respect it differs from barley and oats. A grain of wheat is ovoid in shape with a large groove running longitudinally, the bottom of the groove being sharply defined. On the convex side of the grain and near one end is a depression which marks the position of the germ or embryo.

Apart from giving indications of weathering, the colour of wheat is no indication of the quality of the grain or its by-products.

Wheat is seldom fed to animals except poultry, though unmarketable grain may be ground and mixed with other concentrates for cattle and pigs. It has occasionally been given to horses when it has been cheap, but the results have not been good as it is very liable to cause eczematous skin eruptions and laminitis. The work of Aberklom has indicated that laminitis may be associated with an overloading of the gut with such food as wheat or rye; under these conditions intestinal bacteria may produce decarboxylation of the amino-acid, histidine, to give the toxic base, histamine.[5] Unground, it is difficult to masticate owing to the small size and hardness of the grain. It tends to form into a pasty, glutinous mass in the mouth. For poultry, however, wheat is one of the staple foods and forms the basis of most poultry mixtures.

Wheat Screenings consist of broken and shrunken wheat kernels mixed with weed seeds which have been removed in the cleaning and grading of wheat. Some of the seeds may be harmful, but these are rarely present in screenings in sufficient quantity to have ill effects. Screenings may be ground and added to the offals, but a greater percentage should not be added than was present in the unscreened grain. They are sometimes used in the manufacture of second-class proprietary foods and are also commonly found in poultry mixtures.[6]

In the milling of wheat the removal of the husk does not require the processing to which oats are subject. Wheat is separated into three main portions by milling (a) the scaly outer part of the kernel, or bran, (b) flour and (c) wheat germ. The three fractions differ markedly in nutritive value.

(b) Wheat bran.

Depending upon the thoroughness with which the bran is separated from the rest of the grain, samples of different nutritive value may be obtained, the finer samples having a greater quantity of adherent endosperm. In the past the quality of a bran sample thus depended upon the precise technique used, so that a variety of products arose under several names. Recently attempts have been made to introduce uniformity of product, and in Table 16 the new names, together with the approximately equivalent old name, are set out.

TABLE 16

New Name	Old Name	Percentage composition					
		Water	Protein	Ether sol. Extr.	N. Free Extr.	Fibre	Ash
Bran	Broad bran	12	14	4	55	10	5
	Medium bran	13	15.5	4	54	8	4
Second Weatings	Pollards or fine bran						
	Sharps	14	16	5	56	5.75	4
	Middlings	13	16	3	64	4.5	2

It should be noted that, as the fineness of the bran increases, its fibre, fat, and ash contents diminish, while its protein and soluble carbohydrate contents increase. The vitamin B potency of wheat is also largely associated with the bran fraction.

Good broad bran should be in the form of large flakes which have a fair coating of flour. Should the flakes adhere to one another it may indicate that the bran has at some time become damp and that it is perhaps musty.

If judged by its chemical composition bran should be nearly equal to oats in feeding value, but Kellner showed many years ago that it takes very nearly one and a half pounds of ordinary bran to equal one pound of oats for fattening purposes or as a substitute for oats to yield energy for working horses. The quantity of fibre and the nature of the particles make bran a fairly bulky food, and hence it is often mixed with more concentrated foods so as to ensure that the grain is thoroughly masticated. Bran is rich in phosphorus and magnesium and poor in calcium, that is, its mineral content is unbalanced, the ratio of CaO to P_2O_5 being about $1:23$ (average).

The continued feeding of large amounts of bran as part of a ration, which contains no rich source of calcium to offset the imbalance of calcium to phosphorus in the bran, may lead to abnormal conditions of the bones (p. 67). Bran is chiefly given to horses mixed with the grain ration to prevent bolting of the grain before it is masticated, and it is also given as a laxative in the form of a mash. The laxative effect, which is slight, appears to be due to the fact that the fibre of the bran is only slightly altered in its passage through the bowel and, as Sheehy[*] pointed out, it retains its water holding capacity until it is passed in fæces; the effect is passive. Bran in the form of a mash is a favourite food for sick horses; when freshly made from good bran the mash gives off an appetising odour and, being moist, is more palatable to fevered animals than dry food, but its digestibility is not increased by steaming. Not more than 3 lb. should be used to make a mash, because if a larger quantity is eaten it is liable to undergo fermentation in the stomach, with resultant gastric tympany. A bran mash is made by putting from 2 to 3 lb. of bran in a bucket, adding a tablespoonful of salt and then pouring sufficient boiling water to moisten it thoroughly but not to make a soup of it. It should then be well stirred, covered over and left to stand until cool enough to eat. Bran is given to horses and cattle (a maximum of 3-4 lb./day in each case), but weatings are better foods for the more limited digestive powers of pigs and poultry; young pigs, in fact, should not be given bran. If fattening cattle or cows are being given concentrates that are apt to be constipating, such as bean meal, cotton cake or maize, the addition of soaked bran to the diet will help to correct the undesirable effect of the other foods. Bran is often recommended as a good food for young growing stock, but as its mineral content is unbalanced, and therefore particularly harmful to young animals, the deficiency of calcium should be carefully corrected by the addition either of leguminous foods rich in calcium, or of appropriate minerals.

The finer wheat offals are chiefly given to cows, pigs, calves and poultry. As they are easily digested they are particularly useful for young pigs at weaning time, but the mineral deficiency should be made good. The finer wheat by-products are favourite constituents of the dry mash for poultry.

(c) Wheat germ.

Wheat germ is a valuable foodstuff, containing about 25% of digestible protein of high biological value, 10% of oil rich in vitamin E, and only 2% of fibre. If kept for more than a few days it is likely to become rancid, through oxidation of the fat: solvent-extracted preparations of low fat content and greater stability are now available.

(4) Barley (*Hordeum sativum*)

(a) General characteristics.

Barley is a cereal which is very widely cultivated throughout the world.

An ear of barley is in the form of a spike, and, according to the variety, the spikelets are arranged in six, four or, most commonly, two rows up the rachis or central stalk. As marketed the grain is spindle-shaped and covered with a harsh, closely adherent husk; down one side is a groove and on the other are five well-marked ridges. In the natural state each grain usually carries a long awn, which, however, is almost invariably broken off in threshing. Barley contains about as much protein as oats (10%), but less than half of the fibre and ether soluble extract.

The best barley is, as a rule, too expensive to feed to stock, but inferior quality grain which would not be suitable for malting is given to cattle and pigs. It may be fed to horses in quantities of 5 or 6 lb. per day and makes a satisfactory food for heavy draught horses, when given either crushed or parched, boiled or soaked, to make it more easily masticated. It has been stated that barley is very liable to cause laminitis when given to horses, but this untoward result is probably due to indiscriminate and irrational feeding. In California and on the Pacific slope of America barley is rolled and extensively used for horses, mixed with other foods.

Barley meal should consist of the whole grain coarsely ground. It is variable in quality, but a good sample is excellent for fattening pigs, producing good growth of the animal, with the firm fat and flesh which go to make prime bacon.

Pot Barley and Pearl Barley.—Pot barley is barley from which the husk and bran have been removed. Pearl barley differs from pot barley in that the grain has been further polished to produce a whiter and cleaner appearance, though actually it is less nutritious. These preparations are only used for human consumption, but some by-products are obtained in their preparation which are used for animal feeding, these are *coarse dust, medium dust* and *fine dust.*

(b) Barley offals.

In the preparation of pearl barley for human consumption, by-products akin to those accruing from oat and wheat milling, are obtained. Their chemical composition is given below:

TABLE 17

By-product	Water	Protein	Ether Sol. extract	Soluble Carbo-hydrate	Fibre	Ash
Coarse dust (Barley bran and husks)	8	6	1	52	26	7
Medium dust	14	12	6	49	13	6
Fine dust	12	12	2	66	5	3
Barley feed	10	13	3	61	9	4

Chemical composition % (spanning the last six columns)

Barley feed is a mixture of the first three offals.

It will be observed that there is a change of composition, mainly one of increasing soluble carbohydrate and diminishing fibre contents, in passing from the coarse to the fine foods, such as is noted for the corresponding products derived from wheat and oats. There are similar relationships with respect to feeding values.

The coarse dust is too fibrous to feed in appreciable amounts to other livestock than cattle and sheep, whereas the finer products, of lower fibre content, find a place in the feeding of pigs and calves.

(c) By-products from brewing.

The chemical changes which occur during brewing are largely those of the conversion of starch and sugars to alcohol. On a dry matter basis, therefore, the solid by-products left after fermentation is complete contain proportionately less soluble carbohydrate and more of the other organic constituents, than the original material. Among the by-products which become available for animal feeding stuffs are (a) the sprouts, which are separated from the germinated grain at an early stage in the process, (b) the "grains" which remain after the completion of the brewing and which may be purchased either wet or dry, and (c) the residues left from the production of spirits, in which process other additional sources of carbohydrate than barley, such as maize, rye, potatoes and molasses, are used.

(i) *Malt sprouts, malt culms.*

These consist of the sprouts of barley which has been allowed to germinate and has then been kiln dried. The product should be light brown in colour and should have a pleasant aromatic odour; the taste is rather bitter. Dark coloured sprouts and those containing much dust should be regarded with suspicion.

Malt sprouts are chiefly used for feeding to dairy cows and horses

(3 lb., and 5-6 lb./day, respectively) and to sheep. As sprouts are liable to swell in the stomach, large quantities should not be given dry, and unless the amount given at one meal is small, it is advisable to soak them some hours before feeding. Some people consider that malt sprouts, if given freely, are liable to cause digestive troubles.

(ii) *Brewers' grains.*

These are available in either wet or dried forms. The wet product is also known as " draff ", and consists of 75% water plus the husks, fibre and protein of the original grain, but minus most of the starch. When warm and fresh it is palatable and may be given to dairy cows in amounts of 20-40 lb./day. Unless it is kept under special conditions it soon becomes sour, mouldy and unfit for food, but packing the material well down, together with the addition of 1% of salt, helps to preserve the freshness of the product.

It should be given to horses and sheep in small quantities as an adjunct to a less watery ration, while, mixed with other foods, it is suitable for fattening cattle and pigs.

Because of the difficulty of preservation and transportation of the wet brewers' grains, the material is dried and sold as " dried grains ", which is a bulky food containing a high proportion of protein (18%), about 6% of fat, and 15% of fibre, with 45% of soluble carbohydrate, chiefly pentosans.

Such a material is a suitable food for cattle and dairy cows, in amounts up to 6 lb./day, and for fattening sheep (1 lb./day). It may also replace half of the oat ration, on a pound for pound basis, of a horse, but, save in small proportions it is unsuitable for pigs.

Porter grains are not appreciably different from brewers' grains either in composition or in nutritive value, and the same is true of an *average* sample of distillers' grains.

(5) Maize (*Zea mays*)

(a) General characteristics.

Maize or Indian Corn is a cereal which thrives and matures only in a hot climate. It is grown to a limited extent in Great Britain for making into silage and for green cropping; when green it is particularly valuable for dairy cows. The grain used in this country is imported chiefly from North and South America, North and South Africa and India.

There are two distinct types of maize—(1) Dent or Flat Maize, and (2) Flint or Round Maize. Flint maize, as its name implies, is the harder variety and is not so suitable for horses; poultry feeders, however, as a rule, prefer the flint to the dent. The grain appears in various colours, among the most common being different shades of yellow and orange, and also white and red, but the colouring, which is confined to the horny starch, has no bearing on nutritive value, except that yellow maize contains cryptozanthine, a precursor of vitamin A, which is not present in white maize. Maize is very liable to attack by weevils, which eat away the soft endosperm leaving the flinty starch and hull.

Maize is a palatable food, readily consumed by livestock, which is rich in soluble carbohydrate (69%) and low in fibre (2%) and in calcium. Moreover, though it contains as much protein as the other cereal grains, it is poor in the essential amino-acid, tryptophane. Because of its low fibre, calcium and tryptophane contents it is not a satisfactory food by itself, but, if it is fed rationally as part of a balanced diet, it gives excellent results.

The supplementing of maize with meatmeal, fishmeal or bloodmeal, or with whole or separated milk, makes good its deficiencies of tryptophane and calcium. Green fodder will also offset the former deficiency, and if leguminous crops are fed, the lack of calcium will be met, too.

Provided that its deficiencies in fibre are remembered and are balanced by the feeding of suitable coarse foods, maize may be given to horses in quantities up to 10 lb./day. The energy value of maize is 25% greater than that of oats, so that proportionately less of the former should be included in the ration where it is being used to replace oats. In the maize belt of America the working horses receive no other cereal grain than maize and thrive well on it, the mineral deficiency being made good with alfalfa hay (*medicago sativa*). Alfalfa hay contains 1.95 per cent. CaO, whereas maize grain has only 0.02 per cent. Winkler[8] found that neither the general health nor working capacity of horses was impaired when 4 kg. of maize were given daily with alfalfa hay; the horses did not sweat inordinately. In this country it is chiefly used for heavy horses doing slow, hard work. The grain should be given in cracked or kibbled form, and not as a fine meal, nor should it ever be given after being steeped in water, either with or without cooking, otherwise digestive upsets may follow.

(b) Maize preparations.

(i) *Maize meal.*

Maize meal or Indian meal consists of the whole grain ground into a meal. It is a useful food, which may be given, not too finely ground, to young stock, provided that its deficiencies are made good. Maize meal is excellent for fattening stock and can also be incorporated in the ration of dairy cows.

(ii) *Flaked maize.*

In spite of its greater cost than the whole raw grain, this product is becoming very popular with stock feeders. The process of manufacture is as follows: the grain is screened and cleaned, kibbled and next softened and then passed through a cooker where it is slowly cooked by steam; later it is passed between hot rollers where it is flattened out to thin flakes and then dried by hot air so that the moisture content is reduced to approximately 11 per cent. During the process nothing is intentionally removed from the grain, though the oil content as well as the fibre and ash are slightly reduced. The heat treatment increases the digestibility of the preparation and consequently weight for weight flaked maize has a higher food value than the untreated grain. Thus Woodman [*] gives flaked maize a starch equivalent of 84 and the average composition of flaked maize as is shown: —

TABLE 18

	Maize Grain per cent.	Flaked Maize per cent.
Moisture	13.0	11.0
Protein	9.9	9.8
Ether Extract	4.4	4.3
N.-free Extractives	69.2	72.5
Fibre	2.2	1.5
Ash	1.3	0.9

Flaked maize is very palatable to stock and is fed to horses, cattle, dairy cows, pigs, poultry, and dogs.

(c) Maize by-products.

Maize is used industrially for the preparation of starch. By a complicated series of operations, the grain is separated into four chief fractions, (a) the starch, (b) maize bran, (c) maize gluten, or maize gluten meal, and (d) maize germ. Very often the second and third fractions are combined and sold as maize gluten feed, while, because of its tendency to become rancid, the wheat germ is treated, either by pressure or by solvent extraction, so as to give maize germ oil and maize germ meal. Though the compositions of these products tend to vary somewhat the following table gives an idea of their relative compositions (starch, being very largely carbohydrate, and maize germ oil, are omitted).

TABLE 19

			Chemical composition %			
Product	Water	Protein	Ether sol. extract	Soluble carbo-hydrate	Fibre	Ash
Maize bran	12	8	4	62	12	2
Maize gluten meal ...	9	36	5	47	2	1
Maize gluten feed ...	10	24	3	57	3	3
Maize germ meal ...	11	22	10	49	6	2

The last three products shown in the table are all good protein concentrates provided they are adequately supplemented. Maize gluten feed can be given to dairy cows, fattening cattle, sheep and pigs, and may also be incorporated in the rations of dogs, but it is too finely divided to give to horses unless included in a mash.

Corn and Cob Meal.—It is common custom ·in maize-growing countries to grind the cob with the grain for cattle-feeding, thus increasing the fibre content so that the grain is not so likely to form into a doughy mass in the intestinal tract. Ground cobs have also been fed successfully to fattening pigs.

Carbone [10] considers that crushed cobs can be included in balanced diets as follows:—pigs 25-50 per cent., according to age and whether for breeding or fattening; heifers 30 per cent. and milch cows 40 per cent.

(6) Rice (*oryza sativa*)

Rice, an annual grass, of which there are many varieties, provides essentially a carbohydrate-rich food, some 76% of the grain consisting of small, easily digested starch granules. The husk, however, is hard, siliceous, and indigestible, and the grain is poor in protein (7%) and in fat (0.5%), though its fibre content is low (1%).

Apart from inferior samples little of the whole grain is fed to livestock, except in the East, where it may be given with some suitable form of protein supplement. The husk, of no known food value, is said to irritate the intestine, and the kernel, being small and hard, is best ground before it is used as a food.

Rice meal consists of the bran coat plus the germ and some amount of the dust which is formed in the polishing of rice for human consumption; a small amount of the hulls may be present. An average sample contains about 13% of protein, 14% of oil, 6% of fibre and 9% of ash, so that rice meal is a useful food, though its high oil content and finely divided state mitigate against its keeping qualities. The compositions of rice bran and of two grades of rice polishings were found by French [11] to be as follows:

TABLE 20

Food	Protein	Ether sol. extract	Soluble carbohydrate	Fibre	Ash
		Chemical composition %			
Rice bran	13	10	46	18	13
First polishings ...	17	15	55	6	7
Second polishings ...	15	18	54	6	7

Digestibility trials of the three materials with sheep showed that in each case about 85% of both protein and fat were digested, together with some 70% of the soluble carbohydrate and 40% of crude fibre. Tests were made with pigs on the two grades of polishings, the digestibility data for protein and fat being comparable with those for sheep and the soluble-carbohydrate digestibilities a little higher. Rice meal is thus a suitable food for cattle and pigs, and a quantity of it is incorporated in compound cakes and meals, to which it also supplies fair amounts of aneurine.

Rice Slump is a material left as a residue from the manufacture of starch from rice; it is used for cattle and pigs in the wet or fresh state, and also pressed and dried. The starch equivalent of dried slump is approximately 62 and the protein equivalent 19.

(7) Dari seed (*Sorghum vulgare. Andropogon sorghum*)

Of the many varieties of sorghum seed used for feeding, that most commonly seen in Britain is the white sorghum or dari seed; a variety called red dari is also on the market, while *Guinea Corn,* a variety of *Sorghum vulgare* which is marketed with the glumes attached, is sometimes found in poultry and chicken mixtures. The crop is grown extensively · in America, and in Africa, Australia and Asia, and the many varieties are known by such names as kaffir corn, durra, dari and milo. In this country dari seed is used chiefly for poultry feeding, but elsewhere the crop is grown for use in place of maize as food for cattle, sheep, horses and pigs. The plant furnishes seeds rather like maize in chemical composition but has the advantage of being more drought resistant. 69% of the grain is soluble carbohydrate, with only 1.5% of fibre. Dari contains about as much fat as maize, 3-4%.

Like the latter food, dari seed can be given in the ground form as part of a concentrate ration, and can replace maize on a pound for pound basis. As is the case with maize, dari needs to be given with an efficient supplement of protein and calcium.

(8) Millet

Various millet seeds are fed to hens and chickens in this country, and both grain and plant form valuable foods in the countries in which they are grown. The use of the grain in Britain is practically restricted to poultry feeding. The millet most commonly used for this purpose is *Panicum miliaceum.*

(9) Rye (*Secale cereale*)

Rye, the principal grain of Northern Europe, is chiefly cultivated in Britain as a forage plant for cattle, being sown for the purpose of soiling as a catch· crop, and for providing green food for ewes and lambs in the spring, although the grain is also used for feeding to stock. Rye is, however, not a very favoured grain with stockfeeders and is considered liable to cause digestive troubles. It should be fed only when it is fully matured and is in good condition, especially with regard to freedom from moulds. In chemical composition and nutritive value it closely resembles wheat, but it appears to be less palatable for stock.

Kellner [12] has recommended that rye should be cooked before it is given to horses, and that even then it should not form more than half of their grain ration.

As a part of the concentrate ration rye is a suitable food for cattle and has been used successfully for pigs and lambs, to which latter animals it is given as coarse meal.

Though rye is viewed with some distrust by livestock feeders, its successful use in Europe suggests that it is a satisfactory foodstuff when it is fed with care.

In the manufacture of rye flour *Rye Bran and Rye Middlings* are obtained as by-products, but they are usually mixed together and sold as *Rye Feed*. These products are more nutritious than the corresponding wheat offals but they are not so palatable.

REFERENCES

1. Lathrop, A., and G. Bohstedt, (1938). U. Wisconsin Agric. Exp. Sta. Bull., No. 441.
2. Sheehy, E., (1935). J. Dept. Agric. Eire, *33*, 167.
3. Winkler, G., (1939). Biedermanns Zentralbl., (B) Tierenährung, *11*, 245.
4. Harrison, D. C., and E. Mellanby, (1939). Biochem. J., *33*, 1660.
5. Akerblom, E., (1934). Skand. Arch. Physiol. Suppl., *68*.
6. Linton, R. G., (1925). Scottish J. Agric., *8*, No. 4.
7. Sheehy, E., (1935). Sci. Proc. Roy. Dub. Soc., *21*, No. 29.
8. Winkler, G., (1940). Biedermanns Zentralbl., (B) Tierenährung, *12*, 22.
9. Woodman, H. E., and J. Stewart, (1927). J. Agric. Sci., *17*, 60.
10. Carbone, E., (1937). Nutrition Abs. Rev., *7*, 476.
11. French, M. H., (1937). Tanganyika Ann. Rep. Vet. Sci., 101.
12. Kellner, O., (1926). " The Scientific Feeding of Animals ", 2nd. Edn.

LEGUMINOUS SEEDS

1. Introduction.
2. Beans and peas.
    (a) Varieties.
    (b) Chemical composition and feeding value.
    (c) Pea and bean hulls.
3. Gram.
4. Lentils.
5. Lupins.

(1) Introduction

The legume seeds constitute a very valuable group of foods for live-stock. As a class they are distinguished by a high content of dry matter, 20 per cent. or more of protein, some 50-70 per cent. of soluble carbo-hydrate, fibre contents of about 8 per cent., and 3 per cent. of mineral matter. The starch equivalent of these foods is of the same order as that of the cereal grains, but the proportion of protein is much higher.

On the whole the legumes contain proteins which appear to supple-ment very well the cereal proteins. This fact, together with their high protein content, and their usual relative richness in calcium, makes them especially useful complements for the cereal grains in concentrate mixtures for productive purposes.

Table 21 shows the approximate compositions of the legume seeds:

TABLE 21

Legume	Dry matter	Crude protein	Oil	Soluble carbo-hydrate	Crude fibre	Ash	N.R.	Starch equiv.
	%	%	%	%	%	%		%
Beans	86	25	2	48	7	3	2	66
Peas	86	23	2	54	5	3	3	69
Gram	89	23	1	54	5	5	3	67
Lentils	86	26	2	52	3	3	3	70
Lupins, sweet								
(yellow) ...	88	42	6	25	10	5	1	71
(blue)	87	34	6	37	7	3	1.5	72

(For locust beans, see " Miscellaneous Foods ", p. 228.)

(2) Beans and peas

As these two groups of feeding stuffs are very similar in nutritive value, they may be considered together when once a description of their respective varieties has been given.

(a) Varieties.

The beans which are fed to stock in Britain include the British field or horse bean, and the New Zealand field, China and Algerian beans, all of them varieties of *Faba Vulgaris*. These beans are all characterised by their flattened shape, and the large, broad, terminal hilum. The red Burma bean and the white Burma, or haricot bean, in its numerous varieties, are also used. (The soya bean is dealt with in the section on oilseeds (p. 209).)

Many varieties of the Phaseolus species are given to livestock, but *Phaseolus lunatus*, a bean which is found, with various markings or mottlings, in black to brown, red or white colours, and which is commonly called the Java bean, is poisonous, 2 lb. of the beans being approximately enough to kill an adult bullock.

The British field, or horse bean is the one most commonly used for stockfeeding.

Edible peas, all of them varieties of *Pisum arvense* or *Pisum sativus*, include the British dun and maple field peas, and grey, China, white Indian or " Calcutta ", and New Zealand kinds.

(b) Chemical composition and feeding value.

These valuable foodstuffs contain 20-25 per cent. of protein, some 50 per cent. of soluble carbohydrate, only 1 per cent. of fatty material, 3 per cent. of ash and some 5 per cent. of fibre. In that it is relatively rich in lysine, the protein of these foods supplements that of the cereals. If the amino-acid compositions of oat and pea proteins are examined it will be seen that in most cases the lack of a particular essential amino-acid in the one is balanced by a relative excess in the other.

As with so many other foodstuffs, new peas and beans should be fed with care to livestock; the foods are easiest to handle when they are about a year old and are mature. They should not be excessively wrinkled, nor should there be any smell, or visible signs, of mould when specimens are split open.

Peas may be fed whole to poultry, but horses, cattle, sheep and pigs should be given peas and beans which have been kibbled or ground. For horses 1-3 lb./day may be given when there is no other nitrogenous concentrate in the ration.

Commercial preparations of bean and pea meals are defined by the Fertilisers and Feeding Stuffs Act, 1926 (Amended Regulations 1932) as " the meal obtained by grinding commercially pure beans of the species (1) *Vicia faba* (synonym *Faba vulgaris*) or any of its varieties, commonly known as ' horse bean,' ' field bean ' or ' broad bean '; or (2) *Phaseolus vulgaris*, the ' true haricot bean ' or any of its varieties, white or coloured " and " the meal obtained by grinding commercially pure peas, as grown, of varieties of *Pisum sativum* or *Pisum arvense* " respectively. Both pea and bean meals may be given to fattening cattle and to dairy cows in amounts of 2-3 lb./day; they are valuable supplements for the cereal concentrates (p. 120).

Flaked Beans.—Beans steamed and rolled into flakes possibly have a higher feeding value than whole beans kibbled or ground, as is the case with maize.

Bean Hulls.—In the preparation of beans, peas and lentils for human consumption the seeds are split and the seed-coats (*testæ*) or husks are removed and are used for animal feeding. An investigation into their nutritive value showed that the protein and fat contents are low and that there is much fibre, but the digestibility of the fibre is high and from feeding trials with sheep the starch equivalents for bean, pea and lentil husks were 56, 67 and 53 respectively; the digestible crude protein was *nil* to 1.5 per cent. A most important point is the distribution of calcium and phosphorus in the seed. It was found that the husks of legumes [1] contain appreciably more calcium than phosphorus, but in the dehulled seed the reverse is the case. In this manner the calcium is removed from legume seeds prepared for human consumption and a preponderance of phosphorus remains, as is shown:

TABLE 22

	Crude Protein	Ether Extract	N-free Extractives	Crude Fibre	Total Ash	CaO	P_2O_5
China Beans (*Faba sp.*) (whole seed)	26.20	2.06	58.73	9.65	3.36	0.25	1.21
China Beans (husk)	5.36	0.22	41.12	49.70	3.60	0.65	0.12
China Beans (kernel)	30.86	2.11	62.53	1.22	3.28	0.09	1.24

Pea Hulls.—This is a favourite food with shepherds in certain districts; it is moderately well digested.

(3) Gram (*Cicer arietinum*)

Gram, also called the *Chick Pea,* is a leguminous seed which is chiefly imported from India. The specific name *arietinum* originates from the resemblance of the seed to a ram's head, and it is called chick pea because the grain is also said to be like the head of a young chick. The seed-coat is light to dark brown and, like that of the other peas and beans, darkens with age. The seed is used for feeding horses and poultry and of late years it has become more extensively used for fattening cattle and for dairy cows. It is a nitrogenous food, containing about 20 per cent. of protein in addition to 4% ether extract, 8% of fibre and 53% of soluble carbohydrate. For all stock, including poultry, it should be crushed or kibbled. It is often imported badly affected with weevils (*Calandra oryzæ* or *Calandra granaria*). Occasionally, samples will be found to contain a few mutter peas, but not in sufficient numbers to cause anxiety. The maximum quantity usually given to horses and cattle in this country is from 2 lb. to 4 lb. per day. In the East it is fed more liberally and is one of the staple concentrated foods for camels. The ground grain is a common constituent of poultry mash of which it may form up to 20 per cent.

(4) Lentils (*Lens esculenta, Ervum lens*)

The lentil, one of the oldest known foods, has a grey-brown or reddish coloured seed-coat. The composition of this grain is like that of gram but it contains slightly more protein (23%) and less fibre (3%). Lentils are chiefly used as lentil meal given to dairy cows, for which animals they form a most valuable concentrate, in quantities of from 2 lb. to 4 lb. per day according to the composition of the rest of the ration. *Lentil husks* or to give it its trade name, *Lentil bran*, is a by-product obtained in the preparation of lentils for human consumption, and it is also marketed as a stock food; naturally its food value is considerably less than that of the whole seed. Lentil ash is rich in iron.

(5) Lupins

Lupins are of nutritional interest as both plants and their seeds are fed. The species Yellow Lupin (*L. luteus*) and Blue Lupin (*L. angustifolius*) are those most commonly grown, particularly the Blue Lupin. The plants are grown for the purpose of supplying fodder, principally for sheep, on light soils to which, as is the case with other legumes, they supply nitrogen.

Seeds of the older kinds sometimes contained alkaloids which were the cause of many serious outbreaks of poisoning, but strains of lupins have been bred ("sweet lupins") which are practically free from alkaloids and which give promise of providing a more valuable fodder crop, as well as protein-rich seeds which can be fed without anxiety.

Sweet lupin seeds have been found to contain only 0.08% of total alkaloids, whereas the ordinary seeds contain 0.7 to 1.3%. Feeding trials with sheep have shown that, on a dry matter basis, the seeds have an energy value equal to that of maize and a digestible crude protein content of 35-43%.[2] Ground sweet lupin seeds may be incorporated in the mash of laying hens, provided that the diet contains a sufficiency of animal protein.

Green sweet lupins.

Experiments with sheep have shown that air-dried green sweet lupins provide 12-15% of digestible crude protein and total food value about equivalent to broad bran;[3] horses are able to consume as much as 15 lb./day,[4] though they are unable to derive quite so much nourishment from the crop as sheep. Lupin silage is also of high nutritive quality.

Green sweet lupins when artificially dried have been used successfully in the feeding of breeding sows. When fed at the rate of 2 lb. daily their value was equivalent to the same amount of cereal meals.

Blue lupins have been grown successfully as a soiling crop for sheep, but owing to the bitter taste of the ordinary lupin the animals must be introduced to the crop gradually. If this precaution is taken, sheep soon become accustomed to them and thrive well.

REFERENCES

1. Linton, R. G., A. N. Wilson, and S. J. Watson, (1934). J. Agric. Sci., *24*, 260.
2. Kirsch, W., and H. Jantzon, (1938). Biedermanns Zentralbl. (B), Tierenährung, *10*, 265.
3. Bünger, H., E. Fissmer, W. Harre, and H. Schmidt, (1939). Ztschr. Tierenährung Futtermittelk, *2*, 134.
4. Gretsch, K., (1939). Biedermanns Zentralbl. (B), Tierenährung, *11*, 435.

HERBAGE

(1) Introduction

It is impossible to over-emphasise the importance of good pasture in the scheme of nutrition of farm stock, forming as it does the natural food of herbivorous animals, cattle, sheep and horses, and contributing to the nutrition of pigs and poultry.

Good pasture during its period of optimum growth supplies all the nourishment needed for normal growth and reproduction of heribivorous animals, and it has been estimated to provide 60-70 per cent. of the total food of animals in Britain. To the agriculturist, pasture has a much wider interest than simply the nutrition of animals, closely connected as it is with soil fertility, and thus with successful agronomy.

Grazing grounds range in productive value from the poor acid moorland or high-lying hillsides carrying herbage of very low feeding value, where three to four acres will barely nourish a small sheep, to rich, carefully and scientifically tended grassland, capable of carrying seven to eight sheep to the acre.

Under natural conditions animals are found on grazing lands that meet their requirements and they move from area to area as necessary. To a certain extent they adapt themselves to their environmental conditions; thus small sheep and ponies are found on hills and moors that would be incapable of carrying bigger boned stock.

Under agronomic conditions, however, such natural selection of grazing ground is not possible, and artificial grazing areas have to a large extent replaced natural grazing ones. Natural or semi-natural grazing grounds have not usually a high stock-feeding capacity, and some are decidedly deficient in certain elements necessary for keeping stock in healthy condition or else contain proportions of some substances high enough to produce toxic effects. The artificial grazing areas are usually called pastures and by maintaining a high state of fertility, suitable cultivation and careful grazing, the herbage is generally far superior to that of natural grasslands and is capable of supporting a larger number of stock in a sound and flourishing condition. As artificial grasslands are due to the work of man and his handling of grazing animals, when neglected they revert to the more natural heath, scrub or wood, or mixtures of these; from such types of vegetation they were originally derived and gradually altered, both as regards vegetation and soil conditions, until they reached their present state. Thus the provision of food for stock from pastures has become more intensive and has yielded a product of higher nutritional value, but the maintenance of this high productivity requires cultivation and manuring and control in the stocking of the pastures.

Since the achievement of a fairly satisfactory solution of the problem of winter feeding, animal husbandry has made tremendous progress in Britain and much of this may be attributed to the favourable climate, which is particularly suitable for grass production. When the temperature falls below a certain level, grasses and clovers cease to grow and the food available to feed stock rapidly diminishes and soon becomes inadequate; a similar result follows prolonged drought or very high temperatures, which cause the grass to wither. In few countries of the world are climatic conditions so favourable as in Britain, from whose grasslands come milk and milk products, meat, wool and hides, and some of the world's finest stock. Hence our artificial grasslands are of supreme importance.

(2) The characteristics of some common herbage plants

As the agricultural value of grassland is very closely related to the botanical composition, it is necessary to consider some of the individual herbage plants before attempting its classification.

(a) Grasses.

The most important grasses of agricultural value are the Rye-grasses, Cocksfoot, Timothy, Meadow Fescue, Rough-stalked Meadow-grass and Crested Dogstail.

Perennial Rye-grass (*Lolium perenne*) is one of the best plants of natural pasture but it demands a highly fertile soil, becoming very coarse and stemmy under poor conditions. It is a long lived plant and provides valuable leafy food in the autumn, although it tends to run to stem in the summer. There are many different strains, showing very considerable differences from one another.

Italian Rye-grass (*Lolium italicum*) is short lived and so is only sown in short leys. It is a very rapid grower and comes away well after cutting, yielding well for hay. This grass is earlier than the perennial rye-grass and gives an earlier aftermath. It is frequently sown as a

" cover " to more permanent grasses, and provides a large bulk of very valuable grazing.

Cocksfoot (*Dactylis glomerata*), another early grass, produces a large amount of fleshy growth but it is very sensitive to management and is easily killed by over-grazing in the spring, although it becomes very coarse and unpalatable if allowed to grow unchecked. With careful rotational grazing it provides a large amount of very valuable food. Cocksfoot provides bulky hay and it is usually sown in large quantities as otherwise it grows in tufts and becomes coarse. This grass, of which there are many different strains, the New Zealand being more valuable for grazing whilst the Danish strains are preferred for hay, will tolerate poorer conditions than perennial rye-grass and it resists drought well.

Timothy (*Phleum pratense*) is a late grass which does best on moist heavy soils and so in western regions of high rainfall it is often used to replace perennial rye-grass. It may be sown alone, although more frequently with clover. Besides being very palatable to stock, it produces very heavy yields of hay and provides valuable winter grazing although it is late to start growing after cutting and is very sensitive to severe competition.

Meadow Fescue (*Festuca pratensis*) is a valuable grass, abundant in many good pastures, which like timothy does not resist competition well, but it produces good grazing in the summer months when perennial rye-grass may be poor and, as it provides valuable aftermath, it may be grown along with timothy.

Rough-stalked Meadow-grass (*Poa trivialis*) is a moisture-loving grass providing a valuable bottom growth of winter green herbage. It is useful to develop a thick sward and suppress weeds; it provides a lot of keep in wet seasons.

Crested Dogstail (*Cynosurus cristatus*) is also a winter green which can provide valuable leafy growth on heavy soils, although it very readily runs to stem and seed unless it is mown when the stems appear. This grass is only sown where conditions are unfavourable for more valuable grasses, but it is persistent and is well eaten by sheep in winter, if it is not stemmy.

Other grasses of agricultural value include Tall Fescue (*Festuca elatior*) Meadow Foxtail (*Alopecurus pratensis*), Golden Oat-grass (*Avena flavescens*) and Tall Oat-grass (*Avena elatior*). These are rarely sown but may be indigenous on certain soils and frequently establish themselves on permanent grassland.

Inferior grasses which are undesirable on good soils include Sweet Vernal (*Anthoxanthum odoratum*) and Yorkshire Fog (*Holcus lanatus*), both common weeds of good land, as well as the numerous grasses typical of poor soils and commonly occurring on the rough and hill grazings.

Sweet Vernal, containing the aromatic substance coumarin, contributes to much of the sweet smell of hay but has a bitter taste and is of very little value. Yorkshire Fog is a very common and objectionable grass, being hairy and unpalatable except when very young; nevertheless it can establish itself from seed under poorer conditions than any other grass and can grow rapidly, which makes it of some value in the reclamation of very poor land. Soft Brome-grass (*Bromus mollis*) is another rapidly spreading weed grass not eaten by stock but common on waste land and frequently occurring in cultivated grass.

Grasses typical of poor soils are the Bents (*Agrostis spp.*), Sheep's Fescue (*Festuca ovina*), Wavy Hair-grass (*Aira flexuosa*), Moor Mat-grass (*Nardus stricta*) and Purple Molinia or Flying Bent (*Molinia cærulea*). There are very many strains of Bent and some are quite valuable, although all are considered undesirable in leys sown on reasonably good land; they have definite value on poor land but are only palatable when young. Sheep's Fescue, growing in tufts at high altitudes and in exposed positions has a value in its natural habitat, the hillside sheep runs. Wavy Hair-grass, also common on infertile hill land, provides some summer food for sheep but is useless for cultivation and produces a lot of stem and flower which browns off in the autumn. Moor Mat-grass and Flying Bent are both extremely common moorland plants of little agricultural value though providing some food for sheep when nothing better is available.

(b) Legumes.

Many types of Legumes are employed in agriculture but clovers are the most important in grassland, although Trefoil and Vetches may also occur. White Clover (*Trifolium repens*) occurs as two quite distinct types, Wild White and Ordinary (or Dutch) White. Wild White Clover is the most useful clover for long leys or permanent grass and is indigenous on most grassland. It spreads over the ground after the first year and provides nitrogen for the grasses growing along with it. It suppresses weeds very effectively and produces a closely-knit sward ideal for grazing and not easily set back by drought. For good pasture it is generally considered indispensable. Dutch White Clover is more useful for a hay crop, being more stemmy and lacking the creeping habit of the wild white. It is earlier but is short lived, dying out after two years.

Red Clover (*Trifolium pratense*). Wild Red Clover is tufted, with a hairy stem and is not much liked by stock. The cultivated red clovers are divided into two types, the Broad Red or Early Flowering Red Clovers, and the Late Flowering Red Clovers. Broad red clover is a very valuable plant in short leys, being early growing and giving a high yield in the first year, but it is short lived, usually disappearing in the third year. Late Flowering Red Clover is more persistent, can stand more heavy grazing and usually carries on into the third year.

Crimson Clover (*Trifolium incarnatum*) is frequently grown in the South of England for sheep folding, being sown as an individual crop or along with Italian rye-grass.

Alsike Clover (*Trifolium hybridum*) which is similar to, but less persistent than, late flowering red clover, does well at high altitudes and under heavy rainfall, wintering well and giving good hay, but a poor aftermath.

Trefoil (*Medicago lupulina*) establishes itself well and is valued for sheep feeding, although it dies out after one year.

Kidney Vetch (*Anthyllis vulneraria*) is also relished by sheep and is very useful for autumn and spring grazing. It is short-lived.

Lucerne is a leguminous plant which enjoys greater popularity abroad than in Britain. It has ability to withstand drought and will leave land in excellent condition for a subsequent cereal crop, although, to derive full benefit from it both as a fodder crop and for its enrichment of the land, it needs to be left for four years or more. Stapledon regards it as an excellent crop on arable and grass-arable farms, particularly where dairy herds are kept and where silage is made. (See p. 179).

(c) Other Herbage Plants.

Other herbage plants which are neither grasses nor legumes include various weeds of little or no feeding value (e.g., thistles) and miscellaneous herbs of greater or lesser utility, some of which are peculiar to limited habitats. Thus, on moorlands occur Heather or Ling (*Calluna vulgaris*), Blæberry (*Vaccinium myrtillus*), Deer " grass " (*Scirpus cæspitosus*) and Cotton " grass " or Draw moss (*Eriphorum polystichum*), whilst in saltings the bulk of the grazing material may often consist of Sea Daisy (*Armeria maritima*), Sea Plantain (*Plantago maritima*) and Ram's Horn Plantain (*Plantago coronopus*). Less localised herbs of agricultural value are Ribgrass or Plantain (*Plantago lanceolata*), Yarrow (*Achillea millefolium*) and Chicory (*Cichorium intybus*). Ribgrass is of high mineral and carotene value and is winter green, yarrow is very tolerant of heat and drought and forms a useful food for sheep, whilst chicory is also relished by sheep and is a valuable source of mineral matter.

(3) The general classification of grasslands

The grasslands of Britain may conveniently be divided into two main groups, namely, natural and artificial grasslands. In turn the artificial grasslands are subdivided into (a) temporary leys and (b) permanent grass, depending upon whether the grass is, or is not, turned in periodically as part of a system of crop rotation. A second method of classification of the artificial grasslands is that based upon the use to which they are put; they may be used as pasture or meadow. As might be expected, however, these subdivisions are not always as clear-cut as the above description sets out.

(a) Natural grasslands.

These vary greatly in extent and type. They include large areas of hill grazings, downs, moors and heaths, together with sections on the peaty districts of the fens and tidal grazings. The last named, which are also known as saltings, often provide valuable sheep pasturage, the merit of which is increased by the unsuitability of the brackish or salt water for the snail (*Limnaea truncatula*) associated with the liver fluke parasite.

The herbage shows considerable variations in botanical type. Typical plants of hill grazings include Molinia, Cotton-grass, Deer-grass, Rushes (*Juncus spp.*), Nardus, Sheep's Fescue and Bent, some areas being dominated by one or two of these species and other districts by quite different ones. Saltings may consist largely of seaside "weeds" with only a small proportion of grasses such as fescue and marram-grass (*Amnophila arundinacea*).

Differences in nutritive value are to be expected from plants growing under such very different conditions. For example the mineral fractions of plants grown on the chalky sub-soil of the downs, the acid soil of peaty districts, and on land subject to periodic tidal flooding, will differ from one another in respect of calcium and iodine contents.

(b) Artificial grasslands.

Grass may be cultivated for two different objects, firstly as a useful or even necessary stage in a system of crop rotation, or secondly because of the value of the crop in its own right. It does not follow *a priori* that the two objects are mutually exclusive. For reasons which will be made apparent later, grass is being cultivated more and more for the sake of its nutritive value as a crop.

(i) *Cultivated permanent pasture.*

Cultivated permanent pasture may be divided into rye-grass pastures (all containing *some* rye-grass) and Agrostis pastures (containing little or no rye-grass). Stapledon and Davies [1] have distinguished three grades of rye-grass pasture and their classification has been followed here.

First grade Rye-grass Pastures contain 30 per cent. or more of rye-grass, together with wild white clover and smaller amounts of bent, fescue, etc. There are only small areas of this type of land in Britain and the productivity is very high. Of this class are the best fattening pastures of the Midlands of England, or of Romney marsh.

Second grade Rye-grass Pastures, which contain about 20 per cent. rye-grass, have a larger proportion of the less valuable plants, are common in the best dairying districts, and can maintain dairy herds in milk without extra feeding.

Third grade Rye-grass Pastures are still more common than the above and form many of the permanent pastures in the dairying districts. Bent predominates but there is about 10 per cent. of rye-grass and a fair proportion of wild white clover. Grasses like Yorkshire fog, crested dogstail and sweet vernal, together with various weeds, are present in considerable quantity and where the fertility is relatively high, meadow foxtail, meadow fescue and rough-stalked meadow grass occur. Third grade rye pastures are capable of maintaining milk production or bullock fattening if a little extra feeding is given.

Agrostis Pastures are of several different types, but all contain only negligible amounts of rye-grass, bent being predominant. The greater part of the pastureland of Britain falls into this class. White clover occurs in the better agrostis pastures, along with meadow foxtail and rough-stalked meadow grass, but where fertility is low, Yorkshire fog, crested dogstail, sweet vernal and fescue are widespread, the principal legumes being Bird's Foot Trefoil (*Lotus corniculatus*) and Mountain Vetchling. (*Lathyrus montana*). The better agrostis pastures will carry store cattle, but extra feeding is necessary for milk production. Poorer agrostis pastures frequently contain a large proportion of fine-leaved fescue and form sheep runs of very low feeding value.

The nutritive value of the herbage falls off in the order which has just been given, and, to quote Stapledon and Davies,[1] " Agrostis pastures must be regarded as units of low production. They are typically rearing pastures for store animals, and it is exceptional to find an agrostis pasture capable of fattening prime lamb or cattle beast without excessive feeding of concentrates ". The same authors produce figures to show that less than 2 per cent. of the permanent pasture is of the first grade, about 6 per cent. is second quality, 27 per cent. is third rate, and the rest, some two-thirds of the whole area, is of the poorest kind. This is a most undesirable state of affairs.

(ii) *Temporary leys.*

A. Introduction.

It has become increasingly the practice during the last two decades to produce grassland by sowing seed for that definite purpose. Such an artificially produced grassland is called a " ley ", when it is intended that sooner or later the grass shall be ploughed in and followed by a different crop. In other words a ley is a deliberately produced and predetermined grass crop which is meant to constitute a stage of crop rotation. If the ley is left so long that the sown species of grass are largely replaced by unsown types, then the term ley can no longer be said to apply to it.

The above reference to the replacement of artificially by naturally sown species implies competition between different types of herbage for the land available. Such competition is also a characteristic feature even of the artificially sown plants, so that it is not advisable to settle the composition of the seeds mixture which it is desired to establish without having in mind the proposed duration of the ley. Leys are divided into sub-groups in accordance with the length of time which the artificially produced grassland is to be kept in being, so that one speaks of one-year leys, two-three-year leys, and of long leys of several years duration.

The power of herbage plants to survive is not, of course, a fixed and definite factor independent of the nature and management of the soil, of the climate, of the time and duration which the plants are grazed, or of the species of livestock which is put to graze on them. Consequently the types of plants which are sown, the proposed duration of the ley and the management of the latter are three inter-related factors, and the value of ley farming lies in the extent to which it makes available for the feeding of livestock young grass of high nutritive value. Before carrying this study further, however, it is necessary to consider the chemical composition and nutritive value of herbage in relation to its stage of growth.

B.   Chemical composition of plants at different stages of growth.

In the latter part of the last century, Wilson[2] examined various grasses at different stages of their growth and came to the important conclusion that " compared with the difference of composition at different stages of growth, the differences between the composition of the various grasses cut at the same stage are small ". He observed that " as the grass advances to maturity, the percentage of water in the green grass diminishes greatly. In the dry matter the percentage of albuminoids diminishes greatly, the ash and oil generally diminish, but less regularly and to smaller extent. The woody fibre and extractive matter free from nitrogen, on the other hand, increase. The greater the amount of albuminoids, the more easily they seem to be digested, so that the digestibility of albuminoids also decreases as the plant grows older ". These conclusions were true of both grasses and clovers, despite the higher protein contents of the latter. Another important discovery was that the leafy portion of the plant is richer in protein and poorer in protein than the stem.

These discoveries were later extended by Woodman. The table below illustrates the changes in the composition and digestibility of the protein of grass in relation to the stage at which it is cut.[3]

TABLE 23

Frequency of cutting	Protein content %	Protein digestibility %
Once per week	25	81
Every 2 weeks	24	80
Every 3 weeks	21	79
Every 4 weeks	19	76
Every 5 weeks	18	74

There was a somewhat smaller fall in the total nutritive value of the grass. Kellner[4] had also shown that clover in the very young, bud, early flowering and late flowering stages, had protein contents of 25, 21, 18 and 16% respectively on the dry matter basis, the corresponding digestibilities being 79, 73, 73 and 65%. Young grass is thus a foodstuff which contains an appreciably higher proportion of protein than does the mature crop; these changes are associated with an increasing ratio of stem to leaf in the plant.[5] As Woodman and his associates have shown, not only is there an increase in the amount of fibre in the plant as growth continues, but the digestibility of the fibre (for sheep) falls.[6]

For productive purposes the protein content of the herbage should be high, so that, provided it does not lead to deterioration of the plants, nor to a diminished annual yield of protein and total nutriment, there is everything to be said for close grazing, by which means the plants are kept in the young leafy stage. The management of the grassland, so that intensive grazing does not lead to deterioration, is very often purely a matter of local conditions; it depends on climate, season, altitude and the nature of the soil. There is no evidence that intensive grazing, under conditions of good management, is less productive than the practice of allowing the herbage to grow and become more mature, for Woodman has shown that although a weekly system of cuts produced only about half of the total dry matter which were obtained by taking a hay crop plus the aftermath, the total nutritive value (starch equivalent) per acre was only slightly less (2,532 lb. against 2,880) while continuous cutting yielded 750 lb. of digestible crude protein against 460 lb. (Quoted by Watson.[7])

The effect of intensive grazing upon the nature of the herbage, as opposed to extensive grazing, where large areas of land are grazed by too few stock, is shown [8] by the analysis given in Table 24.

TABLE 24

Type of Pasture	No. of Samples Exam'd.	Crude Protein %	Ether Ext. %	N-free Exts. %	Fibre %	Ash %	CaO %	P₂O₅ %	S.E.	P.E.
Extensively Grazed	10 { *M †	15.53	3.01	44.80	25.25	11.42	0.93	0.81	57.9	9.65
		(12.63	2.20	42.30	22.18	9.23	0.74	0.62	50.9	8.70
		(18.39	4.67	48.25	33.05	14.47	1.09	0.99	63.1	11.97
Intensively Grazed	1	22.46	2.71	40.17	20.98	13.68	0.91	0.94	59.9	15.40
Aftermath	2	12.87	2.92	49.72	24.72	9.78	0.91	0.72	62.05	-8.96

* Mean   † Limits

The increased value of young pasture, as opposed to that of the more mature, extends also to mineral matter and carotene contents, which are present in higher concentration in young plants and, in the case of the mineral elements, in more easily assimilable form.[9]

C. Seeds mixtures and ley management.

Stapledon [1][14] has written of the seeds mixtures which the present evidence suggests are most suitable for particular conditions of management. Not only do different species of grass and clover grow at different rates and become established in the sward in varying periods of time, but the same is true of several strains of the same species. Such species and strains have been deliberately produced by plant breeders so that they contain a high proportion of leaf to stem, or mature early or late, or are adapted to some particular soil conditions or climate. It is clearly desirable, therefore, that the species put down in a seeds mixture for a ley should not contain types whose habits are not compatible with one another under the conditions of management which it is proposed to use.

The case of hay production will be considered later, and only grazing practice need be mentioned here. In this connection it has been said that " hay and pasture strains and quick- and slow-starting species should not be blended in grazing mixtures unless it is reasonably certain that the grazing will be controlled properly in the seeding year and during the first and second harvest years. No risks should be taken in respect of the longer duration leys, i.e. upwards of three years." [10]

For such a long ley relatively simple seeds mixtures have been suggested, e.g. perennial rye-white clover, or timothy-white clover on good land and cocksfoot-white clover on poorer soils. For calcium-rich soils with little rainfall, the use of lucerne, with a little cocksfoot and white clover is suggested. Different strains are used to suit particular conditions. For very long leys more complex mixtures may be needed.

A ley which is intended to last two to three years may be seeded from a mixture of Italian and perennial rye-grasses, cocksfoot, the red clovers (less persistent than the white) and white clover. The strains to be used and the proportions depend upon whether the mixture is to be sown with a cover crop or not, and whether it is to be moderately or intensively grazed. The following examples are taken from Stapledon,[1] and show the seed requirements in lb./acre.

TABLE 25

Species	Average soils with cover crop	Average soils without cover crop	Light soil	Heavy soil
Italian rye-grass	4	10	4	4
Perennial rye-grass (3 strains mixed)	12	12	10–8	12
Cocksfoot (2 strains mixed)	6	6	8–10	—
Timothy (3 strains mixed) ...	—	—	—	9
English broad red clover ...	2	2	2	2
Late red clover	2	2	2	2
White clover	1	1	1	1
Trefoil on lime-rich soils ...	1	1	1	—

One-year leys are often used largely for the hay crop they provide, but they may be grazed hard so that the dung and urine of the grazing animals improve the quality of the land. Rye-grass and the red clovers provide the basis of the seeds mixture.

Catch crops may also be sown to provide food for stock for times of normal scarcity. For example, a mixture of Italian rye-grass and red clovers may be sown with oats, so that, in the autumn and winter, there will be stubble grazing of enhanced nutritive value.

Because of the increased attention which has been paid to the value of grass in the feeding of livestock, there has followed inevitably some discussion of the difficulties of winter feeding, when, as a rule, the growth of pasture is small. Attempts have been made to provide grass as a winter crop, the name foggage relating to grass which is to be fed *in situ* during the winter. The clovers do not seem to be particularly suitable for this purpose, and, although cocksfoot has been suggested as a suitable grass species, it would seem that the production of foggage is a problem in its own right and one that, however promising its possibilities, still needs a lot of investigation. An interesting account of the sowing of cocksfoot in drills to provide winter feed of this kind, has just been given by Hughes.[11]

(c) Meadows.

Pasture refers to grass which is grazed, the herbage being eaten off as it grows. The word meadow, however, is a very vague term and owing to its wide popular use it is impossible to limit it to any narrow definition. Generally a meadow is grassland set aside, either entirely or partially, for hay. Some meadows are always cut for hay, but in other cases they may occasionally be grazed for a year. In some places they are grazed in the spring and then laid up for hay, but in others they are cut in late spring and the aftermath grazed; often there seems to be no set rule except what the farmer thinks most suitable with due regard to other farming operations. On pastures a short leafy herbage is most desirable, but for making hay, taller growing plants are to be preferred. As all meadows are grazed at some time or other they serve a dual purpose and their composition needs to be a compromise between the tall- and short-growing, or the hay and pasture types of plants. Newly sown grass may suffer very considerable damage from over-grazing, so new pastures are sometimes meadowed in the first year. The hay obtained provides a valuable and nourishing food and after this is removed the field is grazed and allowed to settle down as a pasture. Further consideration will be given to meadows in connection with a study of the nutritive value of hay.

Mention should also be made of *water meadows*, in which the productivity is considerably increased by a periodical flushing with water. Considerable attention is required and a system of drainage trenches has to be dug and kept clear.

(4) Grassland management

Some aspects of grassland management have already been mentioned, and others may now be briefly discussed. Soil cultivation is essential; this may partly be achieved by the livestock on the land, but usually needs to be supplemented by harrowing in order to prevent the formation of a matted sward and to spread the droppings evenly.

For the satisfactory growth of the herbage, manuring is required; for although the dung and urine of the grazing animals return some quantity of nitrogen and potash to the soil, the calcium and phosphorus which are removed from the area in the meat and milk of productive animals usually need to be replaced, especially the phosphorus. The needs for specific nutrients for the herbage vary widely from district to district. This is an important problem and one which is likely to become more so. In the past bad management has often led to the land being stripped of its fertility, with the result that the number of livestock which a given area can support has fallen; in turn there has been a reduction in the number of human beings such land can provide with food.

The animals used for the grazing of pasture land are important, since the different species have different effects on the plants composing the vegetation. Cattle are general grazers, tending to feed on both low- and tall-growing vegetation, but sheep consume the lower plants. Horses are selective feeders also, and, in addition, they tend to graze certain areas and to discharge dung and urine on others. Pigs and poultry are similarly characteristic in their way of feeding. On this account mixed or rotational grazing and the spreading of the dung keep the pasture in best condition.

The amount of grazing to which the pasture should be subject needs to be varied in accordance with the principles which have been formulated in the preceding sections. To maintain good, succulent herbage there must be reasonably intensive grazing, the animals not being allowed to graze selectively, consuming some plant species and leaving others to grow tall and nutritively poorer. If the number of livestock is not sufficient to keep pace with the herbage at its flush period of growth, then there must be supplementary cutting to obtain the same overall effect as fairly intensive grazing. On the other hand over-grazing can be harmful in leading to the delayed recovery, or even the eradication, of some plant species, so that the nature of the whole pasturage is altered and grassland which could otherwise have been relied upon to furnish a steady level of food throughout many months is turned into an irregular and impoverished source of food for livestock. Just how much grazing can be tolerated depends, of course, upon the season and the condition of the soil in addition to other factors. The best kind of intensive grazing is one in which the plot is treated with suitable manures beforehand, and is then grazed by livestock, which then pass on to other similar plots in turn. In this way a steady supply of good quality green food is normally assured, and although each plot in the system may be grazed several times in one season it benefits from the manuring and rest it receives at other times. Clearly, good management is essential for such an undertaking. A favourable climate is also required. The selection of the best grass species for a particular region is a matter for some discrimination.

Although intensive grazing systems cannot be applied to all regions, and although they are said to be expensive, there seems to be little doubt that the need for food for the world's rising population must cause such attempts at increased food production to be more and more

closely studied. In the face of food scarcity the word " uneconomic "
loses much of its meaning; the production of sufficient food for life and
health is the first charge upon the labours of humanity, not the last.
It is a matter of each region providing the maximum possible quantity
of food; and in Britain there is no doubt that grass shows up well in
respect of the amount and kind of nutriment it can provide for stock.
The following data, quoted by Watson,' illustrate the point.

TABLE 26

Crops	Particulars	Dig. crude protein lb./ acre	Dry matter lb./ acre	Crude protein lb./ acre	Starch equivalent	
					lb./ acre	Order of yield
Pasture	New sown	1285	10011	1777	5746	1
Pasture	Permanent, intensive	1123	7745	1538	4484	2
Lucerne		896	6720	1260	2548	11
Leafy crops	Kale, cabbage	873	7257	1180	4435	3
Forage crops	Maize, mustard, rape, sunflower and comfrey	672	7018	1090	3283	6
Forage, mixed	Cereals, vetches, oats, legumes	657	5876	883	3087	7
Grasses	Rye, etc.	582	9150	976	3936	4
Legumes	Ciovers, lupins, sain-foin, etc.	540	3861	758	1709	13
Pasture	Permanent	534	4494	762	2838	9
Pulses	Beans, peas, grain and straw	473	4421	662	1848	12
Root crops	With tops	434	5845	618	3394	5
	Root alone	271	4533	394	2903	8
Cereals	Wheat, barley, oats, grain and straw	264	6520	423	2648	10

Although some variations are to be expected within the groups in the
table, there is little doubt that pasture well repays the work which is
put into it and it spreads its yield over a longer period than do most
other crops. This, however, is not to deny the fact that there are
seasonal variations in yield. On the one hand there is the relative scarcity
of herbage in winter, and on the other the spurts of growth which occur
in the late spring or early autumn. To a degree it is generally true that
the period of active growth is that of May to October. Within that
period, and to some extent at the beginning and end of it, the amount
of growth is partly dependent upon temperature and rainfall. It is in the
overcoming of such difficulties that one of the arts of good management
lies : food which cannot be used immediately by the grazing stock should
be preserved either in the form of hay, dried grass or grass silage, and
steps must be taken to see that the surplus crop is collected before it is
too mature.

Analyses of grass which show the variation in composition during
one season in one particular district, are given in the following table ";

TABLE 27

PERCENTAGE OF SOIL-FREE DRY MATTER

	May 2	May 31	June 29	July 25	Aug. 24	Sept. 17
Crude Protein ...	19.7	16.0	16.5	18.8	20.5	23.3
Ether Extract ...	3.2	3.1	3.0	3.3	4.0	3.7
N-free Extractives	48.7	49.7	51.0	46.1	45.9	42.6
Crude Fibre ...	19.6	23.2	21.6	22.7	20.7	20.9
*Ash	8.9	8.1	7.9	9.1	8.9	9.6
*including—						
Phosphoric						
Acid (P_2O_5)	1.06	1.04	0.99	1.12	1.10	1.25
Lime (CaO) ...	1.30	1.42	1.53	1.60	1.43	1.37

These data, of course, give no indication of the digestibilities of the herbage at the dates specified, but the effect of seasonal changes on the value of pasture for dairy cows in the drier part of Britain may be expressed in the following way: "In late April the grass provides maintenance and complete nutrition for 2.5 gallons of milk and proteins for a further 1.5 gallons. By July the grass provides maintenance and complete nutrients for 1 gallon of milk. By August the grass may provide at most maintenance only".[13]

Quite clearly there are difficulties associated with the production of grass as a food for livestock. Much knowledge of the feeding value of various plant species for livestock still remains to be acquired, and there are other problems concerning the plants themselves and their relationship to the soil and their environment generally which have to be tackled. The standard required steadily increases but it will have to be raised even further to provide sufficient food for the human race; the difficulties, therefore, have got to be overcome, although it will need teams of workers, beginning with geologists and engineers and ending with the actual livestock producer, to do so.

(5) Further relationships of grassland to animal nutrition

So many factors are concerned with grass production and animal nutrition that inevitably some aspects of the feeding value of grass for livestock have been dealt with in the preceding sections. The total feeding value of herbage and its protein content have thus been discussed; it remains to give account of the biological value of the protein, and a more detailed examination of the mineral element of pasture, together with several other matters, knowledge of which is less well founded.

Comparatively little work has been done on the biological value of grass protein. For the rat it was found to have quite a high biological value,[14] while for milk production, as opposed to maintenance, its value appears to be high and above that of the usual oil seed proteins.[15] A lush growth of pasture may produce digestive disturbances in the cattle which are allowed to consume it, some scouring or perhaps bloat resulting. The precise cause of bloat does not yet seem to be fully established;

it is much more troublesome in sheep and cattle than in horses and may be associated with the microbial population of the rumen. This seems the more likely since young herbage or herbage after plentiful rain contains a higher proportion of water soluble nutrients, including " amides ", than at other times. Such material is thus particularly well suited to bacterial fermentation. Whatever the cause, to restrict grazing so that the livestock are introduced gradually to this type of food is the safest answer to the problem. Clover is especially suspect with regard to bloat, but animals of the same species differ from one another in their tendency to the complaint.

The relationship of the mineral content of the soil to that of the plants which grow on it and hence to the livestock which are nourished by the herbage is important. Several factors appear to be operative, including the acidity or alkalinity of the soil, the actual content of certain elements, the ratio of the amounts of certain elements to those of others, and the physical form of the soil. Examples of this have already been quoted in Section 1, and it will suffice to bring together here in tabular form those mineral elements which are known to be associated with nutritional disorders in livestock. It must be emphasised that knowledge is very far from complete, and that there are complex inter-relationships between the different elements.

TABLE 28

Element		Disorder produced by imbalance
Sodium ⎫ Chlorine ⎭	D	Unthriftiness, loss of appetite, lowered milk and egg production, weight loss.
Calcium	D	Rickets in growing stock, bone fragility.
Phosphorus	D	Loss of appetite, emaciation, depraved appetite (pica), stiff joints, rickets, lowered fertility.
Magnesium	D	Possibly grass tetany, but not clearly established.
Iron	D	Anæmia, but simple iron deficiency probably uncommon.
Copper	D	Unthriftiness, depraved appetite, anæmia, loss of fertility, " falling disease " of cattle, " swayback " in lambs.
Cobalt	D	Loss of appetite, unthriftiness, anæmia, " bushsickness " of sheep and cattle, " pine ".
Iodine	D	Goitre, young born goitrous, stillborn or dying soon after birth, lowered fertility.
Manganese	D	" Slipped tendon " in growing chicks, low hatchability of eggs, high proportion of deformed embryos.
Fluorine	E	Defective tooth and bone structure, loss of appetite, poor growth and reproduction.
Molybdenum	E	Scouring disease of cattle, associated with " teart " pastures, loss of weight or milk production.
Selenium	E	Loss of hair, unthriftiness, emaciation, " alkali disease ".
Nitrogen as nitrite	E	Staggering or prostration, methaemoglobinaemia.

D = deficiency   E = excess

Different species vary in their susceptibilities to such disturbances of mineral metabolism, as do individual animals of the same species.

The question of palatability in relation to grassland needs consideration. It does not matter how productive a pasture may be if the palatability of the herbage is not sufficient to cause the livestock to graze it to the full. In this connection the feeding value of many so-called " weeds " has probably been under-rated. This, of course, does not imply that such plants should be allowed to grow at large but simply that their properties require investigation so that whatever benefit their controlled addition to pasture may contribute shall be realised to the full.

(6) The Stocking of Pastures

The carrying capacity of any grassland depends very much upon the season; in a good year the fields may be capable of carrying a larger head of stock than can be provided out of the farmer's capital; in a dry year the herbage may be insufficient for the maintenance of the animals already on the farm. The experienced grazier, however, can commonly tell from the appearance of grass what it is likely to carry in an average year. The figures and example given below are intended to show very briefly how to estimate the stocking of grassland.

A comparison of the food requirements of the various classes of stock show that : —

> 1 calf is equivalent to 2 sheep.
> 1 heifer or store bullock is equivalent to 4 to 5 sheep.
> 1 cow or fattening bullock is equivalent to 6 sheep.
> 1 horse is equivalent to 6 sheep.

These sheep equivalents provide a common basis on which the stocking of pastures may be calculated.

The carrying capacity of various classes of pasture during the grazing season is approximately as follows : —

First year grass on the best land, and the finest permanent pasture	7 to 8 sheep per acre.
First-class permanent pasture	6 ,, ,,
Average pastures	4 to 5 ,, ,,
Poorish pastures	3 ,, ,,
Hill and mountain grazings	$\frac{1}{4}$ to 1 ,, ,,

For example, suppose the following to be the grass available on a mixed farm : —

	Sheep equivalents.
20 acres first year seeds at 7 sheep equivalents per acre ...	140
10 acres first-class permanent pasture at 6 sheep equivalents per acre	60
10 acres good hay aftermath at 2 sheep equivalents per acre	20
40 acres poor pasture at 3 sheep equivalents per acre ...	120
Total carrying capacity of grassland	340

This grassland might therefore be stocked as follows:—

		Sheep equivalents.
4 Horses at 6 sheep equivalents		24
20 Dairy cows at 6 sheep equivalents		120
5 Heifers at 5 sheep equivalents		25
5 Heifers at 4 sheep equivalents		20
9 Calves at 2 sheep equivalents		18
1 Bull at 6 sheep equivalents		6
50 Half-bred ewes and 75 lambs = 125 Sheep		125
Total Stock equal to		338

One final point requires stressing, namely the fact that it is not just sufficient to feed livestock well; there must also be attention to hygiene. So far as grassland is concerned the little field, which has no part in any system of rotation but which is kept for any sick animals as well as for some of the sound ones, merits severe condemnation; it is an example of grassland mismanaged.

REFERENCES

1. Stapledon, G. R., and W. Davies, (1948). "Ley Farming", 18.
2. Wilson, D., (1886). J. Highland and Agric. Soc., 18 (4th series), 148.
3. Woodman, H. E., and D. B. Norman, (1932). J. Agric. Sci., 22, 856 and 862.
4. Kellner, O., (1926). "The Scientific Feeding of Animals", 285.
5. Fagan, T. W., and F. Jones, (1924). Welsh Plant Breeding St. Bul., 3H, 85.
6. Woodman, H. E., D. Blunt, and J. Stewart, (1926). J. Agric. Sci., 16, 205.
7. Watson, S. J., (1939). "The Science and Practice of Conservation: Grass and Forage Crops".
8. Watson, S. J., and E. A. Horton, (1936). J. Agric. Sci., 26, 142.
9. Watson, S. J., (1948). Nutrition Abs. Rev., 18, 1.
10. Stapledon, G. R., (1949). Agriculture, J. Min. Agric. Engl., 55, 415.
11. Hughes, G. P., (1948). Agriculture, J. Min. Agric. Engl., 55, 98.
12. Thomas, B., and B. Boyns, (1936). Empire J. Exp. Agric., 4, 374.
13. Halnan, E. T., and F. H. Garner, (1946). "The Principles and Practice of Feeding Farm Animals."
14. Bartlett, S., K. M. Kon, S. K. Kon, W. L. Osborne, S. Y. Thompson, and J. Tinsley, (1938). Biochem. J., 32, 2024.
15. Morris, S., N. C. Wright, and A. B. Fowler, (1936). J. Dairy Res., 7, 105.

THE CONSERVATION OF GRASS AND FORAGE

1. **Introduction.**
2. **Hay: its production and nutritive value.**
   (a) Hay making.
   (b) Chemical composition of hay in relation to stage of growth of plants.
   (c) Plant species for hay production.
   (d) Overall yield of nutrients provided by hay.
   (e) Storage qualities of hay.
   (f) Feeding hay to livestock.
3. **Dried grass: its production and nutritive value.**
   (a) Methods of drying employed.
   (b) Botanical nature of the crop.
   (c) The nutritive value of dried grass.
   (d) The grading of dried grass.
   (e) Feeding dried grass to livestock.
4. **Silage: its production and nutritive value.**
   (a) Introduction.
   (b) Principles involved in silage production.
   (c) The practice of silage making.
   (d) Losses incurred in silage making.
   (e) Types of silo.
   (f) Crops for ensilage.
   (g) Feeding silage to livestock.
5. **The comparative nutritive values of dried grass, hay and silage.**

(1) Introduction

To assist in the feeding of livestock during the winter period, when the natural growth of herbage is much diminished, and to avoid the wastage of grass during the period of its rapid production, when the livestock grazing upon it may fail to consume it at a sufficiently fast rate, methods of grass preservation and conservation have been developed. There are three ways of achieving this, (a) by drying the grass, (b) by making hay, or (c) by ensiling the crop. The second method is the oldest, the first being broadly speaking a way of using modern technical equipment to achieve a somewhat better result than can be derived from natural drying methods. Silage production is also quite modern and other green crops than grass can be preserved by means of it, although these will be treated separately.

In this section the main purpose will be to compare the three practices from the point of view of animal nutrition. What are usually described as economic factors will be touched upon, but, since the rapidity of technical developments often upsets completely arguments based upon existing practice, they will not be elaborated.

In the case of each method of conservation it is necessary to discuss the following topics, (a) a general outline of the technique employed, (b) the chemical composition and feeding value of herbage at different stages of growth, (c) plant species suitable for the purpose, (d) the overall yield of nutrients, (e) the storage qualities of the product and (f) the feeding of the product to livestock.

(2) Hay: its production and nutritive value
(a) Hay making.

Instead of being grazed grass is left until it is more mature when it is cut, left on the ground for a period of drying and curing, and then, when its moisture is believed to be sufficiently low enough for the crop to keep well, it is stacked.

The best time at which to cut grasses for hay can only be judged by experience. If the weather is bad it is usually better to delay cutting rather than to have the hay spoiled on the ground, as more damage will be done to the crop after it is cut than if it were left standing. In hay making the farmer tries to get the plants dried as rapidly as possible and with as little handling as need be. If, owing to rain or heavy moist weather, the hay has to be turned and tossed frequently and made up into small " coils " in the field and then spread abroad again, much of the nutriment, and that of the more soluble nature, will be lost; if the hay is exposed to rain and sun alternately it will become bleached, and the carotene content greatly reduced by oxidation.

In addition to causing the valuable leaves to fall off, rough handling of the partially dried plants cracks or fractures the stems, so that in later exposure to rain the more soluble constituents are lost. The rapidity with which hay can be made depends upon the nature and thickness or bulk in the swath and also upon the weather; wind, of course, is a valuable aid to the farmer.

Atmospheric humidity, too, is of great importance, especially at the later stages of drying for it has been shown that with humidity of 85 per cent. hay will retain 25 per cent. moisture. With such a water content the hay may be put up into cocks but not into sacks.

Owing to our unstable climate and the difficulty often experienced in early winning good hay, various devices have been adopted to allow of cocking and stacking while the moisture content is still relatively high. Among the most popular of these is the provision of an open vent in the centre of the cock or stack. This can most easily be achieved by the use of light metal tripods on which the cock is built and, in the case of stacks, a series of these may be placed in a row. The same principle can be followed by improvising structures which will allow air to circulate through the stacked hay. In more progressive agricultural countries the practice of cocking hay on tripods in the fields, well clear of the ground, has been the custom for many years.

In very favourable drying weather hay may be made and stacked in two or three days, or the operation may extend to weeks. In Scotland

and the North of England it is the practice to leave the hay standing in pikes in the fields for some weeks before stacking, while over the greater part of England it is stacked as soon as it appears to be dry enough. Hay is carried before it is really dry but, if it is too moist when stacked, excessive fermentation will take place, with conversion of some of the soluble carbohydrates into sugar and alcohol, and the hay will approach ensilage in character. Hay which has undergone much fermentation and heating in the stack is brown in colour, has a characteristic aromatic smell and is sweet; such hay is called " mow-burnt." In some districts in England slightly mow-burnt hay is much preferred to ordinary hay and fermentation up to a point is therefore encouraged in the stack but, if the fermentation and heating proceed too far, the hay will be spoiled.

The conditions which lead to hay becoming mow-burnt may bring about the spontaneous ignition of hay in the stack. Respiration of the plants, which may continue for a time after stacking if the hay has not been thoroughly dried in the field, coupled with bacterial action, may serve to raise the temperature to 70° C., at which temperature carbonisation may begin.

The practice of storing hay in Dutch barns instead of in small stacks has much to recommend it; firstly because a smaller quantity of hay is exposed to weathering on the outside (on the windward side in an exposed position rain and snow will be driven in up to a foot deep with much wastage in consequence); and secondly because the galvanised-iron roof is storm-proof. The hay is carried straight from the field to the barn, where it lies loosely packed, and is dried off by the heat from the galvanised-iron roof during the day, and by the wind which blows through the barn at night. A day is allowed to pass before the next batch of hay is brought from the fields, and then the same process is gone through again.

(b) Chemical composition in relation to stage of growth of plants.

Some indication has already been given (p. 148) of the way in which the chemical composition of herbage changes as the plants become mature. A further example is shown in the table below [1]:

TABLE 29

ANALYSIS OF PASTURE GRASS, ON DRY MATTER BASIS.

	April 26	May 24	June 21	July 19
Crude Protein	14.69	12.73	10.51	8.48
Ether Extract	3.53	3.03	2.85	1.96
N-free Extractives	55.91	56.56	52.02	49.99
Crude Fibre	16.41	20.36	·27.46	31.53
Total Ash	9.45	7.31	7.16	8.05
Silica-free Ash	6.05	5.75	4.57	5.62
CaO	1.19	0.97	0.83	0.73
P_2O_5	0.88	0.80	0.85	0.72

In order to get a crop good both in quantity and quality, grass should be cut when the principal plants have reached the flowering stage. As meadow hay consists of a great variety of plants, it is clear that all will not be cut at the same stage of ripeness. Advantages in early cutting are that the plants are less fibrous and more nutritious. On the other hand, if the crop is cut very early it gives a small yield and contains more moisture; it is difficult to save, since the grass is short and lies closer in the swath. The increased handling which this involves causes a certain amount of wastage, as the young brittle leaves are liable to break away and be lost.

One cannot expect a hay crop which will have so high a protein content, nor so low a proportion of fibre, as young grass and it is usually a matter of fine judgment as to when the hay should be cut. Watson [2] has provided the following data with respect to the average composition of meadow hay from Jealott's Hill. Ordinary meadow hay and early-cut meadow hay contained 7.3 and 12.8 per cent. respectively of crude protein, 3.0 and 6.8 per cent. of protein equivalent, on a dry matter basis, and furnished 38 and 48 lb. of starch equivalent per 100 lb. of dry matter. The differences were due to cutting at an interval of three weeks; other examples of this kind have been reported by many workers and they illustrate very well the difficulties of gauging the right moment, so far as the composition of the herbage is concerned, at which the latter should be cut. Certainly that time is, at latest, the very early flowering stage: seeded hay is very poor.

Quite apart from changes in composition, there may be rather sharp falls in the digestibility of protein, fibre and soluble carbohydrate within fairly small intervals. For example, in one experiment the digestibilities of the crude protein, fibre and soluble carbohydrates were 57, 61 and 62 per cent. respectively on June 25th, and on July 4th had fallen to 42, 39 and 38 per cent. [3] It is not known if there are corresponding changes in the amino-acid composition of the protein.

As previously indicated, the mineral matter of herbage diminishes in quantity with approaching maturity of the crop, but this factor is so bound up with the mineral content of the soil that few generalisations are possible. Legumes as a class are safer sources of calcium than are the grasses, and, with respect to phosphorus content, several workers have shown quite a sharp fall as herbage matures. Though the carotene content of late grass seems to be less than that of the young crop, the differences are slight compared with the effect that hay making has upon it. The curing of hay so much destroys its carotene, that hay should not be looked upon as a safe source of the precursor of vitamin A.

Kellner [4] classified meadow hay from " poor " to " excellent " with an ascending content of protein and total ash and a lessening in the amount of fibre: —

TABLE 30

Meadow Hay	Crude Protein	Total Ash	Fibre	S.E.
Poor	7.5	5.0	33.5	18.9
Medium	9.2	5.4	29.2	23.7
Good	9.7	6.2	26.3	31.0
Very Good	11.7	7.0	21.9	36.2
Excellent	13.5	7.8	19.3	40.6

In general the appearance of hay is not a reliable guide to its chemical composition, and a sample of meadow hay, consisting chiefly of good grasses, which would be graded as good or very good by a farmer, might be found on analysis to be deficient in protein, soluble carbohydrate and ash, with a low feeding value.

On Kellner's classification " good " hay should contain nearly 10 per cent. of protein with not more than 25 per cent. of fibre. The analyses of many samples of hay in Britain show that it is exceptional for hay to have as much protein. Thus Knox and Prowse [5] give a protein content of 8.18 and crude fibre 28.27 per cent., while Watson and Ferguson in 22 samples of well saved hay found a range of 4.81-12.90 (average 8.92) per cent. of protein, with fibre 30.06-40.96 on dry matter basis. The average percentage composition of the 22 samples, assuming a moisture content of 15 per cent., was:—

TABLE 31

Crude Protein	7.58 per cent.
Ether Extract	1.49 per cent.
N-free extractives	40.78 per cent.
Crude Fibre	28.71 per cent.
Ash	6.44 per cent.

The average percentage composition and digestibility coefficients for the various constituents were, when sheep were used, 40, 50, 60. and 60 per cent. (approx.) for protein, ether extract, fibre and soluble carbohydrate respectively.

The starch equivalent, 35, determined from the average values of the 22 samples indicated quite good hay, but the protein was definitely low.

These and similar investigations naturally lead to the question as to how the farmer can assess or have assessed for him, the nutritive value of his hay. Assuming that the hay has been well saved and is of good colour and aroma, then short of complete analysis and digestibility trials, which of course are impossible in ordinary practice, the most satisfactory method is to have the crude protein, fibre and acid-soluble ash determined. These by themselves supply valuable knowledge and it may be taken as a general rule—but there are exceptions—that there exists an inverse correlation between fibre and protein in growing herbage.

When compounding rations, in order to get the best and most

economic results, it is necessary to know not only the chemical composition of the various foods to be incorporated, but also their actual nutritional value, expressed in the simplest—and admittedly incomplete —form as starch equivalent and protein equivalent. To determine these accurately by feeding experiments is a long and costly business and a search for a simpler method for finding these values for hay was made by Watson and Ferguson.[6] They plotted values of starch equivalent (S) against the sum (X) of twice the crude fibre content and the crude protein content (on dry matter basis) and found that a simple relationship existed. From the straight line so obtained they derived the equation:—

$$S = 77.136 - 0.5297 \ X$$

A similar method was adopted for the regression of the protein equivalent (P) on the crude protein (Y) and in this case the equation was found to be:—

$$P = 0.6992Y - 2.148$$

For example, a sample of hay was found by analysis to contain on the dry matter basis 9.5 per cent. crude protein and 30 per cent. crude fibre. Substituting these values in the equation we obtain:—

$$S = 77.136 - 0.5297(2 \times 30 + 9.5)$$
$$= 40.3 \text{ on dry matter basis}$$
$$= 34.2 \text{ with 15 per cent. moisture in hay as fed.}$$

Similarly for the protein equivalent:—

$$P = 0.6992 \times 9.5 - 2.148$$
$$= 4.5 \text{ on dry matter basis}$$
$$= 3.8 \text{ with 15 per cent. moisture in hay as fed.}$$

(c) Plant species for hay production.

In a relatively few cases hay is produced from pure grass species; in a larger number " seeds hay " is obtained from leys, and in most instances " meadow hay " represents an indeterminate mixture of herbage plants over the nature of which there has been comparatively little control.

Watson,[2] who has collected many data on the composition of different classes of hay, finds that the equation previously given for starch and protein equivalents fits fairly well the different samples. In the author's own words:

" Examination of data for grass hays, ' seeds ' mixtures of grass and clovers, leguminous hay, cereal hays, and dried fodders such as maize and sorghums, shows that all exhibit the usual trend of changes with stage of growth.

" The striking fact arises from the mass of data in the literature that all types of hay, whether from grasses, legumes, or cereals—small or large—fall into line and can be calculated from a single equation for protein equivalent and another for starch equivalent.

" Hays should be classified on a knowledge of their crude protein and fibre contents, but hays which have 'heated' in the stack will be of lower feeding value than their composition would indicate."

In view of the above general relationships and the fact that it is the leaf which is rich in protein and low in fibre, the attempts of the plant breeder to produce new hay strains which will show greater leafiness and greater persistence and still show early growth in the spring, will be understood. Hay strains of perennial rye-grass have been produced which differ markedly from the pasture strains. A valuable hay strain of cocksfoot is the New Zealand Certified (Akaroa) and a corresponding strain of timothy the Aberystwyth S 51. As there are different strains to suit different conditions of soil and climate reference should be made to the various authorities in this field. New varieties of red and white clover have also been developed.[7][8] Among the leguminous crops lucerne is reputed to provide far and away the best hay, but its superiority over red clover seems to be due to the fact that it is cut at an earlier stage, when its protein content is therefore higher.

Meadow vegetation tends to vary widely, the number of grass, legume and herb species often approaching 50 to 100, although the bulk of the herbage usually consist of tall grasses and herbs. Cocksfoot, tall or meadow fescue, timothy, tall oat-grass and some rye-grass contribute to the bulk of the hay crop; in the bottom growth, bent, Yorkshire fog and soft brome-grasses are common. There is usually a large collection of weeds.

In good meadow hay there should be a preponderance of the better type of grasses, but the botanical species normally found in meadow hay are dependent primarily on the nature and position of the land. Thus what would be regarded as a very second-rate grass on the best lowland pastures might well be of considerable value, comparatively, on high lying moorland. On the best pastures one would expect to find a preponderance of the grasses and other forage plants which have already been indicated as of high nutritional value and suitable for haymaking as well as grazing. A large proportion of weeds and second-rate grasses indicate that the hay has been gathered from poor ground unable through poverty in nitrogen and salts to sustain the better class of plants. Weeds especially objectionable are horse tail (equisetum), thistle, couch grass, Yorkshire fog and tufted hair-grass. A large proportion of withered fibrous bottom growth is also to be deprecated.

Various forage crops and mixtures of them are also grown for making into hay. These include winter oats and tares, spring oats and peas, rye and tares, rye and peas, winter barley and winter tares, and oats alone. The best results are obtained if the crops are cut when some of the legume pods have formed, and before seed formation is advanced. Probably the greatest value is obtained from the oats when they are cut in the "milky" stage, or when the seed is just beginning to become doughy. The cut crops require careful handling; they are much slower to wilt than grass, are therefore more difficult to make into hay and after the hay is "made" the brittle but very nutritious leaves of legumes are liable to be broken off and lost. Oat and tare hay or oat and pea hay contain more protein than "seeds" hay but the percentage varies, of course, with the proportion of legume in the crop, the state of growth at cutting and the manner in which the crop has been saved. When well made, these crops form valuable roughage, especially for the feeding of dairy cows, but they tend to be rather high in fibre. The inclusion of legumes in the crop increases the calcium content of the hay.

(d) Overall yield of nutrients provided by hay.

In discussing the overall yield of nutrients provided by hay one must consider (a) the total weight of dry matter obtained as hay, (b) the percentage composition of the crop, (c) the digestibility of the various constituents and (d) the value of the aftermath when the hay has been taken.

On the average the early-cut hay provides less dry matter, rather less starch equivalent, but more protein equivalent per acre than the later-cut crop. However, the sharp fall in percentage digestibility with increasing age of the herbage, to which some reference has already been made, is an important factor in this respect. Calculations by Watson' of some of the available data show that a week or ten days delay in taking the crop may cause a 50 per cent. fall in its total nutritive value and quite a sharp fall in the yield of protein equivalent per acre. There are indications that weather conditions have a big influence in this respect.

If the value of the aftermath is included together with that of the hay, then there is evidence to show that an early cut of hay plus a late aftermath is likely to furnish as much starch equivalent and more protein equivalent than any other combination of early, middle or late hay making with early or late aftermaths. In all, therefore, the best policy seems to be to take an early hay crop together with the late aftermath. Certainly some of the hay samples which are submitted for analysis show that their feeding value cannot be greater than good straw. The low protein content of more mature herbage may be sufficient for maintenance purposes but for high levels of production something better is needed.

(e) The storage qualities of hay.

To store well the moisture content of hay should be low when it is stacked, otherwise there is the risk of heating in the stack and consequent loss of nutritive value. On the other hand since a leafy type of product has the highest feeding value, it should not be kept too dry, for in any case there is likely to be some loss of the fairly brittle leaves and the loss will be increased by excessive drying. The bleaching which hay undergoes in the field destroys most of its carotene and the subsequent fall is thus of no great consequence. Good hay should not be dirty, dusty, mouldy, or burnt; it should be soft and pliable, green in colour and pleasantly aromatic in smell; a fairly high proportion of leaf should be present.

(f) Feeding hay to livestock.

Because of its high fibre content hay is most suitable for ruminant species and secondly for non-ruminant herbivorous animals. First-class hay is thus a good food for cattle and sheep : it can be gradually added to the ration of calves for whom it will provide food and also the fibre for the development of the rumen. Horses will also do well on good hay, though their capacity for the digestion of fibrous food is less than that of ruminants and therefore a hard-working horse may require less hay and more concentrates than an idle one.

The position is rather different where inferior grades of hay are concerned; their protein content is low and their fibre is high so that their value for productive purposes falls, although they may have some use for fattening. Such poor hay can be used to provide fibre for an otherwise too concentrated ration, but in that case it may have very little more food value than good straw. Time, labour and land have been wasted when the hay crop is of that kind.

Hay is an undependable source of carotene and where livestock are being given rations consisting of hay and straw, or hay and roots, or hay and such · protein concentrates as linseed or groundnut cakes or meals, it is advisable to include some small daily ration of green food. For preference fresh green food should be added, but, failing that, good quality dried grass or silage is needed. Carotene or fish liver oil concentrates will provide carotene or vitamin A, but there are excellent reasons for believing that all the good qualities of fresh green foods are not resident in their protein or carotene contents.

Hay is also a variable source of minerals, as previously indicated, and since herbivorous animals are principally dependent upon hay during the winter months, and in the case of town horses all the year round, to obtain their supply of calcium, the chemical composition of this food is of great importance. This is so not only because hay is the principal source of supply of calcium, though its percentage in different types of hay varies considerably, but because all the cereals and oil cakes supplying the concentrated portion of the diet are deficient in calcium and contain a marked preponderance of phosphorus; thus a good supply of calcium in hay would help to correct such unbalanced calcium-phosphorus ratios.

Generally, but not invariably, with hay grown in Britain a high silica-free ash indicates a high calcium content; thus hay with 2.43 per cent. of ash had 0.51 per cent. of CaO and 0.33 per cent. of P_2O_5, while that with 7.33 per cent. had 1.78 and 0.69 per cent. of CaO and P_2O_5 respectively. The percentage of calcium in hay varies considerably.'

Hay made from leguminous crops contains the greater amount of calcium, clover hays having from 1.5 to 2 per cent. or even more, whereas timothy hay appears to have the least calcium. The choice of hay in feeding dairy cows, where there is a great drain of calcium from the body during lactation, is important in relation to its mineral content as well as its general nutritional value.

The intake of calcium with a daily ration of 15 lb. of timothy hay would be in the region of 40 gm. CaO; meadow hay 70 and clover hay 130 gm. Such differences in the intake of calcium over a lactation period must be of considerable importance. It is suggested that a good *meadow hay* should have at least 4 per cent. of silica-free ash and 9.5 per cent. crude protein, with not much more than 30 per cent. of crude fibre; on dry matter basis such a hay should have a starch equivalent of approximately 34.

The question of mineral intake is important and one which should not be left to chance, for, as Woodman and Evans have shown, serious mineral deficiencies are to be expected in livestock fed on hay derived from mineral impoverished land.[10]

(3) Dried grass; its production and nutritive value

In previous pages the point has been made that young herbage is a better foodstuff, certainly for the production of meat, eggs and milk, than the mature crop. Furthermore, several cuttings of the herbage can furnish as much total energy value and more protein than one single hay crop. On these accounts the production of dried grass has greatly increased during the last two decades.

(a) Methods of drying employed.

Several types of plant have been developed for the production of dried grass. In the simplest units the crop is spread out in trays and a current of hot air flows over it and removes the greater portion of the moisture; in other cases the cut grass is fed on to a travelling belt which passes through a chamber in which hot gas is flowing, this process being a continuous one; in yet a third kind of apparatus the grass is agitated in a drum during the passage of the hot gas. There are advantages and disadvantages with respect to fuel consumption, amount of labour required, size and cost, etc., for each type.

The process is more efficient the higher the temperature of the gas used for the drying; provided that the material which is exposed to the hot air flow is not already dry, a gas stream at a temperature as high as 800° C. may be used without harm to the product. In practice this means that the time of exposure in the drying chamber, and the temperatures of the incoming and outflowing gas streams have to be adjusted in accordance with the moisture content of the grass crop. Some field drying (wilting) may first be used.

(b) Botanical nature of the crop.

Watson[11] uses the term dried grass for " the products of the drying of all those grasses and legumes which may be used for grazing by animals ". Apart from lucerne, sainfoin and timothy most of the crops used for this purpose are mixtures of grasses and legumes.

It has been stressed elsewhere that as grass matures the proportion of protein falls, and that of fibre rises, while the digestibilities of the constituents also tend to fall. The value of a grass crop thus depends primarily upon the stage at which the plants are cut, for efficient drying apparatus changes but slightly the food value of the fresh material. If the crop is cut at the stage just before seeding then the final product will not be any better than good hay, but, since the cost of the evaporation of water is high, it will have been produced much more expensively.

(c) The nutritive value of dried grass.

The development of dried grass production has been due very largely to the careful work by Woodman and his collaborators, in which not only the composition of the fresh and dried foods was studied, but also the digestibility of the product for cattle and pigs.[12] In considering the nutritive value of dried grass its total energy value, its protein, vitamin and mineral contents require attention as well as its storage qualities.

The total nutritive value of dried grass will necessarily vary with the species of livestock to which it is fed. The following table [11] shows the composition of dried grass and its starch equivalent for ruminants.

TABLE 32

Crop	Dry matter %	Crude protein %	Starch equiv. %	Protein equiv. %
Grass				
Very leafy	90	18.7	54.1	13.6
Leafy	90	15.0	51.7	9.3
Early flowering ...	90	12.1	51.2	6.8
Flowering	90	10.4	49.5	5.5
Lucerne				
Bud	91	22.3	50.1	13.6
Early flowering ...	91	16.2	44.1	10.5

The data show that, other factors being constant, there is a slight fall in the nutritive value of the material with increasing age of the crop; this fact has been stressed previously and it remains to point out that good quality dried grass has about two-thirds the starch equivalent of the cereal grains and nearly twice that of hay on the dry matter basis. It must not be assumed, however, that the dried food has quite the same nutritive value as the fresh grass. Even though the chemical composition of the two products is the same, and though the digestibility coefficients do not differ, experiments have shown that the dried grass requires more energy to be expended on its mastication and digestion than does the fresh crop on a dry matter basis.[13] The use of dried grass instead of the green crop at the same stage of growth involves a loss of about one-sixth of the nutritive value of the latter.

Where there is overheating of the material in the drier an extra loss of nutritive value is the result, the magnitude of the loss depending upon the extent of the maltreatment of the grass.

The data in the following table show the respective compositions and digestibilities of fresh and dried grass as reported by Watson,[2] the data of the first six rows relating to dry matter basis.

TABLE 33

| | Low-protein grass | | | | High-protein grass | | | |
| | Fresh | | Dried | | Fresh | | Dried | |
	Comp. %	Dig. %	Comp. %	Dig. %	Comp. %	Dig. %	Comp. %	Dig. %
Ether ext. ...	2.11	55.9	2.40	55.4	2.09	38.9	2.79	53.1
Fibre ...	30.43	70.3	28.20	72.3	21.95	80.4	21.92	78.1
Sol. carb. ...	47.55	69.6	49.27	70.6	44.86	77.5	45.92	77.0
Crude prot.	10.62	63.1	10.86	56.1	17.58	77.6	17.83	72.6
True protein	7.58	55.6	10.08	58.4	13.13	70.8	16.90	72.2
Organic matter	90.71	69.0	90.73	69.1	86.48	77.3	88.46	75.7
Dry matter	21.10	66.6	90.30	67.3	17.21	74.4	86.42	72.3

The digestibility of the protein fraction is very slightly diminished by the drying of grass but fairly harsh treatment is needed to cause a large fall. The biological value of the dried grass protein is high for milk production.[14] Drying appears to increase the amount of "true protein", perhaps through the condensation of amino-acids or simple peptides.

One of the advantages of the efficient drying of grass is the relatively small loss of carotene which ensues, and, in view of the poverty of most of the concentrates, straws and roots in this factor, this is a most important characteristic of the food.

Comparatively little work has been done on the effects of drying upon the availability of the mineral fraction of grass, but there seems to be little reason to suppose that there is any significant deterioration.

The data which have been presented reveal that dried grass can be a very good food for livestock, for it contains large proportions of good quality protein, easily digested fibre, some 50 per cent. of soluble carbohydrate, a good mineral content and ample carotene (and, with the exception of vitamin C, other vitamins). Since the food has to be stored it is important to know whether there is significant deterioration upon storage.

Provided that it has been dried to a moisture content of about 10 per cent. and it is stored under satisfactory conditions (p. 234), there is likely to be no deterioration of any factor other than carotene during normal periods of storage. Ferguson[15] has summarised the evidence relating to carotene stability. Dried grass which has been cooled properly after passing through the drier, and is then bagged and stored in a dark, cool place, may be expected to retain 50 per cent. of its carotene for periods up to about a year. Warmth, exposure to light, the free access of air and fine grinding instead of high pressure baling of long material, all tend to cause additional loss of the vitamin.

(d) The grading of dried grass.

A good deal of confusion has arisen because of the manner in which dried grass has been graded for sale, the classification being based on its carotene content, and the rather modest figure of 0.025 per cent. of carotene being accepted for the first grade.

Unless small amounts of dried grass are being used to supplement an otherwise carotene-deficient ration, in which case there is some reason for using carotene content as a basis of assessment, the above method is open to criticism and alternative methods have been proposed. The critics have pointed out that the carotene content of dried grass provides little indication of the general feeding value of the material. A given sample may have been produced from grass which has been cut at the right stage and which has then been satisfactorily processed, when its feeding value and protein contents will be high; alternatively—and carotene content is a poor guide in this respect—the sample may be little better than hay.

It is as well to spend some time in considering this matter, for it involves an imporant principle, namely, how far one may assess the full nutritive value of a foodstuff on the basis of the best chemical analysis which scientific knowledge can provide at the time. Despite the fact that new food factors are discovered one after another there is always the tendency to fail to consider the value of some product as a food and not as a source of such factors as happen to be fashionable at the moment.

Dried grass is capable of providing good quality protein, easily digested fibre and soluble carbohydrate, useful mineral elements, carotene and, in all probability, a number of other factors which are present in traces only but are nutritionally important. So far as animal foodstuffs are concerned good quality protein is relatively scarce, although there is no scarcity of foods which are rich in carbohydrate; but good silage, good dried grass and fresh green foods are the only reliable sources of carotene, the bulk of the concentrates, roots and coarse foods containing very little of this substance. Although the vitamin A of fish liver oils can replace carotene in a diet, there are other factors present in dried grass which it cannot so replace. At this stage the carotene content of dried grass, in relation to the needs of livestock for carotene, requires examination.

Ferguson [15] has recently investigated the problem. In the following table are shown the daily carotene requirements of cattle of different body weights, the requirements being set at five times the known minimum requirements, together with the weights of dried grass which would meet their needs.

TABLE 34

Live weight lb.	Daily carotene requirement mg.	Dried grass supplying carotene gm.	lb.
200	11 – 15	75	0.17
600	33 – 45	225	0.50
1000	55 – 75	375	0.83
1200	66 – 90	450	1.00

Ferguson suggests that valuation on carotene content is unjustified, since cattle would be fed at higher levels of dried grass intake than are set out in the above table, and since, at the beginning of the winter feeding period, cattle normally have a bodily reserve of vitamin A.

For these reasons he argues that there should be valuation on the basis of protein content. The carotene content of dried grass, however, does give some idea of the treatment to which the product may have been subjected and, since cattle are by no means ideally fed in all districts even in summer, there is a good case for the publication of both protein and carotene contents of dried grass. This at least would leave a purchaser free to buy the material best suited to his purpose.

Lewis and Eden [16] have also criticised adversely the adoption of carotene content for the grading of dried grass and have suggested that in Britain this practice has led to the production of *quantity* of dried grass at the expense of overall nutritional *quality*. On the basis of Watson's equations relating protein equivalent, starch equivalent and protein content (on a dry matter basis) the above workers have suggested the following grading of dried grass in relation to milk production.

TABLE 35

Category	Crude protein (90% dry matter basis)	Amounts of dried grass to feed per gallon of average milk
A	17 or over	5 lb.
B	15 to 16.9	5.5 lb.
C	13 to 14.9	5 lb. plus 0.5 lb. high protein cake, or 4 lb. plus 1 lb. medium cake or beans.
D	11 to 12.9	4 lb. plus 1 lb. high protein cake, or 3.5 lb. plus 1.5 medium cake or beans.
Ungraded	Less than 11	Maintenance only.

Lewis and Eden described, in addition, a system of management of grass which has yielded a food of such quality that two thirds of the material was in grades A and B, and therefore approximately balanced for milk production, about 25 per cent. was of grade C and only 10 per cent. was inferior material. Their system of management yielded a good tonnage of grass silage containing 12 to 15 per cent. of protein on a dry matter basis.

(e) Feeding dried grass to livestock.

To cattle, sheep and horses dried grass may be fed in fair quantity, though there is some evidence that the finely ground material is not very suitable, being apparently unpalatable and liable to lead to some digestive trouble.

The basis upon which the material may be given to dairy cows has been set out in the preceding table. Its cost is one of the factors which limits the amounts which it is economic to use. There is no doubt, however, that it is a most useful addition to the usual mixed concentrates. Ferguson [15] has suggested the following scale of replacement of hay or concentrates by dried grass:

TABLE 36

| Protein content of grass | 10 lb. dried grass replaces— | | |
	Concentrates lb.		Average meadow hay* lb.
15+	8.5 - 9.5		—
14	7	plus	4
13	5	„	7
12	2.75	„	10
11	1.5	„	12
10	—	„	14

* Starch equivalent 35; protein equivalent 3.1.

For dairy cows kept in during winter months and fed under artificial conditions, high grade dried grass is a most valuable food to include in the diet. Apart from the fact that the carotene improves the colour of the milk and butter, it stimulates appetite and supplies food constituents not generally found in the class of concentrates usually given to these animals.

The quantities fed to fattening cattle and dairy cows should generally not exceed half a stone a day, but much depends of course on the composition of the rest of the diet.

Dried grass can with advantage be included in the diet of calves, the quantity naturally depending upon their age.

For box-fed sheep dried grass can profitably replace concentrates in equal amount and it is not necessary to use the highest grades. When the growth of grass is backward it is an excellent food for early lambing ewes, both before and after lambing.

Town-kept horses could with great advantage have high-grade dried grass included in their diet at all times, except when they are given fresh cut grass under the soiling system. Other horses which would benefit appreciably by such an addition to the diet are pit ponies and also polo ponies being maintained indoors between seasons. For brood mares foaling very early in the year, especially if kept indoors, good dried grass should be considered a necessary adjunct to the diet.

Dried grass can also be given to all classes of pigs, but particularly to brood sows; 5 per cent. is a useful amount to include in the daily ration.

Poultry not on free range may have a small amount of dried grass which, apart from its nutritional value, improves the colour of the yolk. It should, however, be noted that the protein of grass cannot altogether replace the animal protein so desirable in the diets of pigs and poultry. Halnan [17] considers that normal chicks', growers' and layers' rations may contain up to .7 per cent.; in times of food shortage the level may be as high as 18 per cent. of the dried grass.

(4) Silage: its production and nutritive value

(a) Introduction.

Ensilage is a method of fodder conservation which has been known for over a century, but which had made little progress in this country until recent years. Where silage was formerly made it was generally used as an alternative food to roots, although its fibre content is much higher and, when leguminous crops are ensiled, the protein content is also considerably greater than in roots. Since the demonstration of the high nutritive value of young pasture grass, however, much attention has been given to the problems of grass conservation and the possibilities of ensilage have been re-examined. As a result of very considerable investigational work much more is now known about ensilage and several new methods of making silage have been evolved. The greatly increased popularity of ensilage which has resulted from this work has led to the introduction of many types of temporary and portable silos, which are considerably cheaper than the more substantial permanent towers and which have made possible a very rapid expansion of this method of fodder conservation.

(b) Principles involved in silage production.

When fodder plants are cut they remain living for some time and, as a result of their respiration, carbohydrates are used up, being converted to carbon dioxide and water, while much energy is liberated as heat. In a silo, where the plants are closely packed, this heat does not readily escape, so that there is a considerable rise in temperature, and unless the respiration is controlled, losses of valuable nutrients may become considerable, the temperature rising so high that the nutritive value is still further impaired. One of the most important aims of silage manufacture is to reduce respiration by pressing the crop to a compact mass and thus excluding air. By this means, complete oxidation of carbohydrates to carbon dioxide and water is prevented and only anærobic respiration is permitted. In anærobic respiration the oxygen is obtained from the crop itself, very much less energy is evolved as heat, and, in addition to carbon dioxide, the products of respiration include alcohol and many organic acids. Even with anærobic respiration, however, sufficient energy is liberated to yield a considerable amount of heat, the effects of which become quite marked in a silo.

As a result of high temperature, or exhaustion of respirable material, the plants eventually die and the cellular protoplasm no longer retains its semi-permeability. The cell contents diffuse out and are acted upon by the numerous bacteria which are always present in a crop. Bacterial action in silage is very important, the quality of the product depending very largely upon the exact nature of the bacterial activity. The general effect of bacterial action is to break down the complex organic substances, particularly carbohydrates, by which process they obtain the energy and matter they need for growth. Nitrogen is usually obtained from amino-acids, although more complex protein compounds may be attacked. Although bacteria usually do not break down protein readily, under suitable conditions many anærobes can hydrolyse very complex proteins and the addition of fermentable carbohydrates, with its stimulus to growth, results in a marked increase in protein cleavage. In good silage many of the proteins are broken down to their constituent amino-acids but further degradation should not occur and it is only in very poor silage that the amino-acids are decomposed to form volatile bases. Carbohydrate breakdown leads to the formation of many organic acids and in good silage the non-volatile acids, particularly lactic acid, should be greater in amount than the volatile acids acetic, propionic and butyric.

Lactic acid is the organic acid most desirable in silage and the aim in silage-making is to favour the development of lactic bacteria, which soon produce an acidity sufficient to suppress undesirable bacteria of the butyric type. Butyric fermentation, besides producing undesirable end products, causes a considerable energy loss. In order to control butyric fermentation, rapid acidification is essential and this may be achieved by adjusting conditions so that there is very rapid growth of the lactic bacteria. At a pH of 4.5 the activities of the undesirable bacteria are eliminated and at a pH of 4 or less, lactic bacteria are able to flourish at the expense of other organisms; the best silage is produced when this degree of acidity can be quickly achieved.

Temperature control is of special importance in promoting lactic development. Undesirable organisms producing butyric and propionic acids cannot flourish at temperatures above 122° F. (50° C.), although the lactic acid bacteria are able to do so. But high temperatures can be reached only by the expensive oxidation of considerable quantities of carbohydrates, and although a palatable food may be produced under these conditions there is inevitably a reduction in the nutritive value of the crop. Although the lactic acid bacteria flourish at high temperatures, they grow well at about 100° F. (38° C.), a temperature which can be attained without undue respiratory loss. It is at moderate temperatures, in the region of 100° F., therefore, that silage can be produced most economically and the access of air to silage should be controlled so that the temperature never exceeds 120° F. The warm fermentation process, using the higher temperature of 122° F., has been used, especially for the production of stack silage, in Holland and Switzerland, and the cold fermentation process, carried out below 80° F., with the material closely packed and the silo rapidly filled, has found considerable favour in Germany.

A palatable nutritious silage is most easily produced when the supply of oxygen is restricted, the amount of fermentable carbohydrates is plentiful and the bacterial activity is predominantly that of lactic acid organisms. The chemical changes which occur chiefly concern the carbohydrate fraction of the ensiled material, some four-fifths of the material lost during silage making consisting of carbohydrates and less than one-fifth of nitrogenous substances. Some mineral matter may be lost from the silage by drainage of the liquor, while too high a temperature during the fermentation usually means that conditions are favourable for the destruction of carotene. From the carbohydrates of the ensiled material the lower fatty alcohols are formed, plus a group of organic acids; it is this last group which is so important. The acids

which are to be found in the different qualities of silage are indicated
in table 37, from data of Kirsch and Hildebrandt, and quoted by
Watson.[2]

TABLE 37

Class	Content of acid in silage of 18-22% dry matter content			Proportions of total acid as:		
	Lactic %	Acetic %	Butyric - %	Lactic %	Acetic %	Butyric %
1 Very good ...	1.77	0.68	———	72	28	—
2 Good	0.76	0.95	———	44	56	—
3 Intermed. ...	1.14	0.55	0.14	62	30	8
4 Poor	0.59	0.26	1.65	24	10	66
5 Inedible ...	0.09	0.10	0.03	—	—	—

Most of the butyric acid in grades 3 and 4 is in combined form.
Such silage would not be suitable for dairy cattle and grade 5 is not
fit for feeding at all.

The nature of the activity which has predominated in a silage can
usually be estimated by the acidity. A pH of 4 - 4.5 indicates a predominance of lactic bacteria whilst 'a value greater than 5 suggests a
considerable development of butyric acid bacteria. The acidity is determined to a large extent by the chemical nature of the crop and by the
control of the temperature, as well as by the nature of any materials
(e.g., molasses or mineral acids) which may be added during the manufacture of the silage.

The extent of the breakdown of protein material is rather variable;
in the first stages of fermentation there is some breakdown of protein
to amino-acids but any subsequent decomposition is checked by the
development of an acid reaction.

If the supply of oxygen is unlimited, the temperature moderate and
sufficient moisture present, moulds flourish, alkalinity develops instead
of acidity, and the crop becomes useless. Wasted material of this type
is invariably produced in situations where the exclusion of air is difficult,
as on the sides of stack silos.

(c) The practice of silage making.

The condition of the crop to be ensiled is most important and
particular attention must be paid to its moisture content and its bulkiness.
At the time of cutting a green crop will contain about 75 per cent. of
water, so that if carted and packed immediately it tends to settle closely
owing to the weight of water. There will be comparatively few air
spaces and consequently oxidation cannot proceed far and the temperature does not rise to a desirable height, remaining far below 80° F.
Undesirable bacteria flourish and putrefaction tends to develop. Better
results are therefore obtained by allowing the crop to wilt slightly in
the field before carting. The time allowed for this to occur must of
course be governed by the atmospheric conditions—in dry windy weather

two or three hours may suffice, whereas in wet weather there may be little alteration in the moisture content at the end of a day.

The amount of treading which is required depends on the bulkiness of the crop, long grass and mature crops generally requiring more treading than short young material which packs easily. Tight packing brought about by ensiling not too dry crops and pressing this well down by even and thorough treading, particularly in the centre, naturally compacts the mass with the exclusion of air. It is very important to see that the centre is well trodden and then kept higher than the sides so that the greater pressure at this point will force the material out and fill the spaces round the sides; otherwise settlement at the centre would draw the crop away from the sides and allow access of air. Good silage is made by avoiding extremes; thus too tight packing is undesirable, as is too loose packing, but the novice is more likely to err by leaving the material too loose, particularly at the top, though naturally it might be tight enough at the bottom. If the crop is stored as it is cut, i.e., in the long state, it will pack more loosely than if it is chopped. Chopping into lengths of 4 to 6 inches allows of easier distribution in some types of silo (e.g., tower silos) and also permits of tighter packing. In the case of a tower silo chopping is necessary in order to get the material blown up to the top of the tower and it is in any case necessary when thick-stemmed plants such as maize are dealt with.

Rate of packing also has very great influence on the access of air and on the extent of heating. With continuous and uninterrupted packing too great a weight is superimposed on the mass of material at the base; consequently air is excluded to an undesirable extent and in the lower layers of material the temperature does not rise to the optimum degree. Thus uneven heating takes place. Experience has shown it is the better practice to pack up to a depth of about 5 feet each day. The object is to allow the mass to heat sufficiently before additional weight is superimposed. The temperature aimed at is in the region of 100° F.

The rapidity with which lactic acid develops in newly made silage depends to some extent on the composition of the crop, and particularly on its content of readily fermentable carbohydrates. A highly nitrogenous crop, e.g., one containing a high proportion of legumes, will hold insufficient carbohydrate for the desirable multiplication of the right type of bacteria. This deficiency of carbohydrate can be made good by the addition of molasses, which is an excellent medium for the bacterial growth. The quantity usually recommended is from 20 to 30 lb. per ton of material to be ensiled. 20 lb. per ton is sufficient for grass or clover, while more—up to 30 lb. per ton—is necessary for crops such as lucerne containing a higher percentage of protein. The molasses is diluted with 3 to 5 times its volume of water, depending on the dryness of the crop, and is sprinkled on with a watering can or hand-spray pump, each succeeding 6 inch layer of material being evenly treated.

When the ensiled fodder has settled, more fresh material may be added until the silo is filled to capacity, and the final loads are usually filled in very rapidly as there is relatively little pressure at the top of the silo and overheating may readily occur. The top of a full silo, which should be dome shaped and well trodden, must be carefully sealed off to reduce wastage. It is covered with sacks or paper and then given an air-seal of 4 inches of soil. In order to give adequate pressure on the top layers of silage, weights must be added, or the layer of soil increased to at least 12 inches. Protection from rain may be provided by a rough thatch or by any other available means, unless the silo is provided with a permanent roof.

Special Silage Methods.

Although the use of molasses is really a special method of silage making, its value is so widely recognised and its use is so widespread that it has been described above as a normal procedure in ensilage. It is not, of course, necessary with crops of relatively low protein content and high carbohydrate value. The use of whey or sugar extracted from whey has also been employed in a similar manner with satisfactory results.

Although the manufacture of molassed silage has become widespread in this country, the first of the modern silage processes was evolved and patented by A. I. Virtanen and is popularly known as the A.I.V. method. In this process the acidity of the silage is controlled directly by the actual addition of acid to the crop as it is ensiled. The object is to bring the acidity of the crop to a pH of 3 - 4 and this is done by sprinkling each successive 4 - 6 inch layer of crop in the silo with a solution consisting essentially of hydrochloric acid, containing some sulphuric acid, made to twice normal strength. About 15 gallons of the solution are required per ton of fresh material, less in the case of a very succulent unwilted crop. In Britain it is not a popular method of making silage because, though efficient, great care has to be exercised to avoid burning accidents. The solution must be made in a wooden barrel and decanted into rubber lined watering cans. The men, who must be duly cautioned concerning the care necessary to be taken, must wear rubber thigh boots and rubber gloves and aprons. Virtanen recommends that the top layer of the ensiled crop be sprayed with an anti-mould preparation, the basis of which is oil of mustard. This is now considered to be unnecessary if the material at the top of the silo is well compacted and covered with paper or sacking and soil well beaten down.

The Defu process and the Penthesta process, which are examples of some other types of acid treatment, are modifications of Virtanen's original method. With the former a dilute solution of hydrochloric and phosphoric acids is added, with sometimes the addition of molasses. In the Penthesta process a solution of phosphorus pentachloride is used.

In the acid treatment of ensiled crops there is some danger of over-acidification, particularly towards the bottom, and in feeding this material it may be necessary to add chalk before giving it to the animals to eat if untoward results are to be avoided. Approximately 4 lb. of chalk per ton of silage is required.

(d) Losses incurred in silage making.

Besides those already indicated, e.g., those due to respiration and other oxidative activity, the following losses occur to a greater or less degree in silage.

Putrefactive changes, brought about by the activity of proteolytic and cellulose splitting bacteria, occur when acidity has been restricted and heating up has not been adequate, when the crop has been too succulent, or when tight packing has resulted from seepage or collection of rain. In good silage the loss of digestible crude protein may be about 10 per cent. or even less, but on the other hand in bad silage it may be as high as 40 per cent. Reduction of starch equivalent value may vary from 20 to 40 per cent. or more.

The most common gross loss, however, is occasioned by the action of moulds and that mostly takes place at the top and sides of the packed material, or any place where there is likely to be free access to air. In a stack silo, where it is practically impossible to avoid loss from this cause, it may be of the order of 45 per cent. It may also occur in a tower silo if the top has been inadequately covered or if the crop has sagged to the centre because of insufficient treading there allowing access of air to the sides. Moulding also commonly occurs at the top and sides of pit silos. In any type of silo, however, insufficient treading results in pockets of air being left throughout the crop and at these sites moulds will certainly develop. Favourable conditions for the growth of moulds are also provided while the silage is being cut out. Thus if a large face is exposed that will not be cut again for some days, moulds will have established themselves to a considerable depth before the next layer is removed and hence inevitable wastage will result. This can be avoided by cutting out the silage in such a manner that the least possible surface is exposed and by removing that surface at comparatively short intervals, that is every day or two (maximum five days).

Another common cause of loss is the drainage which occurs as a result of the pressure which falls on the material of a packed crop. The more succulent the crop, the greater will be the amount of moisture expressed and the greater the loss of nutrients. Not only is a considerable amount of soluble nitrogenous substance lost in this way, as well as soluble carbohydrates, but quite large quantities of phosphates, calcium and potash are also drained off. The drainage may be caused by rain or other water taken in with the crop, especially if wet material is put on the top of the silo so that it seeps through the whole stack.

Excessive losses may arise from a process of slow combustion if the ensiled crop is too dry, or filled too slowly or with insufficient treading. Overheating may even cause a total loss of the ensiled crop.

(e) Types of silo.

Silage may be made in stacks, in tower silos, in pits or trenches. or in clamps.

Difficulties in the packing and compression of the silage in stacks often lead to too vigorous fermentation. The rela⁺ively high temperatures that follow produce " sweet " dark brown silage, which has a pleasant, appetising smell and is readily consumed by stock, but which may have lost a considerable amount of its food value through overheating. In particular the digestibility of the protein may be very adversely affected.

Various types of tower have been used for silage preparation. Their main disadvantages have been found to be the cost of their construction and of the accessory equipment needed for loading them. Much better control of the course of the fermentation can be achieved by the use of towers than by stacking. The " warm method " which results in the kind of product described above can be followed, or by employing lower temperatures, acid, light-brown or yellow-brown silage, still pleasant smelling and palatable, can be obtained. Alternatively the crop may be chaffed, rapidly packed and trodden well down, so that cold fermentation ensues, a green fruity silage being obtained.

In Britain the production of silage in pits seems once again to be becoming more popular, on the score of cheapness and ease of management. Good management of the crop will lead to the production of any of the desired types of silage. The use of the clamp is a compromise between the stack and the pit; where there are difficulties with respect to the soil which prevent a deep pit being made, this method is useful.

(f) Crops for ensilage.

Almost any green crop can be made into ensilage but a food of high value cannot be withdrawn from a silo if inferior material or material of a low food value is used. Foods other than green crops can also be ensiled satisfactorily, e.g., potatoes if steamed and mashed can be preserved by this method, and surplus products, such as sugar beet tops, may be made into very valuable silage. The modern object in making ensilage is to provide a succulent food which has a fairly good percentage of protein and which is highly digestible to the animals for which it is pr⁚narily intended, i.e., dairy cows and bullocks. That other animals can utilise silage, though to a less extent, is a secondary consideration. While grass, if cut young enough, makes good silage and while fully grown grass, which would have been made into hay but for hopelessly adverse conditions, can also be ensiled, many crops are specially grown for silage so as to provide a high grade food as well as yield a big bulk per acre. Choice of crop is governed largely by the suitability of the land.

Owing to their high protein content *clover* crops *alone* do not make first class silage, and the same applies to *lucerne* and other highly nitrogenous legumes. This fault can be corrected by the addition of molasses so as to provide the carbohydrate necessary for bacterial activity of the right type.

Tares (vetches) when grown with a suitable supporting crop, such as oats, make excellent ensilage. A supporting crop is necessary owing to the nature of the plant, which will not stand by itself. Beans are also used as a supporting crop with or without the inclusion of oats in the seeding mixture.

Maize is grown extensively in warmer climates for making into ensilage and to a lesser extent in Britain. It can be grown satisfactorily here in certain localities if the right type of seed—a quick maturing variety—is used. If well grown and cut at the right time, maize provides a great bulk of very nutritious food that can easily be ensiled.

Kale is a crop which has been ensiled, but as it is harvested at a time of the year when green food is scarce most of it is fed directly. Nevertheless, for use in the early months of the year there is much to recommend the growing of a larger acreage of kale and putting the surplus into silage before frost damage begins. Kale will yield about two-thirds as much dry matter and crude protein as newly sown pasture, but requires only a single harvesting, whereas for maximum results pasture must be cut several times in the year. Other leafy crops, like cabbage, give yields similar to kale and will also make very useful ensilage, but because of the nature of such plants the process is carried out with difficulty.

So far as grassland herbage is concerned, the use of the warm fermentation process requires a rather mature crop, though not one which has been taken as far as the hay stage. Wilting of the crop until the moisture content has fallen below 75 per cent. is also advantageous. Young herbage will not heat readily.

If the low temperature process is to be employed, then the herbage may be cut rather earlier than for the above method and it should not be allowed to wilt. As the crop matures the packing of the silo should be speeded up and the material well compressed so that there shall not be too high a temperature rise.

The cold fermentation process requires tight packing and the presence of a fair amount of legume in the crop, which is taken at a fair stage of maturity so that, although the protein content will be reasonably high, there will be sufficient carbohydrate to achieve a rapid fermentation with the production of the requisite amount of lactic acid. Too young a crop is likely to produce sour silage under these conditions.

(g) Feeding silage to livestock.

While silage can be described as a succulent food it differs in many important respects from all the other succulents. It is similar to the roots and other succulent foods in that it contains from 60 to 80 per cent. of water, 70 per cent. probably being near the average. But compared with roots it contains about 3 times as much fibre, as well as more protein and ether extract; the carbohydrate fraction is about half that found in roots. A clearer picture of the chemical composition of silage can be obtained by comparing its dry matter content with that of other foods:

TABLE 38

		Swedes	Meadow Hay (Good)	Oat and Tare Silage	Grass and Clover Silage	Dried Grass
Crude Protein	...	11.3	11.3	14.3	17.8	17.9
Ether Extract	...	1.7	2.9	4.1	2.9	3.8
N-free extractives	...	70.5	47.9	40.1	45.9	38.8
Crude Fibre ...	...	10.4	30.7	31.9	21.9	31.6
Total Ash	... ...	6.1	7.2	9.6	11.5	7.9

Though silage crops are often grown very largely to replace roots clearly silage is not, strictly speaking, a replacement food, though it may be fed either wholly or partly instead of roots. /Neither is it a substitute for hay though it may be used to replace hay to a considerable extent in the ration. Silage, and by this one implies good quality silage, is a food that possesses all the advantages of succulence coupled with a fairly high percentage of protein and fibre. Furthermore its carotene content may be practically the same as that of artificially dried grass—20 to 50 mg./100 gm. of dry matter—fresh grass containing from 30 to 60 and meadow hay practically none, or at the best, 4 or 5 mg./100 gm. Owing to the nature of the food and to the fact that some experience is necessary in its production, the quality and nutritive value of silage are not constant, a fact which is illustrated by the data collected by Watson [2] and given in the table below; for comparison some of the data have been re-calculated on a dry matter basis.

TABLE 39

		As féd				Dry matter basis	
Crop	Dry matter	Crude protein	Starch equiv.	Dig. crude protein	Protein equiv.	Starch equiv.	Dig. crude protein
1 Clover	20	4.1	8.9	2.7	2.1	45	13.5
2 Grass, leafy ...	20	3.5	12.4	2.8	2.0	62	14.0
3 Grass, early flowering	25	3.2	14.5	2.1	1.4	58	8.4
4 Grass, full flower	25	2.9	11.4	1.2	0.9	46	4.8
5 Kale, marrowstem	16	2.0	9.8	1.5	1.3	61	9.4
6 Lucerne ...	17	3.7	7.0	2.5	2.0	41	14.7
7 Vetch and oat	25	3.4	10.8	1.9	1.4	43	7.6

Provided that the crops have been well ensiled, leafy grass and the leguminous foods, clover and lucerne, contain a sufficiently high proportion of protein to be used for productive purposes, while the rest of those given in the above list, save for grass in full flower which is suitable for maintenance alone, are of slightly less value.

The figures for digestible crude protein are of much greater value
than protein equivalent in assessing the value of silage, as in this type of
food much breakdown of protein occurs without causing any actual
loss of protein feeding value. Much of the protein in an ensiled crop is
broken down by the action of bacteria and enzymes into its component
amino-acids so that analysis shows a high proportion of free amino-
acids and a correspondingly low content of true protein. If the feeding
value of the crop is estimated on the usual basis of protein equivalent, a
wrong impression is obtained, because in this instance the amino-acids
are the direct derivatives of the proteins originally present in the food
and have merely been liberated in a very similar manner to that of
the process of digestion by the animal; if recombined, these amino-
acids would again form complete proteins, with a feeding value identical
with that of the protein precursor. Thus the non-protein nitrogenous
compounds of silage are totally different in feeding value from those of
other foods, and should be accorded a value equal to that of the true
proteins by assessing all the nitrogenous substances in terms of digestible
crude protein.

A very useful report on the average composition of different crop
silages in Britain was published in 1947.[18] Some three thousand samples
were examined from widely different areas, and the general conclusions
arrived at were, (a) silages made from any one crop varied widely in
composition, (b) the composition varied from year to year, (c) the fermentation quality of the silage, which could be judged fairly satisfactorily
on the smell and colour, influenced the composition of the silage; stage
of growth had a somewhat smaller effect, (d) there was no evidence
that any one type of silo was superior to another as regards the fermentation of the silage. Where an accurate estimation of the composition of
the silage is needed, chemical analysis is essential, although a guide to
the probable feeding value of the silage may be obtained from the
average values for dry matter and protein.

The report assessed fermentation quality on the basis of colour, smell
and acidity, as follows:

TABLE 40

Fermentation class	Colour	Smell	pH
Satisfactory	Greenish-brown, yellow-green or light brown.	Fruity or vinegary, moderate or mild.	4.0 - 5.0
Overheated	Dark or light brown.	Tobacco-like or caramel-like, strong.	4.0 - 5.0
Underheated	Light greenish brown, olive or dark green.	Butyric or, less often, vinegary, strong.	5.0 - 6.0

In the tables which they present, the Committee believe that the
probable errors in the estimation of the dry matter and protein value,
respectively, are 3.0 and 0.4 per cent. in the fresh silage, except for
" Other Crop Silages ", where the data provide only a rough guide.

TABLE 41

AVERAGE SILAGE COMPOSITION

[N.B. Protein value = $\frac{1}{2}$(crude protein in fresh + crude protein in dried silage)]

Crop	Fermentation quality	Stage of growth	Dry matter %	Protein value %	pH	Protein value in dry matter
POOR QUALITY PERMANENT GRASS	Satisfactory	Young leafy	22	3.3	4.5	15.0
		Mod. mature	22	3.1	4.6	14.2
		Ful. mature	24	2.9	4.6	12.0
	Overheated	Young leafy	25	3.2	4.8	13.0
		Mod. mature	31	3.8	4.6	12.4
		Ful. mature	31	3.8	4.7	12.4
	Underheated	All stages	19	3.0	5.2	15.6
GOOD QUALITY PERMANENT GRASS	Satisfactory	Young leafy	23	3.4	4.4	14.8
		Mod. mature	23	3.3	4.7	14.5
		Ful. mature	23	3.3	4.7	14.5
	Overheated	Young leafy	24	3.5	4.4	14.4
		Mod. mature	29	3.7	4.8	12.8
		Ful. mature	29	3.3	4.2	11.4
	Underheated	All stages	19	3.0	5.8	15.7
TEMPORARY SEEDS: GRASS AND CLOVER	Satisfactory	Young leafy	23	3.8	4.8	16.4
		Mod. mature	23	3.6	4.7	15.5
		Ful. mature	24	3.7	4.6	15.3
	Overheated	Young leafy	24	4.0	4.5	16.8
		Mod. mature	29	4.2	4.4	14.6
		Ful. mature	29	4.0	4.3	13.7
	Underheated	All stages	20	3.4	5.1	17.1
CEREAL-LEGUME MIXTURES	Satisfactory	Young leafy	20	2.8	4.6	14.2
		Mod. mature	22	2.8	4.4	12.9
		Ful. mature	26	2.9	4.5	11.3
	Overheated	Young leafy	24	3.2	4.3	13.5
		Mod. mature	29	3.4	4.2	11.8
		Ful. mature	29	3.4	4.4	11.6
	Underheated	All stages	19	2.9	5.2	15.0
OTHER CROP SILAGES	LUCERNE, 1st CUT		22	3.2	5.3	15.3
	LUCERNE, 2nd CUT		23	4.1	5.5	17.7
	LUCERNE, 3rd CUT		27	4.9	5.8	18.5
	KALE		16	2.3	4.3	14.9
	MAIZE		15	1.4	4.8	9.4
	SUGAR-BEET TOPS		23	2.8	4.8	12.2
	PEA HAULMS		24	3.4	4.8	14.1
	RYEGRASS AND RAPE		20	2.8	4.3	13.9
	OATS (BADLY LAID)		24	2.4	4.5	10.1

Cows.—Silage made from good grass or specially grown crops is an excellent food for dairy cows during the winter months, the animals being attracted by its succulence and soon acquiring a liking for its flavour. Experience has shown that it can be fed in amounts up to 70-80 lb./day, and, provided that the food is of good quality this level of intake does not adversely affect the flavour of the milk produced. From what has been said above, however, the food may vary and it is useless to expect to feed poor quality silage and get as good results from it as from first-class material. Quite apart from general hygienic grounds, it should be obvious in view of the nature of the fermentation processes that when silage is being fed the food troughs should always be kept clean, with no residues left to become sour and evil smelling.

The feeding of silage has a profound influence upon the quality and appearance of the milk, especially during the later part of the season, largely because of the carotene it provides. Silage has also been found to improve the general health of housed cattle during this trying period of the year.

Another benefit associated with the feeding of silage during the winter and early spring is that when cattle are turned out to grass in spring they do not suffer from the laxative effects of young grass which are often so troublesome with in-wintered beasts that have been kept on dry food.

Calves.—In the absence of fresh grass, silage forms a useful introduction to solid food and helps to develop the rumen.

Bullocks.—A decade or so ago silage was not a popular food for fattening bullocks owing to the prejudice of butchers who maintained that there was excessive shrinkage after slaughter. Nevertheless it can rightly be considered a valuable food for the winter fattening of cattle. It keeps up their appetite, maintains the bowel contents in a suitable physical condition and imparts to the animals the bloom that is associated with health. The quantity which it is advisable to feed daily naturally depends upon the composition of the rest of the diet, but half a hundredweight a day is probably the maximum for profitable use.

Sheep.—To an increasing extent silage is being fed to sheep, good reports of its value coming from many parts of the world. In New Zealand up to 5 lb. per head per day has been fed when grass has been scarce. Provided that this food is introduced gradually into the ration there is no doubt that it produces good growth and is suitable for fattening.

Pigs.—Owing to its high fibre content, the use of silage is practically restricted to full-grown stock, but small quantities may also be given to growing and fattening animals, because of its succulent nature. Only certain forms of silage—those with low fibre content—are suitable for these animals: potatoes, sugar beet tops, and really young grass may be used.

Horses.—In reviewing the use of conservation products for horses, Watson[2] describes silage as a safe food for horses if it is of good quality and is carefully fed: in this respect he emphasises the susceptibility of the horse to moulds. Subject to the gradual introduction of the food into the ration, oat-and-vetch or maize silage has been fed in different countries up to about 14·lb./day. From the point of view of its carotene content it might with advantage replace part of the hay in the conventional hay and oats ration.

(5) *The comparative nutritive values of dried grass, hay and silage*

In concluding this section some attempt must be made to compare the three methods of grass conservation as they are currently practised.

Knowledge concerning any one of them is still incomplete so that the research which the demand for animal food will evoke during the next decade may require some slight modification of present views. It seems unlikely, however, that any major change will be necessary.

From what has been said of the nature of the changes in the chemical composition of herbage as it matures, the conclusion seems unavoidable that hay is made from plant material, the nutritive value of which is relatively low, under conditions which lead to the destruction of most of its carotene and perhaps of other labile factors also. Hay is inevitably a roughage with a ratio of starch equivalent to protein equivalent which makes it suitable for maintenance purposes but not, by itself, for the production of protein rich material, whether that be milk or eggs or the new tissue of young growing stock. Dried grass and silage, on the other hand, can be—and certainly should be—made from herbage of a better type, richer in protein and containing, not only less fibre but fibre of a more digestible kind. In both types of food almost the full value of the original carotene content of the plants can be preserved. Against this must be put the necessity for more expensive technical equipment, although this objection cannot well be sustained when there is a world shortage of food; increased attention to the land, with the aim of greater productivity, will probably have to be paid for.

Using the food value of the original herbage as a standard, the evidence suggests that 5 per cent. of the starch equivalent is lost if the crop be dried artificially, about 40 per cent. when it is made into hay, 35 per cent. if ordinary silage is produced, but only 20 per cent. if molasses or acid is employed in the silage process. The corresponding losses of digestible crude protein are approximately 8, 30, 40 and 10 per cent.[7] Dried grass and silage will each lead to about twice as much starch equivalent and 2 - 3 times as much protein equivalent per acre as hay and the aftermath on the recent estimates of Featherstone,[10] provided that the crops are properly handled.

On this basis should one argue against the production of hay? At the moment the answer should probably be in the negative. From the most logical point of view it seems that, so far as the general management of livestock will permit, the value of herbage *in situ* should be utilised to the full. Because, however, of the need for winter feed and of the seasonal failures of livestock to keep pace with the productivity of the land, the production of dried grass from herbage at a suitable stage of growth comes next. Then, if for some reason the drying plant is unable to dry all of the grass which is being produced, it should be used for the best quality material, while the slightly more mature and more fibrous fraction should be made into good silage. And finally, any surplus grass should be converted into hay, and, as far as possible, this should be done before the crop has become too mature. In this way, as described by Lewis and Eden,[16] the three methods of conservation are made to dovetail with one another so that, from a given area of land, the maximum yield of nutrients is obtained. The problem is thus partly one of efficient management.

The solution suggested above probably has one other advantage, in that it offers some chance of varying the palatability of rations. No matter how high the starch equivalent or the protein content of a given foodstuff, if it is not palatable for livestock, much of its virtue may disappear. In the production of suitable strains of herbage plants, palatability has so far had little consideration but its importance is now being stressed. Stapledon[20] has described the habit of sheep which, during the daytime and especially on fine dry days, would graze seeded grassland, but chose to make their first meal of the day on rough, natural grazing. There are many plants, now regarded as weeds, which may well prove to have some part, perhaps only a minor one from the quantitative aspect, in the balanced feeding of livestock. Stapledon, indeed, has advocated the sowing of " herb-strips " in association with modern leys, from which "weeds" are almost excluded.

REFERENCES

1. Moon, F., (1939). Empire J. Exp. Agric., 7, 27.
2. Watson, S. J., (1939). "The science and practice of conservation: grass and forage crops."
3. Brüne, F., K. Richter, K. E. Ferber and H. Brüggemann, (1932 and 1935), quoted by Watson, 2 above.
4. Kellner, O., (1926). "The scientific feeding of animals."
5. Knox, M., and I. Prowse, (1934). J. S-E. Agric. Coll., Wye, 34, 227.
6. Watson, S. J., and W. S. Ferguson, (1937). Agriculture, J. Min. Agric. Engl., 44, 247.
7. Stapledon, G. R., (1948). "Ley farming."
8. Stapledon, G. R., (1949). Agriculture, J. Min. Agric. Engl., 55, 415.
9. Linton, R. G., (1931). Proc. Nat. Vet. Med. Assoc.
10. Woodman, H. E., and R. Evans, (1930). J. Agric. Sci., 20, 587.
11. Watson, S. J., (1948). Nutrition Abs. Rev., 18, 1.
12. Woodman, H. E., and R. Evans, (1948). J. Agric. Sci., 38, 51.
13. Crasemann, E., and O. Heinzl, (1943). Ber. schweiz. Bot. Ges., 53A, 449.
14. Morris, S., N. C. Wright and A. B. Fowler, (1936). J. Dairy Res., 7, 105.
15. Ferguson, W. S., (1949). Agriculture, J. Min. Agric. Engl., 55, 517.
16. Lewis, W., and A. Eden, (1949). Agriculture, J. Min. Agric. Engl., 56, 12.
17. Halnan, E. T., and F. H. Garner, (1946). "Principles and practice of feeding farm animals."
18. Agriculture, J. Min. Agric. Engl., 54, 305.
19. Featherstone, J., (1947). Agriculture, J. Min. Agric. Engl., 54, 68.
20. Stapledon, G. R., (1947). Agriculture, J. Min. Agric. Engl., 53, 428.

THE STRAWS

1. Introduction
2. Straws.
3. Chaff and cavings.

(1) Introduction

After the seeds, such as oats, wheat, barley, rye, beans, peas, etc., have been removed from the ripened and harvested plant by threshing, three products remain:—*straw, chaff* and *cavings*. As the crop is not harvested until the grain is ripe (or nearly ripe as in the case of oats) it follows that the straw—that is the stems, leaves and other parts concerned with the nourishment of the seed—will be less nutritious than if the crop were to be cut during the actual growing period of the plant. Thus it is that, in general, the nutritive value of straws is very small.

The *straw* consists of the stems and leaves of the plant; the *chaff* of the glumes; the pales, if these fall away from the grain (as in wheat) together with fragments of stems and leaves constitute the *cavings*.

(2) Straws

Straws consist very largely of relatively indigestible lignified fibre, a variable amount of soluble carbohydrate, very little protein or fat, and a considerable amount of ash or mineral matter, although this is chiefly composed of silica, phosphates and calcium being deficient. The chemical composition of the straws is very variable, depending upon the nature of the ground on which the crop is grown, the nature and extent of the manuring, the stage at which it is cut, the manner in which it is harvested and the period for which it has been stored. The variation is perhaps most marked in the protein, nitrogen-free extractive, and crude fibre contents. The chemical composition of straw, and thus its nutritive value, depends upon the extent to which the nutritive constituents have passed from the plant to its seed. Variation caused by season or weather has less effect upon the protein of straws than upon grass with its greater concentration of organic constituents, but it remains a fact that straw from spring sown cereals contains less crude fibre than straw from autumn sown grain, and that its starch equivalent is appreciably higher. The quicker the plant has grown, the richer as a food is its straw. Probably the different feeding values of straw, which have long been recognised by the cattle feeder to exist according to the district in which the straw was grown, may to some extent be due to the variation in protein content, so that where it is contained at the higher level it is possible to fatten cattle on a diet of oat straw and swedes, while in other districts these foods must be supplemented with concentrates.

The nutritive value of the straws is limited by the amount of fibre in them, their bulk being too great to allow the quantity which would meet the requirements of the animal to be eaten in a given time. Generally speaking the fibre is of such a nature that only ruminants can deal with it effectively. Even cattle, however, are unable to digest it completely—in fact in the case of oat straw, which of all the straws is the most digestible, just one-third of the energy it contains can be liberated by a bullock, and almost two-thirds of this amount is utilised by the animal in the process of digestion, etc. The digestibility is of course closely connected with the degree and manner of lignification. In old matured plants where lignification is widespread, cellulose-splitting bacteria do not easily gain contact with the material upon which they can work because of the encrusting coat, and thus digestion is rendered difficult. It has been shown that lignification is encouraged by a deficiency of potassium in the soil.

The more nutritious part of straw is the upper part, despite the fact that it tends to contain more silica and less soluble inorganic matter than the lower. Cattle seem to find it more palatable; animals given whole uncut straw to " pick over " invariably eat the upper portions. Straw is given to stock, such as cattle and horses, mainly for the purpose of supplying bulk to the diet; nevertheless good oat straw, in particular, supplies a moderate amount of nutriment, and as has been stated, excellent results are obtained in some districts with feeding cattle on a diet composed mainly of straw and roots and suitably supplemented. But for animals in a forward condition of fattening, heavy milking cows and working horses, particularly if working at a fast pace, the use of straw of any kind should be restricted and the roughage part of the ration supplied by more digestible food, such as hay, yielding a greater amount of net energy. Good oat straw is better than inferior hay, however.

Straw and particularly barley straw deteriorates if it is not carefully stored. After a year in the stack, the effect of weathering and the action of moulds, forage acari and other organisms are generally apparent. Such straw usually has a musty, stale smell, is more brittle and is less palatable as a food for stock than fresh, clean material.

The practice of forcing animals to consume large quantities of straw, particularly wheat straw, by chaffing it and mixing it with more palatable foods is one that requires careful consideration on the part of the feeder. If he does not require his animals to fatten rapidly or, in the case of horses, to do much work, then a fairly liberal use may be made of straw as in the case, for example, of carrying over store cattle on little more than a maintenance ration during the winter months to the spring. In this connection straw should be used with discretion. One meets cases of dairy cattle being given rations consisting largely of straw and dried sugar beet pulp, eked out with a very small amount of inferior pasturage. Such a ration is deficient in so many factors that it is inadequate by any standards and most of all where the food is—presumably—being given for productive purposes. The custom, which still lingers, of feeding bulls on rations of straw and roots, with little or no green fodder, is also to be deprecated; there is little wonder that the animals do not maintain the level of fertility which their owners desire. Straws may also be made more nutritious by predigestion by the method, described under " Food Storage and Preparation ".

Oat Straw.—Of the cereal straws, oat straw is the most valuable for feeding purposes, the chief reason for this being that oats are cut before they are fully ripe—before the growing plant has ceased its function of carrying soluble food material to the seed. Oat straw is also the most palatable of all the straws, being sweeter and containing less fibre. It is the only straw that should be used for horses, and then only in moderation.

Wheat Straw.—The utilisation of wheat straw should be restricted to bedding, and it should never be fed to horses because it actually causes the expenditure of more energy in its digestion than it supplies. Wheat straw may be fed to cattle in order to supply bulk; it should not be chopped, but fed in bunches, so that the cattle can be left to pick out the more nutritious parts.

Barley Straw.—The composition of barley straw is very similar to that of oat straw, but because of its use as a nurse crop it sometimes contains a fair proportion of clover leaves which enhance its feeding value. It is extensively used for feeding to cattle in some districts.

Rye Straw is very harsh and, like wheat straw, carries a lot of lignin. It is not suitable for feeding to stock.

The Legume Straws.—The straws or haulms from beans, peas and vetches have a better chemical composition than the cereal straws and are richer in protein. The actual stems are less digestible than oat straw but the upper parts, holding the pods and leaves, yield a considerable amount of nutriment. Legume straws are often more difficult to harvest and store in a dry condition than the straws from cereals and for this reason are sometimes liable to be mouldy. They generally have a constipating effect. Unlike the cereal straws those from legumes are rich in calcium and magnesium. Legume straws make an excellent substitute for hay for store or resting animals.

The straws of *buckwheat* and *rape* are of low feeding value and are used only in emergencies. The same applies to *rice* and *linseed straw*. If any of these are fed indiscriminately they will cause serious digestive trouble. On the other hand, *sorghum* and *millet straw* form a very large part of the diet of cattle raised in countries where these crops are grown.

(3) Chaff and Cavings

Cereal Chaff has a nutritive value very similar to that of cereal straw, but it usually contains a lot of silica. Oat chaff is the most nutritious, and is probably of higher value than the oat straw itself. Chaff containing many barley awns does not make a good food because the awns are liable to penetrate the mucous membrane of the mouth and thus allow access to the organisms of actinomycosis. Chaff if given in large quantity has a binding effect on the food in the alimentary tract, causing impaction in the stomachs of ruminants. The most satisfactory way in which to feed it is to mix it with pulped roots.

Linseed Chaff differs from the cereal chaffs in that it consists of the dried fractured leaves and the broken brittle pods with some of the unseparated seeds. Thus both its protein and oil content are relatively high—as much as 3.5 per cent. of protein and 5 per cent. of oil may be present. As one would expect, it contains a large amount of indigestible fibre and therefore is only suitable for adult ruminants.

Cavings.—The nutritive value of cavings is often higher than that of the straw, but cavings are sometimes dirty and their use for feeding requires discretion. Like chaff they give the best results when mixed with pulped roots. On the majority of farms cavings are not used for feeding but are used in the bullock yards as a bedding material.

SUCCULENT FOODS

1. **Roots and tubers.**
    (a) Turnips and swedes.
    (b) Mangolds.
    (c) Carrots.
    (d) Parsnips.
    (e) Beet.
    (f) Potatoes.
    (g) Jerusalem artichoke.

2. **Green foods.**
    (a) Cabbages.
    (b) Kohl rabi.
    (c) Kale.

(1) Roots and tubers

The roots and tubers, which belong to the class of succulent foods, may conveniently be divided into three subgroups (a) turnips, swedes and mangolds, (b) carrots and parsnips, and (c) potatoes, beet and artichokes. The chief difference between the three groups is in soluble carbohydrate content, the respective averages for the three groups being 8, 10 and about 18 per cent. respectively, with turnips lowest of all the individual foodstuffs. In all cases the ash content is about 1 per cent. of the fresh weight of the food, while the crude fibre percentages vary from 0.7 to 1.4 and those of crude protein from 1 to 2; in the case of fibre and protein the variations are as much within the groups as between them. All of the foodstuffs are poor in fatty matter (0.1-0.3 per cent.).

The roots and tubers are thus essentially suppliers of soluble carbohydrate, and, provided that the comparison is not carried too far, they may be likened to " watered down " cereal grains. The members of group (c) have about one quarter of the nutritive (energy) value of cereal grains, and, on the same weight for weight basis, between two and three times as much as that of turnips, swedes and mangolds. Replacements of one class of foods by another should be made with these differences in mind.

The fibre of roots and tubers is practically limited to the outer skin, and, though the protein contains a rather large proportion of amides, there seems to be no doubt, when the fully matured roots are used for feeding under suitable conditions, that it can be well utilised. Where proper feeding systems are in operation, the biological value of the protein of potatoes, for example, seems to be equal to that of the cereals even for pig feeding.

Carrots are outstanding among the roots and tubers because of their high and valuable carotene content.

All of these foodstuffs have a definite laxative action, which, during the period of winter house-feeding, helps to balance the effects of dietary hay, straw and other dry fodders.

The leaves are rather fibrous, contain but little nutriment, and shrivel up and fall off if the plants are left in the ground long enough; they are rarely fed to stock, being cut off with the crown and root and ploughed into the soil, but in the case of sugar beet the crown with the leaves is of distinct nutritive value.

Mangolds, swedes and turnips are valuable food for all stock, including poultry, but the crop is expensive to handle and feed after it is ripe. Roots are sometimes given to fattening cattle, up to a hundredweight or more a day, while 70 to 80 lb. a day is a common ration for both fattening cattle and dairy cows. Feeding with heavy quantities of roots is not, however, a practice to be encouraged, and while 80 lb. or so may be given to fattening cattle, the quantity for dairy cows should be limited to 30 to 40 lb. per day.

Under certain conditions of farming, cattle are sometimes fattened on little more than roots and straw, but it is doubtful whether this method of feeding makes the best use of such foods.

Horses are fond of roots, especially carrots, and if the quantity is limited to about 10 lb. a day, they are undoubtedly useful when the remainder of the diet consists of dry foods. Roots are beneficial to colts and may be given pulped and mixed with chopped hay and straw and crushed grain, but they should not be given in excessive quantities.

For pigs, particularly if sty-fed, roots form a valuable addition to the diet. They should always be given raw and not boiled as is sometimes the case, and should be pulped or sliced and mixed with the dry meals. Roughly about 5 lb. a day is as much as is good for a fattening pig, although the quantity, of course, varies with the size and age of the animal. During the last stages of fattening the allowance should be greatly reduced and merely given as a laxative. For breeding animals, except near the time of farrowing, roots may be given more liberally.

Roots are used both for fattening and milk production in sheep husbandry. The amount eaten daily is about 15 per cent. of their live weight, or the requirements can be put at 1 cwt. per head per week for gimmers or wethers, and rather more for in-lamb ewes in the early stages of pregnancy. The crop can best be eaten standing and thus the expense of handling is avoided and wastage eliminated; folding the sheep on the roots in this manner is also very beneficial to the land. If the roots are not eaten off the land they are best pulped and fed with concentrates.

For poultry, which are confined and not allowed free range on grass, roots of any kind, particularly if given raw, are a valuable addition to the ration, though they cannot in general replace grass as a source of fat and fat-soluble vitamins.

(a) Turnips and swedes.

There are two species of the genus *Brassica*:—(1) *Brassica campestris*, of which the variety *rapa* includes the common turnip and the rough-leaved summer rape; and (2) *Brassica campestris* var. *rutabaga*, including the swede (American " rutabaga ") and the smooth-leaved summer rape.

Many varieties of swedes and turnips are cultivated, the swedes usually being the earlier sown crop. When these foods are stored there follows an increase in their sugar content, and a fall in the percentage of nitrates, particularly in the case of swedes, which, in consequence, have greatest value in the late winter and spring, the freshly pulled crop having a tendency to produce scouring. Swedes have a greater content of soluble carbohydrate than turnips, are harder, and keep better. Turnips are consumed before swedes and they may be eaten off the ground by sheep, lifted and stored, or left in the ground and lifted as required.

If turnips and swedes are fed only after milking is completed, and in limited quantities, they do not taint milk.

(b) Mangolds (*Beta vulgaris*).

For reasons similar to those described above in the case of swedes but rather more urgent, mangolds should be stored for two or three months after harvesting, e.g. until Christmas, so that they may become mature.

Mangolds are less liable to taint milk than turnips and swedes. They are often given to ewes and lambs in the spring, and the belief that mangolds cause the deposition of urinary calculi in male sheep is unsubstantiated.

(c) Carrots (*Daucus carota*).

Like the foregoing roots, the carrot is a biennial plant and stores its food reserve in a long tap root. Apart from the other nutrients which give carrots superior feeding value to turnips, swedes and mangolds, their carotene makes them valuable winter feed, both for directly contributing to the well-being of the livestock consuming them and for improving the quality and colour of the milk or eggs they may produce. To cattle 40-50 lb./day may be given and pigs can utilise 3-4 lb./day. Their feeding value relative to other roots has already been stressed (p. 191).

Raw carrots are more valuable than raw potatoes, and they have always been a favourite succulent food for horses, and especially for sick and debilitated animals. It is frequently the case that a sick horse will eat a few carrots from the attendant when he will eat nothing else; it is desirable to wash the carrots well and to slice them lengthways. 10 lb. a day is a suitable allowance, and they should be given raw, and not cut up into very small pieces for horses because they are then liable to cause choking.

Carrots are also dried and ground to a coarse meal for incorporation in some commercial supplementary foods, in particular for valuable stock being prepared for show.

(d) Parsnips (*Pastinaca sativa*).

Parsnips are not used to such an extent as carrots for feeding to stock, as they are less palatable, although their nutritive value is somewhat higher. They are sometimes fed to fattening cattle and to dairy cows, and occasionally to horses, but are little used in this country for any stock, chiefly owing to the expense of cultivation.

(e) Beet (*Beta vulgaris*).

The sugar beet is a cultivated variety of *Beta vulgaris* which reaches its best in well worked soil deeply cultivated and yields from 15 to 20 per cent. of sugar. While most of the cultivated beet is sent to the factories for sugar extraction, it is sometimes fed to stock, particularly to cows and pigs. The hard nature of the root makes it imperative that it should be pulped or grated, particularly for pigs, to which it can be fed up to 20 per cent. of the ration without adversely affecting the carcase quality. Approximately 4 lb. of topped beet are equal to 8 lb. of mangolds. Excessive quantities are liable to cause scouring.

Sugar Beet Tops.—When sugar beet is harvested the leaves together with the crown are topped off. Though the crown contains less sugar than the main root, it still holds an appreciable amount, which Woodman puts at one-tenth to one-fifth of the total dry matter of crown and leaves, according to the proportion of leaves. The leaves contain 2-3 per cent. of protein and 1-2 per cent. of fibre, both of which are readily digested by sheep. Caution is necessary in their use owing to the fact that the leaves of beet as well as of mangolds contain oxalic acid; with ruminants there is less danger than with pigs and horses, though dairy cattle have been poisoned by them. The risk of oxalic acid poisoning can be greatly reduced, if not entirely eliminated, by the addition of chalk in the proportion of $\frac{1}{4}$ lb. chalk to 250 lb. of leaves.

Freshly cut beet tops contain about 15 per cent. of dry matter, of which 15-20 per cent. consists of protein. They may be fed to fattening cattle, dairy cows, horses, sheep, and older pigs, but hungry animals should not be allowed to gorge themselves with them.

The tops may be eaten by folding stock on the fields, the tops being arranged in rows, or they may be carted to grass fields or to housed cattle. An excess of beet tops over that which can be eaten fresh may be ensiled, or artificially dried; dried beet tops have been used successfully, in amounts up to 13 lb./day, for the feeding of dairy cows and of horses. With rational feeding systems these foodstuffs need not give rise to tainted milk.

Sugar beet pulp.—In the extraction of sugar beet, the washed roots are cut up into long thin slices to facilitate the diffusion of the sugar during the process. The sugar-free residues are available, under the name of sugar beet pulp, for livestock feeding.

The wet material, which contains 1-2 per cent. of protein, 10 per cent. of soluble carbohydrate, 3 per cent. of fibre, and 85 per cent. of water, is a useful foodstuff, roughly comparable, on a dry matter basis, with turnips, though of distinctly higher fibre content. It's high water content, both from the point of view of transport and storage, limits its free adoption for animal feeding, however. Dairy cows may be given 30 lb./day and bullocks twice that quantity.

Most of the beet pulp is dried and is sold as dried sugar beet pulp, and, of this material, a big proportion of it has had molasses (p. 230) incorporated in it. The product contains some 10 per cent. of water, an equal amount of protein of not very high biological value, 60 per cent. of soluble carbohydrate and 18-15 per cent. of fibre, depending upon whether molasses has been added or not.

Dried sugar beet pulp is not only inadequate in protein value but it contains too much fibre for it to be used alone as a substitute for cereal concentrates. Since the food readily absorbs water, and swells greatly in so doing, it should be invariably soaked in two or three times its weight of water for some time before it is fed to livestock, especially horses.

One pound of dried sugar beet pulp may be used to replace 7 lb. of mangolds for cows, to which up to 8 lb. of pulp may be given daily; an excess of this food in the ration of dairy cows tends to yield butter which is hard, white and of poor flavour. Fattening bullocks may receive some 12 lb./day.

Although the fibre and soluble carbohydrates of sugar beet pulp are quite well digested by pigs, this is not the case for the protein, three-quarters of which is excreted. Consequently this food should be given to pigs in no greater amounts than about 10 per cent. of their ration.

Horses may be given dried sugar beet pulp as a substitute for about a quarter of their grain ration, and the material can also be employed for fattening sheep and lambs, provided that it constitutes part of a balanced ration.

(f) Potatoes (*Solanum tuberosum*).

Of the "roots" the potato and the sugar beet contain least water, the potato being essentially a carbonaceous food.

The potato is composed of the following parts: —(1) An outer rind, or skin, forming about 2 per cent. of the whole tuber; (2) under the skin a fibro-vascular layer comprising approximately 8.5 per cent. of the tuber; and (3) the flesh which makes up the remaining 89 per cent.

The skin or rind is of little nutritive value but when it is removed in the ordinary way by peeling, the greater part of the subjacent or fibro-vascular layer is taken with it. This fibro-vascular layer contains proportionately more mineral matter and protein than the body of the potato.

Most of the protein of potatoes is of the "amide" type, but it has a biological value almost as high as those of the cereal foods. The 21 per cent. of soluble carbohydrate in potatoes is present mainly as large characteristic starch granules, which are well digested when the raw food is given to herbivorous animals, but are more efficiently utilised by omnivorous and carnivorous animals after the tubers have been cooked.

When potatoes are plentiful they are often fed to dairy cows and fattening cattle; the former may receive up to 2 stones a day, while in potato growing districts large numbers of cattle are fattened on chats and brock in quantities up to 100 lb. daily. The secret of success lies in increasing the quantities of the tubers *gradually* in the diet.

When cooked potatoes are given to pigs in quantity the increase in liveweight is generally satisfactory, but the dressing percentage of the carcase is lower than when the animals are fattened on a diet of cereal meals.

Dried Potatoes.—Surplus stocks of potatoes, " chats " and " brock," may be dried after they have been washed and then sliced into cosettes: These are highly digestible by ruminants and have been used with great success for the fattening of cattle and sheep. It has been found, however, by Woodman and Evans [1] that when potatoes are fed to pigs either as cosettes or as potato meal, in anything but small quantities, digestive disturbance is caused with prejudicial effect to liveweight gain. Potato flakes and potato slices, on the other hand, can be used liberally for pig feeding in the replacement of cereals. In the production of both these products the tubers are subjected to preliminary steaming or to exposure to a high temperature which raises the digestibility of the soluble carbohydrate from about 85 per cent. to almost 100 per cent. for pigs, and causes a corresponding increase in protein digestibility from some 50 per cent. to 80 per cent. The slices can be produced on the plant normally used for drying sugar beet in the factories, and can be turned out much quicker than either cosettes or flakes.

The relative food value of potatoes compared with cereal meals, such as barley meal, for pigs is approximately 4 lb. of cooked potatoes to 1 lb. of meal.

Potato Silage.—Satisfactory silage, of particular use in pig feeding, can be made from potatoes, such as bruised and damaged tubers which, converted into silage while still fresh, will keep indefinitely and will be available when other succulent foods are scarce. One method recommended is to wash the tubers thoroughly, steam them for 30 to 45 minutes, mashing to pulp while still hot, and then to pack them tightly in a suitable pit. After packing, the pulp is covered with sacking on the top of which is placed 9 inches of clay to exclude air entirely. About 20 per cent. of the weight is lost but total dry matter is increased to 31 per cent.

Moist steamed potatoes form a good medium for some mould and bacterial growth; it is therefore important not to expose more silage than is necessary when cutting out for use.

Another method of conserving potatoes is to incorporate the raw potatoes in alternate layers with three times their weight of ordinary ensiling fodder. During the process of heating in the stack the potatoes are partially cooked. If a high temperature is not reached in the pit, the potatoes are not cooked and a low-grade product results instead of a palatable, highly nutritious food.

Raw potatoes should be given more sparingly to horses than to cattle, a normal limit being about 6 lb./day, though this limit may probably be exceeded provided that due attention is paid to the condition of the animals and the increase is made gradually.

To sheep not more than 6 lb. per day of washed, sliced potatoes should be fed.

The most important point to remember in feeding potatoes raw, even when they are sound tubers, is to begin with a very small quantity, gradually increase, and to avoid stopping the supply too suddenly. This rule applies, of course, to all changes of food, but is of especial importance in this particular case.

(g) Jerusalem Artichokes (*Helianthus tuberosus*).

The tubers of the Jerusalem artichoke contain 17 per cent. of soluble carbohydrate, principally in the form of inulin, and 1.5 per cent. of protein. They are sometimes fed to pigs and, less commonly, to cattle and horses. The leafy stem is occasionally cut just before the leaves begin to shrivel and fed as green forage to cattle. As a rule artichokes are grown in this country for human consumption and it is generally only those that are surplus to requirements which are used for stock feeding. It would seem, however, to be a profitable undertaking to plant artichokes in waste land and to turn pigs in to root the tubers. Artichokes do not contain sufficient protein for the complete nourishment of either store or fattening pigs, and some nitrogenous concentrate must be given in addition.

(2) Green foods

Since the nutritive values of grass and other similar crops are discussed elsewhere (p. 141), the chief foods for consideration here are cabbage and kale. Like many green fodders, they are valuable foods, for, though their dry matter content is only about 14 per cent., it includes more than 2 per cent. of protein, over 0.5 per cent. of ether extract, 7-8 per cent. of soluble carbohydrate, 2-3 per cent. of fibre and about 2 per cent. of ash. These foods are therefore better balanced with respect to the ratio of protein to carbohydrate than the roots are. Moreover, they are usually rich in carotene (which is chiefly in the outer, deep-green leaves) and probably contain other valuable fat-soluble factors, but not vitamin D. In proportion to their dry-matter content these foods contain useful amounts of members of the vitamin B group; they are also rich in vitamin C. The ash includes an appreciable amount of calcium (0.4 per cent. for kale), quite well balanced with respect to phosphorus, and of the trace elements. Lastly the foods are very palatable, are laxative, and become available from the autumn onwards at a time when grass is beginning to fail. In succession they can be used to provide valuable food during the otherwise difficult period before the spring growth of pasture commences. As some of these foods contain goitrogenic substances, i.e., compounds which favour the incidence of goitre, they should not be fed in excessively large amounts for prolonged periods but should, like any other food, be used with discretion and good management.

(a) Cabbages (*Brassica oleracea*).

Cabbages are fed to all classes of cattle, dairy cows, pigs and poultry. They should be cut as soon as mature, but may be consumed before then, as they do not keep well after they have fully ripened, although they have been ensiled with success when special precautions have been taken. A usual allowance for dairy cows is from 40 to 60 lb. per day, and, to prevent the tainting of milk, cabbages should not be stored near a cow-shed or milking parlour, and all uneaten leaves must be removed from the mangers and standings. When cabbages are cut so as to leave a few basal leaves, a secondary growth will take place which will provide nutritious food for sheep.

(b) Kohl Rabi (*Brassica oleracea* var. *caulorapa*).

This succulent, very palatable, thick-stemmed plant, has a feeding value, as a root, which is akin to that of swedes, since it contains 9 per cent. of soluble carbohydrate, and about 1 per cent. each of fibre and ash; it contains more protein, however (2 per cent.).

As it has rather a tough and fibrous skin, it should be sliced before it is fed to stock. It does not taint the milk when it is given to dairy cows.

The leaves of this plant have a nutritive value similar to those of kale.

(c) Kale (*Brassica oleracea* var. *acephala*).

Marrow-Stem Kale, a cross between thousand-headed kale and kohl rabi, is cultivated either thinned out or left unsingled, and yields a heavy crop of nutritious succulent food. To milch cows, 100 lb, or even more may be given daily; for them and for fattening cattle it can be cut and fed in sheds or strewn on the fields. Sheep may be folded on the crop, which is not readily soiled by treading, owing to the nature of its growth. In-lamb and milking ewes do very well on it; but while sheep grow well, they do not seem to fatten satisfactorily when folded on it. When the thick stem has become fibrous animals, including cattle, will eat it more readily if it is chopped.

Thousand-Headed Kale.—This crop withstands the cold winter weather better than marrow-stem kale and when sown late provides valuable green food for cattle and sheep in the early spring. It is useful after lambing, when ewes and lambs may be folded on it.

REFERENCE

1. Woodman, H. E., and R. E. Evans, (1942). Agriculture, J. Min. Agric., England, *49*, 165.

OIL-SEED CAKES AND MEALS

1. Introduction.
2. Types of oilcake and meal.
    (a) Methods of preparation.
    (b) Decorticated and undecorticated cakes.
3. The nutritive value of oil-seed cakes and meals.
    (a) Oil-seed proteins.
    (b) Oil.
    (c) Fibre.
    (d) Storage and toxic effects.
    (e) Amounts to feed to livestock.
4. The individual foodstuffs.
    (a) Coconut.
    (b) Cottonseed.
    (c) Groundnut.
    (d) Kapok seed.
    (e) Linseed.
    (f) Maize germ cake.
    (g) Palm kernel.
    (h) Rape seed.
    (i) Safflower seed.
    (j) Sesame seed.
    (k) Soya bean.
    (l) Sunflower seed.
5. Compound cakes and meals.

(1) Introduction

Oil-seed cakes and meals are the residues left after the oil has been removed from certain seeds and fruits. They play a very important part in the feeding of farm livestock.

(2) Types of oilcake and meal

Oilcakes can be classified in at least two ways, firstly depending upon the method which has been used for the removal of the oil, and secondly as " decorticated " or " undecorticated ".

(a) Methods of preparation.

Two methods of preparation of oilcakes and meals ·involve the expulsion of the oil from the raw material by mechanical pressure while, in the third method, it is extracted by organic solvents.

In the first method the familiar, flat, rectangular slabs of oilcake are produced by squeezing cloth-wrapped layers of the oil-seeds, previously heated by steam, in large presses. Most of the oil runs out and sheets of "press cake", which may later be broken into pieces of convenient size or ground into a meal, remain.

In the expeller method the material is forced through an annular space of gradually diminishing cross-sectional area, so that the steadily increasing pressure and friction expel the oil from the seed, the residue of which is usually cast out of the expeller in the form of small, polished pieces of "expeller cake" showing the curvature of the rotating shaft of the machine. Production by this method is increasing at the expense of the simple press technique.

The last method is that in which the oil in the crushed raw material is washed out of it by the use of a suitable organic solvent, such as low-boiling petroleum. After the extraction of the fat and the draining of the greater part of the solvent, the final traces of the latter are removed by treatment with steam, the meal being simultaneously cooked to some extent.

Which process is used affects the nutritive value of the product in two ways. Firstly, the pressure methods leave 6-8 per cent. of residual oil, while the solvent process removes all but 1-3 per cent., yielding a food of lower energy value; secondly, the three different methods are capable of heating the oil-seeds to different extents and hence of altering the nutritive value of the protein. Mild heat treatment benefits soya bean (p. 41), while the low temperature of the solvent process appears to give an improved coconut meal as compared with the other methods. Even a 5 per cent. increase in nutritive value, due to improved milling techniques, would constitute a distinct improvement, but studies of this kind are still lacking.

(b) Decorticated and undecorticated cakes.

In the case of cottonseed, groundnut, safflower and sunflower cakes, two different products are available, the "undecorticated", which is made from the entire seed, and the "decorticated", prepared from seeds whose coats or husks have been removed prior to the milling process.

When comparisons are drawn between products made by the same extraction process, the undecorticated cakes usually contain less protein and more soluble carbohydrate, in addition to more fibre, than the corresponding decorticated cake or meal, as table 42 shows.

Such differences greatly influence the nutritive values of the two kinds of cake and their practical application to the feeding of livestock. Undecorticated cakes, for example, are not suitable for young stock, nor for pigs.

TABLE 42

Oil-seed	Water	Chemical composition %				
		Protein	Ether extract	Soluble carbohydrate	Fibre	Ash
Cotton, undec.	12	23	5	33	21	6
Cotton, semi-dec.	11	35	11	26	11	6
Cotton, dec.	10	41	8	27	8	6
Groundnut, undec.	10	30	9	22	23	6
Groundnut, dec.	10	47	8	23	6	6
Safflower, undec.	8	20	10	25	33	4
Safflower, dec.	12	48	8	20	6	6
Sunflower, undec.	7	19	7	29	30	8
Sunflower, dec.	10	37	14	20	12	7

(3) The nutritive value of oil-seed cakes and meals

Oil-seed cakes and meals are essentially protein concentrates, but many of them, especially the decorticated ones and those which contain 5-10 per cent. of residual oil, are foods of high energy value. For example coconut, decorticated groundnut, linseed (pressed), palm kernel, sesame and decorticated sunflower seed cakes are equal in this respect to barley, wheat or rye.

(a) Oil-seed proteins.

As the oilcakes are used primarily for their protein contents and for feeding in those cases where there is need for abundant good quality protein, namely for growth, reproduction and lactation, it is important to examine carefully their efficiencies in this respect.

The protein contents of the common oil-seed cakes range from about 20-45 per cent., the digestibilities of the protein, for cattle, varying from 75-90 per cent. Full data for the amino-acid compositions and biological values of oil-seed proteins are not available, but the following figures are probably representative.

TABLE 43

Oil-seed	Data relating to protein				
	Chemical score	Protein eff. ratio	Biological value	Net utilization	Net protein† value
Coconut	—	1.2	70	61	13
Cotton	37	1.3–2.0	80	68	27*
Groundnut	24	1.7	58	56	25*
Linseed	35	1.9	78	73	22
Soya, heated	49	2.3	75	72	30
Sunflower	53	—	64	61	24*
Sesame	39	2.6	78	66	29

† Net utilization multiplied by protein content of food.
* decorticated

The above data are for the rat, but, in the absence of more precise and specific results, they give some idea of the comparative values of these foods for young stock and for omnivorous species, but not for adult ruminants. No indication of possible supplementary effects, either of the proteins of these foods with one another, or with other types of food, are provided by these figures, but, bearing these limitations in mind, it is still possible to make useful conclusions concerning the oil-seed cakes.

In the first place, with the exception of groundnut and sunflower seed the biological values of these food proteins are all fairly high and stand between those of milk and egg proteins and the cereal grains; they are almost as good as many animal proteins.

Secondly, the net utilization data which, in taking into account both protein digestibility and biological value, are of greater practical value than the latter factor alone, show linseed and (heated) soya cakes to be somewhat superior to the rest.

Thirdly, none of the oilcake proteins has a high chemical score, so that they are rather badly balanced protein foods. Soya bean protein is, indeed, the outstanding protein in this class of foodstuffs probably because of its relatively high lysine content, but the whole group tend to be deficient in the sulphur-containing amino-acids, although sun-flower seed and sesame seed are richer in methionine than many animal proteins. Most of these foods have amino-acid compositions which suggest that they would be well supplemented by milk proteins, which are rich in lysine, leucine, and iso-leucine, amino-acids in which the oil-seeds tend to be lacking. Good supplementation between this class of proteins and dried yeast is to be expected, while meat meal, wheat germ and maize germ proteins, which contain moderate quantities only of cystine and methionine, appear to be of less use, and the cereal proteins are as deficient in lysine as the oil-seeds themselves.

For the developed ruminant the problem of assessment is more difficult, and, for simple maintenance needs, no very deep enquiry is perhaps needed, but the satisfaction of the high protein needs of the good yielding dairy cow is another matter of a different order. Very little of the necessary research, having as its object rations containing oil-seed cakes and taking amino-acid composition into consideration, has yet been attempted. Morris and Wright did not find groundnut cake to be a very efficient supplement for oats for milk production,[1] but as both foods are deficient in lysine one would not now expect such action.

For poultry soya bean (heated) and sunflower seed meals have proved good sources of dietary protein, but sesame seed is less efficient.

(b) Oil.

The fatty material of oilcakes is important in that it may provide a good source of dietary energy, or it may affect the palatability of the food as a whole, or influence the body fat of the stock which are fed on it.

Much the greater part of the oil consists of glycerides, having an energy value for stock more than twice that of corresponding weights of starch or protein. The oil content of seedcakes is thus a significant quantity to be considered in assessing the nutritive values of these foods.

In the case of cotton, groundnut, linseed, safflower, sesame, soya and sunflower cakes, the fatty acids combined in their oils are largely of the unsaturated series. If such cakes are fed in too large amounts to stock they are likely to produce a soft and undesirable type of body fat. Particularly is this the case with linseed cake. The effect produced varies of course with the amount of residual oil in the cake. In the oils of coconut and palm kernel cakes, the fatty acids are mainly saturated and the above effects are not produced. Coconut oil is comparatively easily hydrolysed, so that storage of the cake in a damp place may give rise to a rancid product of objectionable flavour and probably diminished nutritive value.

The oil present in seed cakes and meals of this simple kind contains no carotene.

(c) Fibre.

The fibre of oil-seeds in some instances limits their use in livestock feeding. In general, undecorticated products should not be fed to young stock at all while samples of seed cakes containing more than some 10 per cent. of fibre are not suitable for pigs, unless they are used to offset the lack of fibre of the rest of the ration. The fibre can be of use, however, in checking scouring in cows on fresh pasture.

(d) Storage and toxic effects.

Oil-seed cakes can provide good food for micro-organisms as well as for livestock. Unless commonsense precautions are taken to keep cakes and meals in a dry place, with good ventilation, they may well become mouldy. The undesirable effect which may then follow the feeding of such unsound food is too often blamed on the food itself and not on the faulty management which is really responsible.

Apart from the question of negligent storage, attention should be paid to the possible undesirable effects which may ensue if linseed, cottonseed, and rapeseed cakes are not used properly. The probable difficulties are described under the appropriate headings.

(e) Amounts to feed to livestock.

The amounts of the different oil-seed cakes and meals, which may be fed to livestock, depend upon many factors, such as the nature of the cake or meal itself, the nature and especially the protein content of the rest of the ration, and the animal to which the food is being given. With regard to the last point, the species, age and productive condition of the animal are all matters which must be considered. The following table can thus be no more than a very general guide as to the amounts of cakes and meals which it is advisable to feed to farm livestock.

TABLE 44

Cake	Cattle Dairy	Cattle Fattening	Sheep	Horses	Pigs	Young stock of all kinds	Page Ref.
1. Coconut ...	3–4	4–5	Yes	Yes	1	Yes	
2. Cottonseed	4–8	4–8 ⊁	0.5 ⊁	1	No	Calves only and then more than 9 mth. of age	

(These figures represent maximum quantities to be fed and then only
   when first-class roughage, with adequate carotene, is also provided.)

3. Groundnut	3	3–4	0.5	2	1	Yes	
4. Linseed ...	2–3	2–3	0.5	0.5–1	1	Yes	

(Linseed meal may be fed to pigs in larger amounts in early growth
   but it is advisable to cut down the quantity or omit the food
   altogether later because of its adverse effects on body-fat.)

5. Palm kernel	3–6	3–6	Yes	0–2	Yes	Yes	
6. Rape ...	⊁ 2	⊁ 4	⊁ 0.5	No	No	No	

(Rapeseed cake should not be fed to young stock, nor to pregnant
   animals; it is liable to cause serious digestive troubles in all
   species.)

7. Soya bean	2–4	2–4	0.5	0.5–1	1	Yes	

(Similar reservations as for linseed cake, above.)

NOTE: The above figures are suggested intakes in lb./day. Where data are
otherwise lacking or where the amount of cake needed would vary with size and
weight, etc., the word " Yes " has been inserted to indicate the general suitability
of the material. For further details the relevant section should be consulted.

(4) The individual foodstuffs

(a) Coconut (Cocos nucifera).

The coconut is the fruit of the coconut palm which grows in
tropical and sub-tropical countries. After the nut is split open the kernel
is extracted and dried; the dried kernel is called copra.

There is a considerable variation in the quality of exported copra,
and if it has been badly dried and become rancid the residual cake or
meal will, in consequence, be of inferior feeding value. A good sample
of coconut cake has a slight reddish or brownish-grey colour with a
pleasant characteristic smell and an aromatic, nutty flavour. When the
cake absorbs moisture it swells greatly and for this reason the cake and
meal is often soaked in water some time before feeding. Though both
cake and meal are palatable, animals do not take to them immediately,
though they soon acquire a liking for the coconut flavour.

The cake is well digested and is a valuable food, especially for
dairy cows, helping to produce a firmer and a better flavoured butter
than is the case with linseed cake. In the form of a meal it may be
included in the rations of pigs as it produces a firm fat. It has also been
fed to horses with good results. For fattening cattle it may form up
to 50 per cent. of the concentrated ration and it may be fed if the cattle
are on grass or on dry-feeding.

(b) Cottonseed (*Gossypium sp.*)

The cotton plant yields a seed which has long, white fibres (cotton) attached to the outer coat or hull, which are more or less easily removed from the seed, depending on the variety. Those varieties from which the lint is easily and completely removed are called black seed, while others, such as some Indian types, owing to the adherent fluff or lint, are called white seed. The seed is about the size of a garden pea and is ovoid in shape and of a brown to black colour. The seed-coat is hard and fibrous and encloses an oily kernel.

Cottonseed Cakes and Meals.—Decorticated cottonseed cake is readily distinguished from the undecorticated variety by its distinct yellow colour, absence or practical absence of black hulls, and freedom from lint. It should have a pleasant nutty flavour and agreeable smell. Both the decorticated and undecorticated varieties of cotton cake are among the best known and most commonly used nitrogenous concentrates for feeding to cattle and sheep, and are valuable foods which give good results if fed rationally. It is possible, however, to use too much of the decorticated product, and the undecorticated cake, owing to its fibre content, is not suitable for young stock.

It has for long been known that cottonseed contains a toxic substance—gossypol—and that if cottonseed products are fed in large quantity, toxic symptoms may occur. The exact nature of gossypol poisoning is not yet known. It appears in some cases to be associated with a vitamin A deficiency and in others with a general low level of nutrition coupled with an excessive intake of cottonseed or its by-products. Pigs and calves appear to be most susceptible. In general, no harm is likely to result from feeding the cakes to adult cattle or milch cows, but both varieties of the cake should be fed very sparingly, with plenty of good quality green fodder, to young stock.

Both kinds of cake have a constipating effect on cattle, that of the undecorticated being the more pronounced. Undecorticated cotton cake is usually given to cattle when at grass, or when they are getting a heavy root allowance, while the decorticated is chiefly used for milking cows and stock not getting such laxative food.

Cotton cake is sometimes given to horses when on hard work, but other cakes and meals are probably more suitable. Cottonseed products are not suitable for poultry.

Undecorticated cotton cake usually forms the basis of compound cakes, sheep mixtures, etc.

(c) Groundnut (Earth nut) (*Arachis hypogœa*).

The groundnut, also called the earth nut, monkey nut, or pea nut, is the fruit of a leguminous plant which grows in most tropical and subtropical countries, and is peculiar in that it matures underground, the pod being devoid of chlorophyl and of a yellowish colour. The dry pod, brittle and easily broken with the fingers, usually contains from two to five kernels, which hold about 48 per cent. of oil.

The semi-decorticated cakes more nearly approach the undecorticated than the decorticated cakes, but the qualification "semi" gives little or no indication of the amount of fibre present. There is great variation in the colour and appearance of groundnut cakes. Some decorticated samples are nearly white, with particles of the reddish-brown bran coat or pellicle dispersed through it, while others, particularly the imported Rangoon cake (sometimes called "Jungle Nut Cake") is of a chocolate-brown colour. The undecorticated and semi-decorticated cakes are brown and fragments of the husk can be seen.

The decorticated cake is particularly valuable for supplying protein to dairy cows, for fattening cattle, sheep, and for incorporating in the ration of growing pigs when a nitrogenous concentrate is needed. Both the decorticated and undecorticated varieties of the cake have been fed to horses doing hard work, about 4 lb. of oats being replaced by 2 lb. of the decorticated cake when no other nitrogenous food, such as beans, is given. The decorticated meal is suitable for young growing stock, and a satisfactory calf food may be made by mixing it with separated milk and warm water. If too large a quantity is given to fattening pigs it produces soft fat of a low melting-point and inferior pork and bacon.

A good sample of groundnut cake should have a pleasant smell and taste; a sharp, bitter taste indicates rancidity and decomposition.

(d) Kapok seed (N.O. *Bombacaceæ*).

Kapok seeds contain 19 per cent. of oil and have some resemblance to cottonseed in that they are covered with woolly hairs. The residual cake is rich in protein but contains much fibre.

(e) Linseed (*Linum usitatissimum*).

Linseed is the seed from the flax plant. The seed-coat is very hard and the seeds, small and smooth and provided with a membraneous covering which swells up (gelatinises) when wetted, tend to escape mastication when eaten in a natural state and pass through the intestines unaltered. For this reason when the entire seed is fed to stock it is invariably crushed or cooked. Linseed is chiefly fed to animals in the form of cake or meal after the oil has been abstracted, but is also given as crushed, boiled or steamed seed (without the oil being removed) to sick animals. When it is given together with skimmed milk to calves, its fat helps to compensate for the butter fat which has been removed from the milk.

The seeds contain on an average about 36 per cent. of oil and a fair proportion of minerals, and they are also rich in nitrogenous matter, but for milk production its value is probably not high owing to its low lysine content. The carbohydrates are chiefly in the form of mucilage and the seeds contain no starch.

Owing to the hardness of the seed coat, linseed should be prepared in one of the following ways before feeding:—(1) by boiling or stewing; (2) by prolonged steeping in hot water; (3) by grinding the whole seed to form linseed meal; and (4) by soaking in cold water for two or three days until it becomes soft and jelly-like. If given in large quantities it is nauseating.

Linseed and its products contain a cyanogenetic glucoside, linamarin, which by the action of an enzyme produces prussic acid. Practically the only animals which are poisoned by it are calves, and then only when the material is improperly prepared. It is necessary to point out that if the food is prepared by merely steeping it in either hot or cold water, the enzyme is activated and a large proportion of free HCN may be liberated rapidly in the gut of the animal; a toxic dose may then be absorbed. It is therefore desirable in preparing linseed products for calves that the food should be sufficiently heated (boiled for 10 minutes) to destroy the enzyme. If this precaution is taken linseed and linseed cake are safe and valuable foods.

Linseed Cake.—A good sample of this cake should have a reddish-brown colour, be free from starch, sugar, sand and weed seeds. The presence of starch indicates adulteration with some cheap carbonaceous food, such as milling offals. The cake should be hard and give off a characteristic, pleasant smell when steeped in hot water. It is a very popular food with farmers, since it is considered to be one of the safest cattle foods, and there are few others that will put such a bloom on fattening cattle as linseed; it makes the skin soft and pliable and the coat sleek, and for this reason it is very commonly used during the last stages of fattening, as cattle finished on this cake are always favoured by butchers. Linseed cake or the cake ground to a meal are also suitable for young growing animals and, like the whole seed meal, are extensively used in the feeding of calves. Owing to its laxative nature it is most valuable when the diet is otherwise of a constipating nature, but if given in large amounts to cows it is liable to make the butter soft and greasy. On account of a similar effect on the body-fat, it should be fed with discretion to pigs. A half to one pound a day may be given with advantage to hard-working horses or to debilitated animals, such as those recovering from sickness, but sometimes horses find the modern hard-pressed cake rather difficult to masticate.

Linseed Meal.—This is made by grinding the whole seeds to a meal and it contains all the oil naturally present in the seed; in this respect, therefore, it is very different from linseed cake meal. It is extensively used for calf-feeding (with suitable precautions) and for sick animals but should not be given too liberally.

(f) Maize germ cake.

This has been discussed as a by-product of maize (p. 132).

(g) Palm kernel (*Elæis guineensis*).

Palm fruits are gathered from the palm tree, *Elæis guineensis*, and are chiefly imported into this country from West Africa. The nut, which has a black, rather thick and very hard shell, encloses an ivory white kernel with a black skin. The cake is of a grey colour, with particles of black skin scattered throughout it, and has a smell similar to coconut cake but not so pronounced. Samples of palm kernel cake vary considerably in composition, especially in the percentage of oil and fibre.

It is certainly true that the cake is not so palatable as other cakes, being gritty and dry and causing considerable salivation during mastication. Animals are disinclined to eat it at first, but if it is introduced to them carefully and in small quantities they soon become accustomed to its unusual character. As it is a cheap and nutritious food and one that is well digested, it is worth while taking some trouble in making use of it.

As with any other newly introduced food, palm kernel cake should be introduced gradually into the ration, and preferably blended with some such food as molasses or locust bean meal. Not more than one third of the concentrate ration should consist of this cake.

Numerous experiments have been made with this food on dairy cows and the results seem to suggest that it has a favourable effect on the production of butter-fat and gives butter of a firm consistency. Palm kernel cake is not very rich in protein compared with other cakes, but still 3½ lb. will supply both the starch and protein equivalents for one gallon of milk. This cake can therefore be added to a balanced milk ration without further adjustments being necessary. Either the cake or the meal will give good results when fed to fattening and store cattle. As a partial substitute for oats, palm kernel cake has been given to working horses up to 2 lb. per day, and is said to be especially good for horses which are out of condition. The author has had no difficulty in persuading horses to eat a limited quantity of the cake, but it invariably caused considerable salivation.

It is a good food for pigs but it must be given in very small quantities at a time to begin with, otherwise they will decline to eat it. An excessive quantity is liable to cause diarrhœa, but for sty-fed fattening pigs it is rather an advantage than otherwise to give a food that has a laxative effect.

(h) Rape seed (*Brassica napus*).

Rape or colza seed is grown chiefly in Germany, Austria, Russia and India. Its value is due to its oil content, which is removed by the same processes as are employed for other oleaginous seeds. The residual cake or meal is used for feeding stock.

Some rape seed cakes made from black seed resemble linseed cake in appearance, especially old samples, but the one can be easily distinguished from the other if the cakes are broken, when rape cake shows on the freshly-exposed surface a characteristic greenish colour; the smell also is different.

Rape seed cakes and meals are not regarded as good foods for animals because the seed, like mustard, contains the glucoside potassium myronate, which, by the action of the ferment myrosin occurring in mustard seed, is decomposed into allyl isothiocyanate, glucose and potassium hydrogen sulphate. Mustard seed is usually present with the rape seeds but rape seed cake sold as " feeding rape " is generally considered to be more or less free from mustard. Steaming or boiling rape seed or rape seed cake causes the dispersion of allyl isothiocyanate (essential oil of mustard) as it is volatile and is carried away by the steam, and so the cake or extracted meal is rendered harmless and more palatable.

Some rape seed is more dangerous than others, and Indian seed is considered to be the most harmful. In some parts of the world mustard seed cake is regularly fed to cattle. In Britain rape cake is not a favourite food for stock; it is rather bitter and distasteful. Large amounts of inferior quality cake may cause enteritis and irritation of the kidneys. It should not be used for dairy cows.

Kellner recommends that if used for stock it should be fed dry and that the maximum allowance for cows should be 2 lb. per day, 4 lb. per day for fattening bullocks, and less than 0.5 lb. per day for sheep. It should never be given to young animals.

Rape cake is often incorporated in compound cakes and meals.

(i) Safflower seed (*Carthamus tinctorious*).

Only small quantities of safflower cake are used for stock-feeding in this country. The undecorticated variety—which is the more common— contains a high percentage of fibre, but it is sometimes used in compound cakes and meals.

(j) Sesame seed (*Sesamum indicum*).

Sesame is a tropical seed, which is white, reddish or black, yields a large quantity of oil, and leaves a residual cake which is used as a food for cattle. Sesame or " Gingelly " cake may be of a whitish colour with bran-like specks throughout, or black if made from the black seed. It is a nutritious and palatable food of good keeping qualities.

This cake is particularly rich in crude protein and calcium, and it compares very favourably with better known feeding cakes. It has given satisfactory results when fed to dairy cows, fattening cattle and sheep.

(k) Soya Bean (*Soya hispida. Glycine hispida*).

Soya beans differ from ordinary peas and beans in several respects; they contain nearly twice as much protein, about twelve times as much fat, and very little, only about 2 to 4 per cent., of the carbohydrate is in the form of starch. The pressed cake is one of the richest protein concentrates that we have, containing over 40 per cent. of protein and only 4 per cent. of fibre—approximately 75 per cent. of the carbohydrate is sucrose and 25 per cent. raffinose. The proteins of soya beans are of high biological value for growth and production. The most common colour is a pale yellow—a colour very similar to that of white Calcutta or China peas. White, black, brown and green varieties are also known. The common yellow variety can be distinguished from yellow and white peas by the slightly ovoid and flattened shape and by the presence of a distinct brown hilum. There are a pressed cake, a cake meal and an extracted soya meal on the market. Soya bean cake and meal can safely be used for all classes of stock if their highly concentrated nature is kept in mind. It is rarely that a greater quantity than 2 lb. per day need be given for fattening cattle or dairy cows, and the limit should be 4 lb. per day. Horses may be given from 0.5 lb. to 1 lb. per day if hard-working and the ration is otherwise carbonaceous. The cake is somewhat laxative so that care should be taken that the other ingredients are suitably chosen.

Soya bean meal is used successfully as a substitute for fish meal in the feeding of poultry and pigs, provided that its deficiency in minerals is made good and that it does not form the sole source of protein.

(1) Sunflower seed cake (*Helianthus annus*).

Sunflower seed cake is available in two forms, the decorticated variety containing 40 per cent. or more of protein and the undecorticated product about half of that.

The protein contains about 4 per cent. of lysine, in which respect it is second only to soya bean cake, and 4 per cent. of methionine, in which it is much richer than all of the other cakes, with the exception of sesame cake. Its methionine content is more than three times that of peas and beans and is exceeded only by egg proteins among foods of animal origin. Sunflower seed protein seems to be very well balanced with regard to the proportions of the essential amino-acids present in it.

Although the fibre content of sunflower seed cake (about 12 per cent. for decorticated and up to 40 per cent. for undecorticated types) limits the amounts of it which can be used in the rations of certain species of livestock, there is no doubt that it is a very valuable foodstuff.

(5) Compound cakes and meals

Compound cakes and meals are so called because they are made up of a variety of materials. Each manufacturer has his own set of formulæ but these may vary from time to time, according to the relative availability of the main ingredients.

The earlier compound cakes served a very useful purpose in providing palatable food and using up material which, while wholesome and of high feeding value, was either not sufficiently palatable or was in some other way unsuited for use as an individual food. In the manufacture of the modern compound cake or meal, the choice of raw materials is influenced by the use to which the food is to be put, and compound foods therefore indicate their purpose by being named fattening, dairy, calf or pig meals, etc. The proportions of the ingredients are adjusted so as to give a suitable nutritive ratio and most manufacturers include a proper proportion of minerals and, to some extent, vitamins. The manufacturing process offers an opportunity for precision and distribution of small quantities throughout the mass, which is difficult to attain in home-mixed food.

In addition to the ordinary raw materials familiar to the stock owner, compound cakes usually include a certain amount of locust beans and molasses. The high content of sugar in these helps to make the mixture more palatable and in the case of cakes and cubes or nuts, helps to bind the material together.

The steady growth in popularity and importance of compound foods tends to maintain a high standard of quality. Quality is also maintained by the working of the Fertilisers and Feeding Stuffs Act, the growing knowledge concerning the nature and value of various foods, and by competition between manufacturers.

One difficulty that may arise in the use of compound cakes is that the real nutritive value cannot be assessed like that of the so-called " straight " materials when making up a ration. An approximate figure can be got by assuming that about 75 per cent. of the declared albuminoids are digestible, and if a cake has 20 per cent. of albuminoids or crude protein and about 6 per cent. of fibre, its production starch equivalent will be about 64 to 68.

The palatability and texture of compound foods makes them acceptable to cattle and in addition to this advantage, stock owners find them convenient to store and handle, and also of some assistance in more exact rationing. The avoidance of unsuitable materials for the different kinds of livestock or of the excessive use of any one material is one of the advantages of using compound cakes produced by reputable firms. It is moreover cheaper for the manufacturer to compound a number of foods satisfactorily than it is for the farmer, who must of necessity buy in much smaller quantities and therefore at dearer rates.

FOODS OF ANIMAL ORIGIN

1. Introduction.
2. Meat, bone and blood meals.
   (a) Meat meal.
   (b) Meat-and-bone meal.
   (c) Bone meal.
   (d) Sterilized bone flour.
   (e) Low-temperature bone meal.
   (f) Fibrinogen meal.
3. Fish meals.
4. Whale meat meal.
5. Cod liver oil.
6. Milk and its by-products.
   (a) Composition and nutritive value of whole milk.
   (b) Separated milk, buttermilk and whey.
   (c) The drying of milk and milk products.
   (d) Colostrum.

(1) Introduction

The principal animal products used for feeding to stock include meat meal, tripe meal, meat-and-bone meal, bone meal and bone flour, fish meal, whale meat, dried blood, milk and milk products.

The raw by-products obtained from the flesh and bones of animals or fish are heated so as to separate out the fat and also to cook thermostatically to the point of sterilisation. Provided that putrid material, which is useful as manure, is not included the products obtained are most valuable complementary foods for all classes of stock. The biological value of animal protein is high but when the flesh is subjected to high temperatures for the purpose of sterilisation its nutritive value is reduced. The Foot-and-Mouth (Boiling of Foodstuffs) Order, 1932, requires that all material of animal origin must be exposed for a period of at least one hour to a temperature of not less than 100° C. But exemption from this requirement may be granted by the Ministry of Agriculture under certain stringent conditions, and what are called *low-temperature* meat meal, bone meal or blood meal are produced. These have a much higher nutritive or biological value than products obtained following exposure to higher temperatures. It follows that purchasers of these foods should ascertain which class of material they are buying. In the low temperature process the maximum temperature reached is 72° C.

The fundamental process in the production of meat meals and meat-and-bone meals from animal tissue is the removal of the moisture and

part of the fat content by the application of heat or solvent, thus producing a concentrated product of fairly long keeping qualities. Three
processes are possible—dry rendering, digestor, or solvent extraction.

In the first method the steam which is used for heating does not
come into contact with the food, whereas in the second it does. The
differences in technique have as one of their consequences a higher fat
content in the products of the former process. As is the case with oil
meals, the solvent extraction method yields the food of lowest fat content.

(2) Meat, bone and blood meals

(a) Meat meal.

Owing to the nature of by-products obtained from carcase residues,
there is liable to be a considerable degree of variation in the composition
of the products. Therefore these are defined in the Fertilisers and
Feeding Stuffs Act, 1926. Thus *feeding meat meal* is defined as " the
product, containing not less than 55 per cent. of albuminoids (protein)
and not more than 4 per cent. of salt, obtained by drying and grinding
animal carcases or portions thereof (excluding hoof and horn) to which
no other matter has been added." Good quality meat meal usually
contains 60-70 per cent. of protein.

The fat content of meat meal varies, depending upon the method
of preparation and the nature of the raw material, from about 15 - 3 per
cent., a useful sample for general feeding purposes containing about
9 per cent.

(b) Meat-and-bone meal.

Feeding meat-and-bone meal, which is made from condemned
carcases of food animals or from slaughtered animals not intended for
human food, is defined as " the product, containing not less than 40 per
cent. of albuminoids (protein) and not more than 4 per cent. of salt,
obtained by drying and grinding animal carcases or portions thereof
(excluding hoof and horn) and bone, to which no other matter has been
added." It is to be noted that while the proportion of bone to flesh is
not specified, an excess of bone is prevented by the minimum limit of
protein. The bone yields from 20 to 35 per cent. of calcium phosphate,
and magnesium is also present.

Good quality meat-and-bone meal is a very valuable complementary
food for all classes of stock, particularly breeding and young growing
animals, supplying as it does not only protein of good biological value
but the constituents for bone building.

(c) Bone meal.

Feeding bone meal, defined as " ground bone—commercially pure
bone, raw or degreased, which has been ground or crushed ", should be
distinguished from sterilised bone flour and also from low temperature
bone meal produced from healthy animals. Unless sold under certifica-
tion of sterilisation it should not be used for feeding to animals owing
to the risk of its carrying infection.

(d) Sterilised bone flour.

After boiling to remove the fat and nitrogenous matter the bones are ground and then sterilised by steam under pressure (Digestor process). The product is a fine powder containing 45 - 48 per cent. CaO and 30 - 33 per cent. P_2O_5. Standard products have a consistently reliable composition. Sterilised bone flour is now widely used as a source of calcium and phosphorus for including in the rations for practically all classes of animals; it is commonly incorporated in commercial compound foods, especially for pigs, poultry and calves and other young stock.

(e) Low-temperature bone meal.

This is a special product made, under licence,† from the shanks of healthy sheep. It has a definitely higher value than sterilised bone meal and its composition is (Table 45):

TABLE 45

					Per cent.
Fat	...	...	...	...	8 to 11
Protein	...	...	...	...	29.0
P_2O_5 ...	...	...	...	...	21.8
CaO ...	...	...	...	...	27.6
Fe_2O_3 ...	...	...	...	...	0.17
Lysine	...	...	...	...	1.69
Cystine	...	...	...	...	2.18

(f) Fibrinogen meal.

This valuable material is made in Scotland from the blood of healthy sheep. It consists of the blood fibrin and corpuscles dried at a low temperature (under licence). Its composition is given in Tables 46 and 47.

TABLE 46

					Per cent.
Moisture	...	...	...	...	8
Protein	...	...	...	...	78
Fe_2O_3 ...	...	...	...	...	0.8
Cu	...	...	...	...	0.0
CaO	...	...	...	...	0.14
P_2O_5 ...	...	...	...	...	0.3

TABLE 47

Amino-Nitrogen Analysis

(As percentage of total N)

					Per cent.
Lysine	...	...	...	...	11.0
Tryptophane ...	...	...	...	6.5
Cystine	...	...	...	...	2.6
Arginine + Histidine	...	...	...	17.9

Blood fibrinogen or fibrinogen meal possesses a definite advantage over blood dried at higher temperatures in that the protein value is not decreased to the same extent (p. 56).

† W. & J. Dunlop, Dumfries.

Dried blood meal and in particular low temperature fibrinogen meal are very valuable protein foods, suitable for all classes of stock, and particularly useful for breeding animals and for their young at weaning time. If large amounts are given to start with they are liable to cause troublesome intestinal disturbance with diarrhœa, but the ration may contain as much as 20 per cent. when milk is replaced by solid food; this amount must be considerably reduced as the animal gets older.

Quantity Fed.—When making use of any of the above products it should be understood that they are complementary foods, the primary purpose of which is to make good deficiencies in ordinary mixed rations. Therefore it is neither necessary nor advisable to give large quantities. The following are the amounts, expressed as percentages of the total ration, which can be considered as the normal maximum needed for different classes of livestock.

TABLE 48

Food	Livestock	Per cent.
1. Meat-and-bone meal and meat meal	Chicks and heavy laying hens and young pigs	15
	Pullets and laying hens, store pigs and fattening pigs ...	10
	Pregnant or lactating cows and sows	8
	Other stock	5
2. Sterilised bone flour	Laying poultry	4
	Lactating cows	3
	Pigs and other stock	2
3. Fibrinogen meal plus twice the weight of low tempera- ture bone meal	Dogs	10
	Sows, foals, lambs, tups, ewes	5
	Fattening pigs, horses	2

(3) Fish meal

The Schedules to the Fertilisers and Feeding Stuffs Act, 1926, recognise three forms of fish meals, the first of which, *Fish Guano* or *Fish Manure*, is unsuitable for use as a foodstuff. The foods derived from fish are defined as follows: —

Fish Residue Meal is a product obtained by drying and grinding or otherwise treating waste fish to which no other matter has been added.

White Fish Meal is a product (containing not more than 6 per cent. of oil and not more than 4 per cent. of salt) obtained by drying and grinding or otherwise treating waste of white fish to which no other matter has been added.

Fish meal, prepared from the skeletons of fish, fish skin, and a good deal of adherent flesh, all of them by-products of the preparation of food for human consumption, is a first-class source of animal protein.

Modern plants for the production of white fish meal are designed to dry the meal at a low temperature. After the raw material has been steamed, sterilised, softened, disintegrated and partially dried under vacuum it is gently propelled backwards and forwards through long tunnel driers from which the moisture is extracted as it vaporises. The dried meal as it emerges from the drier is milled to reduce it to the necessary degree of fineness but receives little or no further processing apart from such blending as may be necessary to secure uniformity.

From the official definitions already quoted the only recognised analytical differences between white fish meal and fish residue meal is that the former must not contain more than 6 per cent. of oil and 4 per cent. of salt. The purpose of the definition is to exclude from the white fish meal category those fish meals that contain large amounts either of oil or salt, such as herring meal, which would, if the oil were not removed, contain up to 50 per cent. of oil. Other fish such as dog fish, mackerel, etc., also contain significant but smaller amounts of oil and require treatment other than simple drying if the final meals prepared from them are to contain less than what might be regarded as the desirable maximum of oil, approximately 10 per cent.

To produce meals reasonably suitable for feeding properties from raw materials of the oily type some or all of the oil must be removed. This is normally effected in one of two chief ways, either by solvent extraction, which can produce an almost fat-free fish meal, or by pressing the steam-cooked fish, a method which may yield a product containing 10 per cent. or less of oil. The second method has had wide application to the production of " herring " meal (" Menhaden " meal in the U.S.A.).

Feeding Properties.—The things of greatest value in fish meal are the animal protein and the bone and ash constituents (mostly calcium and phosphorus) which accompany it. The oil of fish meal may be discounted or indeed regarded as of negative value for reasons which will be explained later. Animal proteins are of particular value in the nutrition of livestock because they are admirably designed to make good the admitted deficiencies of cereal proteins in certain essential amino acids, notably lysine and tryptophane.

From the point of view of bone or mineral constituents, cereals are outstandingly deficient in calcium, and fish meals are especially suitable for making good this deficiency. Additional mineral advantages may well arise from the presence of trace elements, such as iodine, which are undoubtedly present in fish meals in quantities sufficient for nutritional needs. Fish meals are very uncertain sources of vitamins A and D, however, and they should not be relied on to furnish those factors.

Fish meal, like the protein of meat meal or milk, should be used with discretion. By virtue of the supplementary relationships (p. 53) between the proteins, relatively small amounts of fish meal will, in combination with cereal proteins, yield a ration, the biological value of whose proteins may approach that of the animal protein alone. Herbivorous animals can use the proteins of green foods to good effect, so that fish meal tends to be reserved for pig and poultry feeding. In whatever species of animal there is a need for relatively large amounts of protein in the ration, as for example pregnant animals, or those in heavy lactation, or young growing stock, fish meal is a valuable food.

The use of excessive quantities of fish meal, especially those which contain relatively large amounts of fat, or the feeding of unsound samples, can lead to fish taint in finished products, such as eggs or bacon. Other foodstuffs, however, such as beet-tops, can also give rise to such undesirable results if they are used without discretion. Both protein and highly unsaturated fatty acids may be responsible, as well as organic bases. Provided that fish meal is in reasonable proportions in concentrate rations, it is unlikely to cause trouble.

Quantity to use.—Assuming that only high grade white fish meal is to be used, a suitable amount is 5 per cent. of the concentrate ration. For young growing pigs, young chicks and all animals making rapid growth or in high production, the quantity may with advantage be increased to 10 per cent. Smaller quantities may be used, however, where the rest of the ration provides a good blend of vegetable proteins.

(4) Whale meat meal

About 30 per cent. of the whale carcase is red meat resembling ordinary beef, but somewhat coarser in texture, yet not more fat than the meat of land animals. The fat (whale oil) is concentrated in the blubber (an expanded tough ivory coloured skin structure), the bones and the tongue.

Processing.—In modern processing large double rotary digestors are used in which the meat is cooked by steam and disintegrated by the simultaneous rotation of the digestor cylinders.

Bones are treated in the same way and in similar disintegrators. Lean meat yields little, and bones a great deal of oil when processed in this way, but the residues in both cases make excellent foods if they are dried expeditiously and at low temperatures. The meat and bone residues from the digestors should be dried in plant of the same general type as for the best grades of fish meal. In both cases violent and prolonged heating must be avoided, and if such heating is employed, the resulting products should be classed as guanos and used as fertiliser.

Feeding Values.—The processing of whale meat and bone is primarily designed to bring about release of oil by transforming the connective collagen and ossein tissues of the bone, and to some extent the meat, to soluble glue (gelatine) waters which are run to waste. This enhances the feeding value of the residual proteins and is precisely the opposite of what occurs with normal residues from land animals. Meals from these sources are normally disproportionately rich in collagen and ossein, i.e., gelatine proteins derived from cracklings or from bones. It is this relative excess of gelatine proteins of lower biological value which makes ordinary meat and bone meals and tankage on the whole less valuable and less dependable in feeding practice than the corresponding grades of whale meals. Good whale meals have in this respect an advantage even over fish meals, although they may contain 5-10 per cent. of indigestible "fibre".

Whale meat meal, if true to name, i.e., derived only from meat, should contain at least 80 per cent. of protein and not more than 10 per cent. of oil. Such a meal is deficient in minerals, and normally it is blended with the bone meal of the whale carcase to give the 60 - 65 per cent. protein and 20 - 25 per cent. ash most useful for feeding purposes.

The oil of whale meals, though of mammalian origin, is quite highly unsaturated, i.e., it is of the same general nature as fish oils. It seems to be less liable to produce fish taints in animal products and there is apparently no reason to insist on a lower limit than 10 per cent., but meals which are excessively oily should be avoided. In general, the same care should be exercised in the purchase and use of whale meat meals as in the case of fish meals or other meals of animal origin, and they should in practice be used in the same way.

(5) Cod liver oil

The use of cod liver oil in feeding practice is as old as, or even older than, its use medicinally. The especial values of cod liver oil were recognised both in veterinary practice and medicine long before the scientist discovered the presence of vitamins A and D in high concentration.

Cod liver oil owes its pre-eminent position in general practice to two main factors—it is outstandingly rich as compared with any other normal food in the two fat-soluble vitamins, A and D, and under normal conditions it is available in practically unlimited supply.

Under present-day commercial conditions the better cod liver oils are extracted rapidly and without deterioration from the freshly caught fish. The use of damaged oil, e.g., oil from half-empty containers left long exposed to the air, in substantial amounts in the feeding of animals can undoubtedly lead to very undesirable flavours in farm produce, but such results do not attend the use of good oil even in quantities many times greater than is necessary to provide for all essential nutritional needs.

Chemical and Physical Characteristics of Cod Liver Oil.—The only specification of an official nature for veterinary cod liver oil at present in existence is the British Standards Institution Specification No. 839 "Veterinary Cod Liver Oil (1939)".

The vitamin potency of the oil must not be less than 500 units of vitamin A per gram and 50 units of vitamin D per gram.

Feeding Properties.—Oils used in veterinary practice should conform at least to the minimum requirements of the B.S.I. Specification No. 839 given above. A lower free acidity than 1 per cent. is desirable, since the lower the figure the more carefully has the oil been prepared. Similarly the lowness of the figure for unsaponifiable matter is an index of the purity of origin from fish of the cod family, oil from which never exceeds 1.5 per cent. of such matter.

The minimum values of 500 International Units of vitamin A and 50 International Units of vitamin D are more than is necessary to meet nutritional needs when the oil is used in normal quantities of 1 to 2 pints per cwt. calculated on the dry concentrated food consumed by the animal. The vitamin A and D concentrations in cod liver oil vary from season to season and from one fishing ground to another. The range is from 5000 to 500 units of vitamin A and from 500 to 50 units of vitamin D per gram of oil. Averaged over a considerable output the ratio between A and D is approximately 10 units of vitamin A for each 1 unit of vitamin D, but there can be considerable deviations from this ratio.

Cod liver oil is a useful complementary food for all animals kept under conditions where they are deprived of green food and sunlight. These conditions are typically found in pig husbandry carried out on the intensive system indoors, or where poultry are kept in batteries or otherwise continuously housed, or where dogs are given only lean or poor-quality meat.

Under such conditions cod liver oil is beneficial when included in the diet of young growing stock and their dams, both before and after parturition, but it is unnecessary for herbivorous animals grazing good pasturage. Cod liver oil can also be given with advantage to milking cows that are kept indoors, provided that the quantity does not exceed 2 oz. per day; larger quantities are liable to cause a depression in the secretion of butter fat, but the addition of even such a small quantity as 2 oz. daily will materially increase the vitamins A and D in the milk and improve the health of the cow and calf.

When the oil is mixed in with the bulk of the concentrate ration, the greatest care is necessary to see that it is evenly distributed throughout the food and owing to the great difficulty of ensuring that this is done, it is much better to give each animal its allowance individually.

In the feeding of cod liver oil to pigs its greatest use is for nursing sows and for young growing pigs. It is undesirable to give cod liver oil to porkers and baconers during the *later* stages of fattening. One per cent. in the food is sufficient, for apart from the unnecessary expense of giving larger quantities than are necessary, cod liver oil if given in excess tends to soften carcase fat.

So far as poultry are concerned, it is practically impossible to rear and maintain birds satisfactorily under housed conditions without the inclusion of fish liver oil in the diet. The desirable percentage in the diet is the same as for pigs, but high-producing laying hens and chicks may be given up to 2 per cent. In laying hens the cod liver oil ensures proper utilisation of the calcium for egg shell formation, which has an important bearing on the hatchability of the egg.

Cod liver oil oxidises readily when exposed to the air and in course of time there is a considerable increase in the free fatty acid content, and the vitamin A may be reduced to negligible proportions. When farmers buy cod liver oil in bulk they should decant it from the tins into clean bottles which should be tightly corked and kept in a dark cool place until required. The common practice of opening a tin and leaving it lying about the steading is to be deprecated.

The demand for a mixed food or meal fortified by the inclusion of cod liver oil for feeding to sheep, pigs or poultry cannot satisfactorily be met, from the feeder's point of view, because of the rapidity with which the vitamin is destroyed on exposure to the air, though the inclusion of antioxidants in the food may to some extent prevent this.

A good carefully prepared cod liver oil can be regarded as a fully digestible oil and as such has a calorific value $2\frac{1}{4}$ times that of an equal weight of pure digestible carbohydrate. This is a matter of considerable importance in evaluating the food value of the oil as a whole, since although cod liver oil is a rich source of vitamins A and D, nevertheless the actual weight of vitamins present is only a small fraction of 1 per cent. of the total, the greater part of the material consisting of glycerides.

(6) Milk and its by-products

(a) Composition and nutritive value of whole milk.

The milks of the various domesticated animals, though containing the same chemical constituents, differ from one another in that the constituents are in different proportions and the biological value of the milk of each species of animal is highest for that species. Nevertheless, the milk of any one species of animal may be used, if suitably modified, for rearing the young of any other species, but it seldom, if ever, gives such good results as are obtained by the more natural method. Cow's milk, for example, is often used for rearing foals, puppies, kittens, pigs and sheep. While one might assume that on the termination of the suckling period the young animal should no longer require milk, it is nevertheless true that its addition to the food of growing animals, or even of animals that have reached maturity, effects an improvement in the diet and has a beneficial effect on the animal greater than might be expected; this is probably chiefly due to the high biological value of milk protein.

Whole milk or any of its by-products may with advantage be fed to any animal at any age. It is of particular value for young growing stock, especially for pigs, not only because of its high nutritive value during the difficult weaning period, but also because it has such a good effect on carcase quality.

When given to chickens[1] it has an astonishingly beneficial action, stimulating growth to a marked degree. Its best results are obtained when it is fed from hatching up to 6 or 7 weeks of age. It appears in some way to increase the utilisation of other foods. .

Milk is also very beneficial for sick animals, owing to its high nutritive value and the ease and completeness with which it is digested.

The average composition of the milk of various mammals is shown in Table 49.

TABLE 49

PERCENTAGE COMPOSITION OF MILK FROM VARIOUS SPECIES OF MAMMALS

	Water	Fat	Sugar	Casein	Other Protein	Ash
Human	87.50	3.75	6.35	0.90	1.20	0.30
Cow	87.40	3.70	4.75	2.70	0.70	0.75
Mare	89.10	1.60	6.15	2.65		0.50
Sheep	79.50	9.00	4.70	4.65	1.15	1.00
Pig	84.05	6.50	3.25	3.70	1.50	1.00
Goat	82.35	7.50	4.90	3.65	0.75	0.85
Cat	82.35	4.95	4.90	3.80	3.35	0.65
Dog	75.50	11.80	3.25	5.55	3.10	0.80
Rabbit	...	16.71	1.98	8.17	2.21	...
Rat	68.35	15.00	2.85	9.50	2.70	1.60
Ass	89.90	1.45	6.15	0.75	1.25	0.50
Camel	86.65	3.05	5.50	3.50	0.50	0.80
Elephant	67.85	19.57	8.84	3.09		0.65
Whale	48.67	43.67	...	7.11	...	0.46
Reindeer	68.55	17.10	2.65	8.40	1.75	1.55
Hippopotamus	...	4.51	...	...	...	...

The high nutritive value of cow's milk can perhaps best be appreciated if its constituents are expressed on a dry matter basis:

TABLE 50

	Normal	Dry Basis	Ounces per gallon (approx.)
	per cent.	per cent.	
Water	87.40	...	...
Protein	3.40	27.00	43
Fat	3.70	29.37	47
Lactose	4.75	37.70	60
Ash	0.75	6.00	9.5

Milk Protein.—In cow's milk the protein consists of approximately casein 76, albumin 12, globulin 6, and other nitrogen compounds 6 per cent. The casein occurs in the form of a colloid and is very closely associated with the calcium in the milk. The albumin has a particularly high feeding value.

Milk Fat or Butter Fat.—Milk fat exists as minute globules in the form of an emulsion with the milk plasma. Each fat globule is surrounded by a very thin film of protein which is responsible for the stability of the butter fat emulsion in milk. The fat globules are fewest in number and greatest in size early in lactation; later the number increases and the size decreases. Size also varies with the breed, being much greater in the Channel Islands breeds.

Milk fat consists of the mixed glycerides of about 12 different fatty acids, together with small quantities of lecithin, cholesterol, and carotenoid pigments. The most important fatty acids occurring in butter fat are:—the volatile butyric acid and the non-volatile oleic, palmitic, stearic and myristic. The proportion of volatile to non-volatile fatty acids varies, but the amounts of volatile constituents are always higher than in other natural fats. The proportions of the various fatty acids in milk fat may be affected by several factors. Cold temperatures and other discomforting climatic conditions, or a lack of succulent green foods, or general poor feeding, cause a lowering of the volatile fatty acids and also a lowering of the unsaturated acids (e.g., oleic and linoleic). Heavy feeding with oilcake gives an increase in non-volatile acids.

Milk Carbohydrate.—This is almost entirely lactose, which occurs in true solution in milk. Milk is the only natural product containing lactose. Although blood sugar is a precursor of lactose, recent work suggests that other blood constituents may also be concerned in lactose synthesis. Lactose is not sweet and is of poor solubility but has a high feeding value. It is more effective than other sugars in stimulating the growth of young animals and it encourages the development of a beneficial intestinal flora, and favourably influences the assimilation of calcium and phosphorus salts.

Milk Ash.—This represents the total mineral matter of milk, only part of which occurs in true solution. Sodium and potassium salts, citrates and chlorides are completely in solution in milk, but calcium and magnesium salts and phosphates occur partly in solution and partly in the colloidal state associated with the milk protein. The amounts of minerals found in normal cow's milk are shown below:

TABLE 51

	per cent. in milk	per cent. of ash		per cent. in milk	per cent. of ash
Na_2O	0.075	10	SO_3	0.020	2.5
K_2O	0.200	25	P_2O_5	0.200	25
CaO	0.160	20	Cl	0.100	15
MgO	0.020	2.5			
Fe_2O_3	0.0002	—			

While milk is rich in most of the minerals required for the metabolism of the young, the amount of iron, copper, manganese or cobalt is very low, but these essential trace elements are normally stored in the foetus in sufficient amount to last until the young animal consumes extra-maternal nourishment. When the animal is born without a sufficient reserve store or for some reason is denied access to foods containing these elements, symptoms of deficiency may become manifest.

In addition to numerous enzymes, milk contains various vitamins. Vitamin A is present in amounts which depend upon the nature of the diet, while vitamin D occurs in quantities which reflect the nature of the diet or of the exposure of the animal to sunlight, the amounts usually being small. The water soluble vitamins are represented by small proportions of aneurin and rather more riboflavin. Vitamin C is present but is rapidly destroyed by exposure of the milk to light.

One should not conclude that the properties of milk have been fully described as soon as a list of its chemical constituents has been compiled. The casein from human milk is precipitated with greater difficulty and in a more finely divided and flocculent state in the stomach of a child than is casein from cow's milk. In such a manner differences of digestibility between the two proteins may arise. Not a great deal is known relating this phenomenon to the feeding of domestic animals, but one application with reference to calves is given on p. 328. The possibility should always be remembered.

(b) Separated milk, buttermilk and whey.

There are several by-products obtained from milk which are of considerable importance in the feeding of animals, and Table 52 gives their composition:

TABLE 52

	Cream	Separated Milk		Buttermilk		Whey		
		Normal	Dried	Normal	Dried	Normal	Paste	Dried
Water . .	70.00	90.60	10.30	90.97	10.00	93.06	54.00	7.8
Protein :	2.71	3.52	32.8	3.60	35.30	0.73	6.20	12.6
Fat .	22.86	0.07	1.5	0.80	7.00	0.24	0.80	1.4
Lactose	3.86	5.02	47.00	4.06	40.00	4.87	35.00	70.5
Ash .	0.57	0.78	7.5	0.75	7.70	0.44	0.40	7.7
Sp. Gr. .	1.010	1.037	...	1.030	...	...	...	...
S.E. . .	...	8.3	82	9.2	91	6.1	43	86

Separated Milk; Skim Milk.—This is milk from which the greater part of the cream has been removed, the percentage of residual fat depending upon the method of separation. Mechanically separated milk contains less fat than skim milk because the method of separation is more efficient. The composition of skim milk also varies—depending upon whether the milk is " shallow set " or "deep set ". Deep set milk takes away more cream than does shallow set milk. The composition of separated and skim milk is given in the above table. As only the cream is removed, it follows that the other constituents of the original milk are left in the by-products; thus separated and skim milks are valuable foods and may be freely used for all animals, especially if fortified with cod liver oil.

Owing to its bulky nature and to the fact that it does not keep sweet for long, most of the liquid product is used at or near creameries or on the farm. As such large quantities are available during the summer at the peak of milk production, during normal times much of it is dried.

Buttermilk.—This is the residue of whole milk after it has been churned and the butter-fat removed. The percentage of cream left in buttermilk depends upon the efficiency of churning; with good churning it should be less than 1 per cent. Buttermilk usually contains less milk-sugar than is present in either skim or separated milks, but in other respects the composition of these products is similar. The reduction in the percentage of milk-sugar is due to the formation of lactic acid. If buttermilk contains salt, as it sometimes does during the summer months, it should be used with great caution for animals. Buttermilk is, as a rule, given to pigs and chickens.

Whey.—This is the fluid left behind after the clotting of milk for cheese manufacture and it differs from other milk residues in that most of the nitrogenous matter is removed for conversion into cheese. Its food value is not high, as compared with buttermilk or skim milks, but it should be noted that it contains nine-tenths of the aneurin of the original milk, three-fourths of the riboflavin, and up to 90 per cent. of the calcium. Liquid whey must be fed fresh as it quickly sours and decomposes. Early scalding followed by rapid cooling checks this tendency. Its great use is for pigs and poultry. Whey is also evaporated to form *Whey Paste,* containing about 50 per cent. of dry matter, with a controlled acidity. This product allows of easier distribution and its keeping qualities are greatly enhanced—for several months—so that it can be fed during winter and early spring.

Whey is also dried over heated rollers from which it comes as a gummy solid which dries to a hard cake on cooling and can then be easily ground to a powder. The colour may be quite brown due to caramelisation. It is very hygroscopic but keeps well if properly packed. Suitably combined with other foods it is useful for pigs and poultry.

(c) The drying of milk and milk products.

(i) Introduction.

Milk powder may be prepared by drying whole, skimmed or separated milk. If it is carefully made, the resultant flaky powder has much of the nutritive value of the original food. Moreover, when water is added to it, a reconstituted milk, possessing almost the same physico-chemical stability as the natural emulsion, may be obtained.

The bacterial content is naturally of considerable importance, as it is in fluid milk, and it must be recognised that while the heat treatment does very materially reduce the number of bacteria—including pathogens —there is no certainty that *mycobacterium tuberculosis* is in all cases destroyed, though its virulence may be reduced. Nevertheless there are no authentic records of living tubercle bacilli having been found in powdered milk. Feeding experiments with milk deliberately infected with tubercle bacilli and dried by the *roller* process have been made on calves without producing infection in the animals. In the case of spray drying the actual dehydrating process is not so reliable in its germicidal effect, but provided the milk is pasteurised before spray drying the risk even here should be negligible. The possibility of tubercle surviving the drying process is a matter of very great importance as large quantities of dried milk are used for the nourishment of the young.

(ii) Methods of producing dried milk.

In the production of dried milk by roller drying, the milk is run in a thin film over rollers whose internal temperature is between 100° C. and 160° C. The time of contact with the moving rollers, though short, is sufficient to drive off the water, the dried milk film being then removed by knives. A more rapid evaporation of the moisture and at a lower temperature (55° C.) is achieved by carrying out the operation under diminished pressure.

Spray-dried milk is produced by spraying the milk into a current of hot air; rapid vapourisation of the water results and the dried material falls as a fine powder. The temperature of the drying chamber may be as high as 115° C., but the substance itself probably does not reach as high a temperature.

(iii) The effect of drying on the nutritive value of milk.

The conditions for the production of dried milk are such that the nutritional value of the proteins is almost unaffected, although their solubility in water may have been slightly diminished. Vitamin C is about one third destroyed, but the amount of destruction of the other vitamins is small and in any case the fat soluble vitamins should be derived from other constitutents of a ration and not from milk.

Powdered milk may be considered to be reasonably free from bacteria and especially from pathogenic organisms since these as a rule are more susceptible to the devitalising action of heat. It is also the case that the numbers of bacteria decrease on storage.

Keeping qualities.—Powdered milk of good quality, carefully packed, has about 8 per cent. of moisture and a low bacterial content; consequently it might be expected to keep in an unaltered state for an indefinite period. Generally speaking this is the case, but there are factors, all of which are not fully understood, which may tend towards deterioration; its solubility may be somewhat decreased, the fat may become rancid, or a stale flavour and discolouration may arise.

Dried milk is now commonly incorporated in many high quality commercial calf and pig foods.

(d) Colostrum.

This is the first milk secreted after parturition and differs fundamentally from " normal " milk. Its purpose is to form a bridge between intrauterine and extra-uterine nourishment. The colostral period lasts from 3 to 7 days and the change to normal milk is gradual, as is shown in Table 53.[2]

From the above analyses of colostrum it will be seen that the first milk to be secreted is very much richer in total solids than normal milk, chiefly due to the large amount of protein, the major portion of which is in the form of albumin and globulin, which take the place of the serum albumin and globulin of the maternal blood during the transition period mentioned above. For this reason, apart from others, colostrum has a very great value for the newborn. Colostrum is also richer in

TABLE 53

Time after Calving	Sp. gr.	Total Solids	Total Protein	Casein	Albumin and Globulin	Lactose	Fat	Ash
Hours		per cent.	per cent.	per cent.	per cent.	per cent.	per cent.	per cent.
0	1.067	36.99	17.57	5.08	11.34	2.19	5.10	1.01
6	1.044	20.46	10.00	3.51	6.30	2.71	6.85	0.91
12	1.037	14.53	6.05	3.00	2.96	3.71	3.80	0.89
24	1.034	12.77	4.52	2.76	1.48	3.98	3.40	0.86
30	1.032	13.63	4.01	2.56	1.20	4.27	4.90	0.83
36	1.032	12.22	3.98	2.77	1.03	3.97	3.55	0.84
48	1.032	11.44	3.74	2.63	0.99	3.97	2.80	0.83
72	1.033	11.86	3.86	2.70	0.97	4.37	3.10	0.84
96	1.034	11.85	3.76	2.68	0.82	4.72	2.80	0.83
120	1.033	12.67	3.86	2.68	0.87	4.76	3.75	0.85
168	1.032	12.13	3.31	2.42	0.69	4.96	3.45	0.84

mineral matter, while the lactose in the earlier stage of colostrum is about half that found in normal milk. The percentage of fat is variable; in some cases colostrum may be rich in fat, but usually it does not differ to any extent from the normal.

Colostrum contains a great deal more carotene and vitamin A than is found in normal milk and also more vitamin D, but under bad conditions of animal husbandry its vitamin A content may be low.

Since the young animal is born with but very low reserves of vitamin A in the liver, the supply of this vitamin via the colostrum may be regarded as essential for the well-being of the newborn and there are indications that the prevalence of calfhood diseases may be associated with a deprivation of colostrum or that the colostrum when available only contains a relatively small supply of vitamin A. Furthermore, it has been established that the early secretions of milk carry maternal antibodies in the globulin solution and that the suckling can absorb these directly during early life.

REFERENCES

1. Newbigin, H. F., & R. G. Linton, (1931). Scot. J. Agric., *14*, 2.
2. Engel & Schlag, (1924). Milchw. Forsch., 1924, *2*, 1.

MISCELLANEOUS FOODS

1. Acorns.
2. Buckwheat.
3. Cocoa residues.
4. Locust beans.
5. Molasses.
6. Seaweed.
7. Swill.
8. Tapioca flour and sago pith meal.
9. Yeast.

(1) Acorns

While acorns have been used from time immemorial as food for stock there is no doubt that they are often responsible for heavy mortalities, particularly among young cattle.

Notwithstanding the frequency with which cattle are poisoned when at pasture, acorns are commonly gathered and fed to cattle, sheep, pigs and poultry, but it is generally agreed that the safest way to make use of them is to spread them over the floor of a barn, allow them to sprout and then to check further growth by exposing them freely to the air, or better still by drying in a kiln. After they are dried they should be kibbled or ground to a meal and mixed in reasonable quantities among other food. Either fresh or dried acorns have a bitter taste and are not immediately acceptable to stock, and for this reason if for no other they should be introduced gradually into the ration. They are essentially a carbohydrate food, containing, in their 50 per cent. of dry matter, 3 per cent. of protein, 7 per cent. of fibre and 36 per cent. of soluble carbohydrate.[1]

Acorns should not be fed to cattle under two years old and only in emergencies is it worth while feeding them to older beasts. They are not suitable for cows, although sheep seem to be able to eat them with impunity, a suitable amount for fattening sheep being about half-a-pound daily. Pigs thrive on them; 1-2 lb./day can be fed with advantage to pigs over 70 lb. Stock pigs may be given up to 3 or 4 lb./day but it is inadvisable to feed acorns to sows advanced in pregnancy. They may be fed to poultry, either whole or kibbled, and both hens and ducks appear to relish them, but they are said to make the eggs dirty in colour.

When it is evident that there will be a heavy crop of acorns stock-owners would be well advised to take precautionary measures, such as removing the cattle from pastures containing oak trees when the acorns are about to fall, placing temporary fences where practicable around the trees, removing the fallen fruits, and providing the stock with additional food if the pastures are getting bare.

In East Anglia it is a common practice to put sheep over the parks early every morning before the cattle are let out to graze, and in the heavy-wooded areas where acorn-poisoning of cattle once was comparatively frequent, it is now unusual. During windy autumn weather oak pastures are kept free from cattle until sheep have eaten the majority of the windfalls.

(2) Buckwheat (*Fagopyrum esculentum*)

This is chiefly used for poultry feeding and, less often, for dairy cows. The dark brown or black hulls are hard and fibrous and the endosperm is white. The chemical composition is similar to that of oats but there is more fibre. This grain produces firm white flesh if fed to poultry. If given in excessive quantity to dairy cows it is liable to make the butter tallowy. In countries where buckwheat is given freely to pigs and other animals it causes a dermatitis (*fagopyrismus*) when the skin is unpigmented and the animals are exposed to the sun.

(3) Cocoa residues

In the manufacture of cocoa and chocolate and cocoa butter, the fermented seeds of the cacao tree (*Theobroma cacao*) are roasted, dehusked and pressed. The cocoa shells, or husk meal as it is called when ground, as well as the residual cake have on occasions been used for stock feeding.

Both by-products are unpalatable and both contain the poisonous alkaloid, theobromine, in amounts varying to 1 - 3 per cent., so that cocoa by-products should at all times be considered a dangerous food.

The use of the husks as a source of vitamin D has already been referred to, but, although they [2] and cocoa meal [3] both contain appreciable amounts of protein much of it is indigestible, and this factor, together with their unpalatability and their theobromine content, limits the amount which should be given to stock.

Poultry, pigs and horses appear to be particularly susceptible and these animals should never be given cocoa by-products, even in small amounts.

It is said that the feeding of 2 lb. of the shells daily to dairy cows is not only free from risk, but increases the butter fat in the milk as well as increasing its vitamin D content. The small amount may be fed to fattening cattle but none should be given to calves. [4] [5]

(4) Locust beans

The locust or Carob bean (*Ceratonia siliqua*), which belongs to the N.O. Leguminosæ, consists of a thick, fleshy pod containing approximately a dozen seeds, the pods being about 89 per cent. of the total weight. The average chemical analysis of pods, seeds, and pods together with seeds have been given by Jaffa and Albro (Table 54):

TABLE 54

	Seeds	Pods	Pods and Seeds
Water	11.74	11.50	13.28
Protein	16.46	4.50	6.75
Ether Extract	2.50	2.37	2.17
Reducing Sugar	...	11.24	11.08
Sucrose	...	23.17	19.44
Nitrogen-free Extractives	58.61*	36.30*	39.80*
Crude Fibre	7.50	8.78	9.29
Ash	3.18	2.72	2.57

* Nitrogen-free extractives other than sugar.

Seeds.—These are somewhat oval in shape and flattened, and are very hard and tough with a fibrous red-brown covering and a yellowish kernel. Owing to their peculiar toughness they are not masticated by animals and, if fed uncrushed, pass through the intestines unchanged; they have been known to accumulate in the stomach and intestines with fatal results. Thus, though they contain a considerable amount of protein, their actual feeding value is very little unless they are well crushed. The seeds are devoid of starch and contain but little sugar, but as a nitrogenous concentrate they are worth using, if previously crushed, and prepared in this way they have been given to dairy cows with good results.

Pods.—The chief value of the fleshy pod is its sugar content, which consists of both invert sugar and sucrose; as a rule sucrose appears to predominate. The pods contain very little starch, about 1 per cent., and are deficient in protein, ash and fat, though containing more fat than ordinary field beans.

The pods are sweet and very palatable and, with or without the seeds, are given to horses, cattle, sheep and pigs. The large amount of sugar present makes them suitable for fattening, but care must be taken to see that the diet contains a sufficiency of protein. In addition to their actual nutritive value, the pods are favoured because, being themselves so sweet and palatable, when added to a mixture of other *sound* but insipid concentrates they make the whole more appetising. The most economical method of feeding the pods is to give them in the form of a meal prepared after the seeds have been removed. The quantity to be given depends on the constitution of the remainder of the diet. The dried pods have a tendency to absorb moisture from the air, which would favour mould growth, therefore care should be taken to store them in a dry place.

(5) Molasses

Molasses is the name given to the by-product of the sugar extraction process. It may be derived either from sugar cane or sugar beet and its compòsition varies somewhat for that reason.

In the extraction processes most of the sucrose is removed and the concentrated beet or sugar-cane juices which remain contain about 25 per cent. of dry matter, most of which consists of a mixture of sugars of varying complexity. Raffinose, as well as uncrystallised sucrose, occurs in the mixture.

The nitrogen content is usually low and represents, for the most part, substances of low-molecular weight, including the important base, choline.

Apart from its sweetness and its palatability for livestock, molasses is a useful constituent of foods because of its binding qualities for mixtures of powdered or ground foodstuffs and for its supply of choline and pantothenic acid.

(6) Seaweed

Along the sea boards of many countries where food for stock is hard to obtain, recourse has long been had to the feeding of seaweed. Cattle and sheep in such districts take to the seaweed readily; where they are at liberty to roam they will invade a seaweed-strewn beach and gorge themselves on the plants thrown up by the sea. Besides-ruminants, both pigs and horses have been fed on seaweed. It has been reported that pigs have been profitably fattened on it in Northern Ireland, and in 1917 a number of French Army horses were successfully maintained on it when it was substituted for oats in their ration.

In Britain the greatest abundance of seaweed belongs either to the genus *Fucus* (Natural Order *Fucaceæ*), known as " Black " or " Bladder Wrack," and which grows beyond tide marks; or to the genus *Laminaria* (Natural Order *Laminariaceæ*), commonly called drift weed or tangles, which grows below low-water mark. Both are popularly considered to be palatable to animals, but sheep and cattle which Hendrick[6] was able to observe closely, ate only two varieties, namely *L. stenophylla* and *Alarin esculenta,* and that in spite of the fact that these two varieties had often to be searched for and picked from many others. Only the fronds were eaten. The same authority found tne composition of *Laminacea stenophylla* to be as given in Table 55.

TABLE 55

Water	81.41%	N-free Extractives	10.74%
Crude Protein	1.69%	Fibre	1.19%
Ether Extract	0.21%	Ash	4.76%

Although the normal food constituents on a dry matter basis somewhat resemble those of the cereals, the ash content is extremely high and may in fact be from 20 to 30 per cent. of the total dry matter, and as the ash is mostly composed of the salts of potassium and sodium,' it must be a limiting factor of the amount normally consumed.

(7) Swill

Swill is the name given to the waste products of human foods, and consists of scraps of meat, fish, bones, fat, vegetable parings, stale bread, etc. Winter swill is more digestible for pigs than summer swill, since it contains a higher percentage of bread and potato peelings, whereas summer swill contains more raw green vegetable scraps, which are less easily digested by pigs.

Swill often contains undesirable ingredients, such as tea leaves, salt, washing soda, and nutshells. Nevertheless, when properly prepared, swill forms a valuable food for pigs and poultry. Under the Foot-and-Mouth Disease (Boiling of Animal Foodstuffs) Order of 1932, swill is not only defined, but regulations are made requiring it to be boiled before it is fed to animals.*

This very important Order is for the purpose of preventing the spread of Foot-and-Mouth disease, and it is obviously essential that the greatest care be taken to see that it is properly carried out. Furthermore, swill which contains unsterilised bacon rinds is very liable to cause swine fever, so that the careful boiling of such material is a wise precaution.

During the boiling process the fat rises and can be skimmed off, the bones are boiled bare and separate out, and the fibrous material is broken down. If too much fat is left in the swill, indigestion may result from its being fed to livestock. The usual practice is to steam the whole for several hours; this ensures thorough mixing, sterilisation, and the loss of undesirable volatile matter; but on the other hand, too long cooking destroys the heat-labile vitamins.

If a purchaser intends to contract for large quantities of swill he may find it worthwhile to have it properly sampled and analysed. This will give him a better idea of its nutritive properties and monetary value.

Swill for pigs.—Pigs may be fed on swill after they have reached 50 lb. live weight (at 12 to 14 weeks of age), but if it is fed to pigs over a prolonged period or in very large quantities, it produces an excessively fat carcase of poor quality, containing much moisture, and thus liable to shrinkage. To counteract this disadvantage, barley meal and/or skim

* " Every person having in his possession or under his charge—
    (a) Any meat, bones, offal or other part of the carcase of an animal; or
    (b) Any swill; or
    (c) Any other broken or waste foodstuffs which have been in contact with meat, bones, offal or other part of the carcase of an animal, shall cause such articles to be boiled before they are fed to animals, and until they are so boiled, shall keep the articles so that no animals shall have access thereto.
" ' *Boiled* ' means exposed for a period of at least one hour by any process to a temperature of not less than 212° F., and the expression ' boiling ' shall be construed accordingly."

milk (if seasonally available) should be fed during the last month, and no food given for 48 hours before slaughter. For pigs, the chief constituents to be avoided are excess of fat, salt and soda.

Swill for poultry.—Swill can be mixed with meal in equal quantities, or fed by itself after a minimum of boiling. The poultry should be allowed to help themselves—they will pick out what suits them best.

Processed Urban Swill.—This is the name given to swill collected by urban authorities and sterilised by them. It is produced by filling the swill into a cylindrical drum surrounded by a steam jacket carrying steam under pressure, the material being kept agitated by means of revolving paddles. The heat process lasts about 2 hours. The cooked material on cooling forms a stiff pasty mass which can be transported in bags.

Woodman[8] found that concentrated swill, the main ingredients of which were potato peelings and cabbage leaves, with smaller amounts of a variety of root peelings and still smaller quantities of waste bread, pudding and bacon rind, contained 30 per cent. of dry matter, of which 3.9, 2.3, 17.6 and 1.5 per cent. consisted of protein, fat, soluble carbohydrate and fibre respectively. Sheep were able to digest 82 per cent. of the food, the digestibilities of the four constituents named above being, in order, 61, 81, 90 and 46 per cent.

In an earlier investigation Woodman[9] and Evans found that when fed to pigs, 1 ton of concentrated swill with a slightly higher dry matter content (31.9 per cent.) supplied as much digestible food nutrient as 0.37 ton of the mixture of 2 : 1 by weight barley meal and middlings.

Dried Swill.—Swill may be sterilised by cooking and drying, and the advantages in storage, transport and sterility are obvious. The dried swill is rich in protein (25 per cent.), lime, phosphoric acid and salt, as Woodman[10] showed.

No protein or mineral supplement is required.

Swill has a constipating effect, so middlings should be fed to prevent binding and to provide vitamin B. As dried swill is practically devoid of vitamin A, fresh green food or cod liver oil should be fed with it.

(8) Tapioca Flour (*Manioc Meal, Cassava Meal*) and Sago Pith Meal

Tapioca flour is derived from the tubers of the tropical plants *Manihot utilissima* (bitter cassava) and *Manihot palmata* (sweet cassava). There are four grades of tapioca flour, of which the best is the " B " tapioca.

Sago pith meal is the fruit of the sago palm (*Metroxylon sagu*). Woodman, *et alia*,[11] found that both " B " tapioca flour and sago pith meal contain about 2 per cent. of protein, some 0.5 per cent. of fat, and 90 per cent. soluble carbohydrate; the former contains rather less fibre than the meal, namely 3 per cent. against 5 per cent. Both foods are rich in starch and are useful in replacing cereals such as maize and barley meal in the fattening of pigs. Woodman and his colleagues have shown that both meals, but tapioca in particular, are not only very highly digestible but make excellent carcase fat and prime bacon. Tapioca flour can form up to 40 per cent. of the ration for fattening pigs and sago pith meal up to 20 per cent. when the animals are over 100 lb. in weight.

(9) Yeast

Yeast as a by-product of the brewing industry is a valuable food for animals. The wet material can only be used in the vicinity of the brewery, so that the yeast is skimmed off, dried by the same process as is used in the milk trade, and pressed. Yeast is rather unpalatable to dairy stock because of its bitter taste, but if it is introduced gradually, the cows take to it and will eventually eat it readily.

Yeast contains some 40 per cent. of protein, 35 per cent. of soluble carbohydrate, very little oil or fibre, and about 10 per cent. of mineral matter. It is a rich source of vitamins of the B-complex and a valuable food from that point of view, but its protein, though only of medium biological value (63) has a useful amino-acid composition. The protein is far richer in lysine than any of the cereal foods, appreciably richer than peas or soya beans, and about twice as rich as the best of the oil-seed proteins; it is equalled only by egg, milk and the better animal foods. In threonine and isoleucine content it is exceeded by none of the common vegetable foods, but, on the other hand, it tends to be deficient in the sulphur containing amino-acids.

Its amino-acid composition is such that dried yeast is a useful supplement for other protein concentrates, especially the oil-seed cakes and meals, in a ration. As a supplement, of course, it should not constitute more than a small percentage of the ration, and 10 per cent. by weight probably represents the upper limit that it is desirable to feed to stock.

An extremely useful summary of the feeding value of this foodstuff has been provided by Braude.[12]

It is very useful in quantities up to 3 - 5 per cent. of the ration for poultry, pigs and other small animals, but it is advisable to use dried yeast because quite serious digestive disturbances have been produced in pigs fed on fresh material which has caused fermentation of the constituents of the ration.

REFERENCES

1. Woodman, H. E., (1948). "Rations for livestock," Min. Agric. Bull. No. 48.
2. Knapp, A., and A. Churchman, (1937). J. Soc. Chem. Ind., *61*, 29.
3. Asplin, and H. Ellenberger, (1927). Vermont Agric. Exp. Sta. Bull., *272*, 1.
4. Blakemore, F., and G. Shearer, (1943). Vet. Rec., *55*, 15 and 165.
5. Black, D., and N. Barron, (1943). Vet. Rec., *55*, 166.
6. Hendrick, J., (1916). J. Brit. Agric., *12*, No. 11.
7. Beharrell, J., (1942). Nature, *149*, 306.
8. Woodman, H. E., and R. E. Evans, (1944). J. Agric. Sci., *34*, 110.
9. Woodman, H. E., and R. E. Evans, (1941). Agriculture, J. Min. Agric. England, *48*, 1 and 42.
10. Woodman, H. E. (1941). Agriculture, J. Min. Agric. England, *48*, 104.
11. Woodman, H. E., A. W. Menzies Kitchen, and R. E. Evans, (1931). J. Agric. Sci., *21*, 531.
12. Braude, R., (1942). J. Inst. Brewing, *29*, (New series), 206.

CHAPTER 16

FOOD STORAGE AND PREPARATION

1. The storage of food.
   (a) Introduction.
   (b) The storage of different classes of food.
2. The preparation of food.
   (a) Palatability and food preparation.
   (b) Grinding and crushing.
   (c) Cutting or chaffing.
   (d) Soaking or damping foodstuffs.
   (e) Cooking food.
   (f) The treatment of straw with alkali.
   (g) Sprouted grain.
   (h) Cleanliness in food preparation.

(1) The storage of food

(a) Introduction.

Foods which contain more than some 15 per cent. of water are especially liable to attack by micro-organisms when they are stored, with the result that at the least they may become less palatable through acquiring a mouldy smell or taste, while in the more serious cases they may lose some of their nutritive value for the livestock which are to consume them or even acquire toxic properties, as in the case of rye (p. 134).

In order that a temporary surplus of food may be stored without loss of nutritive properties through such causes, several alternative methods of treatment may be used. The food may be dried, either naturally as for hay, or artificially as in the case of dried grass, brewer's grains, beet pulp, or potatoes, until the water content falls below 15 per cent. Alternatively it may be so treated as to make it less easily attacked by micro-organisms; the increase in acidity during the preparation of silage is an example of this type. In the case of roots the food is kept in pits or clamps in a manner which experience has shown is least likely to produce deterioration.

In the case of foods which are low in moisture content, such as hay, dried grass, cereal grains, oilcakes, etc., storage conditions should be such that there is no permanent increase in moisture content. When the humidity of the atmosphere is high such foods tend to pick up moisture and then become more liable to attack by micro-organisms. Efficient ventilation of the storage room, so that a current of dry air may later offset any previous increase in moisture content of the food, is thus desirable. Cool storage conditions assist in the preservation of the food by keeping down the rate of multiplication of bacteria.

There are many other factors which are concerned in food storage. If the food is dirty its moisture and bacterial contents are likely to be increased and the rate of deterioration thereby enhanced; if it is finely ground it offers a larger surface area both for the absorption of moisture from the atmosphere and for attack by bacteria. Furthermore, during the process of grinding some portion of the material may be exposed to microbial attack whereas it is not so in the untreated material. When cereals are ground, for example, the soft starchy portion of the grain is much more vulnerable than it is in the whole grain, where it is protected by the outer, fibrous part.

Quite apart from the effects of micro-organisms when the latter are subjected to conditions favourable for their growth, two other causes may lead to the rapid deterioration of food in storage. Firstly, plant pests may multiply rapidly under favourable conditions; for example, when maize is stored, the presence of weevils may lead to a serious loss of nutritive value of the food during the course of a few weeks, the soft portion of the grain being eaten away. Secondly, the result of grinding is an increase in the proportion of the food which is exposed to light and air, thereby increasing the rates of hydrolytic and oxidative deterioration of fats. The fatty portion of the food tends to become rancid and unpleasant in taste and of lessened nutritive value, while such labile factors as vitamin A are partly or wholly destroyed.

Foodstuffs of this class should thus be clean and free from insect pests when stored; they should be dry and sound, and should be kept in a cool, damp-proof, well-ventilated store. No more ground foodstuffs should be stored than are sufficient for a few days feeding. Stores should not only be clean, but as nearly vermin-free as possible.

(b) The storage of different classes of foods.

In the storage of threshed grains on a farm the most important thing is to see that the grains do not contain an excessive amount of moisture at the time they are stored in bulk. All grain should be turned over from time to time, particularly that which has been threshed and stored soon after harvesting, as it may contain a high percentage of moisture, for moist grain, stored in bulk without frequent turning, is sure to heat and ferment and become musty. Badly weathered grain should not be stored in close proximity to that which has been well harvested and is sound. Stored foods, particularly grains and meals, are liable to be attacked by the various forage mites during warm weather. Nearly all wooden bins harbour these mites and they should therefore be cleaned out regularly and scrubbed with a hot strong solution of soda.

Cakes and Meals.

It is inadvisable for the farmer to lay in a bigger supply of cakes and meals than he is likely to use up in reasonable time, as some of them do not keep well even under the best of conditions. Dangerous decomposition may occur if cakes are stored in a damp place or if they have been allowed to get wet in transit. Occasionally a few bags may get wet in a railway or motor waggon and be stored away with the remainder; the author knows of such a case where two wet bags of cake were responsible for the death of five cows out of a herd of twenty before the fault was detected. When storing a fresh consignment the barn or store-house should first be cleaned out, and each bag of cake should then be carefully inspected before it is put away. If meal or broken cake is stored in bags these should not be packed close, but spaces should be left here and there through which air can circulate. If the floor is of concrete, and therefore liable to sweat, battens should be placed under the bags. Cakes should not be piled closely on top of each other but should be built up cross-wise so as to leave air spaces. All bags or piles of cake, etc., should be kept a little way from the walls as this not only allows of better ventilation, thus increasing the keeping property of the food, but permits freedom of movement to cats when hunting rats.

Roots and Tubers.

These are commonly put into a clamp or pit as soon as they are lifted, to protect them from rain and frost. The clamp should be built on ground that has good drainage so that the tubers are kept dry. Good hard straw, wheat or rye, is laid over the top and on this is spread a layer of soil. As the roots and tubers are living when pitted, the clamp is ventilated by flues, commonly made by allowing bunches of straw to project here and there beyond the earth covering. When the respiration has to a great extent ceased, and there is less heat formed within the pit, the depth of the covering is increased by adding more soil, or in some cases by adding a second layer of straw on the soil and then covering up the whole with more soil. Damaged and diseased potatoes and roots should not be pitted.

Roots, such as turnips and swedes, after topping and tailing, are pitted in a similar manner in order to protect them from frost. All roots and tubers undergo chemical changes during storage, the chief of these being the conversion of some of the starch into sugar. As a result of respiration there is a loss of dry matter and also the conversion of nitrates to harmless amide nitrogen. Overheating during storage results in rot and putrefaction, and so does exposure to very low temperatures.

The stockowner should periodically inspect the contents of his granaries and stores himself, so as to prevent food wastage or damaged and unsafe food being given to his animals.

(2) The preparation of food

The preparation of food has in general three main objects, firstly, to increase its palatability so that livestock will consume more of it and produce meat, milk or eggs more rapidly, secondly, to increase its nutritive value, and thirdly to make it safer for livestock. Under the last heading are included such treatments as may be designed to prevent stock from bolting food and thereby suffering from digestive troubles, or to destroy harmful substances which may occur in the natural, raw food.

(a) Palatability and food preparation.

The evidence now available regarding palatability suggests that rations are most palatable when the constituents are fresh, i.e., in good condition, and when the balance of protein, fat, carbohydrate, minerals and vitamins is right for the particular species and condition of animal being fed. Loss of appetite will often follow rapidly when some simple constituent of the ration has been omitted or is present in insufficient amount. Though only minute traces of vitamin A or of members of the vitamin B complex are required to be fed to maintain normal health in livestock, one of the most characteristic symptoms of their omission from the diet is a loss of appetite.

The processing of foods may sometimes lead to destructive changes in the various constituents of the food; for example, much of the carotene of grass is lost during hay making, or may be lost during bad storage.[1] Food preparation should aim at the retention of as much as possible of the nutritive value of the material, bearing in mind what is known of the effects of air, light, heat and other factors on the different constituents of foods. There is everything to be said, for example, for including some *fresh* green foods *regularly* in the rations of farm livestock.

(b) Grinding and crushing of foods.

Hard foods, such as maize, wheat, beans, and peas, are crushed or ground when they are fed to certain species of livestock. While such processes may facilitate mastication and may increase the amount of food which can be consumed by stock or raise its digestibility, discretion needs to be exercised, otherwise the slight improvement in feeding value may be offset by the extra cost of preparation.

Some benefit is to be gained by grinding hard foods for very young animals, or for sick or old ones; omnivorous animals like the pig also gain by such treatment. Fine grinding is undesirable, as it makes food less palatable and more liable to deteriorate on keeping. The requirements of the various species of animals are dealt with more fully in Section IV.

(c) Cutting or chaffing.

When long hay is fed from racks a quantity is usually lost when it falls to the ground and is trodden under foot; if the hay is cut into short pieces this loss may be prevented, the work of mastication reduced, and, by giving the cut hay with grain, greedy-feeding horses may be stopped from bolting their food. It is now general practice to feed cut hay.

For idle animals a certain amount of long hay is desirable as it keeps them contented, while straw, which is not relished by beasts as much as hay, can be mixed with the cut hay and grain. Nevertheless stock should not thus be compelled to eat more straw than is desirable, and the giving of cut straw, particularly wheat straw, to cows is a bad practice. It is better to allow the animals to satisfy their appetites, as they feel inclined, by picking out the tops and leaves of the straw and leaving the less palatable and less nutritious lower parts of the stems, than to require them to fill themselves with material of low nutritive value.

Chaffed hay is not more digestible than long hay, and there is no advantage in cutting it into very small pieces but rather the reverse, because, if it is cut very small (less than 1 inch) or ground, a certain amount may be swallowed without having undergone sufficient mastication and the material tends to pack in the stomach or rumen. Furthermore, ground hay or straw is definitely less palatable than longer material which the animals have to masticate. If it forms the sole source of fibrous food for ruminants, rumination ceases, and the total intake of the roughage is less.

Roots, such as turnips, swedes and mangolds, may be eaten direct off the ground as they grow, or lifted and stored after topping and tailing and later fed to cattle and sheep on the ground, or they may be fed in the house or court either whole or after slicing or pulping. Pulping is a term used to indicate two methods of cutting roots—(a) cutting into " fingers " by means of semi-circular knives; and (b) cutting into small square pieces by specially shaped knives. Roots are sliced or pulped before feeding to stock for a variety of reasons. Young animals changing their teeth, and animals at an advanced age when the teeth are worn down, as, for example, old ewes, are unable to eat uncut roots, especially if they have become woody and hard. Under these circumstances roots should always be cut. Meals and light chaffy foods can be fed with less wastage if sprinkled on cut roots than if fed dry. A favourite method of feeding cattle and young horses in straw yards and cattle courts during the winter is to feed a mixture of cut roots, chaff and meal from boxes. The animals relish the mixture, and colts are found to thrive well on the system. Treacle diluted with water is often added to the mixture, thereby increasing its palatability.

(d) Soaking or damping foodstuffs.

Hard foods such as flint maize, hard wheat or barley, which tend to escape complete mastication and digestion when they are given to livestock, may be soaked beforehand in order to soften them, although they are better fed in coarsely ground, or kibbled, form.

Soaked food of this type is not suitable for poultry nor, save in very small amounts, for horses. Provided that the animals have access to ample water, as all stock should have, it is unnecessary to soak barley meal and other meals for pigs, though the practice may prevent scattering and wastage.

Soaked foods should not be kept for long periods, especially during warm weather, otherwise they are very liable to go sour. For the same reason the utensils in which they are prepared and from which they are fed must be kept scrupulously clean.

Dusty foods, which tend to be unpalatable or to blow away when fed in the open, and light chaffy foods can be damped before they are fed to livestock. Some discretion should be exercised in this respect. Meals, for example, should be coarsely ground and not fine and dusty, while foodstuffs which have become dry and dusty through long storage are likely to have other nutritional faults than simple dustiness (p. 235).

Woodman and Evans [2] found that it was advantageous to feed dried grass meal in the form of a thick slop when it was being used for bacon pigs. Under such conditions it was possible to use rations containing 25-33 per cent. of this foodstuff, some slight diminution in the amount to be fed being needed only after the pigs were above 150 lb. live-weight.

Ample water should be available for sick animals, and it is doubtful whether there is any logical basis for feeding moistened foods to stock in such a condition. A well-nourished beast ought to have sufficient bodily reserves to tide it over a short period of sickness; if it cannot provide enough fluid for the mastication of food then other digestive secretions may be equally scanty.

(e) Cooking food.

Food for livestock may be cooked for two reasons, either to improve the digestibility of some constituent of it, or to make it safe to eat.

Except in a few isolated cases, the cooking of food does not increase either its digestibility or its nutritive value; the improvement in nutritive value of soya bean has been discussed elsewhere. Another food, for which cooking improves the digestibility for pigs, is the potato, but, in general, cereals, pulses and the various meals have their digestibilities lowered when they are cooked.

When 464 pigs were divided into two equal groups, one being fed on untreated food and the second being given the food cooked, the average weight gains on the latter were slightly less than on the former, being 1.50 and 1.57 lb./day respectively.[3]

Similar experiments by Patterson and Robb [4] showed that with dry raw meals pigs thrive better, have a better appearance and a cheaper rate of live weight increase than when food is steamed.

Foods which are cooked in order to destroy harmful factors in them include milk, when it is presumed to be tuberculous, and meat, bones, offals and swill, which under the Foot-and-Mouth Disease (Boiling of Foodstuffs) Order, 1932, must not be permitted to come into contact with animals and must be boiled for one hour before being fed to livestock. House garbage is better cooked before it is given to pigs simply because it is usually collected under such conditions as promote decomposition and the growth of micro-organisms. Linseed should also be cooked before it is given to calves (p. 207) and a similar precaution applies to rape seed (p. 209).

It is advisable to cook no more food than is sufficient for the day's needs and to cool *rapidly* the food which has been heated. Foodstuffs which have been cooked and left to cool in large batches may lose their heat so slowly that they subsequently give full opportunity for the growth of fresh micro-organisms.

(f) The treatment of straw with alkali.

Following early observations by Lehmann and later by Kellner, who found that the digestibility of straw could be improved by treating the food with sodium hydroxide solution, attempts have been made to make this a practical proposition for livestock feeding. The process is essentially one of delignification and its simplicity and economy allow it to be carried out on the farm without expensive plant, although it requires some care. Straw to be hydrolysed is chaffed to 2 to 3 inch lengths and soaked for at least three hours in eight times its weight of 1.5 per cent. solution of caustic soda. The fluid is then drained off and the straw is washed with water until it is neutral to litmus or has lost its soapy feel, as judged by handling; as sodium hydroxide rapidly attacks animal tissues good care should be taken to see that the washing is complete. The process of predigestion actually continues beyond three hours if the straw is left in the caustic solution, but whereas the action of the caustic is most intensive up to that time, it continues at a progressively slower rate. In practice it often proves convenient to soak the straw overnight and wash it in the morning. The process will certainly have gone as far as is desirable after 20 hours' soaking with the atmospheric temperature at 45° F., but at lower temperatures even further exposure may be desirable. In any case it should be carried on until the nodes of the straw have become so soft that they can easily be squashed between the forefinger and thumb.

In the simple twin concrete basin in which the process is carried out on the farm, it takes one man three-quarters of an hour to handle 200 lb. of straw; about 4 gallons of water are needed for washing each pound. After washing, the straw pulp is drained until its water content is reduced to about 80 per cent. before feeding.

When stock have become accustomed to the treated straw, and they soon take to it, it is eaten readily. The soda treatment raises the starch equivalent value for ruminants between three and four times, so that straw which before treatment had a starch equivalent of 13 may have a value of 50 after hydrolysis in spite of loss of dry matter during the process; that is, the process brings the energy producing value of oat straw up to that of the cereals, and of wheat straw to that of really good hay. The material is most suitable as a food for fattening bullocks, those weighing about 8 to 9 cwt. being given about 60 lb. of straw pulp, representing some 12 lb. of dry treated straw. Up to 20 lb. of the pulp may be fed to dairy cows, but it is too bulky to form the ration of high-producing stock to any great extent. It is useful for sheep and in limited amounts also for pigs. For horses it is probable that the value of the straw is raised *relatively* more than it is for ruminants. A

digestibility trial with horses showed that a poor barley straw with a
equivalent, for horses, of 5.5 was raised to an equivalent of 20.2,
ing the loss of organic matter in the process, that is to the com-
ive value of poor hay.

Woodman and Evans[6] have investigated the digestibility and nutritive value of fodder cellulose made from wheat straw. For sheep some
82 per cent. of the cellulose and hemicellulose proved to be digestible,
while an even higher proportion of the crude fibre was absorbed. Not
only was the protein content of the material indigestible, however, but
the coarse food had a depressant effect on the protein of the rest of the
ration. Pigs, given a ration of 700 gm. of middlings, 350 gm. of maize
meal and 450 gm. of meat meal, to which 700 gm. of finely ground
fodder cellulose was added, the ration being fed as a thick slop, digested
the cellulose almost as well as the sheep. Although these workers found
that the food was much more suitable for cattle and sheep than for pigs,
they presented evidence that fodder cellulose might be fed to pigs at
the rate of about 1.5 lb./day, provided that the pigs were above some
80 lb. live-weight and the product was part of a balanced ration.

A product of this type should be looked upon as a source of carbohydrate only; it lacks protein, fat, minerals and vitamins, and should
not be given to livestock unless those factors are known to be supplied
in full by the other components of the ration.

(g) Sprouted grain.

Although it has been claimed that sprouted maize is markedly
superior to the commonly used succulent foods, e.g., swedes, as a food
for fattening cattle, giving them a finish and bloom equalled by few
other foods, other work in several countries has shown that sprouted
grain has no advantage over high class succulents for milk production,
nor for the growth of calves and pigs. Similarly it has been shown that
it does not improve the breeding powers of cows and sows, and that as
a food for hens it has just the same stimulating action on egg production
as any other palatable green food.

During the process of sprouting it is claimed that the grain proteins
are hydrolysed into peptones and amino-acids and that these occur in
an increased amount, due to the utilisation of the nitrogen from the
cultural solution. There is, however, a decided loss in carbohydrates
which is not offset by the nitrogen intake. The steeping and washing
does, however, remove dust and dirt and thus makes the grain more
attractive. By adding or withholding various salts from the nutrient
solution it is possible to vary the mineral content of the sprout, but
variations large enough to be of practical importance can be brought
about with only a few of the minerals, one of which is iodine. There
are easier and more effective ways of feeding minerals than this.

During the process of germination the vitamin content is varied in
that although the amounts of vitamin A and E remain stationary, there
is a slight loss of aneurin but a large increase of riboflavin and vitamin

C—an increase of 20 times and 10 times respectively, but on the whole the process does not seem to be worth the trouble which is involved in the preparation of the material; its benefits seem doubtful, while other foodstuffs, requiring less attention, are at least as good.

(h) Cleanliness in food preparation.

It is deemed sufficiently important to repeat what has been mentioned in preceding sections with regard to the cleanliness of food which is to be fed to livestock.

Although, under natural conditions, livestock may consume a good deal of adventitious " dirt ", there is no excuse for the feeding of dirty foodstuffs to them under intensive conditions. At the least such foodstuffs provide unwanted mineral matter at the expense of digestible nutrients and at the worst they may be more prone to deterioration on storage.

More important than contamination of this kind is the introduction of undesirable biological agents into the food. These latter range from insect pests, which may themselves consume appreciable amounts of stored food, to bacteria introduced into the ration either by the feeding of unsound foods, such as infected milk, or to the use of dirty vessels. Young stock, particularly, should not be exposed to risks of this kind. In the case of calves, for example, it is sufficiently great a handicap for them to be removed from the dam and then put on milk substitutes, without further exposing them to infection by the use of unsound foods or dirty utensils. Even adult stock are not exempt from hazards of this kind, as the results of feeding mouldy cakes or rye bear witness.

REFERENCES

1. Watson, S. J., (1939). " Science and practice of conservation: grass and forage crops."
2. Woodman, H. E., and R. E. Evans, (1948). J. Agric. Sci., *38*, 51.
3. Anon., (1916). J. Dept. Agric. Tech. Instr., Eire, *16*, 419.
4. Patterson, and Robb, (1916). W. Scotland Agric. Coll., Bull. No. *75*, 1.
5. Woodman, H. E., and R. E. Evans, (1947). J. Agric. Sci., *37*, 202 and 211.

THE FUNDAMENTAL BASES
OF FEEDING STANDARDS

(1) Introduction

(a) General anatomical and physiological factors in nutrition.

Research during the last hundred years has enabled comparisons to be made between the requirements of animals of different species but of corresponding physiological states on the one hand, or between those of animals of the same species but in different conditions on the other. From such comparisons it is possible to draw conclusions that are of value in the practical feeding of livestock of all classes.

It is helpful to make brief contrasts, anatomical and physiological, between the different classes of livestock and then to discuss the information which is now available concerning nutritional needs for maintenance, growth, milk or egg production, reproduction and work.

Although there are differences within each group, perhaps the most useful comparisons one can make concerning nutrition and anatomical and physiological factors are those between ruminant herbivores, non-ruminant herbivores, omnivorous and carnivorous animals, and birds. There is no space here to deal fully with this subject, so that further information must be sought in suitable works of reference,[1][2] but it will be profitable to compare cattle, horses, pigs, dogs and domestic fowls generally, as representatives of each of the above classes.

Considering, (a) the numbers, types and positions of the teeth, (b) power to move the lower jaw laterally as well as up and down, (c) the length and range of movement of the tongue, and (d) the provision of salivary glands in the mouth, one may say that the cow, horse, pig, dog and fowl are progressively less suited for the grinding and mechanical disruption of food in the mouth. Mastication plays a major part in the feeding habits of herbivorous animals, but is only of minor importance in carnivores like the dog. None of these creatures seems well fitted to the ingestion of fine, powdery food, in fact the mouth part of the fowl is best suited for the rapid picking up and swallowing of small particles such as grains, and in this instance palatability, so far as it concerns taste and smell, is of little importance, the bird being attracted mainly by colour and lustre.

In mammals the food which has been swallowed passes quickly along the œsophagus into the stomach, whereas in the fowl it is first taken into the crop—an enlargement of the œsophagus—where it is stored until the digestive system is ready to deal with it and where, to some extent, it is softened by the fluids which are secreted.

The alimentary tract of each of the animal types under consideration consists of three main portions, namely, the stomach, small intestine and large intestine, whose ancilliary organs, such as the liver, gall bladder and pancreas, secrete fluids containing the enzymes necessary to hydro-lyse fats, proteins, carbohydrates and other food constituents prior to their absorption from the gut; the nature of the chemical changes which occur has been considered in Section I. Although the general pattern of the digestive system is common to the different species, there are important differences of detail, both anatomical and physiological, between them.

The relative volumes of the stomach, small intestine and large intestine are very different in some of the five classes of animal, as shown by the following data, which are roughly comparative rather than accurate:

TABLE 56

Species	Stomach	Small Intestine	Cæca	Large Intestine
Cow	100*	26	4	11
Horse	100	356	185	535
Pig	100	116	13	109
Dog	100	37	1	9

* Rumen, reticulum, omasum and abomasum.

In each instance the true stomach, whose function is to secrete hydrochloric acid and pepsin for the initial breakdown of protein, is relatively small. Associated with the stomach (proventriculus) of the fowl is the gizzard, a muscular enlargement of the alimentary canal for grinding hard foods to fine material.

In the adult ruminant ingested food passes first into the rumen and not into the true stomach or abomasum. The rumen and reticulum are greatly enlarged portions of the gut where the roughly masticated food meets with digestive juices and also becomes subjected to the actions of microbial agents of diverse types. The temperature of the mass and its almost neutral reaction are very favourable for the growth of bacteria and, depending upon the type of food material available, varying amounts of protein and carbohydrate breakdown and re-synthesis occur. Extensive breakdown of cellulose usually occurs, the conditions for which have already been discussed (p. 15). Lower fatty acids are also produced and absorbed in this region.

Muscular movements of the rumen not only agitate the mass and assist the breakdown of its components, but return the food to the mouth for more mastication, after which it passes back to the rumen for further breakdown. From there it is passed into the reticulum, and thence to the omasum and abomasum. This description over-simplifies the events, but the processes which go on prior to the passage of the food into the true stomach can be said to have two main functions, firstly the optimum amount of mechanical disruption of the ingested food material, and secondly incubation with microbial agents so as to secure a high degree of breakdown of plant cellular substances. The two processes are inter-related and not separate.[3]

In all species the food products pass from the stomach into the small intestine. Into the mass flows a variety of secretions containing enzymes for the breakdown of fats, proteins, sugars and starches, but not of cellulosic substances. Absorption of the products of digestion takes place rapidly in the lower part of the small intestine. Generally speaking the pattern of digestion and absorption in this region seems to be common to the several species, though there are minor differences. It has been said, for example, that lipase is absent from the gut of the cat.[4]

There are great differences between the relative sizes and functions of the large intestine in the different species. In all cases it serves for the absorption, and hence conservation, of water from the products of digestion. There are differences in the number and sizes of the diverticulæ, the cæca, which open on to the colon.

From the point of view of digestion in ruminant herbivora, the large intestine is of relatively minor importance; its main function in them, as in omnivora and carnivora, seems to be largely one of water absorption, but in non-ruminant herbivora further digestion of plant material seems to continue. The ruminant appears to make better use of microbial agents by employing them *before* the main processes of digestion, so that the starch and protein which the bacteria synthesise for themselves can be digested by the host; but non-ruminant herbivora have not the advantage of rumination, and, though they are able to enlist the services of bacteria in the breakdown of cellulose, the operation seems in consequence to be less efficient.

In carnivora the large intestine is relatively unimportant for the digestion of plant material, while in omnivorous animals like the pig its function seems to be a minor one. The digestibility of cellulose by pigs varies in such a way as to suggest that there are several operative factors, one of them no doubt the nature of the microbial population. Cellulose digestion in the fowl also tends to be very limited.

Hitherto in this section the anatomy of the digestive tract has been stressed in relation to the ability of the animal to utilise plant material. Though one may look upon this function as being the principle one in the nutrition of herbivorous species, the considerable powers of certain bacteria to produce members of the vitamin B-complex is only slightly less useful.

What has been said so far has concerned adult stock. Animals of all species have very limited powers of digestion in the early post-natal period. For mammals milk is the food provided by nature, the young chick has the residual yolk sac to assist it during its first few days of life and the young ruminant in fact, is neither functionally nor anatomically a ruminant during its early existence.

While much study has been made of the nutritional habits of cattle, less attention has been paid to sheep and far less to goats. Of the non-ruminant herbivora the horse has received most attention, but even so the amount of work done has been far less than for cattle and sheep. In the class of omnivorous animals, the pig has been most closely studied, while, of the carnivora, relatively little work has been done at all, though a number of researches dealing with the dog and fox have been published. During the last two decades many hundreds of research papers dealing with the food habits and requirements of poultry have appeared, and a great volume of work on the needs of rodents has been published.

(b) Balances of matter and energy.

A full description of the experimental techniques used in nutritional studies would fill several volumes, so that the following section is a résumé only, further details of which will be found in the reference work quoted.[5]

The simplest of all techniques, that of trial and error, has been carried on throughout the ages. One feeds livestock on whatever foods are available and notes their effects; with a sufficiency of time, food and livestock a certain amount of information can be gained, but the method is uncontrolled and extremely inefficient.

Modern research work on the nutritional needs of livestock rests on the law of the conservation of matter and energy. It is taken for granted that whatever matter is fed to an animal during a given period of time will subsequently be distributed, in a manner typical of the food and the animal, between, (a) the fæces and urine corresponding, (b) the excretions from the lungs and skin, (c) the products of the animal, such as milk or eggs, and (d) the body substances of the animal itself. If, for example, the organic portion of the ration fed during a certain length of time contains 20 gm. of carbon in combination as fat, protein, etc., then the 20 gm. must be present in its entirety in the various fractions mentioned above. A " balance " is thus made.

The measurement of food intake, as of milk or eggs produced, is relatively easy, and in most instances the chemical analysis presents few difficulties, but the detection of the fæces and urine corresponding to the food ingested is more difficult. One way of solving the difficulty is to mix the food with some insoluble coloured substance, which colours the fæces; such a marker may be used to denote the beginning and end of a period of feeding, but the method often falls far short of perfection, even with omnivorous animals, and it is useless with herbivorous species. The most satisfactory way is to feed the animal at a fixed rate for a long period of time so as to enable a uniform rate of excretion of fæces and urine to become established. Once a steady condition has been established—a matter of several days, even in the simplest of cases—the food intake and corresponding excretions for a suitable number of consecutive days may be determined.

Balances of the above type are called " material balances ", but energy balances are often carried out, either alone, or in association with material balances. The energy referred to in this way is either actual heat as such or the potential heat of oxidation of metabolic substances. It is assumed, for example, that the whole of the potential heat of oxidation of any food ingested must be found in (a) the heats of oxidation of fæces, urine and skin secretions corresponding, (b) the heats of oxidation of any useful products obtained, such as milk or eggs, (c) the actual heat loss of the body to its surroundings in the form of radiation, conduction and convection, (d) the heat equivalent of any work done and (e) the heat of oxidation of any increase of body tissue. Of these items those grouped in (a) and (b) are relatively easy to determine, whereas item (d) is difficult to measure except under rigid conditions which are hard to apply to actual practice, while the determination of (c) requires fundamentally the enclosure of the animal in a calorimeter so that its heat loss may be found. Animal calorimeters for large animals are expensive to build and operate, so that indirect methods are often used for the determination of heat loss. Item (e) often has to be found as a difference figure, although weight gains under carefully controlled conditions may give an estimate of its magnitude. Alternatively, numbers of animals being treated in a similar way throughout a standardised feeding experiment may be slaughtered in successive small subgroups at regular intervals of time. In each case the whole carcase of the animal is chemically analysed to determine its contents of organic and inorganic constituents. By this method information as to the amounts of fat, protein, etc., which have been deposited in the body during regular intervals of time, may be found. For small animals this method is not too difficult, but it involves a great deal of work with the larger species.

(2) The maintenance requirements of animals

(a) Basal metabolism of mature animals.

The purpose of nutritional research is not the pursuit of rigid feeding standards to be applied to all types of livestock without critical appreciation, but the separation, so far as it is possible, of the different factors which cause the food requirements of one animal to be different from those of another, or the needs of the same animal to be different at different stages of its life. The qualitative recognition of such factors is not enough; it is desirable that they should be capable of quantitative expression.

Despite the limitations of the method, which have been stressed elsewhere (p. 279), it is convenient to try to summarise the needs of livestock with respect to the total energy they need and the proportions of that energy which should be derived from protein, fat, carbohydrates, and other nutrients. In Section I a study of the kinds of protein, fat and other constituents which are needed in a ration has already been given.

The heat output (usually expressed in Cal./day) of an animal which is engaged in performing the bodily functions that constitute the bare necessities of life, is described as its basic metabolic rate. If the animal is lying still and is therefore in need of no food energy for muscular work, if its digestive tract is empty, so that no digestive processes are occurring and there is no stimulation of the heat production of the body due to absorbed nutrients, and if the temperature of its environment is such that the animal does not have to increase its metabolism to withstand cold nor change its physiological state to offset excessive heat, then whatever energy it requires for the work of the heart and lungs, the preservation of muscular tone and the maintenance of other vital processes is the energy of basal metabolism. The animal must receive *digestible* food energy at least equal to that rate in order to live.

Many determinations of the basal metabolism of different species have been made, and it has been shown conclusively that if the heat requirements are expressed in terms of Calories/Kg. of bodyweight, then, with increasing body size, the values vary from about 200 for the mouse to 8 for the elephant, i.e., the needs of small animals are greater in proportion to their bodyweights than those of large ones.

For reasons which are not of importance here it seems that the basal metabolic rates of all mammals are reasonably well given by the equation

$$B.M.(Cal.) = 39.5W^{0.7}$$

where " W " is the weight of the animal in pounds.[5] For birds the power of " W " is more nearly 0.64.

A selection of the data compiled by Brody is given in the table below:

TABLE 57

Species and sex	Bodywt. (lb.)	B.M. (Cal./day)	Deviation of calculated from observed values %
Elephant, M & F	8,450	30,924	+ 2
Beef steer (Hereford)	2,033	9,996	— 6
Horse, Percheron, F	1,488	9,743	+15
Dairy cow, Holstein	1,120	7,958	+16
Dairy cow, Jersey	926	5,865	— 2
Shetland ponies	619	4,683	+ 6
Swine, M	441	3,660	+ 6
Pigs, M & F	159	1,342	—18
Sheep, merino F	103	1,168	— 1
Dogs, M & F	66	807	— 7
Rabbit, M & F	7.7	189	+ 7
Rat, M & F	0.5	23.6	— 4

Although the agreements are good in view of the extreme range of body-weights, one must still expect an *individual* deviation of ±20% to be within the limits of normal variation.

(b) Maintenance energy.

Animals kept under the conditions described above would be of no use in practical animal husbandry. The data, however, are of great use in so far as they provide a basis for estimating what the energy needs are of an animal when it carries out the normal standing and muscular movements associated with fairly close confinement, when it assimilates food sufficient to maintain its bodyweight and when it has to meet normal environmental conditions.

Because of variations in the nature of the food consumed, of the exact amount of exercise performed and of environmental conditions, it must be emphasised at the outset that only the most general significance can be given to the term " maintenance energy needs."

The importance of the nature of the food may be shown by the hypothetical case of two maintenance rations of equal calorific value but one consisting entirely of carbohydrate and the other of carbohydrate plus protein of high biological value. Bodyweight could never be maintained by the first ration, which could not meet the normal catabolism of body protein (p. 42); the second ration might, but its ability to do so would depend upon the proportion of protein in the ration.

Environmental conditions may vary enormously; a very cold and exposed situation will involve a greater heat loss in the maintenance of body temperature and normal bodily functions than will a temperate and sheltered position.

Similarly the amount of energy required for standing, walking and performing the simple muscular movements associated, not with violent exercise, but the simplest of activities concerned with the ingestion of food, etc., is very variable. Energy for this purpose must be greater for large animals than for small, but it does not follow that it will be directly in proportion to the first power of the bodyweight.

Though maintenance standards have been drawn up by various authorities, they differ quite widely from one another. The maintenance needs for a cow of 1,000 lb. bodyweight, for example, have been variously fixed at 7.9,[6] 6.7,[7] 6.5,[8] 6.0,[9] 5.9,[10] and 5.7[11] lb. of digestible nutrients per day. Brody,[5] who quotes the above figures, found that various specialists in this field were uncertain of the fundamental relationships between bodyweight and the respective energy increments needed, over and above basal metabolic needs, for activity, etc.

The fact must be faced that existing maintenance energy standards are empirical; they may be applied rigorously only to the conditions under which the experiments were made and to the kind of livestock employed. The individual needs of animals may well be 20% above or below the standards laid down, which, indeed, are no more than a guide, the extent of the necessary departures from which must be judged by the husbandman. Nor must this statement be taken as an argument in favour of the neglect of feeding standards; it simply implies that intelligent discrimination must be used in their application.

So far as any generalisations may be made, Brody has shown that the assumption that needs for maintenance energy are twice those of basal metabolism fits in fairly well with existing standards for sheep, dairy cows and horses.[5]

(c) Protein.

Since dietary protein is of varying biological value, the maintenance requirements of livestock for protein cannot be accurately expressed in terms of food protein; all that one may hope to do is to frame a general rule which is likely to cover average needs. As in the case of total energy, it is most convenient to use digestible food constituents as a basis for computation.

Smuts's[12] experiments showing that the endogenous loss of nitrogen under basal conditions is approximately 2 mg./Cal. require now to be mentioned. His experiments covered the wide range of bodyweights from mice to pigs, and his empirical relationship forms the basis of calculations for the protein needs for maintenance. Clearly the intake of digestible protein must make good the endogenous loss, and the questions to be settled are, firstly, the choice of conversion factor for the transformation of weights of nitrogen to those of protein, and, secondly, the factor by which the endogenous loss must be multiplied to allow for the biological value of ordinary dietary protein. For average protein the multiplication of percentage of endogenous nitrogen loss by 6.25 gives with sufficient accuracy the quantity of body protein catabolised, and, on the basis of Smuts's findings and a survey of existing feeding standards for sheep, horses and dairy cows, Brody[5] quadruples the catabolised protein to give the corresponding necessary intake of digestible protein for maintenance. The suggested standard is thus 2 x 6.25 x 4 mg. of protein for every Calorie of basal metabolism, and since maintenance energy needs are twice those of basal metabolism, 2 x 6.25 x 4 mg. of digestible protein for every 2 Cal. of maintenance energy. Since 1 gm. of digestible nutrients supplies, to a sufficient accuracy, 4 Cal., the conclusion is reached that in each 0.5 gm. of digestible nutrients for maintenance, there must be 0.05 gm. of digestible protein. On a dry matter basis the common cereal grains, legumes, fresh green crops, oil seeds, hays and silage more than satisfy this standard for cattle, but the straws and roots do not. While, therefore, the protein quota of the maintenance rations suggested makes ample allowance for the dietary protein being of low biological value, it is clear that lower standards would not be very practicable, for there are several reasons why livestock should not be kept for any lengthy period on roots and straw alone.

The feeding standards which have been variously proposed for farm animals differ from one another. In some cases the quantity of nutrients recommended varies directly as the bodyweight of the animal,[7] but the Brody,[5] Morrison,[13] and British[14] standards assume a greater need by the small animal than by the large one. These differences need cause no confusion to the livestock owner, however, who realises that differences due to varying local conditions are quite likely to be at least as great. The standards are guides; the final appeal is to the condition of the animal.

No mention has yet been made of the possibility that the maintenance needs of an animal may vary with its physiological state. The standards described do not apply to young growing stock, firstly, because their needs differ from those of mature animals of the same bodyweight, and, secondly, because one does not seek to maintain the bodyweight of a growing creature. Brody and other workers have concluded that the maintenance needs of a cow in lactation are higher than for a beast of equal weight in the dry condition.

(d) Fats, minerals and vitamins.

No very exact information is available as to the extent to which fat should form a part of the diet for maintenance. Carotene or vitamin A is needed in proportion to the bodyweight of the animal, approximately 100,000 International Units of vitamin A being required per 1,000 lb. live weight. This important factor is likely to be lacking when the conventional straw, roots and poorer quality hay are used for livestock feeding. Members of the vitamin B-complex are needed in proportion to the amount of food given; this stipulation requires most attention being paid to omnivorous and carnivorous animals. Of the inorganic elements sodium, chlorine, calcium and phosphorus, and the trace elements must be supplied.

(3) Needs for growth

(a) The general pattern of growth in young stock.

Though the change in its conditions affects the nutritional needs of the newly born mammal, there are many points of similarity between the immediate pre-natal and the post-natal requirements of such a creature. Post-natal life adds to the demands which have to be met, but there are many advantages from the nutritional standpoint of trying to view the period just before birth and that following it as one of continuous development.

It is generally true to say that the growth patterns of normal mammals and of poultry are of a similar type, regardless of species. The weight of the body increases in a fairly characteristic way and there are changes in the body's chemical composition as well as those of anatomical configuration.

If the actual weight of the animal is plotted against time, the resultant curve usually shows three fairly clearly differentiated portions, (a) a short initial period when the weight rises rather slowly, (b) a period when there is a rapid increase in weight, and (c) a final period, as the animal is approaching maturity, when the increase in weight steadily falls away to nothing. Since the young of the different species differ so much in their absolute weights, general comparisons are most easy to make if the weights of the animals are given, not in pounds, but as a percentage of their mature bodyweight.

Brody [5] has collected empirical data showing the ages, reckoned from the time of conception, at which animals ranging in size from a cow to a mouse, attain weights corresponding to various percentages of their mature bodyweights. If the times themselves are calculated as percentages of the time taken to reach maturity then the figures take the form shown in the following table:

TABLE 58

| Species. | Weight as percentage of mature bodyweight. | | | | | | |
| | 20 | 30 | 40 | 50 | 60 | 70 | 80 |
	Times as percentages of time from conception to maturity.						
Cow	15	18	22	26	31	38	47
Pig	12	15	19	23	29	36	46
Sheep	15	25	29	32	37	43	52
Guinea pig ...	18	21	24	28	33	40	49
Rat	22	25	28	31	37	43	51
Mouse	18	21	25	29	33	40	48
Averages ...	17	21	25	28	33	40	49

These figures show how growth, as indicated by bodyweight, is crowded into a relatively short time in early life; for example, the animal body attains 50% of its mature bodyweight in some 28% of the time which it needs to become mature—and that 28% includes the period of gestation.

Not only does growth take place at different rates at different times, but the nature of the body substance changes. Although the details of this phenomenon are best discussed later in this section, it may be said *generally* that the first task is the provision of an adequate framework (skeleton) upon which the muscular structures may then be built, this operation constituting the second phase of growth. The third stage is the deposition of body fat.

(b) Energy requirements during growth.

Many experiments have been made to determine the basal metabolic rates of growing animals. In the very early stages of growth the basal metabolic rate must be much less than is given by the equation relating heat production to bodyweight in mature animals. Afterwards, however, the heat production increases and for a time appears to be higher than it would be in mature stock; this period corresponds with the post-weaning stage in many mammals. Towards the end of growth heat production diminishes gradually to that characteristic of the adult. From data which have been compiled by Brody [5] one may see that the basal metabolic rates of half-grown sheep, pigs, cattle and horses are already close to the values relevant to mature animals of the same bodyweights. Table 58 shows that such species are half-grown in about a quarter of the time they take to reach maturity. Prior to that time the ratio of the basal metabolism of the growing animal to that of the mature one of the same weight may reach a value of about 1.3. This figure serves to give a general idea of the extra needs of the growing animal and to re-emphasise the importance of the earlier stages of growth.

Information with regard to the *total* requirements of dietary energy during growth is relatively scanty. A large amount of it has been derived from ad hoc feeding trials in which the number of pounds of digestible nutrients (in arbitrary rations) which will produce satisfactory weight gains has been determined. Without information as to the nature of the ration and of the corresponding " growth " this method is of limited application.

To overcome the difficulties one may attempt to compute separately the energies which are needed for the maintenance and the actual weight gains of growing stock. An excellent example of this method of approach is that of Mitchell, quoted by Maynard.[15] In this case cattle were the object of study. By slaughtering a number of them at intervals and analysing the carcases, Mitchell obtained information regarding the amounts of protein, fat, carbohydrate, etc., present in the bodies of the animals at different ages. These quantities of food constituents could be converted to the equivalent gross energy values and hence it was possible to measure the increase in growth during various intervals of time in terms of energy. Mitchell then calculated the basal metabolic requirements for the animals at each age, and assumed that 45% of this value would have to be added for simple muscular movements. At each age, by adding together the energies required for basal metabolism, exercise and the appropriate growth increment, he obtained the net energy for the process. Using data which were available regarding the relationship of net energy to metabolisable† energy for average cattle rations, Mitchell converted his net energy values to metabolisable energy and thence to pounds of digestible nutrients. At lower bodyweights the figures he thus obtained were appreciably higher than the standards set up on the basis of feeding trials, but as pointed out in other sections it is in the earlier phases when growth is most rapid, and there is evidence that when animals are free to help themselves they do so more liberally during that phase than the conventional standards allow.[16] (†Chapter 18).

It is of fundamental interest to relate the metabolisable energy which Mitchell calculates is needed at different ages to the estimated needs for basal metabolism. The actual ages of the animals, the percentages those ages constitute of the age to attain maturity and the ratios of metabolisable to basal energy are given below:

TABLE 59

Age, months	2.2	3.0	6.6	10.6	15.4	21.3	28.9
Age, % equivalent ...	13	14	18	22	27	34	42
Ratio, total energy needed to basal metabolism ...	3.7	3.6	2.9	2.7	2.6	2.5	2.5

From the general similarity of the growth curves for the different species, from considerations of basal metabolism, and from Mitchell's work, it would appear that the very young animal needs metabolisable energy equal to about four times its basal metabolic requirements.*

By the time the animal has gone through some 25% of its adolescent life the ratio has fallen to 3, after which there is a slow decline to the value of 2, corresponding to the maintenance needs of the mature beast.

Evidence from many other sources suggests that it is the early phase of growth which is the exacting one. One of the most critical papers which has yet appeared is that of Wallace, from which the following quotation is especially pertinent here.

" No better example could be provided of the paramount importance of the level of the diet in the rearing of lambs than our finding that 96% of the variation in the weight gains made by the individual lambs between birth and 112 days can be accounted for by the differences between them in respect to their consumption of milk and supplements.[17] "

Experiments which have been described by Steensberg[18] were carried out over a considerable period, using young cattle of three different breeds and in such numbers as to make the observed differences trustworthy. Here again the gains in weight of the animals were higher in the early stages of growth under the influence of higher planes of nutrition. The following table shows the average increments of weight under the different conditions.

* It would appear that Brody's equation for mature beasts would also be accurate enough for growing stock after weaning.

TABLE 60

Period for which growth increase is given. (Age in months)		Weight gains in pounds.		
		Low plane of nutrition	Average plane of nutrition.	High plane of nutrition.
3.5 to 5.5		70	88	106
5.5 to 8.5		73	103	121
8.5 to 11.5		86	119	132
11.5 to 15.5		134	134	145
15.5 to 18.5		95	95	70

Although there are no data available concerning the body compositions of these animals, the results suggest that young stock benefit by higher planes of nutrition during the early phase of growth, but it must be repeated that the more exact specification of the nutritional requirements during the period of growth await more comprehensive information as to what changes of body composition constitute " growth ".

(c) Protein needs.

When the needs of livestock for protein during the period of growth are considered, it is no longer possible to be content with weight gains as indications of growth. So far as the organic constituents of the body are concerned the main change in body composition is the increased deposition of protein. This, however, is accompanied by the production and deposition of body fat to a degree which varies with the nature and age of the animal itself and the plane and kind of nutrition. In most cases it is possible to control the amount of fattening which occurs and in practice it is usually left until a comparatively late stage of development. By altering the plane of nutrition of pigs, Hammond and McMeekan[19] were able to show that, with a given ration, regardless of the rate of feeding, the needs for the development of the skeleton and vital organs were met first, then those of the musculature, and finally for the deposition of fat. Plane of nutrition affected the rate at which these processes occurred but not their order.

Observations of this kind make it hazardous to attempt to study the protein requirements of growing stock on the basis of weight increases, although this method can be used where different rations, made up to include different but known proportions of protein, are then fed to groups of animals of the same species, sex, age and condition, the respective weight gains over equal intervals of time being determined. The minimal proportion of protein in the ration, which gives the optimal growth rate, is a measure of the requirements of the stock at that particular age. Repetition of the process for groups of animals of a different age will, in time, provide the information, as to the animal's need, but only in terms of dietary intake of a particular kind.

As Mitchell[20] has stated, however, " protein requirements may be conveniently and rationally expressed in terms referable to the animal rather than to its feed ". Such a method of expression necessarily involves the acquisition of information as to the actual amounts of protein present in the body at various stages of growth, and details of this kind may be obtained in two ways, (a) by slaughtering groups of animals at different ages and analysing the carcases, or (b) using nitrogen balance data. The latter method is as tedious as the direct use of weight gains and will not be considered further.

The slaughter technique has a long history, the early part of which has been surveyed by Armsby,[21] who attempted to devise a mathematical formula which would cover the protein needs of growing cattle and other species. His attempt was founded on uncertain premises and did not yield accurate predictions of the protein deposition in young cattle save over a limited middle portion of the growth period.

Slaughter experiments carried out by Mitchell and quoted by Maynard[15] showed the amounts of body protein which were laid down in normal heifers at ages ranging from approximately 2 to 29 months and for corresponding bodyweights of 150 to 1,200 lb. The amounts range from approximately 0.45 lb./day in the youngest animal to one-sixth of that quantity in the oldest. At the appropriate ages, therefore, this quantity of digestible protein of biological value 100 would have to be provided per day for growth alone. There is, however, a maintenance need, which Mitchell calculated on the basis set out on p. 250. In the early stages of growth he found that the ratio of the protein needed for the formation of new tissue to that needed for the maintenance was about 8 : 1, whereas, near maturity, it had fallen to 1 : 3. The overall needs for protein ranged from 0.5 lb. to about 0.25 lb. per day with increasing bodyweight. Average daily needs of digestible dietary protein of biological value 50 would imply twice these quantities.

Data of this kind may be of greater value if the total needs for protein are converted into the equivalent energy values and then expressed as a percentage of the total digestible energy needed for the corresponding stage of growth. For the early stages of growth, some 14.4% of the energy would thus be needed from protein of biological value 100; towards maturity the proportion would sink to 3.2%. In terms of average dietary protein of biological value 50 these proportions would have to be doubled. These requirements may only be applied quantitatively to cattle, but the general principle applies to other species.

In considering the protein needs of young stock useful information should be provided by a study of the natural first food of mammals, namely milk. The milk provided by the dam seems to be highly digestible and to have a high biological value for the young of the species. Discounting for the moment the variations of composition due to breed and stage of lactation, the table below shows the protein content of the milk of various species, the fraction of the total energy which is provided by milk protein, together with relevant physiological data.

TABLE 61

No.	Species.	Time during which birth weight is doubled (days).	Protein content of milk. Weight %	Protein calories, as percentage of total calories.
1.	Man	180	2.1	18
2.	Ape		1.4	12
3.	Monkey		2.1	17
4.	Horse	60	2.1	26
5.	Ass		2.0	22
6.	Mule		1.6	21
7.	Zebra		3.0	21
8.	Cow	47	3.4	27
9.	Buffalo		4.1	21
10.	Goat	22	2.9	21
11.	Sheep	15	4.2	21
12.	Reindeer		10.1	26
13.	Pig	14	5.8	26
14.	Llama		3.9	31
15.	Camel		4.0	31
16.	Elephant		3.1	8
17.	Cat	9.5	7-9	39-51
18.	Dog	9	7-11	25-39
19.	Fox		6.2	32
20.	Rabbit	6	10-15	27-46
21.	Rat		11.8	31

Not all of the data in the table are equally trustworthy, especially those for the less commonly studied species, such as the elephant, for the more retractive ones, such as the carnivores, and for the smaller and less easily managed ones, such as the rat, but, even so, some useful general conclusions may be drawn, namely:

(a) On the whole, rodents and carnivorous animals produce milk richer in protein than herbivorous animals; the milk of primates is poorest in protein.

(b) Rodents and carnivorous animals produce a type of milk of which protein provides well over 30% of the total calories.

(c) Herbivorous animals, especially the domesticated ones, secrete milk containing about 25% of the total energy in the form of protein.

(d) The corresponding figure for primates is about 15%.

(e) So far as it is possible to tell from the incomplete data, the more rapid the growth of the young of a species, the higher is the proportion of protein in the milk appropriate to the species.

Milk substitutes for young stock must contain something like the equivalent of the above percentages of digestible protein of high biological value, or, if possible, its equivalent. During the very early growth period, the difficulty of meeting this requirement alone almost necessitates the use of milk to produce optimal growth.

Many herbivorous species produce their young at such a time of the year that young green crops would normally be the food on to which they would' be gradually weaned. Such crops provide some 20% of their digestible energy in the form of protein.

Although experiments with calves have shown that they gain weight when given rations, adequate in quantity, but low in protein (up to 0.17 lb. protein per 100 lb. of live weight), it should not be assumed that this is a satisfactory type of growth. Long-term experiments have shown that the growth of calves is much improved by high protein intakes [22] and the standards suggested by the prolonged experiments of Steensberg [23] approach the values proposed by Mitchell.[15]

From what has been said in this section, despite the lack of detailed information, it may be seen that the protein needs of young growing stock are high, especially during the early phase of growth. It is to the advantage of the animal and the livestock owner to use this rapid growth rate to the full, for, if the animal does not make satisfactory gain at this time, then most of the food which is actually being given is being used for non-productive maintenance.

(d) Requirements for fat during growth.

Studies of the nutritive values of fats have been far more neglected than those of total energy, carbohydrate or protein. There seems to be a common belief that many species of livestock do not tolerate large proportions of fat in their diets. If the word protein were used as regardlessly of amino-acid composition as the word fat is employed without regard for the kinds and proportions of fatty acids which may be combined in such material, there would now be no logical account of the essential amino-acids.

The fat content of milk tends to parallel the protein content. Whereas the sugar content of milk usually lies within the range of 3-6 per cent. by weight, the percentage of fat may rise to 10-15 per cent. in rodents and carnivora, and to much higher values in mammals which have to withstand severe environmental conditions. Reindeer milk, for example, is said to contain over 20 per cent. of fat, while the milk of aquatic mammals may include more than 40 per cent. A high percentage of fat in milk is thus quite a normal phenomenon, and only in the camel, llama and members of the equine group does fat provide less than 50 per cent. of the total calories, the usual value being, indeed, around 70 per cent.

The nature of the fat appears to be important, at least in some species. For example, when calves were given various fats, added to skim-milk, so as to form " milk " of 3.5 per cent. fat content, it was found that animal fats produced better results than vegetable oils and that butter-fat gave the best result.[24]

Although much more study is needed of the nutritional value of fats, one may conclude from the available evidence that they play an important part in the growth of the young animal.

(e) Carbohydrate in the nutrition of growing animals.

On this subject attention must briefly be directed to a study of fibre, starch and the sugars. Lactose is the unique sugar received by all mammals in the milk appropriate to the species and it provides a good proportion (25 - 50 per cent.) of the total energy in the milk of the common herbivorous animals of temperate climates. It appears to produce suitable types of bacteria in the alimentary tract, with conditions favourable for the absorption of calcium and phosphorus.

Starch and fibre are probably best considered together. Some fibre is necessary for the complete development of the rumen of the young ruminant, and it is best to provide good quality fibrous foods and to allow young ruminants to take their pick of them. The metabolism of starch, cellulose and protein are so inter-related in the ruminant and, despite the excellent reviews of this field which have recently appeared, are so little understood, that generalisations need to be made cautiously. Evidence in relation to the non-ruminant, especially the omnivorous and carnivorous animals, is even more scanty. One may say that for the very young stock of all species the crude fibre content of the ration should be kept very low and then increased gradually, at first in accordance with the free choice of the animal, up to the amount which the mature beast can handle (p. 15).

(f) Mineral needs during growth.

Consideration of the ash content of milk gives the first indication of the possible needs of young stock for minerals. In most instances some 5 per cent. or more of the total solids of milk consist of inorganic elements, chiefly calcium, phosphorus, sodium, potassium and chlorine.

Although milk contains a number of other elements in smaller amounts, it is the above five which are largely concerned in the formation of bone and in the regulation of the balance of the blood. Hammond and his collaborators [19] have shown that it is skeletal development which is the first achievement of the normal growing animal. Unless the necessary elements are provided in the food of such creatures, they are likely to be unthrifty, stunted and subject to bone defects. It is only the worst cases of calcium and phosphorus deficiencies which produce the bad clinical cases of rickets; for every such an example there must be many more where the bone formation is sub-optimal but the fault is not visible to the eye, and may only make itself felt during the additional strain of pregnancy or lactation in later life.

In few foods are calcium and phosphorus present in such a suitable form as in milk; young growing stock which are not receiving milk benefit, therefore, from the inclusion in the ration of foods such as bone meal and fish meal, which do contain substantial proportions of both elements.

The quantities of calcium and phosphorus which must be present in a ration to satisfy the demands of a growing animal depend upon its stage of growth, the relative proportions of the two elements, and the nature of the ration, especially its vitamin D content. This subject has been stressed elsewhere, (p. 67) but it deserves mention again here.

A salt lick will provide sufficient sodium and chlorine, and, in the case of the crude salt, will also furnish sufficient iodine, although in certain areas, iodide supplements may have to be provided. Attention has already been drawn to mineral deficiency diseases which affect some species of young stock (p. 66).

(g) Vitamin requirements.

Vitamin A, or its precursors, is needed by all species in much higher proportion for growth than for simple maintenance. The first source for the mammal is the colostrum and milk which constitute the natural food of the young. In the case of growing herbivorous species this is then supplemented and finally replaced by fresh green foods. Well-made silage and good quality, dried grass are potent sources of carotene, but hay is an uncertain and, in very many cases, a poor source of carotene. For feeding omnivorous and carnivorous animals, it is safer to rely on cod liver oil to provide vitamin A; such animals as the growing pig will consume limited amounts of green foods but in practice, except where they have free range, small supplements of fish liver oil should be given regularly.

For mammals of all species Hart[25] suggests a daily need of about 50 μg. of carotene, or about one-fourth of that weight of vitamin A, per Kg. of bodyweight. There is some evidence that the needs of poultry may be higher than this.

Elsewhere the importance of the "balance" of a diet has been stressed and vitamin A provides a good example of this point, for a diet which provides enough total energy and digestible protein but is lacking in vitamin A is less efficient than one containing the vitamin. Various groups of workers have shown that in growing, vitamin A - deficient animals the utilisation of absorbed protein is poorer than in the normal animal,[26] and this impaired use of absorbed nutrients is measurable long before some of the symptoms of prolonged deficiency may be detected. As in the case of so many other factors in the diet, sub-optimal intake of vitamin A may lead to diminished appetite with a correspondingly lower growth rate. Other results of such rations are impaired bone formation with, in some instances, consequential nerve lesions.[27] In all, therefore, it is of the greatest practical importance that the young animal should not be deficient in vitamin A.

Sufficient has been said in Section I to indicate the need of young stock for adequate vitamin D in the diet. The suckling will derive enough of this factor from the milk of the dam, if the conditions under which the latter has been maintained have permitted, i.e., the dam or her food has been exposed to adequate amounts of sunlight. Apart from such instances it is better to make sure of vitamin D intake by giving fish liver oil in graded doses, or by feeding well-cured hay to appropriate species. The former has the advantage of supplying vitamins A and D together. The young mammal, on a diet which is adequate with respect to calcium and phosphorus, requires about 3 I.U. of vitamin D per lb. liveweight per day, either D_2 or D_3 being adequate, but growing chicks, probably because of their more rapid growth rates, require about 180 I.U./lb. of feed, in the form of the natural vitamin D_3. Higher levels will be needed in cases of diets imbalanced with respect to calcium and phosphorus (p. 68). In the absence of sufficient vitamin D, young animals are likely to show retarded growth as well as bone deformations which may diminish their productive efficiencies in mature life.

In the earliest stages of growth all growing animals need preformed members of the vitamin B group in their diet and such factors seem to be present in adequate amounts in milk. As growth proceeds the herbivorous animals establish with the micro-organisms of their alimentary tracts symbiotic relationships which make the *normal* animal largely independent of dietary sources of members of the B-complex. Omnivorous and carnivorous species continue to need dietary supplies of these vitamins, however, so that it is such animals as the growing pig and dog which require most attention in practice. Nevertheless calves which are being artificially reared may benefit by being given supplements of foods which are rich in the vitamin B-complex, such as dried yeast, since the establishment of a satisfactory intestinal flora is a complex matter, related to the diet in a manner by no means fully understood. Favourable results of the feeding of dried yeast to calves have several times been reported. Where young pigs are reared under fairly natural conditions, with access to fresh green foods, vitamin B deficiency is unlikely to arise, but very often the animals are put on to diets containing large amounts of kitchen waste. Such material, by virtue of its origin or subsequent treatment, may not be satisfactory: here again, yeast supplements are beneficial. Young growing poultry under intensive rearing systems are liable to suffer from deficiencies of members of the vitamin B-complex, especially of riboflavin. Mild deficiencies may produce nothing more obvious than retarded growth, but a severe lack of riboflavin produces the characteristic "curled-toe paralysis". Dried yeast, wheat germ or dried milk in the ration will offset such deficiencies. There is no doubt, however, that a good supply of fresh green foods will supply for young stock not only carotene, but also many members of the vitamin B group and other trace materials, as well as good protein: where it is possible to do so such greenstuff should be supplied regularly.

(4) Nutritional requirements during pregnancy

(a) Introduction.

Nutritional needs for satisfactory reproduction do not begin when the male and female of a species are mated, but much earlier than this. At such a time the animals should be in good condition but not fat: they should have received balanced rations adequate with respect to total energy, protein content and quality, fat, vitamins and minerals. Poor feeding during growth should not have led to deformations of the pelvis in the female for example, nor too low a vitamin A intake to reduced fertility in both sexes. From very many points of view it is highly desirable that a reasonable amount of fresh green food should have been a regular component of the rations of ordinary farm livestock at all times. Rations consisting of the usual roots, straw and hay of doubtful quality are lacking in too many factors to be satisfactory for long-term feeding, and the same criticism applies to some of the household waste given to pigs or fowls. Feeding prior to mating, therefore, should be fairly generous with respect to quality but not so far as quantity is concerned. The result of an unsuccessful mating is that, until the next successful one an animal is having to be fed for maintenance purposes alone and its value as a production unit is lost. Since maintenance costs are nearly always a rather large proportion of the total cost of keeping livestock, it is false economy to bring about the state of affairs described above purely by negligent or niggardly feeding.

In the case of the mammal the fertilised egg is small and, although it undergoes extensive anatomical changes during the early stages of its growth, following its attachment to the uterine wall, in terms of actual weight increase its changes are quite small. During the early stages of pregnancy it is the development of the placenta and of the maternal organs generally, in readiness for the demands that will have to be met during the last third of the period of gestation, which is most responsible for any increase in the quantity of nutrients for the pregnant animal. During this time, the additional need for food is, indeed, relatively small.

During the last third of pregnancy the weight of the fœtus increases rapidly and some additional nutrients must be supplied for it. Even at birth, however, the weight of the young is but a small fraction of the weight of the dam and the problem is still one of quality rather than of quantity of feed. The ration must meet the requirements of the fœtus and be such as will give rise to a good lactation after parturition.

The maintenance of a high level of egg production in the fowl also requires careful attention to the quality of the food given; poor feeding will lead to diminished egg production, so that for a greater proportion of its life than need be the case the bird is receiving food for maintenance only.

(b) Requirements for energy.

Some indication of the energy requirements of pregnancy may be obtained from slaughter experiments, groups of females of a given species and initial weight being killed at regular intervals during pregnancy and the carcases analysed. By this means the changing composition of the whole body and of its constituent organs, as well as that of the growing fœtus, may be observed. An example of this kind of experiment is one which was carried out on pregnant gilts.[28]

So far as the growth of the uterine products was concerned, it was found that the gross energy increases were as shown in the table below:

TABLE 62

Week of gestation	2	4	6	8	10	12	14	16
Increase, Cal./day	6	21	45	76	115	160	213	272
Increase, as per cent. of final week's increase	2	8	17	28	42	59	78	100

These figures illustrate the relatively high demands of the last third of the period of gestation.

Over the whole period the average increase in gross energy was 104 Cal./day, as compared with the final value of 272. These values represent the net energy of pregnancy, and they would have to be multiplied by some factor in order to convert them into corresponding metabolisable energy values and thence into digestible energies. As is shown in Chapter 18, the exact value of the factor would depend upon the nature of the ration; it would probably lie somewhere between 1 and 2, and, if the upper value is taken for comparative purposes, then it is probably large enough to allow for the fact that other parts of the female body than the uterus are concerned in tissue formation during pregnancy. In round numbers the average requirement in Cal./day thus becomes 200, with the corresponding maximal value of 550. For animals of the size used in the above experiments, basal metabolic requirements are approximately 2,000 Cal./day and maintenance needs about twice that figure. The extra food requirements of pregnancy are thus of the order of 5 per cent. of the maternal maintenance needs, while the maximum demand is some three times as much.

There is no question of feeding at very high levels during reproduction, but the food intake should be adjusted in quantity and quality to the condition of the animal.

Where the female is being bred before she herself has reached maturity, then a higher plane of nutrition still is to be aimed at. One cannot lay down precise rules for this since the extra nutrients needed will depend upon the stage of growth which has been reached. It cannot be too clearly stressed, however, that preparation for the subsequent lactation is being made during this period and that feeding practice must be sound. Knowledge is still incomplete as to the exact amounts of the different nutrients which are needed at different stages during pregnancy but it is certain that close attention must be paid to the total energy, protein, vitamin and mineral fractions. These last are dealt with below, but before leaving this section, which concerns the overall plane of nutrition more than any other, one cannot do better than turn to some of the experiments which have been reported by Wallace in connection with the feeding of sheep."

Many workers (see Hammond[29]) have shown that the plane of nutrition of the mother affects the birth weight of the young. The increased weight of the young is important in so far as it indicates a greater degree of development at birth and a better chance of survival. In the case of a poorly fed ewe the single foetus may draw upon the maternal reserves, but this is not so with twin lambs and under such conditions a high mortality among twin lambs can be expected and is actually encountered. A still lower plane of nutrition, even for single lambs, produces weak lambs.

Wallace carried out experiments of this type in greater detail than previous workers had done. He concluded:

". . . both the birth weight of the lamb and the milk yield of the ewe are profoundly affected by the level of nutrition of the ewe during the last 6 weeks of pregnancy. By extreme ill-feeding during this period the birth weight of twin lambs may be approximately halved. . . . The vigour of the lambs is much diminished where the ewes have been inadequately fed before lambing, and the likelihood of losses of both lambs and ewes at lambing time is much increased.

" It is suggested that the weight and vigour of the lambs at birth is important, not merely for avoiding losses, but also in enabling the lambs to take full advantage of the potential milk supply of their dams."

This ability to take a greater quantity of milk leads in turn to an enhanced capacity for dealing with supplementary food at a later date.

Wallace showed that it is the feeding of the ewe during the latter part of pregnancy which is critical. When the ewes were well fed during this period " the gains made by the gravid uteri were equally great whether the animals had started this period with well stocked or depleted bodily reserves ". On the other hand good feeding during the early part of pregnancy achieved no better results than poor feeding if the plane of nutrition was low during the last part.

There is no reason whatever to believe that these stipulations apply to sheep and not to other species.

(c) Protein needs.

Many experiments have shown that the chemical composition of the carcase of young stock differs from that of mature animals of the same species in containing a higher proportion of protein and much less fat.[19] [30] During development of the foetus protein is needed; such protein can either be furnished by the maternal diet or, if the feeding be unsatisfactory, will be derived from the maternal tissues, provided that the pregnant animal has previously been sufficiently well nourished.

Mitchell's data for pigs again suffice to illustrate the way in which the quantity of protein stored in the uteri changes as gestation proceeds. If the amounts of protein stored each day are plotted graphically against the time since conception, then, as for total energy, a curve is produced which shows a much increased demand for the last third of the period. The following table shows the nature of the changes:

TABLE 63

Week of gestation		2	4	6	8	10	12	14	16
Protein increase, gm./day		1.5	4.2	7.7	12	16	21	27	33
Increase as percentage of final week's increase		5	13	23	36	48	63	81	100

The above amounts of protein are best expressed in terms of the maternal maintenance requirements, which are 0.216 lb. or approximately 100 gm./day on the basis described on p. 250. The ratio of protein deposited in the uteri each day thus varies from 1.5 per cent. of the maternal maintenance needs at the beginning of gestation to 33 per cent. at the end. As, however, the standards fixed for maintenance presuppose the use of dietary protein of rather low biological value, the above percentages must be multiplied by a factor of about four to correspond. This adjustment implies that the average protein requirement during pregnancy is about 60 per cent. of the maternal maintenance needs, the actual amount towards the end of gestation rising to over 100 per cent. These figures make no allowance for any protein deposition other than in the uteri but the rather low biological value which has been assumed for the dietary protein will probably compensate for this.

It is of interest to pursue the line of reasoning and to consider how the ratio of protein to non-protein calories in the diet ought perhaps to be varied during pregnancy. On the basis of 100 Cal. of digestible energy representing the maintenance level, it has been shown that some 10 Cal. should be derived from digestible protein. Average total energy requirements during pregnancy may now be fixed at the higher level of 105 Cal., the maximum of 115 being reached during the last period. Average protein requirements, however, are some 160 per. cent. of the maintenance needs, and must thus be fixed at 16 Cal. during pregnancy instead of the 10 Cal. needed for maintenance, while the highest figure becomes about 23 Cal. The data are conveniently summarised in the table below:

TABLE 64

	Maintenance	Pregnancy (av.)	Pregnancy (late)
Total digestible energy	100	105	115
Digestible protein, Cal.	10	16	23
Digestible protein, per cent.	10	(app.) 15	(app.) 20

At the end of gestation about 20 per cent. of the digestible energy should thus be furnished by protein.

Comparatively few slaughter data are available for other species, but there is little ground for the assumption that the position is materially different, while such work as that of Wallace, though not specifically directed towards a consideration of protein needs, supports the general thesis. The amount required by gilts, arrived at on the basis of the above reasoning, is in line with standards suggested by Morrison,[30] namely 0.43 to 0.47 lb. of digestible protein per day. It is somewhat higher than the suggested rations for cattle and sheep, although provision is made for the feeding of more concentrates to them during the last period of pregnancy. Halnan and Garner, in England, have suggested a high level of feeding for cows during this period, as much as 10 to 20 lb. of production concentrates per day being given.[31] On physiological grounds there seems to be every reason to believe that this is sound practice. Halnan's revised estimates of the requirements of poultry for egg production also imply a high level of protein in the ration.[32]

(d) Mineral requirements.

In this case also it has been shown by slaughter experiments that there is a rising demand for minerals, in particular for calcium, phosphorus and iron, during the latter part of gestation. The available data are few, however, so that it is possible to express needs for these elements only in the most general terms. Foods which are rich in calcium, phosphorus and iron should form a part of the ration during pregnancy: if they are not so provided there is every chance that the needs of the fœtus may be met by withdrawal of maternal reserves. In the case of the dairy cow, where the demand also remains high during the subsequent lactation, such a lack is likely to produce very undesirable results.

One factor which tends to make it difficult to lay down standards with regard to the most suitable levels of intake of mineral elements is their varying availabilities in different foods. In good fish or bone meals, for example, calcium and phosphorus are present in good proportions for bone formation and in a form which is easily assimilated. The presence of soluble oxalate in certain green foods or of phytic acid in cereals, however, tends to carry through the gut calcium which may be supplied by other components of a ration. Similarly the solubility of ferric oxide is so low that it is almost useless as a source of iron in a mineral supplement. Another factor which complicates the position, so far as home produced foodstuffs are concerned, is that there are likely to be deficiencies of particular mineral elements or cases of mineral imbalance which are characteristic of certain regions. There are wide areas of the world where the soil and therefore the forage is lacking in phosphorus, and where nutritional deficiency diseases follow; there are other regions where iodine is lacking, or cobalt, or copper. In such areas poor fertility or faulty reproduction will be found in livestock which live on the natural produce of the district. The following table, showing the daily mineral needs of pregnant animals, is thus no more than a rough guide to the needs of the different species. (Data for the laying hen have also been included.)

TABLE 65

Element	Horse	Cow	Pig	Sheep	Dog	Laying hen
Calcium						
Gm., average ...	—	12	16	3	1–2	—
Gm., maximum ...	—	28	—	5	—	—
As % of ration ...	0.4	0.2	0.4	—	0.5	2–4
Phosphorus						
Gm., average ...	—	14	11	2–3	0.7	—
Gm., maximum ...	—	20	—	3–4	—	—
As % of ration ...	0.3	0.2	—	—	—,	0.6–0.8
Sodium chloride						
Gm., average ...	—	— »	15	14	1–2	0.5 (added)
As % of ration ...	0.3 (added)	0.5 (added)	—	—	—	0.5

The above data have been taken from several sources.[33][34][35][36]. In the case of the larger animals requirements for common salt are perhaps best met by the provision of a salt lick.

(e) The needs for vitamins.

The needs for vitamin A or its precursors during pregnancy are three or four times those which are sufficient for simple maintenance. When the vitamin A content of a ration is high enough for the beast to appear to be in excellent condition, it can still be too low, for satisfactory reproduction.

In the case of herbivorous animals there is no doubt that these needs are best satisfied, not on an arithmetical basis, but by the provision of fresh or preserved green foods. Fresh green foods satisfy many needs, in addition to those for carotene; well produced dried grass, or silage, is also very efficient. Hay, however, is not a reliable source of carotene, nor is dried grass if it has been stored for a long time under adverse conditions.

Vitamin A is needed both by the male and the female for good reproduction, and on this score the feeding of bulls is by no means always quite so good as it might be. A ration which may consist of oat straw, roots, plus second quality hay, even when it is fortified with some of the protein concentrates, provides very moderate amounts of carotene: it requires improvement.

The lack of sufficient carotene or vitamin A may lead to the young being blind at birth, it may cause the production of deformed or still-born young, or it can lead to fœtal resorption, or retained placenta and other undesirable abnormalities. What is more, the need for satisfactory feeding, including the provision of vitamin A, begins even before the animal is served. Low fertility is a heavy price to pay for niggardly or foolish feeding practice since an animal which fails to conceive after service is an unproductive one and therefore an uneconomic proposition by any standards. In the case of fowls, egg production will be sub-optimal if the diet is deficient in vitamin A or its precursors.

Green foods provide a solution to the problem so far as the herbivorous animals are concerned; the pig, too, will benefit from such feeding,
for the actual intake which is necessary is not great, but it is often a safer
plan to include fish liver oils or carotene concentrates in the diets of
pigs and dogs and other carnivorous animals.

Vitamin D is also required by pregnant animals for the effective
utilisation of calcium and phosphorus, especially in the last stage of
gestation. Well cured hay—which may thereby be deficient in carote-
noids—will provide limited amounts of vitamin D, but under the present
tendencies towards intensive animal production it is probably safer to
rely on fish liver oils or some of the concentrates containing synthetic
vitamin D. Fowls require vitamin D_3, vitamin D_2 being much less
effective.

Members of the vitamin B-complex are also needed in rather greater
amounts for pregnancy than for maintenance purposes, but relatively few
data are yet available as to precise needs. The ruminant and, to a lesser
extent, other non-ruminant herbivorous animals are independent of
dietary supplies of these vitamins. There would be little point in giving
lists of the requirements of the different components of the B-complex
when knowledge is still so incomplete. For animals such as the sow and
the bitch, as for the laying hen, potent sources of the complex as a whole
should find their place in the ration.

(5) The nutritional requirements of lactating animals

(a) The chemical composition of milk.

Where the bodyweight and condition of the animal are not to be
changed, the law of the conservation of mass implies that the necessary
food to be supplied for milk production in lactating animals cannot be
less than the content of nutrients in the milk yield obtained.

Many analyses of the milk produced by the different species of
animals have been made and, though the greater part of them have been
concerned with cow's milk only, there seems to be little doubt that the
physiological processes which occur in all lactating animals are fundamentally the same.

The composition of a sample of milk depends upon many factors,
including, (a) the species and breed of the animal concerned (b) the
individual characteristics of the particular beast within a species or
breed, (c) the stage of lactation at which the sample was taken, (d) the
time of day when the milking was done and the time during a single
milking when the sample was collected and (e) the nature of the diet
which the animal has been given. For the present it will be sufficient
to consider only such variations as come under the first heading, smooth-
ing out the remaining effects by taking the averages for large numbers
of samples.

The major constituents of milk are four, protein, fat, lactose and
mineral matter. In the following table are set out the compositions of
the milks produced by animals of several different species and of three

typical breeds of cow: in addition to the contents of the four food constituents mentioned, the weights of total digestible nutrients per pound and the corresponding gross energies are given.

TABLE 66

Species	Protein	Composition Lactose	Fat	Ash	Total dig. nutr. per lb.	Gross energy per lb.
	%	%	%	%	lb.	Cal.
Cow (Average) ...	3.4	4.75	3.75	0.75	0.183	330
Ewe	4.2	4.8	7.4	0.9	0.285	513
Mare	2.1	6.9	0.8	0.4	0.119	215
Goat	2.9	4.8	4.5	0.8	0.196	352
Sow	5.8	5.1	8.2	0.9	0.321	596
Rabbit	13	2	13	3	0.55	1000 (Approx.)
Bitch	10	3	11	2	0.42	750 (Approx.)
Rat	10.4	2.8	13.3	1.4	0.486	877
Cow, Jersey ...	3.9	4.9	5.2	0.7	0.227	410
Cow, Ayrshire ...	3.6	4.7	4.1	0.7	0.196	355
Cow, Friesian ...	3.4	4.9	3.5	0.7	0.174	315

Other species than the cow have not been extensively studied. The following arguments, therefore, are strictly applicable to cow's milk, but with suitable modifications may be used for the other species.

(b) Energy requirements for milk production.

Discounting for the moment any differences which may occur between breeds, or between individuals of the same breed, many experiments have been carried out to determine what relationship exists between the amount of food given, over and above the maintenance needs of the animal, and the weight of milk which is produced. Calculations made by Brody,[5] for example, show that the ratio of milk energy produced to productive energy consumed (the " net " or " partial " efficiency) tends to fall with increasing milk production.

Milk protein, like other protein, requires suitable nitrogenous compounds to be provided for its synthesis, so that the net efficiency of milk production must depend upon the amount and nature of the protein in the production ration. With no such protein given for milk production a cow might still continue for some time to give milk at the expense of her own body protein; the same position could arise if the dietary protein were of very low biological value, but instances of this kind are clearly of no practical value save as examples of the wisdom of keeping the animals in good condition against future, temporary, food shortages. The highest attainable efficiency of conversion of food energy to milk energy is not known, but under ordinary practical feeding conditions it is about 60%[5] and tends to fall towards 40% as the volume of milk produced increases; with normal rations, for every 100 Cal. of energy in the milk, on the average 170 to 200 Cal. of digestible food energy must be supplied.

For the purpose of calculating food requirements for lactation in cattle, a particular type of milk is taken as the standard and, by means of fairly simple conversion factors, the milk actually produced is converted into the corresponding volume or weight of "standard milk." In Britain the standard type contains 3.7% of fat and has an energy value of 330 Cal./lb.; for milk of differing fat content, the energy allowance is increased or decreased 20% for each 1% rise or fall in fat content. In the United States, the standard milk is of 4% fat content, milk of any other type being converted into the equivalent amount of the standard by means of Gaines' formula;[37]

$$\text{Equivalent weight of 4\% milk} = 0.4W + 15F$$

where "W" is the weight of milk being considered and "F" the weight of fat contained in it.

For species other than the cow, there are very few experimental data available concerning net efficiency of milk production. From the figures quoted by Leitch and Godden[38] one may assume that the net efficiency of milk production in the ewe is about 45% (gross efficiency 30%) and there are grounds for believing that this is true of the sow.[39]

With regard to the gross efficiency of milk production, in which factor the needs for both maintenance and production are included, the efficiencies of dairy cows consuming the conventional types of ration range from about 22% in beasts which are producing about 600 lb. per year to 41% when the milk yield rises to 60 lb. per day.[38] In the case of a ewe producing 3 gallons of milk per week, the gross energy of conversion was 30%.

For comparing the efficiencies of lactating animals of the same species, Gaines[40] introduced the conception of the "dairy-merit index", this being the ratio of the quantity of standard milk produced per day to the bodyweight, "W", of the animal producing it. Although it is a matter on which a great deal more research needs to be done, Brody[5] examined the question of production in relation to bodyweight and came to the conclusion that for creatures differing as widely in size as the cow, goat and rat, the use of "W" to the power 0.7 for the determination of dairy-merit index, gives an almost constant value of 25 when weight and milk yield are measured in the same units. The constancy applies to the "good average" type of animal among dairy cattle; for champion cows may show indices of 50-75; nevertheless the fact that the average should be about 25 does suggest that the modes of milk production in different species are very similar.

Calculation shows that a 1000 lb. cow producing about 4 gallons of standard milk per day, a ewe of 100 lb. bodyweight producing 3 gallons of milk per week, and a 350 lb. sow producing 6 gallons of milk per week are all secreting milk energy at rates approximately equal to their own daily maintenance needs.

(c) Protein needs during lactation.

Using the same type of argument as in the case of energy needs it is possible to put forward minimum possible protein needs for the production of 1 lb. of milk of known composition. Despite the differences between the various breeds of cattle, the ratio of the total energy of the protein in a given quantity of milk to the energy of the milk solids contained therein is fairly constant and covers the range from about 24-26%. In the case of milk of 3.7% fat content, the protein content of one gallon is approximately 0.35 lb.

The quantity of digestible dietary protein which would form such an amount of milk protein is determined partly by its amino-acid composition in relation to that of the milk protein. In ruminants, where bacteria exert considerable powers for protein synthesis, this matter is perhaps of less importance than in the case of non-ruminant species; nevertheless, there are indications that the rumen bacteria may not be able to cope fully with the protein requirements of high yielding dairy cows so that the nature of the protein fed is not without significance. The ultimate efficiency for milk protein production is not known with any certainty, but for the ordinary type of winter production ration and for cattle fed on grass only, the net or partial efficiency seems to be about 55%. In the feeding of dairy cattle this is a matter of considerable importance, since dietary protein is relatively scarce and dear.

Formerly the suggested allowance in Britain was 0.6 lb. of digestible protein per gallon of milk produced, a standard which agreed fairly well with the U.S. (Morrison) recommendations and with Møllgard's allowance as used in Denmark. In Britain, however, a series of trials in 1935-7 gave rise to the belief that two-thirds of this quantity should be sufficient.[41] To give some margin of allowance for safety, however, a value mid-way between the old value of 0.6 lb. and the apparently sufficient 0.4 lb. was chosen. The figure of 0.5 lb. per gallon of standard milk allows for an efficiency of conversion of 70%, which is rather higher than most of the evidence justifies; especially as Halnan,[42] after a survey of the work which had been done previously, concluded that 70% was the best figure that could be expected under practical feeding conditions.

A simple calculation shows that if the milk production ration suffered 100% conversion to milk, both in respect of total energy and protein energy, then the following relationships should hold good (a) digestible food protein should contribute not less than 15% of the total digestible energy of a complete (maintenance and production) ration for a 1000 lb. cow producing 2 gallons of milk per day, or approximately 20% for a production of 6 gallons, (b) for the ewe and sow quoted above, the values would both be about 17%. For conversion efficiencies of 60%, the values would need to approach more closely to 21-30%. On ordinary rations efficiencies are about 60% for dairy cattle. In the case of laboratory animals milk yields were observed to increase as the protein content of the ration was increased to 25-30%, corresponding to about 23-28% of digestible protein.[43]

Hitherto in this section the arguments for the amounts of protein required for lactation have been based on the assumption of constancy of bodyweight in the lactating animal. There are however, two practical cases which need to be mentioned where constancy of weight would indicate inadequate feeding; they are those of animals which are either still growing or are pregnant. In both instances the food supplied should be more than is set out for simple maintenance and lactation. Quite apart from this, however, one group of workers has suggested that on the basis of economic and not just physiological efficiency, there are reasonable grounds for somewhat higher feeding standards than have been suggested here.[44] This is discussed in Chapter 29.

(d) Fat requirements.

On the whole this subject has received much less attention than the two preceding ones. In a long series of experiments on dairy cows, Maynard and his collaborators in America, have shown that milk yield may be increased about 4% by having suitable amounts of fat in the ration, although the percentage composition of the milk remains unchanged.[45] Rations containing 6-7% of fat appear to give optimum results, but the subject requires further investigation.

So far as the quality of dietary fat is concerned, Hansson[46] has suggested that the fats from palm kernels, coconut, linseed and cottonseed increase milk fat production, whereas other oil-seed fats and cod-liver oil have a depressant action. It is claimed that the depressant effect is due to a relatively high content of oleyl glycerides.

(e) The need for minerals during lactation.

The mineral needs of lactating animals are perhaps most easily considered in relation to the amounts of inorganic elements which they secrete in milk. Broadly speaking one may divide the common mammals into four groups, firstly, man and the primates, where the ash content of the milk is low—about 0.3%; secondly, the common herbivores, where the ash content ranges from about 0.5 to 1.0%; thirdly, the smaller carnivorous species, in which the range is approximately 1.0 to 1.5%, and, lastly, the common rodents, where the values lie within the limits 1.5 to 3%.

In few cases has the composition of the milk ash been as well studied as in the cow, although an extended study of sow's milk has recently appeared.[47] The general nature of the ash varies comparatively little, however, and one may say to a fair degree of approximation that calcium (CaO), phosphorus (P_2O_5), sodium (Na_2O), potassium (K_2O) and chlorine (Cl) account for 25, 25-33, 10, 10 and 15% respectively. These five components thus account for a very large part of the ash.

Under any normal feeding conditions potassium may be disregarded as being unlikely to be deficient; calcium, phosphorus and sodium (as common salt) are the chief causes of difficulty. One gallon of cow's milk will contain about 4.5, 3.6, and 3.5 g. of calcium, phosphorus and sodium (all calculated as the elements) respectively. A salt lick, by which the lactating animal may regulate its own intake is probably the best solution of the problem of furnishing sufficient sodium. It should be remembered that the body has little storage capacity for this element, so that it should be provided regularly in the ration. To compensate for the possible unavailability of some of the calcium and phosphorus, the production ration should contain about one and a half to twice as much as occurs in the milk. The production allowances for the average dairy cow, mare, ewe and sow will thus be approximately those given below:

TABLE 67

| Species | | Daily production requirements (g.). | |
		Calcium (Ca)	Phosphorus (P)
Cow, per gallon of milk produced	...	7-10	5-7
Mare, heavy breeds, height of lactn.	...	27-35	·16-22
Ewe, producing about 3 gal./wk. ...	...	4-5.5	3.5-5
Sow, producing about 7 gal./wk.	...	17-22	11-14

In the case of the smaller animals it is desirable that bone-meal should constitute 1-2% of the ration (dry matter basis) or that some suitable food like fish-meal should be included at a reasonable level.

All of the available evidence goes to show that, at the height of lactation, dietary absorption of calcium and phosphorus in particular cannot keep pace with the output in milk. At these times the animal depends upon its skeletal reserves, and, provided that the high level of these elements in the diet is maintained and the animal is given a dry period, no harm occurs, the reserves being built up again after the time of great demand has passed. If, however, intake is neglected and is kept at low levels, bone fragility and other disorders are likely to follow.

(f) Vitamin needs during lactation.

Comparatively little is known of the precise needs for vitamins by lactating animals apart from the fact that a higher level of intake is necessary than for maintenance.

Corresponding perhaps with enhanced rates of protein synthesis about four times as much vitamin A seems to be needed at the height of lactation as for maintenance. Because of the importance of calcium and phosphorus metabolism during this period, the intake of vitamin D also needs to be increased.

Milk production is also dependent upon a good supply of vitamins of the B-complex. In cattle, as was shown in 1915 by workers in South Africa, ordinary milk production can proceed in the absence of dietary supplies;[48] whether very high levels can also be attained in the same way is open to doubt and is a matter that should not be put to the test except for experimental purposes. From what is known of the functions of this group of vitamins one would expect that the amounts needed would be proportional to the total dietary energy intake; as the need for total energy is higher in lactating animals than in non-lactating ones, the amount of vitamin B is correspondingly increased. In the case of the non-ruminant it is good practice to see that such a parallelism is achieved, preferably by the inclusion of 5% or more of foods rich in the vitamin B-complex. In the recommended daily allowances for swine[35] those for thiamine and total digestible nutrients for fairly well-grown animals and lactating sows are 3 I.U. and 2 Kg., and 6.3 I.U. and 3.4-5.1 Kg. respectively.

The vitamin content of milk is important to the suckling, so that the relationship between the concentration of a given vitamin in the diet and that in the milk secreted is not just an academic problem. At low levels of dietary intake the efficiency of transference from food to milk may be relatively high but to double the average milk content of a given vitamin, where this is possible at all, usually means a several-fold increase in dietary intake. The requirements of a dairy cow for vitamin A for milk production are of the order 100,000 I.U./day, at which level of intake the milk fat may contain about 25 I.U./g. When the vitamin A intake is increased to (a) about two and a half million and (b) five million units, the corresponding potencies of the butter fat may be expected to increase ten and fifteen-fold respectively.[49] The respective efficiencies of secretion are about 5% and 3%.

(g) Colostrum and its importance for young stock.

Provided that the animal has been dry beforehand, the first milk secreted after parturition differs very much, both in chemical composition and in physiological properties, from the " normal milk " which is produced during the greater part of the period of lactation.

This first milk is called colostrum or beestings. It usually contains a higher proportion of dry matter than average milk, largely because of an increase in the protein, there being a great increase in the globulin content of the milk and a somewhat smaller one in albumin. Data relating to colostrum from the cow have been given elsewhere; in the case of the mare the globulin, albumin and casein contents of the colostrum are about 11, 2 and 6% respectively, but by the end of the first day the corresponding figures are about 0.4, 0.6 and 1.8%.

The protein fraction is associated with the production of immunity to disease in the young stock. For this reason, and because colostrum is richer than average milk in vitamins and in some of the inorganic elements, it is important that sucklings should not be deprived of colostrum. The difference between the two types of secretion is well illustrated by recent data relating to the sow, Table 68.[47]

TABLE 68

	Total solids %	Fat %	Solids-not-fat. %	Pro-tein %	Lac-tose %	Vit. A I.U.	Vit. B₁ µg.	Vit. B₂ µg.	Vit. C mg.	Ca. %	P %
Colost.	25.2	4.0	21.1	17.8	3.5	71	97	45	31	0.05	0.08
Milk	19.9	8.2	11.7	5.8	4.8	11	68	46	13	0.25	0.17

Although the element is not listed in the above table, the iron content of colostrum is said to be greater than that in milk.

During the course of two or three days, the composition of the fluid secreted gradually changes to that of normal milk.

(6) Nutrition in relation to work

Milk or egg production are two factors which are easily given quantitative assessment, but, except under laboratory conditions, work performance is one of the most difficult phenomena to gauge. In this brief section the only topics which will be covered will be, (a) the nature of the metabolic changes which occur during the performance of muscular work, (b) the kinds of nutrients which must be supplied for its efficient performance, (c) the efficiency of conversion of energy supplied to work performed and (d) the relationship between the amounts of energy for actual work required per day by animals working at arbitrary rates and their maintenance energy needs.

There seems to be little doubt that the breakdown of carbohydrate is the ultimate source of energy for muscular work.[50][51] Provided that a sufficiency of such material is supplied, the amount of protein degradation is negligible; where, however, such a supply is not forthcoming, the body is capable of converting protein into carbohydrate and then using the latter in the normal way.

One may ask if it is better, then, to provide a working animal with a direct supply of carbohydrate for the performance of muscular work or to give it additional protein and fat and allow the body to convert these into suitable substances for providing the energy of muscular contraction. The first method seems the more simple and direct. Long ago Kellner[52] showed that, provided sufficient total energy were supplied for the maintenance of the animal and for the amount of work it had to do, there was no protein breakdown and there appeared to be no advantage therefore in supplying extra dietary protein for the work done. On the other hand modern research has shown that a number of enzyme systems is involved in the series of chemical changes which occur during muscular contraction, and that some inorganic elements and members of the vitamin B-complex are intimately associated with the enzymes in question. In practice the nutritional problem becomes one of supplying good dietary carbohydrate plus the necessary factors for its utilisation. Usually such factors are associated in abundance with protein-rich rather than carbohydrate-rich foods. Where the ruminant is used as a working animal, the rumen bacteria probably provide all of the vitamins which are needed for carbohydrate breakdown; where horses are used the bacteria of the digestive tract supply some of the vitamins, although it is doubtful if they produce enough for the needs of hard work, wherein lies the argument for supplying bran or dried yeast as an integral part of the daily ration for working horses; where dogs are involved, either for work as such or for racing, then the diet must supply all of the desired factors.

The last problem to be discussed is the magnitude of the energy expenditure associated with given amounts of work. On a simple theoretical physical basis the amount of work done by a horse, for example, is the product of the force exerted by the animal and the distance through which the force is employed. A horse exerting a pull of 100 lb.-weight for a distance of one mile, performs work on the object pulled of 100 x 5,280 foot-pounds, which is equivalent to 171 Cal., or about 1% of the daily maintenance needs of a 1,500 lb. beast. This expenditure of energy, however, is that made on the object pulled and merely represents the *minimum*, possible amount of dietary energy which might suffice for the task. Muscles do not convert the nutrient energy with which they are supplied into work with 100% efficiency however, the maximum value being about 40%. In the example quoted the energy needs for work are thus increased to 2.5-3.0% of maintenance requirements. The distance involved is such as a horse might walk in rather less than half an hour, so that a working day of six hours would entail new energy needs of not less than 30-40% of maintenance.

Under ordinary working conditions the efficiency of working falls off somewhat with increase in the magnitude of the pull required, but for a pull of 400 lb.-weight it is still over 30%. There are other factors involved, however, which must now be considered.

So far the problem has been one of assessing the amount of energy needed for a particular task, using nothing but purely physical principles for the purpose, and then, given the efficiency with which muscular tissue can convert nutrient energy supplied into muscular work, of estimating the total amount of energy which is required. Nothing has been said, however, of the amount of energy needed by the horse for its own movement over the distance involved. Brody[5] has referred to three ways of considering efficiency, thus:

$$\text{Gross efficiency} = \frac{\text{Work accomplished}}{\text{Energy expended}}$$

$$\text{Net efficiency} = \frac{\text{Work accomplished}}{\text{Energy expended above that at rest}}$$

$$\text{Absolute efficiency} = \frac{\text{Work accomplished}}{\text{Energy used above that for walking without load.}}$$

Having considered the last of these, which falls to just over 30% for a pull of 400 lb.-weight, it is the second which is now being considered. The maximal value is about 28% for the higher pulls, falling to about 20% for the lower ones. Not only is the magnitude of the pull important, but also the speed at which the horse is moving. As the speed of movement increases the net efficiency increases up to a maximum and then declines;[53] such a maximum is not reached within the walking speeds of draught horses. This does not mean, however, that horses should be worked at high speeds for there would be little point in achieving such rates at the expense of a short life for the animal. The table below gives data quoted by Brody for the gross efficiencies of working under different conditions in a limited number of experiments.

TABLE 69

Speed of walking, m.p.h.	Draught, lb.-wt.				
	50	100	200	300	400
1.15 (horse)	7	12	17.5	20	21
1.15 (pony)	12	19	—	—	—
2.2 (horse)	10	15	20	23	24
2.2 (pony)	17	22	—	—	—
3.1 (horse)	12	18	22	24	24.5

A 1,500 lb. horse exerting a pull of 400 lb.-wt. and moving at a speed of 2.2 m.p.h. during a six hours working day, would require just over twice as much digestible energy as would suffice for maintenance alone. One recommendation which has been made concerning the conditions under which horses may work without resultant damaging fatigue is that of exerting a pull of one-tenth of their bodyweights over a total distance of 20 miles per day. For a horse of 1,500 lb. this involves food intake at about one and a half times maintenance levels.

Variations of weather conditions, of road surfaces, of gradients and of many other factors, make difficult the application of such principles to actual working conditions. With the help of the body of information which has been acquired concerning the purely empirical feeding of working animals and with intelligent observation of the condition of the individual beast, however, the very variable demands may be met quite satisfactorily.

REFERENCES

1. Dukes, H. H., (1947). " The physiology of domestic animals."
2. Marshall, F. H. A., and E. T. Halnan, (1946). " The physiology of farm animals."
3. Baker, F., and S. T. Harriss, (1947). Nutrition Abs. Rev., 17, 3.
4. Mellanby, J., (1927). J. Physiology, 64, Proc. v., xxxiii.
5. Brody, S., (1945). " Bioenergetics and growth."
6. Haecker, T. L., (1914). Minn. Agric. Exp. Sta. Bul. No. 140.
7. Kellner, O., (1926). " The scientific feeding of animals."
8. Armsby, H. P., (1917). " The nutrition of farm animals."
9. Forbes, E. B., and M. Kriss, (1931). Amer. Soc. Animal Prod. Proc., 25, 344.
10. Mollgaard, H., and A. Lund, (1929), quoted by Leitch and Godden, Imp. Bur. Animal Nutrition, Tech. Comm. No. 14.
11. Hansson, N., (1922), quoted by Leitch and Godden, Imp. Bur. Animal Nutrition, Tech. Comm. No. 14.
12. Smuts, D. B., (1935). J. Nutrition, 9, 403.
13. Morrison, F. B., (1947). " Feeds and feeding."
14. Report of the Dep. Com. on rationing of dairy cows (1925). H.M. Stationery Office, London.
15. Maynard, L., (1947). " Animal nutrition."
16. Black, W. H., B. Knapp, and J. R. Douglass, (1939). U.S. Dept. Agric. Yearbook, 519.
17. Wallace, L. R., (1948). J. Agric. Sci., 38, 93, 243 and 367.
18. Steensberg, (1947). Brit. J. Nutrition, 1, 139.
19. McMeekan, C. P., (1940). J. Agric. Sci., 30, 276.
20. Mitchell, H. H., (1929). U.S. Nat. Res. Council Bul. No. 67.
21. Armsby, H. P., (1917). " The nutrition of farm animals."
22. Swett, W. W., C. H. Eccles, and A. C. Ragsdale, (1924). Mo. Agric. Exp. Sta. Bul. No. 66.

23. Steensberg, V., & Ostergaard, P. S, (1945). Beretn. Forsogslab. Kbh. No. 216.
24. Gullickson, T. W., F. C. Fountaine, and J. B. Fitch, (1942). J. Dairy Sci., 25, 117.
25. Hart, G. H., (1940). Nutrition Abs. Rev., 10, 261.
26. Brown, E. F., and A. F. Morgan, (1948). J. Nutrition, 35, 425.
27. Mellanby, E., (1938). J. Physiol., 93, 42.
28. Mitchell, H. H., W. E. Carroll, T. S. Hamilton, and G. E. Hunt, (1931). Ill. Agric. Exp. Sta. Bul. No. 375.
29. Hammond, J., (1943). Proc. Nutrition Soc., (England), 2, 8.
30. Hankins, O. G., and H. W. Titus, (1939). U.S. Dept. Agric. Yearbook, 450.
31. Halnan, E. T., and F. H. Garner, (1946). "Principles and practice of feeding farm animals."
32. Halnan, E. T., (1947). Min. Agric. Fisheries Bul. No. 7.
33. Bohstedt, G., (1942). J. Dairy Sci., 25, 441.
34. Theiler, A., H. H. Green, and P. J. du Toit, (1928). J. Agric. Sci., 18, 369.
35. Allman, R. T., and T. S. Hamilton, (1948). "Nutritional deficiencies of livestock." F.A.O. Agric. Stud. No. 5.
36. Mitchell, H. H., (1947). J. Animal Sci., 6, 365.
37. Overman, O. R., and W. L. Gaines, (1933). J. Agric. Res., 46, 1109.
38. Leitch, I., and W. Godden, (1941). Imp. Bur. Animal Nutrition Tech. Comm. No. 14.
39. Mitchell, H. H., and M. A. R. Kelley, (1938). J. Agric. Res., 56, 811.
40. Gaines, W. L., (1940). J. Dairy Sci., 23, 1031.
41. Bartlett. S., A. S. Foot, S. L. Huthnance and J. Mackintosh, (1940). J. Dairy Res., 30, 121.
42. Halnan, E. T., (1929). J. Dairy Res., 1, 3.
43. Mueller, A. J., and W. M. Cox, (1946). J. Nutrition, 31, 249.
44. Yates. F., D. A. Boyd, and G. H. N. Pettit, (1942). J. Agric. Sci., 32, 428.
45. Maynard, L. A., J. K. Loosli, and C. M. McCay, (1940). Cornell Univ. Agr. Exp. Sta. Bul. No. 753.
46. Hansson, N., (1941). Nutrition Abs. Rev., 11, 345.
47. Braude, R., M. E. Coates, K. M. Henry, S. K. Kon, S. J. Rowland, S. Y. Thompson, and D. M. Walker (1947). Brit. J. Nutrition, 1, 64.
48. Theiler, A., H. H. Green, and P. R. Viljoen (1915). Union S. Africa Dept. Agr., Dir. Vet. Res. Rept. 3 and 4, 3.
49. Blaxter, K. L., S. K. Kon, and S. Y. Thompson, (1946). J. Dairy Res., 14, 225.
50. Baldwin, E., (1947). "Dynamic aspects of biochemistry."
51. Gemmill, C. L., (1942). Physiol. Rev., 22, 32.
52. Kellner, O., (1880). Landw. Jahrb., 9, 651.
53. Lupton, H., (1923). J. Physiol., 57, 337.

THE NUTRITIVE VALUE OF FOODS

(1) Introduction

When the practical feeding of animals is being considered, two main difficulties arise. Firstly, no two foodstuffs are quite alike, for they may differ from one another in both the nature and amounts of protein, fat, carbohydrate, minerals and vitamins they each contain, and, that being so, the problem of the selection of a fit basis of comparison of their respective nutritive values for some particular purpose arises. Secondly, the needs of livestock vary with species, age, sex, and condition, and, even when those factors are equal, they vary from one beast to another.

In a compromise attempt to overcome the first difficulty the foods may be compared with one another on the basis of the amounts of energy which each food can provide under definite conditions. This method applies only to the organic and not to the mineral fraction of the foodstuffs.

A second basis for comparison is that of the respective protein contents of the foods. Actually, in the computation of rations both the energy and protein standards are used, but, when these have been settled, the fat, mineral and vitamin contents of the rations have also to be considered; a ration must be complete in all respects.

So far as the animal itself is concerned, an arbitrary and to some extent misleading division of its food requirements into two portions is made for the purposes of calculation. Its " maintenance needs " (p. 248) are those which are required to keep the animal alive and in normal health, while its additional " production needs " cover nutritional requirements for growth, pregnancy, lactation or egg production, and work.

(2) The energy value of foods

The organic nutrients which are absorbed from the digestive tract are either oxidised by the body to suit its purposes, or else they are stored and can be regarded, therefore, as potentially oxidisable. During such oxidations heat is produced and thus the energy of oxidation (heat production) of foods provides a basis for the comparison of the nutritive values of different foodstuffs.

The amount of heat which is liberated when 1 gm. of a substance is completely oxidised is known variously as its heat of combustion, total energy, or gross energy. It is a quantity which is characteristic of the substance.

However, it is rarely the case that the whole of a food is absorbed from the gut, part of it, together with some of the intestinal secretions, being lost in the fæces, so that the gross energy of a food does not represent the actual energy value of the food to the animal. The digestible energy of a foodstuff is the gross energy less the corresponding fæcal excretion. It is a quantity which depends both upon the nature of the food and upon the animal consuming it.

The fact that some of the absorbed nutrients, through modification by one of the body's many metabolic processes, may give rise to two or more new substances, some of which may remain in the body while others are oxidised at once, does not affect the argument.

To a lesser extent in the case of fats and carbohydrates, but markedly in that of proteins, the digestible energy of foods does not represent their real value to the organism. Traces of combustible products derived from fats and carbohydrates are voided in the urine, but almost the whole of the nitrogen of metabolised proteins is excreted as urea (in mammals) or as uric acid (in birds). Both urea and uric acid have an appreciable heat of combustion which is lost to the animal. If the respective energy losses for both fæces and urine are subtracted from the gross energy, the remainder is called the metabolisable energy of the food.

Mention has been made in the previous paragraph of proteins, fats and carbohydrates as separate entities, but it should be realised that for any type of natural foodstuff, the gross energy is the sum of the separate heats of combustion of the protein, fat, etc., which 1 gm. of it contains. Similarly its digestible energy is equal to the sum of the energies of the digestible protein, digestible fat, etc.

In the case of an animal doing no work and being kept for maintenance only, the metabolisable energy of the food will appear as actual heat which the body will surrender to its environment. Where, however, a young animal, or a pregnant, lactating, egg-producing, or working one is being fed, part of the metabolisable energy may be used for new growth, or for milk or eggs, or work. This portion of the energy of the food is called its net energy. It may represent only a small fraction of the metabolisable energy of the food. In the case of wheat straw, for example, so much energy is lost in the "work of digestion" of this very fibrous food, that when the loss is subtracted from the metabolisable energy of the straw, the balance, i.e., the net energy, is small.

(3) Gross, digestible, metabolisable and net energies
(a) Gross energy.

Determinations of the gross energies of foodstuffs show that, on a dry matter basis, despite the differences between different members of the same group, proteins, fats and carbohydrates yield average values of about 5.6, 9.4 and 4.1 Cal.*/gm. respectively. Most feeding stuffs have gross energies of about 4.5 Cal., especially the coarse foods, but, naturally, such foods as linseed and other oil-seeds, which contain appreciable amounts of fat, yield much higher figures.

(b) Digestible energy.

The corresponding digestible energies vary to the same extent that the digestibilities of foods vary. They are affected by the species, age and sex of the animal involved, the nature of the ration, and the plane of nutrition, factors whose general influence has already been considered (p. 15).

On a dry matter basis, the digestible energies of palm kernel cake for cattle and pigs, respectively, would be as shown below, using the factors previously given for proteins, etc., and considering 100 gm. of the dry food.

TABLE 70

	Digestible matter, %		Digestible energy (Cal.)	
	For cattle	For pigs	For cattle	For pigs
Protein	19	13	106	73
Fat	2	0.6	19	6
Carbohydrate ...	57	48	234	197
Total/100 gm. ...	78	61.6	359	276
Total/gm.	—	—	3.6	2.8

It is unfortunate that some inconsistencies have been introduced into this part of nutritional study. In the U.S.A. for example, two foodstuffs may be compared with one another on the basis of their " total digestible nutrients ". This is a method which makes use of the energy concept, but without using values in actual calories. The gross energy values for proteins, carbohydrates and fats respectively are in the ratio of 5.6 : 4.1 : 9.4, or 1.37 : 1.00 : 2.3 (app.). From the energy point of view one unit of protein is thus equivalent to 1.37 of carbohydrate, the corresponding value for fat being 2.3. Therefore, if one multiplies the percentages of digestible protein, fat and carbohydrate in the two foods by 1.37, 2.30 and 1.0 respectively, the two foods are reduced to a common carbohydrate basis for comparison, there being then no need to use actual calories. Worked out in this way, using digestibility data for cattle, 100 lb. of oats contains 65 lb. of total digestible nutrients, and 100 lb. of linseed cake, 74 lb. Most of the figures which have been calculated on this basis have involved the factor 1.0 for protein, which is the appropriate figure for the metabolisable energy of proteins, not for digestible energy. As carbohydrates have an average gross energy of

* Kilo-calories. ·

about 4 Cal./gm. it is sufficiently near the truth for all practical purposes to say that 1 lb. of total digestible nutrients has an energy value of 1,800 Cal.

In this country the "maintenance starch equivalent" has been used as a basis for comparison of the energy values of foods for maintenance, where no food storage by the animal is involved. The same standard has been used, namely carbohydrate (i.e., starch) and approximately the same factors. It is clear, however, that in this instance it is metabolisable energy which is being considered and therefore the factor which should be used for protein is the one which allows for its incomplete oxidation, approximately 1.0 as for starch itself. The so-called maintenance starch equivalent, as Woodman has pointed out,[1] is actually a fuel value; it is, however, artificial in conception and of little practical value.

(c) Metabolisable energy.

The ratio of the metabolisable to the digestible energy of a food is not a fixed quantity but depends on the nature of the food, the plane of nutrition and the nature of the animal consuming the food. These points may be illustrated by general reference to dietary protein. Up to a certain amount a digestible protein of high biological value may be almost fully utilised by the animal absorbing it, tissue protein being formed and comparatively little urea, representing a urinary loss of energy, being excreted. If more protein is fed than is needed by the animal then the surplus amino-acids are de-aminated, with the subsequent formation of urea, and the urinary loss is thus increased. Thus metabolisable energy may be affected by plane of nutrition. Alternatively one may consider the case of a ration, the protein of which is entirely lacking in one amino-acid essential for the creature concerned. In this instance the protein would be catabolised with a corresponding loss of urea and of energy. The missing amino-acid fed separately to the animal could not be used (or only to a slight degree (p. 49)) for tissue formation and would suffer a similar fate. By feeding the two materials together the formation of body protein could proceed, with corresponding diminished urea excretion—subject to the plane of intake not being too high—and with less energy loss. The metabolisable energy of the mixture would thus be greater than that of its components alone. This phenomenon has been shown by Swift and his collaborators.[2] The third illustration of the factors affecting the metabolisable energy of a ration is provided by a ration of digestible nutrients which contains a sufficient proportion of protein to satisfy the needs of a young growing animal; such a ration would contain more than enough protein for the maintenance needs of the adult beast, and on the basis of equal intakes of digestible nutrients, there would be a greater loss of energy via urea for the mature animal than for the growing one. Thus the metabolisable energy of food is related to the biological function it has to meet.

Data have not yet been collected which will cover all manner of

rations under all conditions, but the following data, from the paper by
Forbes and Thacker[3] provide a reasonable guide for cattle;

TABLE 71

Metabolisable energy/gm. digestible matter

Food	Energy (Cal.)	Food	Energy (Cal.)
Protein of roughage	4.3	Carb. polysaccharide ...	3.76
„ „ concents.	4.5	„ trisaccharide	3.62
Ether ext., roughage	7.8	„ disaccharide	3.56
„ „ grains	8.3	„ monosaccharide ...	3.38
„ „ oil-seeds	8.8	Soluble carb. (av.)	3.7
„ „ animal foods ...	9.3	Fibre	2.9

(d) Net energy.

By definition the net energy of a food is the amount left for productive purposes, the balance of the metabolisable energy being lost as heat.

It has long been known that the feeding of carbohydrate, fat, or
protein to an animal results in increased heat production. If equal
amounts of energy in the form of the various digestible nutrients are
used, the extra heat production, known as the specific dynamic effect, is
much greater for protein than for the other food constituents.

There has been much confusion concerning this effect, largely
because different experimental techniques have been used. The extra
heat output due to the food absorbed must be measured by the use of
a calorimeter (or by indirect methods which are based upon the use of
a calorimeter), and one of the big problems which has to be settled is
what the condition of the animal shall be whose increased heat production is to be measured. Should the food be given to a resting and fasting
animal whose heat output for equal intervals of time is measured before
and after it receives the ration, or should the food be given to supplement
a maintenance ration? Are different results observed in the two cases?

The heat effects are indeed different for different conditions, e.g.,
for simple maintenance, growth, fattening, or milk production; they are
greater the higher the plane of nutrition of the animal. Correspondingly,
therefore, the net energy of foods varies with the bodily function which
they support and with the food intake. Like metabolisable energy, the
net energies of dietary constituents or of single foodstuffs are not
additive.[4] An animal in a given condition, e.g., one which is simply
maintaining its body weight, or being fattened, or growing, producing
milk or working, cannot carry out its necessary functions using any
chance assembly of food constituents which happens to be given to it.
A growing creature which is given a ration lacking protein cannot make
body substance from it; an animal which is given a ration containing
protein sufficient for a certain amount of growth only will abstract the
necessary food constituents, fat, protein, carbohydrates, minerals and
vitamins for that amount of body substance and any surplus materials
will be oxidised. In a ration it is thus desirable that the different dietary

constituents shall be present in appropriate proportions for the purpose in mind. This does not necessarily mean fixed proportions in the case of *each* constituent, since the body can make some of the things it needs out of others, fat from carbohydrate for example, although there are obviously some factors which have to be provided in the proper amounts, as, for example, essential amino-acids. It will be seen from the example quoted in the previous section that the net energy of proteins depends, among other factors, upon their being " complete ". Forbes and his collaborators have shown similarly that for equal energy intakes of food, as the protein content increases from 10 per cent. to 25 per cent.[5], the net energy increases, and the balance of nutrients becomes better suited to the needs of the body. Animals deficient in vitamin A can absorb but not properly utilise amino-acids, so that the net energy of the ration must be less than for normal animals.[6]

Before summarising this section it will be useful to give some of the data which have been obtained by the methods described. In the table below are shown representative data for some common foods when they are given to cattle; the comparisons are made on equal intakes of gross energy.

TABLE 72

(All of the figures represent Cal.)

Food	Gross	Fæcal	Digest.	Urinary	Metabolis-able	Heat	Net
Maize	100	20.5	79.5	4.5	75	29	46
Timothy hay	100	55	45	.4	41	17	24
Wheat straw	100	67	33	2	31	26	5
Wheat bran	100	—	—	—	55	26	29

It will be observed that fæcal losses account for the greatest differences between the foods, the losses of energy in the urine being small (the protein content of the foods is not large and, since the animals are ruminants the essential amino-acid balance is not so important here as it would be for the pig, for example). It is important to notice that the net energy of maize, a fairly typical cereal grain, is about twice that of hay and nine times that of wheat straw for fattening.

An average mixed ration for cattle will have a gross energy of about 2,000 Cal./lb. of dry matter, roughly 1,600 Cal. being digestible energy, 1,200-1,400 Cal. metabolisable energy, and the net energy about 1,000 Cal.[7]

Since the net energy of food varies with species, plane of nutrition, the " balance of the ration " and the condition of the animal to which it is to be fed, it may be asked whether the concept serves any useful purpose. The answer is that, as we have tried to reduce the nutritive values of different foods to a common basis there is little need for surprise that the values do not express all that needs to be known about single foodstuffs or mixtures of them. Within its limits the concept is useful and there are no better words to describe the position than those of a worker who has been one of the keenest investigators and critics of net energy.

"It is true, however, that despite these imperfections, the method of measurement of food values in terms of net energy has much in its favour, especially for limited purposes of close discrimination, under rigid conditions of experimentation." [8]

(4) The " starch equivalent " system

The starch equivalent system is another method of assessing net energies; the method was developed by Kellner.[9] To the maintenance ration of fattening bullocks he added in turn known weights of " pure " protein (wheat gluten), starch, oil, sugar (sucrose), and fibre (straw pulp) and measured the respective amounts of body fat which were produced. He then compared the fat producing powers of the *digestible* nutrients using that of starch as standard.

Actually Kellner measured the dietary carbon retained, but by the use of the average conversion figure for fat, the results can be converted into pounds of body fat produced. The following table shows his results, the data relating to digestible nutrients.

TABLE 73

Nutrient	Net energy Cal./lb. of food	Equivalent body fat in lb./lb. of food	Relative values
Protein (wheat gluten) ...	1016	0.235	0.94
Starch	1071	0.250	1.00
Crude fibre (straw pulp) ...	1071	0.250	1.00
Ether extract			
of roughage	2041	0.474	1.9 ⎫
of cereal grains	2273	0.525	2.1 ⎬ av. 2.1
of oil-seeds	2586	0.600	2.4 ⎭

Instead of using Calories, Kellner preferred to express the relative values of the different nutrients in terms of an equal weight of digestible starch. In this way the starch equivalent system came into being. One pound of starch equivalent has, under the conditions of Kellner's experiments, a net energy value of 1,071 Cal.[9] (For application to actual feeding it is doubtful whether this accuracy of equation is warranted, the factor 1,100 probably being near enough.)

Kellner then proceeded to examine the fattening powers of a number of representative foods, the number actually tested being quite small. In each case he could express the value of the food in terms of the equivalent number of pounds of starch which would produce an identical fattening. It was also possible for Kellner to measure the amounts of digestible fat, protein, starch, etc., in each of these foods and, using the relative values in column 4 of the above table, to calculate what the theoretical fattening power of the food should be.

In a few cases, notably such foods as groundnut, linseed and cotton-seed meals, the practical and calculated figures for the respective foods agreed to within 1 or 2 per cent., but in most cases the actual value was less than the anticipated one, while in the case of hay and straw, it was considerably less. The discrepancy appeared to be related to the fibre contents of coarse food and Kellner calculated what the effects of various amounts of fibre in different classes of coarse foods might be expected to be; on this basis he introduced correction factors for use in conjunction with tables showing the contents of digestible nutrients of foodstuffs. He also calculated, on the basis of the experiments he had done, correction factors for other foods than oil meals or coarse fodders. In the calculation of the true starch equivalent of a food, the value calculated from a knowledge of its percentages of digestible nutrients and the relative worth of such protein, fat, etc., as revealed by Kellner's experiments, is multiplied by the appropriate " value number ". The example below shows the way in which the production starch equivalent of oats is calculated;

TABLE 74

Digestible constituent	% in food	Fattening power in starch units
Protein	8	8 x 0.94 = 7.5
Ether extract	4	4 x 2.3 = 9.2
Sol. carbohydrate	45	45 x 1.0 = 45.0
Fibre	3	3 x 1.0 = 3.0
		Total 64.7

Calculated amount of starch equivalent to 100 lb. oats ...   64.7 lb.
Value number for oats   · 0.95
True starch equivalent for oats   ...   . 64.7 x 0.95 = 62

Some idea of the relative values of the starch equivalents of the different classes of animal foods will be obtained from the table below; it 'must be noted that there are wide variations within each group.

TABLE 75

Food	S.E.	Food	S.E.
Coarse foods: Hay ...	20–50	Cereal grains and legumes	60–80
Straw ...	10–20	Oil-seeds	80–130
Fresh green crops	10	Oil-seed meals	40–80
Silage	10–15	Meat and fish meals ...	60–90

Starch equivalents are used so widely for the computation of rations that it is very necessary to understand their significance. In the first place they were determined for cattle and not for any other species. In many respects sheep are so like cattle in their powers of digestion and metabolism, that starch equivalents can be used for them with a fair approximation to accuracy, but for pigs, horses, poultry and other species, the method either cannot be used or else needs severe modification. A second reservation regarding starch equivalents is that they were determined for fattening purposes; they do not apply without reservation to other physiological states, though they are often used in such a way. Starch equivalents have, in fact, similar limitations to net energies as a means of expression of the nutritive values of foods. Although they are usually employed additively it is doubtful whether the practice is justifiable: reasons for this have been given with reference to net energy.

Kriss [10] has pointed out how few and, in some cases, how variable were the production values for protein, fat and starch upon which Kellner based his calculations. Work by Armsby on starch also tends to be at variance with that of Kellner.

As with net energy similarly with starch equivalents, one may feel inclined to doubt the value of systems which are so ill-defined and so subject to limitations. It can only be said that starch equivalents serve a useful purpose provided that discrimination is used in their application. The subject of nutrition has so developed that first of all the energy values of foods were studied, then followed the examination of the protein problem, but only within the last two decades has it been possible to examine carefully the requirements of different species in different physiological states. Little service is done to the science of nutrition by elaborate mathematical calculations of starch equivalents to one or two decimal places when neither the nutritive value of the food nor the needs of the animals to which it is to be given can be framed with anything approaching such a degree of precision.

(5) Barley equivalents

In the Scandinavian countries the nutritive value of barley, chiefly for milk production, has been taken as a standard, other foods being compared with it on a pound for pound basis with respect to their productive values.

It is a convenient system when there is comparatively little variety of foodstuffs available. The theory may be extended to cover the main groups of foodstuffs, one food in each group serving as the standard for the group so that replacements may be made on an equivalent basis.

Where the method is applied primarily to one physiological function, e.g., lactation, and where the range of foods is not great, the system is useful, but its limitations outside that range are clear.

(6) Summary

In this section four different methods of comparing the nutritive values of foods have been described, namely the total digestible nutrient system of Morrison, the net energy system of Armsby, Kellner's starch equivalents and the use of barley and other reference foods. Not one of them is free from faults, yet each can be used with profit. To summarise the various points which have been made and to indicate the work which still remains to be done, the following section taken from the review by Kriss [10] is valuable. What he says about net energy applies, with suitable modifications, to the other food standards in use.

" The net energy conception is a correct basis of expression of the ultimate energy value of a ration, and commends itself especially for purposes of fundamental research under conditions of intensive and adequate experimental control. However, the net energy value of a ration is not a constant but is subject to considerable variation, depending on the experimental conditions and the methods of determination. The directly observed net energy value of a ration used for maintenance is different from the value of the ration as used for milk production. Also, the net energy value of a ration, and its significance, depend on the base value of heat production used in its determination. Further, the conditions of experimentation for the determination of net energy values are most exacting, and the necessary control of physical activity, thermal environment, and endocrine functions may not be successfully accomplished.

" The net availability of the metabolisable energy of a ration is prominently affected by the plane of nutrition when the fasting heat production is used as the base value in determining the heat increment. This fact has been interpreted as resulting, in the main, from the sparing effect of the food in relation to the catabolism of body tissue nutrients. In this sense heat increments based on the heat production of fast do not express the real energy expense of food utilisation.

" Energy maintenance requirements are directly determined by balance experiment as the quantities necessary for equilibrium; and since the observed heat increments of rations for maintenance are decidedly less than for body increase, the effect of this difference is to render net energy values for maintenance higher than for body increase. For convenience, however, net energy requirements for maintenance may be arbitrarily expressed in terms of net energy for production; but, whatever the plane of nutrition, the energy required for equilibrium will be increased as the environmental temperature is either higher or lower than the zone of thermal neutrality. In other words, under these conditions the total metabolisable energy becomes net energy.

" The utilisation of the metabolisable energy of a ration for body increase, determined from a comparison of maintenance with super-maintenance planes of nutrition, is not much affected by the plane of nutrition within fairly wide limits above maintenance. This is the method of choice, therefore, for comparison of rations on the basis of net energy for production.

" The utilisation of the metabolisable energy of a ration depends much on the nutritive balance of the nutrients, and the net energy of a ration is not necessarily the sum of the separately determined net energies of the component feeding stuffs.

" The net energy values of individual feeding stuffs are fundamentally variable in the sense that their values depend to a considerable extent on the combination in which they are fed with other feeding stuffs. The associative effects of combination are unpredictable in the present state of knowledge.

" There is some evidence to the effect that in nutritively complete rations the utilisation of the metabolisable energy for body increase and for milk production approaches constancy. This subject deserves further investigation.

" The question of the net availability of the metabolisable energy of rations and of feeding stuffs under various conditions is not yet completely solved and should be investigated further.

" The methods of determination of production and replacement values of feeding stuffs which have been advocated by Fraps, Morrison and Kleiber should be given further consideration."

One cannot read the above paragraphs without coming to the wholesome conclusions that much research on animal nutrition still remains to be done and that the science of nutrition concerns the food to be given to an animal, the environment—using the word in its broadest sense—in which the animal is situated, and the nature of the creature itself. Too much emphasis is too often put on the nature of the food alone, the other operative factors being ignored.

REFERENCES

1. Woodman, H. E., (1948). "Rations for Livestock", H. M. Stationery Office.
2. Swift, R. W., O. J. Kahlenberg, L. R. Voris, and E. B. Forbes, (1934) J. Nutrition, 8, 197.
3. Forbes, E. B., and E. J. Thacker, (1943). J. Animal Sci., 2, 226.
4. Forbes, E. .B., J. W. Bratzler, E. J. Thacker, and L. F. Marcy, (1939). J. Nutrition, 18, 57.
5. Forbes, E. B., R. W. Swift, L. F. Marcy and M. T. Davenport, (1944). J. Nutrition, 28, 189.
6. Brown, E. F., and A. F. Morgan, (1948). J. Nutrition, 35, 425.
7. Brody, S., (1945). "Bioenergetics and Growth."
8. Forbes, E. B., R. W. Swift and A. Black, (1938). J. Nutrition, 15, 321.
9. Kellner, O., (1900). Landw. Vers. Stat., 53, 1.
10. Kriss, M., (1943). J. Animal Sci., 2, 62.

THE CONSTRUCTION OF RATIONS

(1) Introduction

In order to construct a satisfactory ration intended for some specific purpose, the feeder must have a fairly clear understanding of the nutritional requirements of the animal as well as a knowledge of the numerous foods available for his use. Food requirements when expressed arithmetically are called *feeding standards*. The expression of feeding standards is an endeavour to state the nutritional requirements of animals as accurately as our present knowledge allows.

Standards have been determined (a) for the maintenance of the animal, and (b) for the amount of food required for conversion into something specific such as growth, work, milk, eggs or wool. This part (b) of a composite ration is called the production part in contradistinction to the maintenance, subsistence or basal portion which may be described approximately as that which will keep a resting, non-producing animal in good health and in constant weight for an indefinite period. The way in which standards have been determined for maintenance and productive purposes is described elsewhere (Chap. 17) and it will suffice at this stage to say that though the clear-cut distinction between the needs of livestock for maintenance and productive purposes is to some degree an artificial one, it has very useful practical advantages.

Feeding standards are not for rigid application; on the contrary, it cannot be too often stated that they are merely general guides for the feeding of livestock. The standards for some particular species of animal simply suggest what the *average* requirements of those animals are likely to be under definite conditions. Where the local conditions differ from those under which the standards were fixed, a modification of the standards will be required, e.g., livestock which are having to withstand abnormal cold will need to be better fed than the usual standards, which have been framed for average environmental conditions, would suggest. Quite apart, however, from local variations which will affect the average level of feeding, it will still be true that a group of animals exposed to the same environment and even of the same sex and weight will still show variations with respect to food requirements between different individuals of the group. In the last resort each animal is a law unto itself; much of the skill in the feeding of livestock is connected with this recognition of the variation of the needs of individuals for food and with modification of the feeding standards to meet it.

In relation to this topic it is instructive to recollect that the earliest studies of nutrition tended to be concerned with total food requirements, based largely on energy concepts alone. Then the attention was directed to the protein needs of the body, and since then the last three or four decades have produced an enormous amount of work relating to minerals and vitamins. Of late there have been signs that the balance of the various nutrients in foods, in relation to its effect on the well-being of men and beasts, is receiving the attention which it merits. The conceptions which must not be allowed to develop, however, are that the subject of nutrition is now fully understood, that the existing feeding standards and practices represent perfection, and that there can be no further improvements.

(2) Factors concerned in the construction of rations

The essentials of a ration may be summarised thus:

 (i) The food supplied must be suitable for the species and condition (age, sex, function, etc.), of the animal.
 (ii) It must be palatable.
 (iii) It must meet the energy requirements of the animal.
 (iv) Similarly, it should provide sufficient protein (or its equivalent) of the right quality.
 (v) In the ration the ratios of protein and fat to total nutrients must fall within a suitable range of values.
 (vi) The ration must furnish a sufficient and balanced supply of mineral elements.
 (vii) All of the required vitamins must be present in adequate quantities.

These requirements are fairly exacting. It must be stressed, however, that there is not necessarily one and only one way of constructing a ration for a particular purpose from a given list of foodstuffs. Several rations may equally well satisfy the conditions set out above, and if there is one thing which nutritional research has served to reveal it is that there is safety in the provision of a variety of foodstuffs. Straw and beet pulp can be useful foods *if* they are judiciously combined with other foodstuffs, e.g., fresh green foods, which contain the factors that the former lack. It is known that the capacity of the animal body for the storage of certain food factors is limited; if, therefore, a first group of nutrients, for the proper utilisation of which the second is essential, is to be used to the greatest benefit, care must be taken to see that the two groups are combined in the same ration. Apart from this there is now ample evidence that the processing of foodstuffs often leads to the destruction of essential food factors.

Each of the above sections, (i) to (vii), covers a great deal of material and has been dealt with elsewhere in the book. In the construction of a ration what is known about the chemical composition and metabolism of foodstuffs must be brought into juxtaposition with knowledge of requirements of the different physiological states, such as reproduction and lactation, in order that food may be used with maximum efficiency. For this reason, therefore, the following brief notes are appended: the full details must be sought in the relevant sections.

(a) The balance of a ration.

A balanced ration is one which contains the nutrients necessary for a particular purpose and in proper proportions. A ration which is balanced for an animal of a given species in some particular condition, e.g., maintenance, may not be satisfactory when the condition is changed, e.g., when the animal is in lactation. Similarly, rations which are balanced for one species may not be so for another species.

(See section III: also the requirements of the different species).

(b) Total dry matter.

The power of an animal to consume food is limited by its abdominal capacity and by the rate at which food can be passed through the gut. Because the high producing animal of a given species and the non-producing one seldom differ widely in abdominal capacity, it follows that their very different nutritive requirements must be met by a difference in the nature of the food. Thus the non-producer can be supplied with a bulky fibrous food which will meet its appetite requirements and is not extravagant in the supply of nutrients   On the other hand, the high producer must have a great part of its food as concentrates, so that its high requirements can be accommodated in its limited capacity. Somewhere between the two extremes of highly concentrated food and pure roughage there is an optimum for each species and class of animal.

It has become customary to express the measure of food intake in terms of weight of dry matter. Strictly, this does not give a true indication—or in some cases even a near approximation—of the space it will occupy within the limiting walls of the stomach. A highly concentrated, relatively heavy food will occupy much less space than such foods as straw or ensilage. Furthermore, the bulk and space-using power of some foods is very greatly increased when they have absorbed water—examples of such are coconut cake, dried beet pulp and linseed cake (see page 18). Nevertheless, utilisation of the dry matter as a measure of dietary bulk still remains the best practical test we have.

If the dry matter of the ration is expressed as a percentage of an animal's live weight, due allowance is thus made for differences in abdominal capacity, which is known to vary proportionately with the size (and therefore weight) of the beast. For fattening cattle and dry or low-yielding cows, if the dry matter in the ration falls between 1.5 and 2 per cent. of the animal's live weight, or for a cow in full milk, 2.5 and 3.5 per cent., it may be taken for granted that the rumen will not be overloaded.

Bulk limitation in balancing a diet for horses is also very important and may be expressed as a total dry matter content of 1–1.25 per cent. of live weight for idle horses and 1.5–2 per cent. for working horses.

Control of limitation of the intake of bulk is no less important in other animals: in balancing a ration it must always be given proper consideration.

(c) Protein needs.

The importance of an adequate supply of protein, and of protein of the right quality, in the diet has already been explained. In the sections dealing with maintenance, growth, reproduction and lactation and in those describing the feeding of animals of the different species detailed requirements are given and here it need only be stated that provision of an optimum amount of protein together with optimum energy and bulk goes a long way towards producing a balanced diet. (See sections I and III).

(d) Requirements for fat.

The diet must not be overburdened with fat for reasons which have already been explained. In actual practice, however, there is little tendency to do this because the economic value of fat is such that it is not generally available for animal feeding. There are few accepted standards for fat requirements and even the optimum proportion of fat in diets is a matter of conjecture, but the effects of certain kinds of dietary fat upon the nature of carcase fat is fairly well established. (See sections I and III.)

(e) Minerals.

As regards the supply of minerals in balancing a diet, although deficiencies must be avoided, the indiscriminate use of compound mineral mixtures may do more harm than good. The importance of the correct proportions as well as minimum amounts must be remembered. (See sections I and III.)

(f) Vitamins.

No ration can really be considered balanced that does not contain a sufficiency of the vitamins necessary for the purpose for which the food is given, though in commonly formulated feeding standards their presence is taken for granted. This is not a safe practice. As a general rule one should make sure that the vitamin A and D intakes of all species are adequate, particularly in the case of young stock. The normal adult herbivore usually requires little attention so far as members of the vitamin B complex are concerned, but these factors should not be taken for granted in the case of the pig, dog and fowl, nor in the *young* of any species. (See sections I and III).

(g) Palatability.

Animals have their likes and dislikes, as every successful animal feeder knows, but many aversions to particular foods on the part of animals are of a purely temporary nature due to the strangeness of the material rather than an actual dislike, e.g., some horses have at first to be coaxed to eat carrots and swedes—foods which they come to like very much. No animals like dry dusty meals and hens in particular dislike both dusty and pasty, sticky meals. Many foods become unpalatable by decomposition and some feeders attempt to cover this defect by admixture with more attractive material, a practice to be condemned. There are individual likes and dislikes as well as marked preferences exhibited by species. The good stock feeder is the man who takes these into consideration.

A diet is more likely to be satisfactory if it is composed of a mixture of different foods than if the choice is restricted; a variety of foods gives a greater selection of amino-acids with an increased probability that the recipient will be getting those needed; a mixed diet also gives a greater assurance of a beneficial mineral supply including that of essential trace elements. As a general statement it may be said that the palatability and, in some instances, the digestibility of a mixture of foods are greater than when the diet is limited to one of the foods. (See sections I and II.)

(3) Calculation of quantities of ingredients

In composing a ration which is to supply the needs of an animal, several methods may be used to determine the amounts of each ingredient of which it is to be formed, in order to make the diet balanced. Often, however, the selection of the foods, and to a certain extent the quantity of each food to be used, are governed by economic and other considerations, such as those of supply. When the feeder has duly decided what foods he is going to use he can form a rough estimate, based upon his practical experience, of the amounts required, and he must then adjust these amounts so that the nutritive value of the composite ration approximates to the feeding standard accepted as necessary for the purpose in view. He may do this by a process of trial and error, using his practical experience as a guide. This method, as well as being tedious, is by its very nature inexact, and a mathematically more accurate method is obviously desirable.

Suppose that a farmer wants to compound a diet for a cow for milk production. Such a diet should have a protein equivalent of 20 per cent. or a starch equivalent/protein equivalent ratio of $5:1$. He might have available the following foods of varying S.E./P.E. ratios—flaked maize $10:1$, rice meal $10.3:1$, oats $8:1$, and decorticated cotton cake $2.3:1$. As three of the foods have a ratio wider than $5:1$ and one of them has a ratio narrower than that, it is apparent that each or all of the first three may be combined with the last to bring the compounded diet to the desired ratio. For simplicity's sake let us suppose that he decides to use only flaked maize and decorticated cotton cake. His problem now is to know how much of each must be used to supply 20 lb. of P.E. and 100 lb. of S.E.

Flaked maize has   P.E.   8 per cent.   S.E. 80 per cent.
Dec. cotton cake has   P.E.   15   „   S.E. 40   „

By the use of simultaneous equations it can be found how much of each it is necessary to mix so that the P.E. of the cake and maize equals 20, and the S.E. equals 100.

$$\text{Let } x = \text{amount of cake}$$
$$y = \text{amount of maize}$$

Then, based on protein equivalents,

$$0.15x + 0.08y = 20 \qquad \dots\dots\dots\dots\dots(a)$$

and, based on starch equivalents,

$$0.40x + 0.80y = 100 \qquad \dots\dots\dots\dots\dots(b)$$

Multiplying (a) throughout by 10

$$1.5x + 0.80y = 200 \qquad \dots\dots\dots\dots\dots(c)$$

and subtracting (b) from (c)

$$1.1x = 100 \text{ whence } x \text{ equals } 90.9$$

and by substitution of this value for x in equation (b)

$$36.4 + 0.80y = 100$$
$$\text{whence } y \text{ equals } 79.5$$

So that to compound a diet containing 20 lb. of P.E. and 100 lb. of S.E. it would be necessary to mix 79.5 lb. of maize with 91 lb. of cake.

If no definite amount is required but it is desired to mix the ingredients in the proper proportion, the correct proportions can be ascertained by the use of a similar method, thus:
Let x and y represent the amounts of cake and maize respectively which will furnish a ratio of starch to protein equivalent in the mixture of 5:1.
Then $0.40x + 0.80y$ is the starch equivalent furnished by x and y
and $0.15x + 0.08y$ is the protein equivalent furnished by x and y
and since

$$(0.40x + 0.80y)/(0.15x + 0.08y) = 5/1$$

So that $0.40x + 0.80y = 0.75x + 0.40y$
whence

$$0.35x = 0.40y \text{ or } x = 1.143y$$

The amounts needed are thus shown to be 1 part of maize to 1.143 of cake.

In theory the method can be extended to cover mixtures of any number of foodstuffs whose starch and protein equivalents are known, but in practice the method is wellnigh valueless for more than two foods. If the above example were extended to include decorticated groundnut cake (S.E. 70; P.E. 40) of which " z " pounds are to be used, the method would furnish the equation

$$8y - 7x = 26z$$

which is almost useless.

In practice the method is simplified. A mixture is made up from the foodstuffs available and its S.E. and P.E. are found as previously described (p. 286). If its S.E./P.E. ratio is higher than is desired then it must be balanced with one with a ratio lower than the required one; and conversely. In these cases " x " is used to denote the proportion of the first mixture of foods and " y " is used for the food or mixture of foods which has to balance "x" in order to produce the needed S.E./P.E. value. Very often, in the case of concentrate mixtures, a mixture of " x " pounds of cereal concentrates is balanced with "y" pounds of protein-rich substance to give a suitable production ration.

The following may be taken as an example of what might occur in practice:

Suppose that a dairyman has for milk production a fair amount of flaked maize and three times as much oats, and is offered limited quantities of dried brewers' grains, but has to buy decorticated ground-nut cake in sufficient quantities to allow the most liberal use of the other foods. The quantity of foods he has in hand suggests that he should use them in the proportion of 6 of oats, 2 of maize, and 1 of grains. 9 lb. of such a mixture would contain 0.74 lb. of P.E. and 5.77 lb. of S.E., made up as follows:

TABLE 76

	P.E.	S.E.
6 lb. of oats	0.45	3.66
2 lb. of maize	0.16	1.60
1 lb. of grains	0.13	0.51
9 lb. of mixture	0.74	5.77
100 lb. of mixture	8.2	64.1
100 lb. of dec. ground nut cake	41.5	71.0

The mixture has too little protein, a deficiency which may be corrected with the highly nitrogenous cake.

$$\text{Let } x = \text{amount of mixture}$$
$$y = \text{amount of cake}$$

Then

$$(64.1x + 71y)/(8.2x + 41.5y) = 5/1$$

i.e.

$$64.1x + 71y = 41x - 207.5y$$

or

$$64.1x - 41x = 207.5y - 71y$$

whence

$$23.1x = 136.5y$$

i.e.

$$x = 5.9y$$

So for each 600 lb. (approx.) of the mixture, 100 lb. of cake would be needed.

Murray,[1] on an algebraic basis, stated a rule for carrying out such calculations. The necessary steps are as follows:

(i) Divide the S.E. of each of the two components of the mixture by the desired ratio.

(ii) For each component either take the quotient determined by (i) above from its protein equivalent, or conversely, depending upon which is the greater. (N.B.—For one component the quotient should be greater than the P.E., while the reverse should be true for the other; if this is not so there is either a fault in the calculation, or two foods have been selected which cannot possibly give the required ratio.)

(iii) The differences are inversely proportional to the amounts of the two foods which will be needed. Thus for the above example:

TABLE 77

	Dec. ground nut cake.	Mixture.
Percentage of S.E.	71.00	64.11
Divide by 5	14.2	12.82
Percentage of P.E.	41.5	8.22
By subtraction	27.3	4.60
and 27.3/4.6 = 5.9/1		

The quantities, as before, are taken inversely, that is, 590 or, in practical terms, 600 lb. of the mixture are balanced by 100 lb. of the cake.

(4) The Nitrogenous Ratio of a Food

The Nitrogenous, or as it is often called the Nutritive or Albuminoid Ratio (N.R.) of a complete ration is a convenient and valuable guide as to whether a diet is or is not well balanced in respect of the proportion of protein to other constituents. It expresses approximately the ratio of the energy present in the digestible protein-equivalent of a food, or mixture of foods, to that which is contained in the digestible non-nitrogenous portion. Because an energy basis is employed, the amount of digestible fat is multiplied by 2.3 to bring it to a common denominator with the protein and carbohydrate (Chap. 18, (3)).

Where the nitrogenous ratio is of the order of 1 to 9 it is described as " wide "; a " medium " ratio is one of about 1 to 6 or 1 to 8; and a " narrow " ratio would be one of 1 to 4 or 1 to 5.

A great deal of confusion exists regarding nitrogenous ratios; this has been caused by workers in animal nutrition using different methods. Thus the N.R. of a food has been estimated by making use of the digestible crude protein, digestible pure protein, the total crude protein as found by chemical analysis irrespective of the percentage digested, and also by using the protein equivalent. It is not therefore surprising that different ratios such as 1 to 5, 1 to 6, or 1 to 7 have been recommended from time to time for the same purpose. The method followed here is to use the protein equivalent, which gives a somewhat wider ratio than would be the case were the total crude protein used.

Thus the N.R. of oats, using " protein equivalent," is 1 to 7.6; if crude digestible protein is used then the ratio is 1 to 7.1. Again, further confusion has been caused by some workers omitting the percentage of digestible fibre. For example, if this is done in the case of oats, and crude protein is used, then the N.R. will be 1 to 6.7, and in the case of foods containing much fibre the omission to include that which is digestible will give a still wider difference.

A narrow nitrogenous ratio is used for young growing animals when it is desired to maintain them in a normal condition of active healthy growth; for example, the N.R. of cow's milk is 1 to 3.6. A narrow ratio, often used for horses doing exceptionally heavy work, would seem to have little justification (p. 385). Most commonly the ratio used for working horses is from 1 : 7 to 1 : 8. Animals in the early stages of fattening, those bearing young, and cows in milk are put on diets having from narrow to medium ratios, while idle horses and store cattle are given diets having rather a wide ratio. If the ratio adopted is too wide it is probable that the digestibility of the food will be lowered, and thus food will be wasted. Further, with a very wide ratio the animal may not get sufficient protein for its physiological needs. On the other hand a diet that contains an unnecessarily large amount of protein in proportion to the other food constituents is wasteful, as protein is usually very expensive, and an excessive amount of protein may cause digestive disturbances and diarrhœa.

The method of determining the N.R. of a single food is as follows :

$$\frac{\text{Digestible Carbohydrate} + \text{Digestible Fibre} + (\text{Digestible Fat} \times 2.3)}{\text{Digestible Protein Equivalent}}$$

These constituents are found in the Table of Food Values at the end of the book. For example, the N.R. of oats is:

$$\frac{45 + 3 + (4 \times 2.3)}{7.5} = \frac{57.2}{7.5}$$

The N.R. of oats is therefore 1 : 7.6.

Many methods have been suggested for calculating the N.R. of a complete diet and some of them are misleading and inaccurate. Two correct methods are described here, a long method and a shorter method. The short method was introduced by E. T. Halnan of the School of Agriculture, Cambridge, and is very convenient.

The diet for a stud of horses doing fairly hard work might be:

Hay 10 lb., Oat Straw 4 lb., Oats 12 lb., Bran (Medium) 2 lb., and Beans 1 lb. The procedure by the first method is as follows:

(i) From tables find the amount of digestible protein, fat, nitrogen-free extract and fibre in each food.

(ii) Add up the totals for each food constituent; multiply that for fat by 2.3.

(iii) Divide the protein total into the sum of the others.*

TABLE 78

Food.	Quantity.	Digestible Protein Equivalent.	Digestible Carbo-hydrate.	Digestible Fibre.	Digestible Fat.
	lb.	lb.	lb.	lb.	lb.
Hay	10	0.45	2.5	1.5	0.1
Oat Straw...	4	0.04	0.8	0.72	0.02
Oats	12	0.9	5.4	0.36	0.48
Bran	2	0.24	0.8	0.04	0.08
Beans ...	1	0.19	0.44	0.04	0.01
		1.8	9.9	2.7	0.7

$$(9.9 + 2.7 + (0.7 \times 2.3))/1.8 = 14.2/1.8 = 7.9.$$

The nutritive ratio of the diet is therefore 1 : 7.9.

Halnan's method of calculation makes use of the fact that the nitrogenous ratios of most foods are already available in Food Tables. The successive steps in his method are:

(i) From the standard tables of food compositions, look up the protein equivalent of each constituent of the ration.

(ii) Multiply this percentage figure by the percentage weight of each of the constituents, thereby determining the quantity of protein supplied by each food.

(iii) Multiply the quantity of protein equivalent supplied by each food by the nitrogenous ratio for that food. This gives the digestible carbohydrate equivalent contributed by the individual components of the ration.

(iv) Divide the sum of the digestible protein equivalents given by (ii) into the sum of the digestible carbohydrate equivalents given by (iii). This gives the reciprocal of the nutritive ratio, as in the previous example.

* Calculations concerning the percentages of organic nutrients of foodstuffs seldom or never warrant the use of the totals of protein, carbohydrate and fat being expressed more closely than to the first decimal place. For one thing one rarely has available the actual analysis of the food being used, but only tables of the *average* composition of foodstuffs; secondly one can even less often express the requirements of livestock with the degree of accuracy that such a practice would justify. Throughout the book, therefore, calculations have been " rounded off " in the manner described.

TABLE 79

Food.	Amount.	Digestible Protein Equivalent per cent.	Digestible Protein Equivalent in Food.	N. Ratio.	N. Ratio × Protein Equivalent =Digestible Carbohydrate Equivalent
	lb.	lb.	lb.		lb.
Hay	10	4.5	0.45	9.4	4.23
Oat Straw ...	4	1.0	0.04	39.0	1.56
Oats	12	7.5	0.9	7.6	6.84
Bran	2	12.0	0.24	4.2	1.0
Beans	1	19.5	0.19	2.5	0.48
			1.8		14.1

$$\frac{14.1}{1.8} = 7.8$$

When " feeding standards " are used for constructing rations, i.e., where the amount of protein in the diet is defined, it is obviously unnecessary to determine the N. Ratio.

FATTY RATIOS

The ratio of digestible fat to the other constituents in the food is probably of some considerable importance, but as yet our knowledge on this point is very meagre and opinions regarding the optimum amount of fat to be given in a diet are conflicting.

REFERENCE

1. Murray, J. A., (1914). " The Chemistry of Cattle Feeding and Dairying."

CHAPTER 20

THE FEEDING OF CATTLE

1. General introduction
2. The feeding of dairy cows
   (a) Introduction.
   (b) Fundamental principles.
   (c) The influence of specific foods on milk.
   (d) Preparation for lactation.
   (e) Feeding standards for dairy cows.
   (f) Construction of winter rations.
   (g) The summer feeding of cows.
   (h) General management in relation to feeding.
3. Calf rearing
   (a) Introduction.
   (b) Importance of the feeding of the cow before calving.
   (c) Treatment of the newly born calf.
   (d) Systems of calf rearing.
4. The fattening of cattle
   (a) Introduction.
   (b) The fattening of store cattle.
   (c) The production of baby beef.

(1) General Introduction

For convenience the feeding of cattle may be described in three main sections dealing with the nutrition of calves, dairy cows and beef cattle respectively. There are, of course, no sharp lines of demarcation, for the feeding of calves may be related to the feeding and management of dairy cows, and there are dual-purpose herds whose function is the production of both meat and milk. Nor must it be thought that there are rigid systems of feeding which must be followed in every detail; successful feeding consists in part of the adaptation of the general principles of nutrition to the particular herd and even to the individual animal. When allowance has been made, however, for these variations, there still remains a fairly systematic body of knowledge partly the result of centuries of farming experience and partly derived from more modern research.

The mature cow is a ruminant, capable, as previously described in this book (p. 15) of utilizing fibrous foods with a greater degree of efficiency than non-ruminant species can. This greater capacity for dealing with the fibre of foods is due to the rumen bacteria, by which cellulose and hemi-cellulose in particular are decomposed. Because of the large numbers of micro-organisms which are present in the digestive tract and their abilities for synthesizing accessory food factors, the normal cow, on pastures which are not deficient in mineral elements nor contain toxic ones, is largely independent of dietary sources of members of the vitamin B complex. The high-producing dairy cow, however, because of the limits which the size of the digestive system puts upon the amount of coarse foods which may be ingested, needs to be fed in a manner more closely resembling that of the non-ruminant herbivore or even the omnivorous species. The nature of the bacterial flora in the ruminant is influenced by the kind of food ingested by the animal, but whether the organisms present in the digestive tract of the high-yielding cow produce vitamins sufficient in all respects for its needs would seem to require investigation. Regardless of the type of animal being considered, however, its needs for the fat soluble vitamins A, D and E must be met by dietary supplies, save for small amounts of vitamin D such as may be formed by the action of sunlight on the skin.

The calf begins life as a non-ruminant, dependent upon dietary sources for both water-soluble and fat-soluble vitamins and unable to digest fibre. At this stage, therefore, it requires skilled feeding if it is to have no check in its growth. Gradually the young animal develops its digestive system and in conformity with this anatomical change its diet may gradually be altered until it is able to use efficiently the rations normal to the true ruminant.

Calves and high-yielding dairy cows may thus present more difficult problems in feeding than beef cattle, or low or moderate yielding cows.

(2) The feeding of dairy cows

(a) Introduction.

The modern method of feeding, where each cow is given a ration carefully adjusted to suit the quality and yield of milk, is fundamentally sound and years of practical experience have proved it reliable, economical and better for the cow as regards milk production, general health and breeding capacity than any haphazard system.

The question of feeding cows economically and well is undoubtedly of great national importance and the necessity of producing more milk cannot be over-emphasised. As the food bill of the cows is the heaviest item of expenditure, usually over 70 per cent. of the total, it requires careful consideration.

The principle of standardised feeding is to calculate a maintenance ration and feed this to all the cows and then to give to each cow an allowance of concentrates according to the weight and quality of the milk produced. For the ration to be successful several fundamental principles must be carefully studied.

(b) Fundamental principles.

(i) *Water requirements.*

In another place in this book the need for an adequate supply of water for all animals has been emphasised. The practice of giving cows a constant supply of fresh water has now become more general and this is the only satisfactory method of watering cows, for the introduction of automatic water bowls into a cowshed often leads to a definite increase in the milk yield and an improvement in the constitutions of the animals. When the milk yield is 2 gallons, from 10 to 12 gallons of water for each cow will be needed; above this yield, 1.5 to 2 gallons of water are necessary for each extra gallon of milk. On an average one may say that including maintenance requirements, a cow needs some 3 to 4 gallons of water per gallon of milk produced.

On farms where there is not an automatic supply of water it has been said that dry cows require watering only once a day. This is a great mistake; milking cows should be offered water three or four times daily, depending upon the quantity and quality of the succulents provided. If stall-tied cows are allowed out to water only once a day during winter, they will try to take in their requirements for twenty-four hours, often an impossibility. Only water that is above suspicion should be given to cows.

(ii) Bulk of food.

The total bulk of a ration must be sufficient or else the animals will be discontented and restless and will probably fail to give a good milk yield. On the other hand it is desirable that the ration should not contain too high a proportion of coarse foods, or else there is the risk of the cattle consuming insufficient nutrients in relation to their milk yield.

Despite the fact that the nature of the food itself, in its relation to water absorption and swelling, is involved, the most convenient method of judging the suitability of the bulk of a ration is to calculate its dry matter content. This is done from the data in the tables at the end of the book. If the total dry matter of the ration, expressed as a percentage of the animal's body weight, falls within certain limits then the position is regarded as fairly satisfactory.

The exact percentages to be adopted as standards are, however, open to dispute. Quite clearly, so far as digestive capacity is concerned, the breed of the animal may well influence the issue; so may the nature of the ration which was given to the cow during the period of development of the rumen. In Britain a dry matter intake of 1.5 to 2.0 per cent. of the body weight is accepted as satisfactory for a dry cow or one giving a low yield. There is less agreement about the desirable upper limit for higher yielding beasts. Wright and Morris [1] have suggested figures for Ayrshire cows and dairy Shorthorns, and for South Devons and large Friesians, which are equivalent to 3.0 to 3.5 per cent. American practice, quoted by Foot,[2] often entails the free use of bulky foods without the use of concentrates. For ordinary purposes, therefore, one may accept 2.5 per cent. as a safe minimum for this class of stock, the rations then being carefully increased so long as there is a corresponding additional milk yield and provided there are no digestive upsets.

The fundamental issue, of course, is the nature of the system of management, both of the land itself and of the cattle which consume the produce of the land, that will provide the largest quantity of food for human consumption. Not only is the type of crop which should be produced involved in this matter, but also the breeds of livestock, which are to consume the crops, and the way in which they are managed. There is no body of systematic evidence upon which conclusions may be drawn, but the changes in food distribution, etc., which have followed the war, suggest that in Britain there may well have to be increased consumption of home produced foods for livestock; this will certainly mean the use of more coarse foods and less imported concentrates. If this will mean greater use of good quality silage, good quality hay and dried grass, together with a transference of attention from quantity of milk produced to efficiency of food utilisation,. as well as to greater interest in general animal health, it will be a good change.

Where the more conventional type of ration is being fed to individual cows in a large herd then, once the ration has been fixed—say to contain 25 - 30 lb. of dry matter for a herd of Ayrshire cows in various stages of lactation—the method is to feed concentrates first, then hay and finally to bed down with straw; those animals not getting a full ration of concentrates will eat some of the straw to satisfy their appetite, while others whose stomach. capacity has been satisfied with more nutritious food will leave the straw alone and also probably eat less hay. In many cases, if very palatable oat straw is used for bedding, the cows will leave very little of it.

If the cows are consuming too much bulky food, that is to say if there is an excessive amount of coarse fodder such as hay and straw in the diet, many of the animals will be found grunting, which is an indication of uncomfortable overloading of the stomach and points to the necessity of readjusting the ration. It should be realised that the figures given are for average cows and that though many heavy milkers have a higher rumen capacity and are thus able to consume more food, there are many for whom the bulky food or roughage must be reduced so as to allow of sufficient intake of total nutriment.

In an attempt to determine what modifications of feeding practice might be essential where more complex and bulky mixtures of foods, such as would be given on farms aiming at a high degree of self-sufficiency were fed, Blaxter and French[3] varied the times, order and frequency at which a standard ration of concentrates, hay, straw and mangolds was fed to a small dairy herd, making sure, however, that hay and straw were not fed just before milking. They came to the conclusion that "providing care is taken to prevent cows eating too large a quantity of highly palatable foods all at once—which might possibly cause digestive disturbances—and providing that care is taken to conform to advice given on the relation of feeding times to the production of milk of high quality, then dividing the ration into a. larger number of meals, or spreading the feeding of the ration over a longer period is without any substantial effect on milk yield." They also concluded that "herd rationing" (where a calculated amount of a basal ration, sufficient for the full herd, is spread out in the field or the yard for the animals to consume, the concentrates for production above the first gallon of milk being given individually) could be satisfactory only when foods of the lowest feeding value were spread, otherwise the faster-eating or larger animals received more than their share of food.

So far as the types of bulky food which might be given under such conditions are concerned, the merits and limits of hay and straw have been discussed elsewhere in this book (p. 159). Foot,[2] concerning succulent bulky foods, has described the need for a fodder which is palatable, high in digestible nutrients per unit of dry matter, requires little hand labour and stores well for use throughout the winter. He regards the two most hopeful crops as grass-clover and marrow-stem kale silages.

(iii) *Minerals*.

The modern dairy cow has heavy demands made upon her in regard to mineral metabolism. The minerals to which special attention must be paid are sodium, chlorine, calcium and phosphorus, and it may be assumed that with the possible exception of iodine the other necessary minerals will usually be present in the food. The most satisfactory method of ensuring an adequate supply of sodium chloride is to provide salt licks, which may have traces of iodine incorporated—one being placed in each stall, or a number of them in courts. Salt should be available at all times, not only when a cow is in full milk, but when she is dry. While the addition of salt to mixed meals may increase the palatibility of some food it is better to allow the animals to take what salt they want, while permitting them free access to water.

The lime and phosphorus supply requires more careful consideration, both as regards the quantity and the proportions of one to the other. As explained on page 68 the desirable ratio of calcium to phosphorus is about 1.3 to 1, but considerable variation may occur in this ratio without detrimental effects, provided that the supplies of vitamin D, calcium and phosphorus are adequate.

It is very difficult to state minimal requirements of calcium and phosphorus because the percentage utilisation of that in the intake varies greatly (p. 64), but in the practical feeding of cows a sufficiency can usually be provided by giving 40 g. (1.6 oz.) CaO and 22 g. (0.8 oz.) P_2O_5 per 1,000 lb. live weight for maintenance, and 17.4 g. CaO and 21.8 g. P_2O_5 per gallon (10 lb.) of milk. Thus an Ayrshire cow giving 4 gallons of milk would require about 112 g. CaO and 109 g. P_2O_5.

With normal *combinations* of foods in the rations of cows it is unlikely that there will be a deficiency of phosphorus, but this may occur when the hay is exceptionally poor in this element. As a rule the phosphorus is in excess, while the lime content is generally below requirements. Timothy hay, which generally has a very low content of lime, is for this reason not suitable for cows that are heavy milkers. It is perhaps not generally realised that some hays contain less lime than is present in the cereal straws.

A deficiency of lime can to a certain extent be corrected by the addition of powdered limestone to the diet, but this must be done with caution because excessive quantities will have a detrimental effect on protein, fat and phosphorus assimilation. So far as possible shortage of lime should be made good by using good quality legume hay or hay containing a fair proportion of clover. If further adjustment is necessary, sterilised bone flour or " low temperature " bone meal should be given at the rate of about 2 ozs. daily.

Whatever mineral supplements are given and however well a heavy milking cow may be fed during the height of lactation, she will most probably be unable to maintain a mineral equilibrium: in consequence there will be a drain upon her reserves. Provided this drain is not too severe and that she is given a reasonably long dry period between calvings, the reserves can be built up again satisfactorily. In the case of sodium chloride, however, there are no reserves, therefore this must be given throughout lactation.

(iv) *Vitamins*.

Carotene or vitamin A must occur in sufficient amounts in the ration. Very often it is assumed that summer pasturage will provide a sufficient bodily store to last through the winter period. This, however, is a most unreliable method and the winter ration should provide the vitamin, using good silage, dried grass, fresh green crops such as kale, or cod liver oil or proprietary carotene concentrates (in commercial dairy cubes) for the purpose.

Vitamin D will be provided by well-cured hay or by cod liver oil, and vitamin E is unlikely to be absent from a good mixed ration.

Water soluble factors are normally provided in sufficient quantities by the rumen bacteria, but whether the latter can furnish sufficient of these factors for the very high rate of turnover of the high-yielding cow is not too clear. For the sake of its minor constituents alone there seems to be good reason for the regular inclusion in the ration of a small quantity of succulent green food or of good silage. The bloom on the coats of animals which receive such a small daily supplement is not fortuitous.

(v) *Palatability*.

To what extent palatability is related to food digestibility is not known, but appetising foods do result in increased food consumption. Since maximum consumption of foodstuffs is desirable in the case of heavy-milking cows, their rations should necessarily be palatable. Furthermore, dairy cows thrive better when they are given food which they like. An unpalatable food—such as, for example, palm kernel cake —can be made more acceptable to the cows by introducing it gradually into their daily ration. Some foods can be made more palatable by steaming and giving them warm, or by pouring over the mixture a little treacle and water, but spoiled foods should never be offered to cows as, apart from the possibility of tainting the milk, such foods are not relished. Salt often increases the palatability of many concentrates and may be given at the rate of 1 to 2 oz. daily. Glutinous and heavy foods, such as maize gluten feed, and pea and bean meal, give better results when suitably mixed with foods which tend to open them up, since they are then better digested and more pleasant to eat.

(c) The influence of specific foods upon milk.

When an increase in milk secretion has followed the introduction of a heavy root ration it is almost certain that the cows have been kept short of water, or that their feeding has been unsatisfactory in some other respect. Excellent results can be obtained when no roots at all are given to dairy cows, but, to animals fed chiefly on dry foods and by-products during the long winter months, a few roots supply succulent food that is very palatable and is obviously relished. It is impossible to assess the real nutritive value of fresh vegetable juices to animals that are housed during the winter and kept and fed under conditions that can only be described as unnatural. For dairy cows the limiting profitable daily intake of roots is about 30 lb./day.

Except for iodinated proteins and perhaps the active factors of young herbage little is known about the ability of specific foodstuffs to influence yield as opposed to the quality of milk. There are a number of " beliefs " about the virtues of various foods but. they have received no systematic tests. Palm kernel cake and meal and coconut cake are said to increase the percentage of butter-fat; cod liver oil, on the other hand, has a depressing effect and for safety should not be given in greater amounts than 2 oz. daily. With these possible exceptions, it is doubtful if any single food has a very definite or lasting effect on either the yield of milk or percentage of fat. A change in the diet, almost in any direction, often brings about a temporary increase both of yield and butter-fat, but these increases are only temporary and do not last long provided that the cow has already been brought up to her maximum sustained yield by suitable feeding and management. Both the quantity and quality of the milk can be raised, however, if a potentially high-yielding cow is given a suitable and adequate ration where previously her diet had been deficient.

Several foods affect the quality of butter-fat. Bean and pea meals, if given in large amounts, make the butter hard and somewhat tallowy, and the same applies, but to a less extent, to cotton cake and cotton seed meal. Linseed cake and meal, large quantities of maize or maize meal, from which the germ has not been removed, and rice meal, all of which contain oil of a low melting point, make the butter-fat soft. Coconut cake and meal make a fairly hard butter. Pasture grass, especially in the early part of the year when it is fresh and succulent, makes soft butter-fat.

Many of these points require further investigation; for example the different effects of cotton and linseed cakes seem extreme if they are to be ascribed to their fat content alone.

Fresh pigmented foods of all kinds give a rich yellow colour to milk and butter (due to the carotenoid pigments). Such succulent foods as turnips, swedes and cabbages are liable to taint milk if given before milking and if they are fed in excess, particularly to start with. They are also likely to produce a taint if the troughs from which they are fed are left dirty or if these foods are stored near the cow-shed or milk-house, because warm milk very readily takes on any aroma that may be in the air.

Many plants taint milk.[4] The Garlics (*Allium* sp.) give to milk a flavour of garlic or onion, and several of the *Ranunculi*, such as *Ranunculus repens* and *R. ficaria*, are blamed for spoiling milk. In addition to the above, the following plants should be looked upon with suspicion as liable to spoil milk by giving it a bad flavour or odour: Butterwort, Corn Chamomile, Hemlock, Henbane, Lesser Sium, Lesser Watercress, Penny Cress, Mayweed, Tansy, Water Parsnip, Wild Chamomile and Wormwood, Cowbane, Fool's Parsley, Hellebore, Ivy, Mint, and Yarrow.

(d) Preparation for lactation.

(i) *Feeding preparatory to calving.*

An effort should be made to have all milch cows dried off not later than six weeks before calving. A cow which has been milking well throughout a lactation period has been subjected to a prolonged strain so that special care is necessary to see that she recovers her tissue losses during the dry period. It is here that the value of a good observant herdsman becomes apparent, because to get the best results each cow should receive individual attention. The diet will have been reduced during the final stages of lactation, especially if there has been difficulty in stopping lactation. After this it should gradually be made more generous, the object being to have the cow in good condition, though not fat, at the time she is due to calve. It is particularly important to see that the mineral supply is adequate to make good the depletion from her reserves, especially if the cow has been a heavy milker. A cow which calves down in good condition will give a bigger total yield of milk than one which has been badly kept and fed on low grade foods. If calving takes place in the spring, which is the normal time, and there is early grass available, this should go a long way towards meeting her requirements; in addition, the exercise and exposure to the sun will be greatly beneficial.

The cows which calve when grass is not available will require special feeding with concentrates and such succulent foods as are available, choosing for preference those yielding vitamin A. The quantity of concentrates allowed will depend upon the condition of the animal at the end of her lactation. If this is poor, a daily ration of 3 to 4 lb. of mixed concentrates of the same nature as that given for milk yield will do to start with at six weeks or so before calving, and this should gradually be increased until at a week before parturition she is receiving 10 lb. daily. Some dairymen feed much more than this; Halnan and Garner[5] suggest from 10 to 20 lb. daily, the maximum quantity being reached a month before calving and maintained until the cow goes off her feed as calving time approaches. It will be appreciated that close personal attention is needed by the herdsman if heavy-milking cows are to be in the best condition at calving time, and sufficient laxative foods should be included in the dietary to keep the bowels in a good state. Only good quality hay should be given, and, if possible, hay containing some clover. It may be advisable to give 2 to 4 oz. of bone flour daily and an allowance of cod liver oil, while salt licks should be provided. The same general considerations must be paid to the in-calf heifer as it is very important to see that she is in good condition at the first calving.

The food given to bring a cow into good condition will be sufficient to meet the needs of the growing calf provided that it contains sufficient protein and mineral matter. Maynard[6] recommends an increase of 17 per cent. in the protein of the cow's maintenance ration if spread over the whole period of pregnancy, or 40 per cent. during the closing stages.

(ii) *Feeding cows just after calving.*

For the first day or two after calving the cow's diet should be of a laxative nature; it depends upon her state how soon liberal feeding can be begun, and this must be left to the judgment of the herdsman. Provided that the cow has cleansed properly and shows a good appetite there is nothing to be gained by keeping her on short rations for very long. On the contrary, as soon as she is fit for it, the cow should be given gradually increasing quantities of concentrates until the amount given corresponds to the standard set down for the milk she yields, and then this amount should be exceeded by about 2 lb. of starch equivalent in anticipation that she will respond to the treatment by still further increasing her output. When it is clear that a cow has reached her maximum output then the ration should be steadied and fixed for the yield that is given.

It is often stated that a cow cannot be expected to give a heavy yield of milk and keep herself in condition at the same time. In general, this statement is not correct, as with adequate and proper feeding not only will the yield of milk be kept high—and often be increased—but the condition of the cow can be kept in a satisfactory state. There are, however, exceptional cows that persistently remain thin so long as they are milking, do what one may; with these animals it is important to see that they have as long a dry period before calving as is possible, otherwise when the calf is born it may be undersized and sickly and the subsequent lactation period of the cow a poor one. On the other hand, some cows seem to convert most of the food that is given to them into flesh instead of making milk; they get fat quickly after calving but give a poor milk yield. While in many cases this is due to an inherent predisposition of the animal it is sometimes the result of bad feeding prior to and immediately after calving.

(e) Feeding standards for dairy cows.

(i) *Maintenance requirements.*

A Departmental Committee which was appointed by the Ministry of Agriculture in 1924 suggested[7] that the maintenance requirements of a 1,000 lb. (9 cwt.) cow, e.g., an Ayrshire, would be met—so far as energy and protein are concerned—by giving 6 lb. of starch equivalent and 0.6 lb. protein equivalent. This has been proved by experience to be quite satisfactory. For cows and bullocks over this weight, 0.4 lb. starch equivalent and 0.06 lb. protein equivalent should be added per 100 lb. body weight increase, and for every 100 lb. body weight less than 1,000 lb. a similar amount should be deducted. Thus the following maintenance requirements apply to various breeds of dairy cows and also to beef cattle of similar weights, taking into consideration energy, protein and bulk:

TABLE 80

Breed of Cattle	Liveweight	Starch Equiv.	Protein Equiv.	Total Dry Matter in Ration	
				at 2%	at 3%
	lb.	lb.	lb.		
Dexter	650	4.6	0.39	13	20
Jersey	800	5.2	0.48	16	24
Kerry	850	5.4	0.51	17	26
Guernsey	950	5.8	0.57	19	29
Ayrshire	1000	6.0	0.60	20	30
Red Poll	1100	6.4	0.66	22	33
N. Devon ... ... Welsh Black ... ... Blue Albion	1150	6.6	0.69	23	35
British Friesian ... ... Dairy Shorthorn ...	1250	7.0	0.75	25	38
Longhorn ... ... Lincoln Red Shorthorn	1300	7.2	0.78	26	39
S. Devon	1450	7.8	0.87	29	44

(ii) *Requirements for Milk Production.*

The amount of food required to produce 10 lb. of milk of average quality, containing 3.7 per cent. of fat, recommended by the Departmental Committee was 2.5 lb. starch equivalent and 0.6 lb. protein equivalent. For many years this standard was adopted with apparent success but after a critical review of the evidence Halnan suggested that this allowance of protein was on the generous side and recommended that it be reduced to 0.5 lb. per 10 lb. of milk. McIntosh[8] came to a similar conclusion as a result of a large-scale test under ordinary practical dairying conditions where 1400 cows were used, half the number being fed on the higher allowance of protein and half on the lower. It therefore seems safe to adopt the lower standard of protein requirements for general purposes, provided that at least a proportion of the protein is of a reasonably high biological value for milk production. When cows are secreting milk that is rich in fat, the allowance of both starch and protein equivalents should be raised and McIntosh recommends an increase at the rate of 0.5 lb. starch equivalent and 0.10 lb. protein equivalent for each one per cent. of fat above 3.7 per cent. secreted in the milk. Standard allowances for maintenance and for milk production for milk containing up to 3.7 per cent. of fat would be:

TABLE 81

Breed of Cattle	Live-weight.	1 Gallon Starch Equiv.	1 Gallon Prot. Equiv.	2 Gallons Starch Equiv.	2 Gallons Prot. Equiv.	3 Gallons Starch Equiv.	3 Gallons Prot. Equiv.	4 Gallons Starch Equiv.	4 Gallons Prot. Equiv
	lb.	lb.	lb.	lb.	lb.	lb.	lb.	lb.	lb.
Dexter ...	650	7.1	0.89	9.6	1.39	12.1	1.89	14.6	2.39
Jersey ...	800	7.7	0.98	10.2	1.48	12.7	1.98	15.2	2.48
Kerry ...	850	7.9	1.01	10.4	1.51	12.9	2.01	15.4	2.51
Guernsey ...	950	8.3	1.07	10.8	1.57	13.3	2.07	15.8	2.57
Ayrshire ...	1000	8.5	1.10	11.0	1.60	13.5	2.10	16.0	2.60
Red Poll ...	1100	8.9	1.16	11.4	1.66	13.9	2.16	16.4	2.66
N. Devon ... Welsh Black Blue Albion	1150	9.1	1.19	11.6	1.69	14.1	2.19	16.6	2.69
British Friesian Dairy Short-horn ...	1250	9.5	1.25	12.0	1.75	14.5	2.25	17.0	2.75
Longhorn ... Lincoln Red Shorthorn	1300	9.7	1.28	12.2	1.78	14.7	2.28	17.2	2.78
S. Devon ...	1450	10.3	1.37	12.8	1.87	15.3	2.37	17.8	2.87

For Breeds which naturally secrete milk containing a high percentage of fat the necessary adjustments to the Table must be made.

The first essential of a rationing system is the recording of each cow's daily yield, for it is only by recording that non-paying " boarders " can be eliminated and good producers can be encouraged to do better.

Assuming that the farmer has knowledge of the daily yield of each of his cows, his simplest method of feeding is to give to all cows their maintenance portion of the diet and then to allocate to each the weight of concentrates known to supply the necessary starch and protein equivalents. This is most conveniently done by measure, the measure used being known to hold a certain weight of the mixture that is being fed. In a very short time this method loses all appearance of complication and difficulty, and the owner will have the satisfaction of knowing that his cows are doing well and that they are producing milk economically. Normally the necessary starch equivalent and protein for a gallon of milk will be provided by 3.5 lb. of the usual mixed concentrates. More will be required, rarely above 4 lb., if the mixture is chiefly composed of foods having low starch and protein values, or if the hay is of poor quality. On the other hand, if the concentrates are rich or the hay is of first class quality, 3 lb. of concentrates will be sufficient.

The general requirements for a satisfactory milk production ration have been described elsewhere (p. 268), and here it is only necessary to give a few examples before passing on to consider the more detailed feeding of cows in lactation.

Dry matter requirements are such that the choice of foods is limited to those which have a starch equivalent of about 60 or more, or which can be balanced against one another to give a mixture of that average value. This restricts the choice of foods to the cereal grains, dried beet pulp, wheat offals and the oil seed cakes and meals, together with somewhat smaller amounts (because of their cost or relative scarcity) of meat meal, fish meal and dried grass.

By the method described previously, (p. 294) for example, a simple mixture of crushed oats and linseed cake, which will have the desired ratio of starch equivalent to protein equivalent of 5 to 1, may easily be made. Such simple mixtures are not generally to be recommended, save for short periods of scarcity. They tend to be lacking in some of the mineral elements or in the vitamins, or to contain protein of relatively low biological value which, without some suitable supplementary protein, will not be so efficiently used as might be the case.

In the case of more complex mixtures, the easiest course is to group the available carbohydrate concentrates together to give a mixture of known S.E. and P.E. This may then be compounded with a similar mixture of protein rich foods, also of known S.E. and P.E. Sometimes the amounts of the various foods which make up one part of the ration— the mixture of cereals, for example—may be determined simply by what the farmer has on hand; at other times he may decide in advance what type of mixture he will have and purchase quantities of the constituent foods to suit his plan. In the latter case he has the opportunity to consider other factors than the starch and protein equivalents of the foods alone, e.g., mineral and vitamin contents, protein quality, and general palatability. A few examples of such rations, with brief comments upon their quality, is given below.

TABLE 82

	Ration 1	Ration 2	Ration 3	Ration 4	Ration 5
Crushed oats ...	250	50	50	50	50
Cracked maize	—	50	50	50	50'
Kibbled beans ...	150	100	50	45	45
Linseed cake ...	—	—	50	45	35
Dried grass ... (Good qual.)	—	—	—	10	10
Fish meal ...	—	—	—	—	10
Quantity to feed per gallon (lb.) (S.E./P.E.=5.)	4.0	3.75	3.75	3.75	3.75

Ration 1.

This is simple and can be made up entirely of home-grown foods. There is some degree of supplementation between the proteins of the two constituents; the fat content is low in relation to that in the milk; the Ca/P ratio is low and the amount of calcium in 4 lb. of the ration small compared with that in one gallon of milk; the carotene content is negligible.

Ration 2.

What has been said of the first ration applies fairly well to this, except that the use of yellow maize may provide a moderate amount of carotene.

Ration 3.

An improvement with respect to ration 2 so far as fat content is concerned.

Ration 4.

Slight improvement in protein quality of the ration compared with ration 3; substantial proportion of the cow's daily needs for carotene provided; possibly other trace food factors provided.

Ration 5.

Further slight improvement in protein quality; 3.75 lb. of ration now contains a substantial proportion of the calcium needed for one gallon of milk, with improved Ca/P ratio.

More complex rations usually require greater care in the mixing of the ingredients. This is especially true of such complicated ones as some of the commercial preparations, where, for example, a single ration may contain wheat offals, maize, barley, oats, maize gluten, and malt culms, plus linseed, palm kernel, undecorticated and decorticated ground nut cakes, fish meal, and mineral and vitamin supplements; for this type of product efficient mixers are needed. (See also "National Foods" described in Appendix 2.)

(f) Construction of winter rations.

The composition of the winter ration (i.e., for a period of about seven months) should be decided upon some time before it is expected to begin house-feeding, in order that contracts may be made with food merchants, since as a rule it is more profitable to contract ahead than to buy from month to month. Satisfactory contracts can be made which will allow for any fall in the market price of foods and the merchant will deliver in quantities as required. In selecting foods the points to which reference has previously been made, such as variety, palatability, specific action, composition, etc., must be considered. Naturally the dairyman, if farming land, will make use of the crops he has unless it is more economical to sell his own crops and buy in other foods. Assuming that the farmer has a supply of hay, oat straw, swedes and turnips, silage and oats, he will probably still require some nitrogenous and carbonaceous concentrates. It is convenient to divide the ration into *maintenance* and *production* parts. For simplicity in feeding the maintenance portion may be combined with sufficient of the production part of the ration to form nutriment for maintenance and one gallon of milk, the purely maintenance part being generally made up of hay, straw, roots and silage; to it will be added a sufficient portion of the concentrates, so that the combined parts will maintain the cow and enable her to produce one or more gallons of milk according to the amount of the production ration given.

Some examples of rations actually fed in practice may usefully be reproduced here. The first is that prescribed (Linton) for a herd of eighty Ayrshire cows (average weight 1000 lb.) kept for the production of certified milk in the east of Scotland. The cows were started on this ration in September and it was not changed, except from swedes to turnips, throughout the winter and until they were put out to grass in the spring. It gave excellent results. The concentrates were given dry, no mashes being used except for cows just about to calve.

TABLE 83

	Quantity	Dry Matter	Starch equivalent	Protein equivalent
BULKY FOODS:—	lb.	lb.	lb.	lb.
Hay	10	8.6	3.6	0.60
Oat Straw	7	6.0	1.2	0.07
Swedes	35	4.2	2.5	0.25
		18.8	7.3	0.9
CONCENTRATES:—				
Bean Meal	2	1.70	1.36	0.38
Bran	1	0.88	0.42	0.10
Sesame Cake	1	0.91	0.73	0.39
Dried Grains	2	1.80	1.02	0.25
Crushed Oats ...	5	4.35	3.05	0.37
Ground Nut Meal ...	1	0.90	0.71	0.41
Paisley Meal	4	3.50	2.96	0.72
	16	14.0	10.2	2.6
Total in Ration		32.8	17.5	3.5
Requirements		30.0	17.0	2.8
Difference		+2.8	+0.5	+0.7

This ration is constructed for maintenance and 4 gallons, or roughly 40 lb. of milk, of 4 per cent. butter-fat.

For 4 gallons of milk the requirements will be (Table 84).

TABLE 84

	Starch equivalent	Protein equivalent
Maintenance	6 lb.	0.60 lb.
Per 40 lb. Milk	11 lb.	2.20 lb.
	17 lb.	2.80 lb.

To determine if the ration agrees with the standards suggested, it should be set out as above, the dry matter, starch equivalent and protein equivalent of each food being calculated from the table given at the end of the book.

The ration is rather liberal, but the situation of the farm is very exposed to cold east winds. Had the situation been more favourable a reasonable economy could have been effected by omitting the ground nut meal. This would have resulted in a difference between requirements and supply of (a) dry matter + 1.7 lb.; (b) starch equivalent—0.2 lb. and (c) protein equivalent of + 0.3 lb.

The next ration (No. 2) is constructed for a mixed herd, chiefly Ayrshires and Shorthorns, (average weight about 1100 lb.). The butter-fat percentage is slightly under 4. The requirements for maintenance will therefore be:—starch equivalent 6.4 lb., protein equivalent 0.65 lb.; and for milk production per 10 lbs. of milk:—starch equivalent 2.5 lb.; and protein equivalent 0.50 lb. Here again the production part is calculated for 4 gallons of milk, so that the cows will be given for maintenance the full quantity of hay, straw and roots set down, and for each 10 lb. of milk one-fourth (4½ lb.) of the mixed concentrates.

RATION No. 2
TABLE 85

Food	Amount	Dry Matter	Starch equiv.	Protein equiv.
	lb.	lb.	lb.	lb.
Hay	12	10.32	3.72	0.54
Oat Straw	7	6.02	1.19	0.07
Swedes	30	3.60	2.10	0.21
Maintenance		19.9	7.0	0.8
Crushed Oats	8	6.96	4.88	0.60
Bean Meal	2	1.72	1.36	0.38
Linseed Cake	4	3.56	2.88	0.98
Undec. Cotton Cake ...	2	1.78	0.76	0.30
Locust Beans	2	1.74	1.40	0.09
Production of 40 lb. Milk	18	15.8	11.3	2.4
Maintenance		19.9	7.0	0.8
Total		35.7	18.3	3.2
Standard requirements ...		33.0	16.40	2.7
Difference	—	+2.7	+1.9	+0.5

This differs from Ration No. 1 in several respects, though the total amount of nutriment for milk production is approximately the same. The hay is ordinary meadow hay instead of Italian rye. A greater quantity of crushed oats is given, and linseed cake and unde-corticated cotton cake replace the ground nut meal and sesame cake. The linseed cake being laxative will balance the somewhat binding effect of the undecorticated cotton cake. Locust beans are included chiefly because of their palatability. The diet is rather deficient in mineral matter, and this might be made good by the inclusion of a small amount of fish meal or meat and bone meal as in the Ration No. 3.

In this case there is practically an excess of 2 lb. of starch equivalent and half a pound of protein over theoretical requirements; the explanatory remarks made in connection with the first ration also apply here, and as the situation was very exposed and cold it was thought advisable to feed slightly in excess of standard requirements. Had the locust bean been omitted there would still have been a surplus of 0.49 lb. S.E. and 0.42 lb. P.E. with consequent financial advantage.

The point at which a cow begins to pay for her food and other costs depends on many things, but in the average herd it is generally considered that unless she is yielding more than 2 gallons a day she scarcely pays for her keep.

RATION No. 3

The following ration was given to a herd of cows chiefly composed of Ayrshires, with a few Shorthorns (average weight 1100 lb.). The farmer divided the diet into three portions—(a) hay, straw, roots and silage, which was given to all the cows; and (b) a wet mash of concentrates, which was also given to all cows and was considered when added to the first part to be sufficient for maintenance and 1 gallon of milk; and (c) a dry feed of concentrates, 3 lb. of which were given for every gallon above the first that the cows yielded. The ration is as follows:

TABLE 86

Food	Amount	Dry Matter	Starch equivalent	Protein equivalent
(a)	lb.	lb.	lb.	lb.
Hay	5.5	4.73	1.70	0.25
Oat Straw	10	8.60	1.70	0.10
Swedes	35	4.20	2.45	0.25
Silage	30	7.50	4.20	0.52
		25.0	10.0	1.1
(b) MASH:—				
Bran (Medium)	2	0.87	0.49	0.12
Oats	1	1.74	1.22	0.15
Cotton Seed Meal ...	0.5	0.46	0.34	0.17
Maize Meal	0.5	0.44	0.40	0.03
Bean Meal	0.5	0.43	0.34	0.10
Meat and Bone Meal ...	0.25	0.23	0.23	0.16
	4.7	4.2	3.0	0.7
(c) DRY FEED:—				
Bran	.1	0.87	0.49	0.12
Oats	1.25	1.08	0.76	0.09
Dried Grains	1	0.90	0.51	0.13
Bean Meal	0.5	0.43	0.34	0.10
Bombay Cotton Cake ...	1	0.89	0.38	0.15
Linseed Cake	1	0.89	0.72	0.25
Meat and Bone Meal ...	0.25	.0.23	0.23	0.16
	6.0	5.3	3.4	1.0

In the above ration the portions (a) and (b), which together were assumed by the farmer to supply nutriment for maintenance and 1 gallon of milk of ordinary quality, are greatly in excess of standard requirements in regard to starch equivalent:

TABLE 87

		Dry Matter	Starch equivalent	Protein equivalent
Standard ...	...	27-30 lb.	8.9 lb.	1.16 lb.
In Ration ...	...	29 lb.	13.0 lb.	1.8 lb.
Difference	... ...		+4.1 lb.	+0.6 lb.

On the other hand, the dry food given at the rate of 3 lb. per gallon of milk falls short with starch equivalent while the protein is correct:

TABLE 88

				Starch equivalent	Protein equivalent
Standard ...	...	...	...	2.5 lb.	0.50 lb.
In Ration ...	...	...	...	1.7 lb.	0.50 lb.
Difference	...	...	...	—0.8 lb.	Nil.

Therefore, assuming that there are cows in the herd only being fed for maintenance and 1 gallon of milk, these will be getting 4 lb. of starch equivalent and 0.6 lb. of protein too much. But for the cows giving 2 gallons a day the excess of starch equivalent will be just over 3 lb. and the protein excess will be the same, 0.6 lb. This diet therefore requires correcting; some of the concentrates given in the mash should be added to the dry feed so as to increase this to the standard, and the maintenance portion could be considerably reduced by leaving out the swedes altogether; the maize meal in the mash could also be dispensed with.

After correction on the lines indicated, the ration would be a good one inasmuch as the concentrates have been well chosen and are varied, and the meat and bone meal besides supplying protein is a valuable source of minerals. The total dry matter in the ration is correct.

The nitrogenous ratio of part (a) of the diet is 1:11.6; of part (b), 1:3.5; and of part (c), 1:3.8. Of the whole composite diet the nitrogenous ratio is 1:6.4.

RATION No. 4

The following ration is given as an example of dry feeding, without roots or mashes; straw is not available, either for bedding or feeding. The ration is for Shorthorn cows weighing about 1250 lb. and producing milk containing 4 per cent. of butter-fat. Italian rye-grass hay forms the maintenance portion, and the concentrates are for 1 gallon of milk, so that for each gallon (or roughly 10 lb.) of milk, 3.5 lb. of the mixture will require to be given. .

TABLE 89

Food	Amount	Dry Matter	Starch equiv.	Protein equiv.
	lb.	lb.	lb.	lb.
Hay	20	17.20	7.20	1.20
Oats	1	0.87	0.61	0.08
Cotton Seed Meal ...	0.25	0.22	0.17	0.09
Ex. Soya Meal ...	0.25	0.22	0.16	0.09
Dried Grains	0.50	0.45	0.62	0.23
Bran (medium)	0.75	0.65	0.38	0.09
Locust Beans	0.50	0.44	0.70	0.05
Meat and Bone Meal	0.25	0.24	0.24	0.19
		20.3	10.1	2.0
Standard for maintenance and 10 lb. milk ...			9.8	1.3
Difference			+0.3	+0.7

RATION No. 5

At the Field Station of the Agricultural Research Council, at Compton, Berks, the dairy herd (Ayrshires) receive an allowance of approximately 10 lb. of hay and 30 lb. of kale per head per day from October until the end of the year, by which time the kale is finished and the allowance is changed to some 7 lb. of hay plus 56 lb. of good silage. In addition to this a production ration of 3.5 to 4 lb. of dairy cubes per gallon of milk is fed.[9]

Woodman[10] has described, for a 1200 lb. Shorthorn—producing 3 gallons of milk per day—a ration which is rather similar to the above. Its composition is given below:

TABLE 90

	lb.
Good Meadow Hay	18
Marrow-stem Kale	56
Crushed Barley	2.25
Dec. Ground Nut Cake ...	1.5

The kale, as usual, is fed after milking.

Such rations as the first, second and fourth could be improved in quality by substituting for a part of the other ingredients, relatively small amounts of such foods as good grass-clover silage, or good dried grass, or, where the local conditions permit its growth, kale. A minimum allowance of 1-2 lb. of dried grass, or its approximate equivalent in terms of kale or silage, per head per day would be sufficient: it should form part of the ration for maintenance and the production of the first gallon of milk.

It should be noted that animals which have become used to a ration containing a good proportion of concentrates, are often slow to adapt themselves to bulky foods in large amounts. The length of time involved will vary with the local conditions, but may be of the order of a year."

Periodically a farmer may be faced with a temporary shortage of foodstuffs. If the herd consists of animals in different stages of lactation, he may then have to decide which of the animals should, for the time being, receive somewhat less food. Blaxter [11] suggests that " as the effect of under feeding the cow during mid-lactation is small, especially if the plane of nutrition is high, concentrate allowances could be reduced at this time and fed to cows before they calve when the response to a higher plane of nutrition is greater ". This illustrates one of the benefits to be derived from earlier good feeding.

(g) The summer feeding of cows.

No hard and fast rules can be laid down for summer feeding as so much depends on the type of farm, quality of the land, the season, and the nature and quantity of the pasture. In general good pasture at the beginning of the season is able to supply a cow with sufficient food for maintenance and approximately 3 gallons of milk, but very good pasture during the Spring flush will supply sufficient for 4 or even 5 gallons. As the season advances concentrates must be used increasingly, and on many farms by the end of July or middle of August the pasture will yield little more nourishment than is needed for maintenance. In September, however, there is usually a short fresh period of growth, but the feeding value of the grass never reaches that of Spring grass. It is here that the eye and judgment of the farmer are greatly needed, because milking cows or those shortly to calve should not be allowed to fill themselves with coarse fibrous grass. Towards the end of the time cattle are kept at grass great care will be needed to keep up their condition and supply them with sufficient nutriment for their milk yield, as once this has gone off it is not an easy matter to get it back. It is no economy to save concentrates when the cows are at grass late in the season. The quantity of concentrates allowed is also governed by the distance the cows have to walk to and from the milking shed in the day. The author has known a marked decrease in yield in a big herd to follow a long enforced walk to pasture from the shed. The weather at the end of the summer has also to be taken into account, as it follows that cold prevailing winds, such as easterly winds on the east coast of Scotland, will call for an additional allowance of food. Suggestions have often been put forward as to the quantity of concentrates to be allowed at grass from week to week approaching the autumn, but, as has been said above, this can be only judged by the farmer himself. A mixture of concentrates of a slight laxative nature should be given at the end of the grass season, because the grass being fibrous is inclined to be binding. At the early part of the season, when the grass is succulent and inclined to scour, a concentrate liable to constipate should be chosen; the most popular of these is Egyptian or Bombay undecorticated cotton cake, though a more carbonaceous food, e.g., maize, would be more suitable as it would balance the high protein content of young grass. Should the grass be lush and rich when the cows are first turned out

they should **invariably** be given a feed of hay or hay and concentrates
to take the edge off the appetite, and so prevent the animals from gorging
themselves on foods which may cause acute tympany; many cattle are
killed each year because due precautions are not taken in this respect.
Clover, especially in the early morning when it still holds the night's
dew, is more dangerous than grass pasture.

(h) General management in relation to feeding.

However good a ration may be in itself its value to the cow will be
lessened if the method of feeding is not good. The dietary must be
distributed throughout the day so that the cows are not kept too long
without food, and, on the other hand, it is of equal importance to see
that the animals have sufficient time between meals, grooming, and
milking times, in which they can have complete rest and quietness.

It is not possible to suggest a time table that would be suitable in all
circumstances, some dairymen finding it convenient to follow a procedure
that would not be suitable elsewhere, so that the following scheme is
intended merely to show the general idea of one convenient method of
management.

5.30 a.m. The cows are washed, half of the production ration is
fed to them and milking is begun.

7.30 a.m. Milking is finished and half the silage or root allowance
is given, followed by hay.

Noon. The remainder of the silage or root allowance is given,
together with a second feed of hay.

3.30 p.m. The cows are washed, the second half of their production
ration is fed to them and the second milking is begun.

5.30 p.m. A final hay ration is fed.

At about 9 o'clock a final evening visit of inspection is made to see
that everything is in order.

The roots and ensilage are given after milking as both these foods
might taint the milk, though there are many farmers who regularly feed
roots before milking, and even during milking, and claim that they never
have had the milk tainted. Probably hygiene is as important as the
nature of the food but, nevertheless, the precaution is a harmless one.

(3) Calf rearing

(a) Introduction.

Under natural conditions calves are born in spring and suckle their
dams throughout the best of the grass season. In the Northern Hemi-
sphere pastures begin to fail in August and the reduced food supply
brings about a falling off in the milk yield of the cows. By October the
herbage is insufficient to maintain the flow of milk and the calves are
weaned naturally. By this time, however, the young animals have accustomed themselves to subsist on grass and weaning comes so gradually
that they suffer no perceptible set-back.

Modern economic conditions have necessitated the adoption of alternative methods of rearing. Compared with these the natural method has several distinct advantages. For example, the labour involved in attending to the herd is reduced to a minimum as the cows and calves may be left to look after themselves. With regard to the food, the calves in sucking get their milk at the correct temperature and in an uncontaminated condition, and they consequently suffer far less from digestive disorders than when reared artificially. Another advantage is that cow's milk contains all the necessary materials and in exactly the right proportions for reconstruction into animal tissue. Milk-fed calves therefore grow more rapidly and have a better " bloom " and a more attractive appearance than those fed in any other way.

The great disadvantage of the purely natural system of rearing is that under all intensive and semi-intensive systems of farming the cost of keeping a cow a whole year in order to rear a single calf is prohibitive. An exception to this is where the calf has an enhanced value owing to its pedigree.

It should be understood at the outset that the naturally fed calf is the standard of excellence by which all calves are judged. The art of rearing calves artificially is principally one of devising cheap methods of feeding which will cause the young animals to make substantial gains in weight and keep them in good health. There are methods of rearing by which, at very low cost, calves can just be kept in health and show growth; but where such means are adopted there is always the danger of going too far in the search for economy, to the detriment of the health and ultimate usefulness of the young stock. On the other hand there are artificial methods that approach the natural method in cost, and yield almost as good results. Circumstances must decide the method of rearing that should be adopted. Where milk is abundant and of low value it may pay to rear calves largely on a whole milk diet, but where market conditions give milk a high value farmers are loath to give calves more than is absolutely necessary for their well-being. In certain systems of dairy farming there is a tendency to arrange the calf feeding in order to consume available supplies of skim milk or whey.

As a young and growing animal, the calf needs to be provided with a ration containing a relatively high level of digestible protein, easily digested carbohydrate and fat, calcium, phosphorus, the fat-soluble vitamins and members of the vitamin B complex. As it grows it develops from a non-ruminant to a true ruminant, during which period it becomes capable of dealing with the fibre of foods, and, provided there are no complications due to disease, independent of dietary sources of some at least of the members of the vitamin B complex. An excellent review of the nutrition of calves has been given by Savage and McCay.[12]

The watering of calves is very important and must not be overlooked. When the young animals are penned, water should be placed so that they can drink when they so desire. Even a calf getting its fill of milk will take water during hot weather.

Exercise is necessary for growing calves and it is therefore inadvisable to tie up the young animals beyond the stage when they are liable to suck each other. All that is necessary is a good sized pen and freedom to move about; a grass paddock is very useful for young calves in summer.

Young stock do much better if turned out daily, weather permitting, for a short while throughout the autumn and winter, than when they are kept continuously indoors, often in a vitiated atmosphere, until the late spring. When turned out then the sudden change of environment and food consequently causes a considerable set-back.

Shelter should be given to calves that are out at grass so that they may avoid the glaring sun in hot weather and obtain protection from winds and rain when the days are rough. Cheap sheds may be erected in the pasture fields but the natural shelter of trees is sufficient. While it is necessary in most districts to in-winter young stock during the first two years, it is as well to leave them out of doors entirely during their third winter.

(b) Importance of the feeding of the cow before calving.

The feeding of a calf begins before it is born, in the sense that a good plane of nutrition during the last third of pregnancy keeps the cow herself in fit condition, helps to ensure a good lactation, and produces a calf sufficiently well developed to make full use of the available food during the early stages of growth. (See Chap. 17 [4].)

While a lack of sufficient vitamin A in the maternal ration prior to parturition may lead to the production of a stillborn calf or of one which is weakly or blind, and a lack of adequate iodine may also have an adverse effect, insufficient protein may give a calf which is about normal in weight, though its chances of survival will probably be seriously diminished. Similarly the feeding of inadequate amounts of calcium and phosphorus will not produce a calf with rickets *at birth*. Poor management, however, usually results in the feeding of rations which are deficient in several factors, the unhappy results of which will include trouble for the cow during the lactation period and a sickly calf, growing at much less than its optimum rate. This means that so far as the calf is concerned, a much greater proportion of its ration is being expended on its simple maintenance than need be the case. The general principles concerned in the feeding of livestock are now known, even though quantitative requirements may not be capable of exact formulation and there can be little excuse for some of the mistakes which are made.

Quite apart from the feeding of the pregnant cow, one may go even further back and say that the feeding of a calf commences before it is conceived. Lack of fertility—and hence useless maintenance costs again —will result if the cow (or bull) is badly fed prior to service. Here " badly " refers not only to the quantitative but also to the qualitative aspects of feeding.

(c) Treatment of the newly born calf.

The treatment of calves for the first few days follows the same general rules no matter what system of rearing is to be adopted.

It is customary to tie up the cow in a byre or stall for a few days before she is due to calf. After birth, the calf may be tied in another stall or taken to a calf pen. Scrupulous care must be employed to ensure that the young animal is given clean surroundings and kept under hygienic conditions. These matters are of very real importance if calves are to be kept in health and losses are to be avoided. In cold weather or in a draughty building the calf may be rubbed down with a few absorbent fabric dusters and then covered with straw or with a blanket until it is dry. If it is physically normal the young animal should be encouraged to take a little of its mother's milk as soon as possible.

Where suckling is to be the method of rearing the subsequent treatment is straightforward, the only care being the prevention of over-gorging for the first few meals. Breeders differ in their management of calves that are to be pail fed. Some allow the young animals to suck for a few meals until they have gained strength and thereafter feed only from the pail. Others allow the calves to suck for four days (until the milk is normal) and then have recourse to the pail.[13] Yet others milk the cow after calving and teach the calf to drink from the pail right away. A calf can be taught with little difficulty to drink from a pail if two fingers are first inserted into its mouth, and, when it begins sucking, the hand is lowered into the pail so as to bring the animal's mouth in contact with the milk.

The manner of feeding may affect the mode of passage of food along the digestive tract.[12] More evidence is needed on this very important point, but Sheehy says that " nutritional scour " in young calves can be caused by their receiving in two—too large—portions the amount of milk that they would normally ingest in a dozen or more feeds under natural feeding conditions. The disorder may be cured by replacing the milk by boiled water, cooled to body temperature; when the symptoms have disappeared feeding is resumed, using milk diluted with water (half a pint of water or more if necessary to each feed). Sheehy recommends this as routine practice for calves which are being fed no more than twice daily.[14]

Consideration must be given to the quantity of milk the calf should be allowed. The sucking calf particularly if it is weakly should not at first be allowed to over-gorge from a deep milking dam. Perhaps the easiest way to exercise control (for a few days) in such a case is to allow the calf to suck two quarters only and to milk out the others. As a rule, however, deep milking cows are either reserved for the dairy or they are made to rear more than one calf. In feeding a newborn calf from a pail no more than a quart should be given for a first meal and considerably less when dealing with a small or weakly animal. Healthy calves will progress satisfactorily on three meals a day, but when dealing with calves that show lack of vitality the best policy is to give small quantities at frequent intervals. In starting commercial calves on the pail a rough rule is to give one pint of milk per day for every 10 lb. of live weight. This may be increased gradually to two pints per 10 lb. by the middle of the second week, when the calf will have reached its maximum milk ration.

On most farms milking is carried out only twice a day, and it is therefore clear that feeding calves three times daily will necessitate the heating of the milk for one of the meals. This should be done by raising the temperature of the milk to blood heat (102° F.). Although freshly drawn milk will have cooled slightly before it can be fed to calves it gives quite satisfactory results and does not have to be raised to full blood temperature.

The calves should be fed at regular hours and if possible at equal day intervals. They become accustomed to a long night interval. In the absence of regularity the young animals become fretful and excessive hunger may cause them to gulp their food too quickly. As the calves get older, however, they may be fed twice daily. This method is not so good as that of feeding three times a day but it may be justified by labour conditions on the farm. Breeders are at variance as to the age at which to effect the change, some making it after a few days, some after a fortnight and others not until the calves are six weeks old.

The first milk produced by a cow after calving is the *colostrum* or " beestings ". It differs from normal milk in being particularly rich in albumen and ash and in the fact that it coagulates readily on heating: other important characteristics have been described in Chap. 8. The first milk gradually loses its special properties and becomes normal after about four days. When deprived of colostrum the young become constipated. It is of the utmost importance that the newborn calf should be given the colostrum of its mother and not the normal milk of other cows; for this reason official milk recording need not be started until after the fourth day from calving.

(d) Systems of calf rearing.

The systems of calf rearing that are dealt with in this chapter may be classified conveniently as follows:

    (i) Rearing in a pedigree herd.
    (ii) Natural rearing in commercial herds.
    (iii) Semi-natural rearing.
    (iv) Artificial rearing.
    (v) Feeding for veal production.

In a number of instances the methods are compromises between what is desirable from nutritional principles and what is economically possible at some particular time and in some particular circumstances.

(i) *Rearing in a pedigree herd.*

In a herd of this type the main object is to produce well-grown and well-fed bulls for sale at the age of one or two years. Surplus heifers will also be sold but the fact that they do not have the potential value of the bulls relegates them to secondary consideration. The cost of rearing is very great but successful breeders reap ample rewards.

The best months for calving are usually February and March, but if the animals are to be brought out for certain shows and sales it may be expedient to have them dropped in December or January.

The calves may be offered a small amount of hay when they are little more than a fortnight old. At first this hay will be nibbled and sucked but not swallowed; it encourages the eating of solid food and is unlikely to harm a healthy animal. If a number of calves are put in one pen they must not be allowed to suck each other; but this can to a large extent be prevented by *regular* and sufficiently frequent feeding. Certain circumstances may necessitate their being muzzled but it is usually possible to halter them and tie them up.

Pedigree animals must be made to grow quickly. When about three weeks old they should be offered a mixture of equal parts of coarse oatmeal and ground linseed, fed dry in a suitable box. In time they learn to eat this, and when they are a little older and accustomed to the food the mixture may be changed to one of equal parts of crushed oats and finely broken linseed cake. They will be able to eat both concentrates and hay before they are turned out to grass in spring.

May is the beginning of the good grass season, and about this time, depending on the situation of the farm, the cows and calves go out to pasture. It is usually best to make the change a gradual one by at first allowing the animals out for a few hours daily, but when the weather improves they may be left out overnight. Some farmers put the cows with bull calves on the young seeds or the best grass that is available and send the heifers and their dams to less productive grassland. Even when this is not done it becomes necessary to separate the bulls from the heifers when they are three to four months old. It is unusual to give the heifers any artificial food while on the grass. In order to keep the bulls in rapidly growing condition, however, it is customary to recommence feeding concentrates towards the end of July, the usual ration per day being $1\frac{1}{2}$ to 2 lb. of linseed cake or good compound cake. If this food is not given the young animals suffer a slight loss of condition when the grass begins to fail in August.

Certain breeds of cattle have been so selected for beef that the cows are unable to yield sufficient milk for the proper nourishment of their own calves. Hence it has become necessary to use nurse cows to supplement the milk of the pedigree mothers. Suckling of this kind is carried out under supervision and it is not unusual for a good bull calf to have milk until he is over a year old. He may be given access to a nurse cow when very young or this extra food may be denied him until he is about five months old. All nurse cows should have passed the tuberculin test.

The calves are weaned when they are about eight to ten months. When the nights begin to become cold they are brought under cover and fed in boxes during the winter, the intensity of the winter feeding depending upon the purpose for which the calves are intended. If for show or sale at the age of one year the feeding is usually very liberal. Indeed the custom is to give as much concentrated and attractive food as the young animals will clean up, and everything is done to keep up their appetite, although there is evidence that very fat animals are neither necessarily very healthy, nor even very fertile. Concentrates are fed thrice daily and are followed by a few sliced roots, while the best clover hay and good clean water are offered *ad libitum*. Animals that are not to be shown until older are fed liberally but not quite to repletion.

The above-mentioned system of intensive feeding applies particularly to bulls and animals of beef breeds. Heifer calves may not breed readily if they are made fat by liberal feeding, and their rations are therefore more in accordance with the practice in commercial herds. The same may be said of pedigree dairy calves which are usually bred on milk-selling farms from recorded cows.

(ii) *Natural rearing in commercial herds.*

This is the method that most nearly approaches the natural rearing of calves by wild cattle. While it is the common system in the great beef exporting countries, in Britain it is as a rule only profitable in certain areas of cheap or particularly suitable grassland.

Highland cattle on their natural grazings provide a typical example of this kind of rearing. The cows are run on the lower and rougher pastures all winter. Their only supplementary food is a little hay given during the hardest of weather and perhaps for a short time before calving. The calves are normally born in April and the risks of parturition are greatly reduced if the cows can be given the protection of some natural shelter for about a fortnight at this time. Cows and calves are kept on the low fields until the grass is sufficiently in evidence on the high ground. After this all the stock goes to the hills and remains there until the calves are weaned in October. The young animals are housed during their first winter and maintained largely on rough fodder. If the calves are by an early maturing beef bull such as a Shorthorn they will respond to more liberal treatment after they are weaned, and they may be sold for finishing on better land.

The system of management in the Galloway area is very similar to that in the Highlands. In England it is common for the Hereford and some other beef breeds to rear their own calves in the natural way, but this only pays on certain pastures where the grazing cost per head is low.

On good land it may be remunerative to rear calves naturally if there are facilities for bringing the young animals on sufficiently rapidly to enable them to be marketed as baby beeves. The management in such a case follows the lines of pedigree breeding but the feeding is less extravagant.

(iii) *Semi-natural rearing.*

The term semi-natural rearing applies to cases where cows are made to bring up more calves than they have borne. In considering the productiveness of grazing land one finds, at one extreme, poor areas that may be stocked with cows rearing their calves in the natural way. The herbage of such land is not sufficiently nutritious to enable a cow to suckle more than one calf. On many medium-class farms it may not be profitable to keep a cow for the rearing of one calf although it is quite satisfactory if she rears a pair. At the other extreme is land capable of carrying large heavy-milking dairy cattle. Under such conditions even two calves could not take full advantage of the milking capacity of a cow, yet calf rearing may still be carried on profitably if the cow is made to suckle four or five calves per lactation, or even nine or ten.

The chief argument against the system of raising a number of calves on each cow is the difficulty of purchasing newborn animals of good quality. In a beef cattle district the calves will practically all be kept to suck their own mothers, while calves born of dairy animals are often not worth raising for beef, and only the best of them are worth feeding for veal. The most promising sources from which the calves may be obtained are the small farmers who keep a few dual-purpose cows. If such calves happen to be by pure beef bulls they will rear into very satisfactory and profitable cattle. The limitations to the acquisition of suitable calves make it clear that this system of rearing can only be adopted by those who have time to go round their own district and pick up animals of the proper type. Another point is that the system is as a rule only satisfactory when the cows calve in early spring and most of the suckling takes place during the grass season. Winter feeding is generally too expensive to enable much profit to be made out of this kind of rearing, but where winter feeding is abundant and cheap it is better to have the cows coming into milk in the autumn, as the spring grass prolongs the milk supply and the total milk secreted during the year is increased. Some people hold the view—for which there is much to be said—that if calves are born during the autumn or winter they can be weaned in the spring and thus get the maximum benefit from the year's growth of grass.

Cow with two calves.

Where a couple of calves are to be put to a cow it is customary to pen the purchased calf with the cow's own calf so that they may acquire the same odour. The young animals are taken three or four times a day to the cow and allowed to suck under supervision. The feeding hour is often a very trying time as many cows do everything in their power to keep the foster calf from drinking. When the cow goes out to grass the calves go with her. If she has not taken to her foster calf by this time it is a common practice to strap the two calves together by the neck so that it is practically impossible for the cow to repel one without being equally severe on the other. The strap is removed as soon as harmony has been established. It is only fair to state that while many cows take an extra calf without giving any trouble, there is likely to be an odd animal that obstinately refuses to fit in with the system and it may be necessary to remove her from the herd before the next season.

The calves remain on the grass all summer and weaning takes place in the fall when the cows are almost dry. The question of whether the calves are to be given artificial food during summer will be determined by whether they are to be kept as stores or brought on for baby beef. In the latter case one must avoid the risk of the animals losing their calf flesh, and it may be wise to start feeding a pound or two of cake per day in August. The usual arrangement for feeding is to put up a special fence which allows the young animals through to the cake boxes but prevents the passage of the cows. The calves are taught to eat roots on the grass before they are housed for the winter. Winter feeding consists of hay, roots and such concentrates as will give the live-weight increase that is desired.

Cow with successive groups of calves.

The second system of semi-natural rearing, where more than two calves are raised per cow, involves more labour because suckling is usually carried out under supervision throughout the entire period. The problem of obtaining the requisite number of calves is also greater.

The theory of this system is that a good cow run on rich grass and properly fed during the housing period will yield much more milk than is needed to rear one or even two calves. A cow yielding 750 gallons should be capable of raising several calves and with a higher output even more. Assuming that the cow is in milk for ten months, she might suckle two or three calves for 3-3½ months, another group for a similar period and finally one or two until the end of her lactation. She may even be given fresh calves every 2½ months.

Sheehy,[14] on the grounds that late lactation milk produces in the calf's stomach a denser curd than milk from the same cow in early lactation and may therefore produce nutritional scour in a newly born calf, suggests that when one lot of calves is being weaned from the nurse and a second group is being introduced, the latter should only be allowed to take the first milk from the udder. Older calves should then follow up and empty the udder. He suggests, further, that it is better to introduce two-week old rather than very young calves.

The most simple application of this method is where a cow is turned out to pasture with two or three calves and remains there until the young animals are weaned at 3½ months old. The cow is then brought back, tied up in a stall and made to accept other calves, after which she is returned to grass with the young animals for the remainder of the season. The more intensive plan is to keep the calves in pens or paddocks and to take them to the cows thrice daily to be suckled under supervision. In summer the cows are brought in from the pasture for feeding time.

As the calves have to be weaned when about three months old it is necessary to teach them to eat concentrated food when very young. This is best accomplished by giving them daily supplies of crushed oats and linseed cake, also hay in the case of animals that are confined to pens.

The sudden weaning is likely to give the young animals a set-back but they recover without serious loss of condition.

Animals that are weaned in early summer may be put on to healthy pasture land for the rest of the grass season. Their winter feeding will depend on whether they are to be fattened early or kept as stores until the following spring. Calves that are not weaned until autumn will have to be given a variety of concentrated food while they are housed during winter. The hay, roots and small quantities of home-grown grain which may serve to winter the older calves will not provide sufficient variety to carry the young animals on to spring in good condition.

(iv) *Artificial rearing.*

Calves are said to be reared artificially when they are fed from a pail instead of being suckled. Artificial rearing requires more labour than the natural method but allows of much more intensive management of the milking herd. Milk recording may proceed without interference, thus enabling the cows to be fed according to their yield and for their maximum economical production. Another benefit is that the calves can be systematically rationed and adjustments of the feeding are easily made to suit their individual requirements.

Artificial Rearing on Whole Milk.—On some farms none of the milk is separated or made into cheese and thus whole milk may be available for calf feeding. Owing to the high value of milk, however, an endeavour is made to wean the calves as early as is possible without detriment to their well-being. Those fed on whole milk may be weaned when two months old, provided that they are taught to eat solids at the earliest opportunity, but in every batch of calves there are a few individuals that cannot be weaned so young because they have not learned to eat sufficient solid foods. Such animals should be given a small daily supply of milk until they are consuming enough hay and concentrates for their maintenance.

The first treatment of the calf has already been described. An average-sized animal gets $1\frac{1}{2}$ gallons of milk per day by the middle of the second week and this allowance should be continued to the end of the sixth week. The milk ration is then gradually reduced until it is stopped when the calf is weaned at two months or later. The young animal should get its first lesson in eating concentrates when between a fortnight and a month old. Just as the calf is finishing its milk a little oatmeal, or oatmeal and crushed linseed, is dropped on to the bottom of its pail. The young animal usually tastes the material, but if it is shy some of the meal may be rubbed on its nose so that it licks it into its mouth. A handful of food is given in this way after each meal until the calf acquires a taste for it, and thereafter the meal is placed in a small feeding box so that the young animal may eat it when it pleases. " Calf starters " may be purchased which consist of ground cereals, with animal proteins, minerals, etc., and which contain stated proportions of protein, fibre and other constituents. Patience and careful study of individual tastes are required in getting young calves to eat meals. Some animals will take to dry foods while others will prefer the meal moistened with milk or warm water; some will like the flavour of oil seed, especially linseed, while others will more readily eat oatmeal alone. Calves should be given access to a salt lick whenever they begin to get concentrated food, and as it is during this period of their lives, that is before they are consuming much roughage, that there may be a shortage of calcium, it should be supplied as well. Later on crushed oats and linseed cake meal may be substituted for oatmeal and linseed meal.

When six weeks old, calves should be eating a half-pound of meal per day, by two months they should consume a pound per day, and thereafter their daily eating capacity increases by about half a pound per fortnight. Nevertheless, cattle under a year old are seldom given more than three pounds of concentrates per day, as, when fed with good roughage, this is ample to give the rate of development that is ordinarily required. At first the calf will consume about the same quantity of hay as of meal, but as its rumen develops it is able to eat three or four times as much hay as its normal ration of concentrates. Early and full development of the rumen and intestinal tract is thought to be desirable as its enables young stores intended for fattening to consume and make the most of a larger amount of roughage than is the case with more pampered animals which have been reared to a greater extent on concentrates.

Almost any palatable grains will do to teach the calf to eat while it is receiving a full daily allowance of milk, but when the time comes for the milk ration to be reduced the concentrates and hay will together have to provide a ration with a nitrogenous ratio not wider than 1 : 5. The oats in the feed should therefore be balanced with easily digested and fairly nitrogenous materials such as linseed products, bean and pea meals, dried grass, bran, etc.; the roughage should consist of the best leafy hay, particularly legume hay, which besides being rich in protein is also rich in calcium.

The daily live-weight increase will be checked for a time after weaning, but the young animals will pick up rapidly as their capacity for digesting solid food improves.

Artificial Rearing on Separated Milk.—On the great majority of dairy farms little whole milk can be spared for calf rearing; indeed its use is restricted to the narrowest possible limits. However, if calves are fed for a short time on whole milk, they may afterwards be developed into perfectly satisfactory and healthy cattle on skim milk and supplementary foods. Compared with calves fed on whole milk they have at first a slower rate of growth and a less sleek appearance, but by the time they are two years old they cannot be distinguished.

The skimming of milk removes nearly all the fat and the fat-soluble vitamins; it also narrows the albuminoid ratio. Therefore, in order to make skim milk a complete and balanced food, these deficiencies will have to be made good by the addition of suitable nutrients. The presence of 3 - 5 per cent. of butter-fat in milk results in its easier passage through the digestive tract than is the case with skimmed milk.[15] For the above reasons attempts have been made to incorporate such foods as cod-liver oil and various animal and vegetable fats into skim milk. Unless, however, a fat of the right physical and chemical properties is selected and unless it is introduced into the milk in finely divided form through the use of a homogeniser, the reconstituted milk will be poorly digested and scouring will occur in the calves which consume it. Some people recommend the use of oily foods consisting largely of linseed, but while linseed products have a remarkable value in calf rearing at later stages, or in cases where no skim milk is available, they are expensive foods which should not be used unnecessarily; moreover, they are very nitrogenous and their use as a fat substitute will add far more protein to the ration than the calf requires. Cereal grains form the cheapest substitute for butter-fat; they are rich in carbohydrates and have been shown to be easy of digestion. Crushed oats, ground barley and maize meal are all very satisfactory if fed in quantities to supply energy equivalent to the value of the fat removed. If an ounce of cod-liver oil is included in the daily ration the requirements of vitamins A and D will be met while the quality of the diet would undoubtedly be raised by the inclusion of this fat.

Milk direct from the separator will probably be warm enough if fed immediately to the calves: that which has been skimmed by hand and separated milk that has been allowed to cool will, of course, have to be raised to blood heat before feeding. Although hand-skimmed milk contains a bigger residue of fat than does separated milk it is disadvantageous in that it is at least a day old and it may be teeming with undesirable bacteria. For preference the calves should only be given milk from cows that have passed the tuberculin test. Separated milk returned from a creamery should be pasteurized before being fed to the young animals.

Many recipes have been given for preparing gruels by scalding or boiling the concentrates. One method which has been recommended is to take 2 lb. of linseed and soak it overnight in 3 gallons of water, and the next day boil it for 20 minutes, stirring vigorously all the time. After it has been boiling for 15 minutes, a creamy paste of 0.5 lb. wheat flour is added to counteract the laxative effect of the linseed. This gruel should be used at the rate of 1 pint of gruel to 2 quarts of separated milk.

Another is made as follows: 1 quart of ground linseed is scalded and stirred into 1 gallon of boiling water. This makes a porridge of good consistency which is quickly and easily prepared. One pint of it should be added to 4 pints of separated milk.[16]

The exact feeding system to be used depends to some extent upon local conditions regardless of the needs of the calf, but one thing which is common to all systems is that of allowing the calf to take the colostrum. How long the young animal should be given the whole milk afterwards is the main difference between the various methods of feeding. American workers have claimed that after the colostrum period Holsteins may be put straight on to skimmed milk, supplemented with cod-liver oil, when they will make as good gains as calves receiving whole milk. Jersey calves, however, did not do quite so well during the first few months."

Where some whole milk is allowed, it is usually fed for two to three weeks; this is probably the best practice under present conditions in this country. During a transition period one pound of whole milk is replaced by one pound of skim milk each day, until the latter is the only milk in the ration. When the change begins the calf will be receiving some 10 pints of whole milk per day; at the end of the transition period it will be given about 12 pints of skim milk. During the same time a dry meal is given. For this purpose mixtures (see below) prepared from crushed oats, or other coarsely ground cereals, with linseed cake and fish meal or meat and bone meal can be used, the amount increasing to some 2 lb./day by the time the calf is two months old. In order to develop the rumen, hay is introduced into the ration; consumption of this food is likely to begin at about 0.25 lb./day at three or four weeks of age and to increase to 1 lb. in the seventh, 2 lb. in the twelfth, 3 lb. in the fifteenth, 4 lb. in the nineteenth and 7 lb. in the 26th weeks." The hay should be the best quality, early-cut material, otherwise it is too fibrous and too poor in protein. Pulped roots, beginning at about 3 lb./ day, may be introduced into the ration at as early an age as six weeks, while good quality silage, on a comparable S.E. and P.E. basis may be used to replace hay and roots together. After the age of eight weeks it is important that changes should be gradual.

The age of weaning also varies from one district to another. In Britain milk feeding usually ceases at three or four months, provided the calves are in good condition. American workers have shown that weaning is possible at somewhat earlier ages, provided, (a) that the animals are in good condition, (b) that they have been encouraged to consume large amounts of dry feed before weaning, and (c) that it is not particularly necessary to have them quite up to average weight before the age of about nine months." Their feeding test was done without the use of high protein foodstuffs of animal origin, and involved the consumption of large amounts of dry feeds after weaning.

If calves go to grass after weaning they may continue to receive 1 to 2 lb. of concentrates per day, depending upon the state of the pasture and the rate of growth which is desired. Robinson [18] has described experiments made to determine the proportion of protein that is desirable in the dry feed to be used to supplement a hay ration for calves which have been weaned at the age of three to four months. The animals received 1 lb. of calf starter, made into a gruel, 2.0 to 2.5 lb. of meal, and hay *ad libitum* (the consumption of hay was about 5 to 7 lb. per day). The composition of the meals used is given below:

TABLE 91

Ingredients	Ration							
	A	B	C	D	E	F	G	H
Oats	11	11	42	50	50	30	60	30
Dec. groundnut cake	2	1	—	—	—	—	10	10
Fish meal	1	0.5	—	—	—	—	—	—
Beans	—	—	28	—	—	—	—	—
Linseed cake ...	—	—	—	20	50	—	—	—
Linseed, ground uncooked	—	—	—	—	—	10	—	10
Dig. protein % ...	16	12	12	12	16	10	12	16
Meal fed, lb. ...	2.5	2.5	2.5	2.5	2.5	2.0	2.5	2.5
Gain/day, lb. ...	1.4	1.6	1.2	1.2	1.4	1.5	1.3	1.5

The gains, made over periods of three months, depended on the quality of the hay; only good, sweet and palatable hay, with a digestible protein content of 11 per cent., proved suitable.

Since even the rations lowest in protein would contain as much digestible protein as seems to be needed by calves of the weights used,[19] [20] the lack of clear-cut differences between the weight gains due to variations of protein content of the ration is not unexpected. The influence of blends of different proteins, perhaps also of fat content of the ration—as in the good results where linseed meal was used—and of the total digestible nutrients furnished by the complete ration, is reflected in the differing weight gains. For the younger calves used, the digestible nutrients furnished by the calf starter and dry meal together would be about sufficient, as judged by the Morrison standards, but for the heavier ones it would not be enough and they would need to depend on the hay. The amount of good quality hay consumed would make up the deficiency whereas poor quality, fibrous material would not provide as much digestible nutrients as the standards suggest is desirable.

Dried grass was also used, but as it was found to be only of the "super-hay" class, with a protein content of about 12 per cent., the ration given was 3.5 lb. of dried grass, 2 lb. of crushed oats, 1 lb. of calf starter and hay ad libitum. Weight gains of 1.4 lb./day were made and the animals were in a very healthy condition, despite their rejection of a considerable amount of the offered hay.

Mixtures of the above kind, with the use of smaller amounts of the more expensive or less easily obtained protein concentrates, can take the place of older formulæ, of which the general type is linseed cake, 30 to 40 per cent.; white fish meal, 10 to 15 per cent.; starchy meals and grains, 40 to 60 per cent. There is, however, a smaller margin for error, while mineral and vitamin intakes need more consideration and the feeding calls for a greater degree of skill in management. Skilled use of small amounts of such foods as dried yeast, for its protein and vitamin B contents, dried grass, for protein, carotene and other trace factors, and meat and bone meal, fish meal or dried milk, for their protein and mineral contents, as well as a judicious blending of the commoner foods to suit the needs of the calf, is required.

Dried Milk, either whole or machine separated (see Chap. 8), is a valuable food for calves, and can be used in the place of liquid milk. The powder may either be fed dry, or as reconstituted milk, when it is mixed in the proportion of 1 lb. per gallon of water; if it is fed dry a maximum of 1 to 1.5 lb. daily should be sufficient. If separated dried milk is used, the usual fat substitutes must be added.

Artificial rearing on Whey.—The farmer who makes his milk into cheese has a special problem with regard to the rearing of his calves. He can neither afford to feed them on whole milk nor has he an available supply of separated milk. He has, however, an abundance of whey, which he should utilise for rearing his young cattle. Whey differs from whole milk in having had all but a fraction of its fat and protein and a good deal of its valuable mineral matter removed, while practically all the milk sugar is retained. It has slight laxative properties. Ordinarily the whey is obtained from the vats, at about blood heat, once a day, and it can be used directly for the mid-day feed. As the quantity that is held over for the other feeds will become increasingly acid in character, and liable to undesirable bacterial decomposition all whey that cannot be used immediately should be scalded and then rapidly cooled. It may be warmed prior to its being fed.

Calves that are to be reared on whey require whole milk for the first four weeks, the quantity being the same as for calves that are to be reared in other ways. They then undergo a transition period during which the milk is replaced by whey plus easily digested concentrates. At six weeks the milk is entirely stopped but the whey is continued until the normal time for weaning.

Foods that are to be given in conjunction with whey must contain not only the necessary energy producing substances but also an adequate supply of minerals and protein. The following mixtures and meal have been found satisfactory for calves when fed at the rate of 1 lb. per gallon of whey :—(1) Oatmeal, 2 parts; white fish meal, 1 part. (2) Bean meal, 5 parts; linseed cake meal, 4 parts. (3) Linseed meal, 3 parts; bean meal, 3 parts; white fish meal, 1 part. First-class leguminous hay should be given to the young animals as soon as they will eat it. As in the case of calves fed on skim milk, an extra supply of concentrates such as linseed cake should be given from the eighth week onwards. The supply of whey may be stopped when the young animals are about sixteen weeks old.

Although calves may be reared on whey according to the above plan they do not thrive so well as when fed on separated milk, and they do not make such satisfactory gains. The materials that must necessarily be added to the whey to make it a complete food contain indigestible matter that tends to give the animals a " pot-bellied " appearance.

Another disadvantage is that calves are not fond of whey and do not consume it readily.

A daily allowance of 1.5 gallons of whey contains about 0.3 oz. less lime and 0.25 oz. less phosphoric acid than does a corresponding amount of skim milk, and if whey is given together with other foods that are deficient in these minerals it may be necessary to add to the ration 0.5 oz. of chalk and 0.75 oz. of steamed bone flour. When fish meal and clover hay are fed with whey there is no danger of deficiency.

Endeavours have been made to rear calves on water plus meal mixtures without employing milk for longer than a few days. Systems which aim at the use of less than some 30 gallons of whole and skim milk per calf are not to be recommended. To the limits of existing knowledge—which is not very far—a milk substitute can be devised which will contain roughly the desired proportions of the major constituents of milk, but the trouble and expense of making such a substitute and the poor average growth of calves fed in such a way may well offset any saving of money on milk.

(v) *Feeding for veal production.*

Veal of the highest class is obtained from calves fed only on milk and then slaughtered between the age of one and two months. The flesh of older animals acquires the characteristics of beef whereas that of newborn animals is lean, watery and lacking in flavour.

The veal calf should be managed in such a way that it grows rapidly and puts on fat. It ought to be encouraged to rest all the time between meals and it should be kept contented by feeding it almost to repletion. Some veal calves are allowed to suck, but it is better to feed them on the pail so that they may be more carefully and regularly rationed. For the first few days ordinary feeding is carried out, but the milk supply should be gradually increased so that the young animals are each consuming 2.5-3 gallons of milk per day, for some time before going to the butcher. The pens in which they are kept have to be frequently strewn with fresh litter so that the animals are made thoroughly comfortable.

The heavy expense of feeding on whole milk is only likely to be justified where there is a special market for the highest class of veal. Sometimes calves are fed on a moderate milk ration together with an allowance of meals, but such animals never develop the pale colour of flesh and fat that is so much desired.

The rate of growth for a veal calf should not be less than 2 lb. live-weight increase per day.

(e) The growth rates of young cattle.

Table 92 shows the usual relationship of age to live-weight for different classes of young cattle. It should be noted, however, that continuous and uniform live-weight increase is not always procurable under farm conditions and that weights show great variations according to the breed and method of feeding.

TABLE 92

Age.	Beef Steer. (Full growth and fattening.)	Beef Steer. (Full growth without fattening.)	Dairy Heifers. (Smaller type.)
Months.	lb.	lb.	lb.
Birth	80	80	70
3	200	170	150
6	400	350	220
9	560	480	290
12	700	600	360
15	830	720	430
18	950	840	510
21	1080	950	580
24	1200	1060	660
27	...	1170	750
30	...	...	850

(4) The fattening of cattle

(a) 'Introduction.

The older method of beef production was largely concerned with the fattening of beasts of two to three years of age, which had been fed rather lightly since weaning. The period of light feeding, or " store period ", involved slow gains of weight, using for the purpose roots and the coarser foods, chiefly straw. Such a method tended to favour a relatively heavy type of animal, producing large joints of meat. A change in public taste with a greater liking for the smaller joints of high quality beef, not too fat, has led to the production of carcases weighing 550 to 600 lb. from animals of 8 to 9 cwt. body weight. This has produced a corresponding change in feeding and management, the store period being omitted, and the young animal fed for growth and fattening, to be killed about a year earlier than under the older method.

There are important differences between the respective nutritive needs of the two kinds of beast. In the case of the " store " much of the required growth has taken place before the fattening period, as a result of which the need at the latter time is for starch equivalent rather than for protein, whereas the younger animal is putting down body protein and fat simultaneously and requires a relatively high protein intake.

Whereas the store beast needed only moderate quantities of concentrates for its fattening, it has been calculated that the attempt to produce simultaneous growth and fattening for baby beef requires twice the food per pound of saleable meat produced as for growth alone.[21] So far as the use of concentrates is concerned, therefore, the advantage seems to lie with the store system, but if one considers the problem from another angle the conclusions must be rather different. When a calf has attained an age of about three months some 25 per cent. of its total requirements of digestible nutrients is used' for the production of new tissue, but at the age of 9 to 12 months the corresponding value is about 10 per cent.; these are the values for normal growth, without fattening. There would seem to be an advantage, therefore, provided feeding systems can be devised which will allow it, in reducing as far as possible the time taken for beasts to be ready for market; the elimination of the store period is the removal of a stage when nine-tenths of the ingested food is being used simply for maintenance and not for production.

The older method of producing beef was based upon straw and roots, plus concentrates during the fattening period; in the production of baby beef, because of their bulk alone, the first two foods cannot find so prominent a place in the ration and the problem becomes one of finding cheap but more concentrated substitutes for them.

In this section the fattening of cattle for beef production will be considered under two main headings, namely the fattening of store cattle and the production of baby beef.

(b) The fattening of store cattle.

The feeding of cattle during the store period is followed by some account of the fattening of the stores on grass and in courts respectively.

(i) *Feeding during the store period.*

An account of the feeding of calves up to the age of about six months has already been given. During the store period, from the age of six to about 30 months, the maximum possible use is made of coarse foods, roots, and second-grade grazings, concentrate consumption being kept as low as possible. Throughout the whole time the animals are expected to gain weight slowly—about 1 lb. per day—without becoming fat.

As in other cases there should be no abrupt changes in the nature of the ration, so that in the early store period the amount of concentrates may slowly be reduced and the quantity of roots and roughages gradually increased. Some 10 to 20 lb. of roots plus 5 to 10 lb. of the poorer hay, together with 3 to 4 lb. of concentrates, may be fed daily, the precise amount depending upon the age and condition of the beasts. At the age of about one year, straw may have replaced the roots and hay to a large extent (on a starch equivalent basis), 1 or 2 lb. of oil-seed cake making up the necessary amount of protein. This, of course, represents winter feeding, the animals being allowed to graze the poorer pastures in summer, with no supplement given unless the condition of the animals warrants it.

To achieve slow growth and still produce a normal animal, capable of responding well to subsequent fattening and yielding a good carcase, is not an easy task. The straws are relatively deficient in protein, calcium and phosphorous, and lack carotene; poor hay is rather low in protein and cannot be relied on to provide carotene, while dried beet pulp, another fairly common food for the store period, contains no carotene and has had most of its soluble inorganic salts leached from it during the sugar-extraction process. Rations based largely upon the above foods thus tend to be deficient in carotene and mineral elements—and perhaps other factors—with the result that the animals may not make the best use of those nutrients which are provided. For this reason it is good practice to replace some of the coarse food and concentrates by silage; the effect on the appearance and condition of the animals is worth it.

The older stores may receive a ration largely consisting of straw, together with 1 or 2 lb. of protein concentrate, but such a dietary is not a good one for the reasons which have already been given, though it will be improved by the inclusion of silage or by relatively small amounts of green fodder. Far too often store cattle are set to consume, not only the coarsest foods but almost entirely those which are known to be lacking in the trace factors, such as vitamins and mineral elements, upon which appetite and the efficient utilisation of the absorbed nutrients depend. Blaxter and Price [22] have dealt with the needs of growing dairy heifers on typical rations high in the coarse foods and low in concentrates and have concluded that " even when the protein deficiency of oat-straw rations is accounted for, oat-straw dietaries are still unsuitable for young cattle ". Furthermore, these conclusions were reached regarding rations which included a mineral supplement and which were presumed to be satisfactory with respect to vitamin A. The heifers varied from one to two years in age and had been receiving rations consisting of straw, without concentrates or hay, as a result of which they were " undergrown by 7-8 months when 18 months to two years old ". Although such a ration is described as a " war-time dietary ", there is no doubt that it is common enough even in times of peace in certain parts of the country.

(ii) *Fattening cattle on pasture.*

The successful fattening of store cattle may be described as an art assisted by science, for it requires good judgment to know what type of cattle will suit a particular district or farm; for example, beasts in forward condition and which have come off good land and, to the inexperienced eye, look as if they would " finish " rapidly and leave a good profit, may consistently lose condition if put on to unsuitable pasture; on the other hand, cattle bought in poorer condition but with good frames, but which have not been badly nourished as calves, may do very well on the same pasture, showing a consistent and reasonable daily gain in weight and leaving a fair profit to the farmer.

Cattle bought in March or April for finishing on grass, range from two to three years of age, weigh on an average 8 to 9 cwt. and take from 16 to 20 weeks to fatten; when ready they probably weigh about 11 cwt., thus gaining 1.5 to 2 lb./day. Some farmers prefer the older bullocks as they fatten quicker—though not necessarily more efficiently—are less liable to hoven or tympanitis when put on to rich grass, and are not so troubled with parasitic bronchitis, as are young ones.

The area required for grazing naturally depends upon the condition of the pasture and the size of the bullocks; the average is about 1 to 1.5 acres per large bullock. Cattle should never be put from good pasture on to poorer land but be changed so that the feed they get is improving in quality. Store cattle are usually turned out to graze in April or May, depending on the season and the condition of the pasture.

Expressed as starch and protein equivalents, the maintenance requirements of fattening cattle are the same as those for dairy cows. They are given on p. 310. A two-year-old bullock for fattening, weighing about 9 cwt. or 1,000 lb., will therefore require for maintenance 6 lb. of starch equivalent and 0.6 lb. of protein equivalent. Kellner's experiments and later confirmatory trials showed that throughout the whole fattening period it takes 3 lb. of starch equivalent to produce 1 lb. of body-weight increase; in the early stages 2 lb., and towards the end of the period as much as 4 lb. will be required to produce the same gain in weight. In addition to the P.E. required for maintenance, 0.15 lb. for each pound of S.E. used for production is necessary. Naturally the amount of starch equivalent and protein equivalent given for maintenance will require to be increased from time to time as the animals get heavier. Moreover, this estimate does not take into account the expenditure of energy involved in cropping the grass nor that used to offset adverse weather conditions, an amount computed to be from 1 lb. to 3 lb. of S.E. per day, depending upon the character of the pasturage and environmental conditions.

A 1,000 lb. bullock, to fatten at the rate of 2 lb. a day, will require 12 lb. of S.E. and 1.5 lb. of P.E., thus:

TABLE 93

	Starch Equivalent.	Protein Equivalent.
	lb.	lb.
Food for maintenance for 1,000 lb.	6	0.6
Food for 2 lb. daily increase ...	4.5	0.9
(at 2.25 lb. S.E. per lb.)		
Food for extra energy expended (say)	1.5	—
Total	12	1.5

A 9 cwt. bullock can eat about 22 lb. of dry matter per day, and its capacity in this direction will increase at the rate of about 1.5 lb. per day for each 100 lb. increase in body weight. Assuming that average " extensively grazed " spring grass has a S.E. of 55 and a P.E. of 10, 22 lb. should supply 12 lb. of S.E. and 2.2 lb. of P.E. In the early part of the season, therefore, there is ample starch equivalent and a surplus of digestible protein in the food of the grazing animal.

When cattle are first turned on to strong growing pasture they commonly scour to such an extent that a temporary loss of weight follows. A method of avoiding this which seems to bring good results is that of feeding roughage on the grass, throughout the lives of the animals.[23] A large amount is consumed during the " early bite " period. It is a practical application of the statement made elsewhere (p. 254) concerning the habits of livestock which are free to make a choice of herbage and foods. Another way of checking scouring, which usually accompanies too sudden a change in diet, is to feed small amounts of undecorticated cotton cake to animals at grass.

By the end of June the value of average extensively grazed pasture might well be about 50 per cent. starch equivalent and 7 per cent. digestible protein. A bullock which has attained a weight of 10 cwt. and is making a gain of 1.5 lb. a day, thus needs a daily intake of 12.5 lb. of S.E. and 1.7 lb. of P.E.:

TABLE 94

	Starch Equivalent.	Protein Equivalent.
	lb.	lb.
Food for maintenance for 1,000 lb.	6.0	0.60
Food for maintenance for 120 lb. ...	0.5	0.07
Food for 1.5 lb. daily increase ... (at 3 lb. S.E. for each lb.)	4.5	1.05
Food for extra energy expended (say)	1.5	—
Total	12.5	1.7

Such a bullock could meet its requirements by consuming 25 lb. (dry matter) of this grass, an amount within its capacity.

Many farmers still feed their grazing cattle too heavily with rich concentrates, and the fact that richer manure reaches the land is no justification for the practice.

While it is possible to fatten cattle and to finish them on the best pastures without the addition of any concentrated food, on the majority of fields it is necessary to provide some extra feeding, especially towards the end of summer. The amount required depends upon the time of the year and the condition of the pasture. After the laxative action of the fresh grass has worn off there is no need to give any concentrates so long as the grass remains good and the cattle are obviously thriving, for every animal has its own limited daily capacity for body increase and it is wasteful to make extravagant use of expensive concentrates. When cattle are at pasture the constant supervision of the farmer is required, for his judgment is needed to decide if and when concentrates are required to prevent cattle losing the increase gained from the grass. The quantity required ranges from 2 lb. per head at the earliest sign of the grass falling off to a maximum of 6 lb. when the shortage is very obvious, and for the last week or so, 8 lb.; more than this quantity is rarely necessary. It is as well to start mainly with carbonaceous foods when the grass is young and rich, and use foods richer in protein as the grass gets older. No particular cake or meal or combination of these seems to possess any outstanding merit. Cakes particularly rich in protein, such as decorticated ground nut cake or decorticated cotton cake should be combined with foods containing less, such as maize meal and other cereals, for example, 1 part soya bean cake or decorticated ground nut cake with 2 or 3 parts of cereals. In the last stages of fattening it may be thought necessary to feed concentrates, e.g., linseed cake of high fat content, but this depends upon the condition of the stock and the state of the pasture. It has been said that the feeding of such concentrates achieves a sleek, finished appearance, but the ability of grass to yield good quality beasts is illustrated by experience such as that of Lloyd[24] whose well wintered cattle, on young leys, made weight gains of 2.2 to 3.0 lb./day, 48 per cent. of the beasts being graded as " special " and 27 per cent. as " A+ "

(iii) *The winter fattening of cattle in courts or stalls.*

For the winter fattening of cattle, the beasts may be kept in a court either partially or entirely roofed in, or may be tied up in stalls, or kept in single or double pens.

Cattle are put up for winter fattening at from 2 to 3 years of age, the objects being to get them to fatten as quickly as possible, and to consume as much roots and straw (assuming there to be a heavy crop of roots) as is consistent with their well-being. Some lots may, of course, be fed less generously, so as to be ready for a later marketing period when it is anticipated that they will command a better price.

On arable or semi-arable farms the basis of the diet will be oat or barley straw and roots, swedes, silage, turnips and mangolds, and as many of these are deficient in protein, foods such as oilcakes may be added to balance the diet. Where the supply of straw is limited the amount is restricted to a stone or a stone and a-half a day, but in many districts it is given *ad libitum,* the rack being kept full, when the beasts eat only the upper, sweeter part of the straw and the leaves, and tread under foot the less palatable and less nutritious lower portions of the stems. All the straw may be given long, or part of it may be chaffed and mixed with pulped roots and meals, thus compelling the animals to eat the straw without having the opportunity to pick out the portions that they like. It is a mistake, however, to do this for the coarser parts of the straw are of such little value as food that it is uneconomical to insist upon the cattle eating it. Inferior quality hay is often given in the place of straw, but towards the end of the fattening period, when hay should be used in part as substitute for straw, only good quality food should be offered to the animals. Of roots, varying quantities are given depending upon the custom of the locality and the nature of the crop: from 40 to 70 lb. a day is a good allowance, but in some districts as much as a hundredweight or a hundredweight and a-half is given to large bullocks. It used to be thought necessary to pulp the roots for cattle when they are shedding their milk teeth, from 18 months to 2 years of age, but many husbandmen now find that the extra labour involved is not warranted. In addition to the roots other succulent foods, particularly kohl rabi and marrow-stem kale, are used with excellent results, while the additional use of waste potatoes, up to 56 lb./day, has also been described,[25] with the warning that care is needed in feeding large amounts of potatoes where kale is also being fed. The same observer provides mineral licks all the year round and finds that a "good quantity" is consumed. Before being housed for feeding, stores which have been maintained on grass should be gradually accustomed to the change of food and surroundings by giving them hay and roots for a week or two in a sheltered field near the steading.

During the time the beasts are penned for fattening, from sixteen to twenty weeks, the average rate of increase is about 2 lb. per day, and for the first four to six weeks a good bullock will gain from 3 to 3.5 lb. per day, although a good deal of this increase is due to the accumulation of moisture in the tissues; this is particularly the case with young stores being fattened for baby beef. At about the middle of the fattening period the gain will not be greater than 2 lb. a day, and towards the finishing period an increase of 1 lb. a day is as much as the average beast will maintain. During the early stages of fattening an equivalent quantity of concentrates added to a maintenance ration will produce a greater gain than is obtained when the beast is nearly fat; thus the last stages of fattening are the most expensive. The first fat which is deposited in the carcase is the kidney fat, which is not directly apparent to the feeder although he knows of its presence by the healthy look of the animal. The next is the subcutaneous fat, laid over the muscle; this he can detect by his eye and by manipulation of the skin. The last fat, deposited during the expensive finishing process, is the intra-muscular fat laid down between the muscle bundles which breaks these up and thus renders the meat of older bullocks juicy, tender and thus more saleable. Excessive fatness is an undesirable extravagance, but sufficient fat must be interspersed among the lean flesh to make it palatable and to give a cut a "marbled" appearance.

In constructing a suitable ration for fattening housed cattle the same allowances are to be used as those applied to the feeding of grazing cattle and stated on page 339, except that there is no need to take into consideration expenditure of energy in obtaining the food. Thus a bullock weighing 9 cwt. when first put up for fattening and which is to fatten at the rate of 2 lb. per day on the average will require a ration containing 12 lb. of starch equivalent and 1.5 lb. of protein equivalent, during the first stages.

At this period the daily increase which may be expected is 3 lb. and this should be produced at the expense of 2.25 lb. of starch equivalent for each pound of body weight increase. The requirements are as follows:

TABLE 95

	Starch Equivalent.	Protein Equivalent.
	lb.	lb.
Food for maintenance for 1,000 lb.	6	0.60
Food for 3 lb. daily increase ...	6.75	1.01
Total	12.7	1.6

At a later stage the rate of gain of body weight slows down and the expenditure as starch equivalent consumption increases to 3 lb. for every pound of weight increase, so that the requirements at the beginning, at the third month and at the fifth month are as follows:

TABLE 96

Period.	Daily body weight increase	Weight	For Maintenance		For Production.		Total	
			Starch Equiv.	Protein Equiv.	Starch Equiv.	Protein Equiv.	Starch Equiv.	Protein Equiv.
	lb.	lb.	lb.	lb.	lb.	lb.	lb.	lb.
At start ...	3	1000	6.0	0.60	6.75	1.0	12.75	1.61
At 12 weeks	2	1200	6.8	0.70	6.00	0.9	12.80	1.60
At 20 weeks	2	1300	7.1	0.77	6.50	0.9	13.60	1.67

It will be noted that the rate of fattening of 2 lb. per day has been maintained, for when the rate of body weight increase has been reduced to 1 lb. per day, the animal is fat and should be disposed of.

Having decided to feed his bullocks on a balanced ration the farmer has to consider what foods he should use. His choice will be controlled in the first place by the nature of his farm and the kind of crops he grows. If his farm is an arable one he will have oat and probably barley straw and roots, and as the cereal straws and roots are deficient in protein he will need to add to these some foods rich in protein, of which there is a great variety. When he begins to fatten his 8 or 9 cwt. bullocks we will assume that he takes as his maintenance ration 16 lb. of oat straw and, say, 70 lb. of turnips. This will supply the following nutriment:

TABLE 97

Food.	Starch Equivalent.	Protein Equivalent.	N. Ratio.	Carbohydrate Equivalent.	Dry Matter.
	lb.	lb.	lb.		lb.	lb.
Oat Straw...	16	2.72	0.16	39	6.24	13.76
Turnips ...	70	2.80	0.28	13.2	3.70	6.30
Total ...		5.5	0.4		9.9	20.1

Now this diet as it stands has neither sufficient starch equivalent nor protein equivalent for the maintenance of a bullock weighing 9 cwt. It has a nitrogenous ratio of 1 to 22 which is obviously far too wide. The ration clearly requires some protein-rich concentrates, for example, 4 lb./head of palm kernel cake. The ration would then be:

TABLE 98

Food.		Starch Equivalent.	Protein Equivalent.	N. Ratio	Carbohydrate Equivalent.	Dry Matter.
	lb.	lʰ.	lb.		lb.	lb.
Oat Straw ...	16	2.72	0.16	39	6.24	13.76
Turnips ...	70	2.80	0.28	13.2	3.70	6.30
Palm Kernel Cake ·	4	3.00	0.62	3.8	2.36	3.56
Total in Ration ...		8.5	1.1		12.3	23.6
Maintenance Requirement		6.00	0.60			
Excess over Maintenance		2.5	0.5			

This surplus food over maintenance requirementš will therefore supply enough nutriment for a daily increase of 1 lb. per head at the commencement of fattening. The nitrogenous ratio is still rather too wide, being 1 to 11.5. The dry matter is at the rate of 2.3 per cent. of the live weight. While this ration is enough at the very commencement of fattening it should be increased as soon as the animals have settled down to their surroundings and change of diet. If the supply of turnips is good a further 10 or 20 lb. per head may be allowed provided that the cattle are not scouring.

Then the concentrates may be increased and swedes can replace the turnips. Palm kernel cake may still be included in the diet and some decorticated cotton cake or some similar food added:

TABLE 99

Food.		Starch Equivalent.	Protein Equivalent.	N. Ratio.	Carbohydrate Equivalent.	Dry Matter.
	lb.	lb.	lb.		lb.	lb.
Oat Straw ...	16	2.72	0.16	39	6.24	13.76
Swedes	75	5.25	0.52	11.4	5.92	9.00
Palm Kernel Cake	2	1.50	0.31	3.8	1.18	1.78
Dec. Cotton Cake	1	0.68	0.34	1.1	0.37	0.91
Oats	4	2.44	0.30	7.6	2.28	3.48
Total in Ration		12.6	1.6		16.0	28.9

The nitrogenous ratio of this diet is 1 to 9.8 and the diet contains enough starch and protein equivalents for a daily gain of nearly 3 lb. per head.

Towards the end of the fattening period the bullocks should be getting fully 13 lb. of starch equivalent: 1.5 to 2 lb. of protein equivalent is probably ample. The quantity of coarse fodder should be slightly reduced, and even though there may be an abundance of oat straw to consume, at least half the allowance of fodder should be hay, which, in the case of an arable farm, may be Italian rye-grass and clover hay. Some linseed cake may be included in the ration of cattle being finished for the butcher, as has been previously stated, with a carbonaceous food, such as maize meal, added to balance the ration. The following is an example of such a diet:

TABLE 100

Food.			Starch Equivalent.	Protein Equivalent.	N. Ratio.	Carbohydrate Equivalent.	Dry Matter.
		lb.	lb.	lb.		lb.	lb.
Seed Hay	...	7	2.55	0.42	7.2	3.03	6.0
Oat Straw	...	7	1.19	0.07	39.0	2.73	6.0
Swedes ...	...	50	3.50	0.35	11.4	4.00	6.0
Linseed Cake	...	2	1.45	0.49	1.0	0.49	1.7
Palm Kernel Cake		2	1.50	0.31	3.8	1.18	1.8
Maize Meal (de-germed)	...	4	3.20	0.22	12.8	2.82	3.4
Total in Ration ...			13.4	1.9		14.2	24.9

The above amounts of starch equivalent and protein equivalent are sufficient to produce as much increase per day as a bullock of 11 cwt. is capable of making. The N.R. is 1 to 7.6 and the dry matter is at the rate of 2 per cent. of the live weight.

The next ration is compounded of a greater variety of foods. In this case the farmer has plenty of hay and not much cereal straw and his root crop is not good. On the assumption that the beasts are about 2.5 years of age and half fat, with an average weight per head of 1,200 lb., for satisfactory increase they will require about 13 lb. of starch equivalent per head and 1.60 lb. of protein equivalent. (See p. 339). If the foods available are beans, locust beans, dried brewers' grains, decorticated ground nut cake, and maize meal, together with meadow hay and swedes, the following mixture may be tried to see if it gives a balanced diet and if the quantity of food is sufficient:

TABLE 101

Food.			Starch Equivalent.	Protein Equivalent.	Nitrogenous Ratio.	Carbohydrate Equivalent.	Dry Matter.
		lb.	lb.	lb.		lb.	lb.
Meadow Hay	..	14	4.35	0.63	9.4	5.90	11.9
Swedes ...	..	30	2.10	0.21	11.4	2.40	3.6
Beans ...	...	1	0.66	0.20	2.5	0.50	0.87
Locust Beans	...	1	0.70	0.04	15.1	0.60	0.87
Dried Grains	...	2	1.02	0.25	3.9	0.97	1.80
Dec. Ground Nut Cake ...		1	0.71	0.41	0.8	0.33	0.90
Maize Meal	...	2	1.60	0.11	12.8	1.41	1.70
Total in Ration ...			11.1	1.8		12.1	21.6

So far from being satisfactory this ration is faulty in several respects. There is not sufficient starch equivalent for satisfactory daily body weight increase. The N.R. is 1 to 6.7 and therefore narrower than it need be. The ration contains less than the amount of bulk that a beast of 1,200 lb. could deal with, the dry matter being only 1.8 per cent. of the live weight, although there is sufficient protein in the diet—in fact a slight excess over requirements. The diet therefore requires to be altered by the addition of another carbonaceous food or the increase in quantity of such as are already in the mixture. The diet being of a sufficiently varied nature, there is no necessity to make it more complicated so that one might double the amount of locust beans and add another pound of maize meal. The adjusted ration will then be:

TABLE 102

Food.		Starch Equivalent.	Protein Equivalent.	N.R.	Carbohydrate Equivalent.	Dry Matter.
	lb.	lb.	lb.		lb.	lb.
Meadow Hay ...	14	4.35	0.63	9.4	5.90	11.90
Swedes	30	2.10	0.21	11.4	2.40	3.60
Beans	1	0.66	0.20	2.5	0.50	0.87
Locust Beans ...	2	1.40	0.08	15.1	1.21	1.74
Dried Grains ...	2	1.02	0.25	3.9	0.97	1.80
Dec. Ground Nut Cake	1	0.71	0.41	0.8	0.33	0.90
Maize Meal ...	3	2.40	0.16	12.8	2.05	2 55
Total in Ration ...		12.6	1.9		13.4	23.4
Standard Requirements		12.8	1.6			
Difference		— 0.2	+0.3			

It will be seen that the adjusted ration contains sufficient starch equivalent and a slight excess of protein. The nitrogenous ratio is 1 to 7, and the dry matter is 1.95 per cent. of the live weight. On these grounds, therefore, the diet can be considered satisfactory.

If there is such a thing as an ideal diet that is superior to all others for fattening cattle, its composition is not yet known; and the details above are given merely to show how rations should be constructed. So long as foods are combined to make a balanced diet which contains sufficient nutriment to fulfil the object it is given for and is acceptable to the animal, the variety of satisfactory combinations is almost unlimited. It is often the case that a farmer has a special preference for a particular food which, he says, experience has shown him to give exceptionally good results. If an examination were to be made of the ration it would probably be found that the addition of the favoured food made the diet properly balanced or possibly more palatable. Apart from the relative cost of different foods the feeder should keep in mind that palatability of the whole ration is of great importance. If cattle are to thrive and grow fat they must be given food that is acceptable to them, and this should be attended to particularly during the later stages of fattening as it is then they are inclined to refuse their food.

Farmers have different views as to the number of feeds to give during the day; it is reasonable practice to avoid keeping the cattle too long without food and yet to allow the beasts a period of complete rest and quietness. Fattening bullocks thrive if kept quiet so that after feeding they may lie down and ruminate. One of the defects of yard feeding is that additional beasts cannot be added to the yard already occupied as the newcomers are often harried and bullied. Indeed, in all cases when fattening is done in courts, care must be taken to see that the aggressive animal is put out of the yard. There is something wrong either with the diet or the management if fattening cattle are always restless and on the move.

A common and satisfactory method of feeding is to give half the concentrates and half the roots the first thing in the morning, then to fill the rack with long fodder, and to repeat the sequence in the after-noon. There should be sufficient fodder in the rack to last through the night. If the roots are pulped the concentrates may be mixed among them, and this is an excellent method of giving meal as it adheres to the wet surface of the roots. The provision of adequate manger space is very important to prevent crowding and bullying when concentrates are fed, and a good cattleman takes care to see that the food is properly distri-buted in the space available.

Regularity in feeding is necessary, for no cattle will do well if their hours of feeding are irregular. The food should not be changed too frequently, though an occasional variation is sometimes desirable when, towards the end of the fattening period, the animals become tired of their food; when a change is made it must be done gradually. If fat animals have to be held back from marketing it is obviously unnecessary to feed the full production ration.

All fattening cattle should be allowed as much water to drink as they need, and in courts the most satisfactory method is to have self-filling water troughs to which the beasts can go when they feel inclined. In certain districts there is an erroneous belief that fattening cattle do better if their water allowance is strictly limited, but it is just the case that cattle which are given heavy feeds of roots, as is the custom in some areas, scarcely ever look at water, having more than they need in the roots. Nevertheless it should still be available. If cattle are stall-tied and automatic water bowls are not fitted they should be offered water twice daily.

When silage is given to fattening cattle it should be used as a part-substitute for some of the coarse fodder, roots and concentrates. Oats and tares silage, for instance, may in itself be balanced for fattening, but it is best fed along with other material, such as in the following diet, which has been widely tested in Norfolk[25]:

TABLE 103

	Amount.	D. M.	S. E.	P. E.
	lb.	lb.	lb.	lb.
Oats and tares silage ...	40	12.80	6.40	1.30
Dried sugar beet ...	7	6.23	3.64	0.25
Bean meal	3	2.58	2.04	0.57
Straw	ad lib.			
Total		21.6	12.1	2.1

This is sufficient for a 1,000 lb. bullock. As the animal increases in weight its greater needs can be met by the addition of cereals. Attention has been drawn to the nutritive value of silage in the section which deals with the question, and the farmer must take care to see that the right supplements are used to produce a properly balanced diet.

(c)   The production of baby beef.

Baby beef is obtained from carcases of cattle that have been well fed continuously from birth until sufficiently fat for butchering at an age of from 16 to 18 months. Cattle so treated have never passed through a " store " period and therefore have not been kept on a maintenance diet for lengthy periods. Since all maintenance food, by itself, is unproductive it may be more economical to feed for baby beef than to run cattle on until they are 2 to 3 years of age on little more than maintenance rations and then to fatten them, as the food required for maintenance for that period is thereby saved. In this connection Hammond [26] has compared the food value of milk and beef with the total quantity of food consumed by the animal (and its dam during pregnancy). The relative values, as percentages, are given in the table below :

TABLE 104

Product						Food content as percentage of that fed.	
						Protein.	Energy.
Milk (3 lactations)	...	...	...	...	...	17.0	30.0
Beef (birth to 7 cwt.) ...	...	...	...	...		11.1	14.0
„ (store, grass-fattened to 10.7 cwt.) ...				...		7.3	15.0
„ (store, stall-fattened to 12 cwt.)			...	...		7.2	15.3

Hammond considers, rightly, that the store period should be eliminated as far as is possible. To obviate the employment of imported high protein cakes he advocates the better use of grassland, and a system of farming which would make use of long leys, oats and beans for the quick rearing of cattle. This, in turn, means that the calf rearing methods must be such as will give the calf a good start. He quotes the case of North Devon steers which at weights of 10 to 11 cwt. at less than 15 months old consumed less actual food than the average steer which becomes a " store " and does not attain the same weight until 30 months of age. But there are conditions of farming where the carrying of store cattle appears to be necessary.

For the production of young beef all that is necessary is to see that the " calf flesh " is not lost and that the animals are well fed without interruption in the process. Forced feeding is neither necessary nor desirable nor need the process of early fattening be an expensive one. The rate of growth of young cattle from birth up to 30 months is given in a table on page 336. Beef steers kept under conditions of full growth and fattening reach an average weight of 950 lb., but there is considerable variation in the weights of cattle ready for the butcher at this age; prime baby beef may weigh from 7 to 10 cwt. or with exceptional animals even more. Some young cattle are ready for the butcher at 15 to 16 months old, depending upon the breed of the cattle and the manner in which they have been treated as calves. Autumn calves destined for baby beef are well kept during the winter, turned out to good grass as soon as it is ready, in May as a rule, and taken off the grass before it begins to fail towards the end of the summer, so that they do not go back in condition. They are then housed and well fed and should be ready for the butcher towards the end of the winter. Spring calves must be liberally fed during the first winter and may or may not be turned out to grass in the summer; they are finished off during the autumn. If they are kept in courts during the summer they require to be fed on soiling crops, such as grass, tares, green oats, etc., together with a couple of pounds or so of nitrogenous concentrates.

In some cases spring calves that have been suckled during calfhood (instead of being pail-fed) are well nourished during the winter and are then ready for the butcher in the following spring, i.e., when about 12 months old.

A practice followed in Perthshire,[27] where best quality baby beef is produced, is as follows: the calves are bred from a Shorthorn-cross heifer by an Aberdeen Angus bull, this combination giving weight as well as quality. As far as possible, calving is timed to occur in February or March, so that the cows are at the right stage of lactation to make full use of the grass when they are turned out and the calves are at an age when they can use the flush of milk. The cows are wintered in courts and are fed on turnips and straw. They are turned out to grass at about the middle of April, at first for short periods which are extended until they are left out night and day. One cow is expected to suckle only one calf, so that she will do it sufficiently well. Young heifers are preferred either to cows or full-grown heifers, because the amount of milk they give is usually just about the right quantity. Weaning takes place in mid-October, the cows and calves being returned to the yards for lengthening periods each day and the calves given small quantities of concentrates. The calves are then permanently housed, when they receive some 2 lb./day of a mixture of bran, crushed oats and linseed cake, a quantity which is gradually increased up to 5-6 lb. in February and 7-8 lb. during the last two months, i.e., May to June, by which time the beasts will weigh 8 to 10 cwt.

As opposed to the system of a cow of a beef breed suckling one calf only, Hammond[26] has suggested the employment of the higher yielding dairy cows to suckle successive groups of calves for two to three months each, the calves being introduced to hay and other solid foods very early on so as to make good growth and then being finished off on grass plus such concentrates as may be needed.

REFERENCES

1. Wright, N. C., and S. Morris, (1939). Agriculture, J. Minist. Agric. Engl., *46*, 21.
2. Foot, A. S., (1946). Agricultural Progress, *21*, 1.
3. Blaxter, K. L., and T. H. French, (1944). J. Agric. Sci., *34*, 217.
4. Davis, J. G., (1940). Food Manufacture, *11*, 272.
5. Halnan, F. T., and F. H. Garner, (1946). " The Principles and Practice of Feeding Farm Animals."
6. Maynard, L. A., (1947). " Animal Nutrition."
7. Report on Departmental Commission on Rationing of Dairy Cows (1925). H. M. Stationery Office, London.
8. Bartlett, S., A. S. Foot, S. L. Huthnance, and J. Mackintosh, (1940). J. Dairy Res., *11*, 121.
9. Private communication from Dr. W. S. Gordon.
10. Woodman, H. E., (1948). " Rations for Livestock," Min. Agric. Fisheries, Bull No. 48.
11. Blaxter, K. L., (1944). J. Agric. Sci., *34*, 213.
12. Savage, E. S., and C. M. McCay, (1942). J. Dairy Sci., *25*, 595.
13. Kenney, R., (1947). Agriculture, J. Minist. Agric. Engl., *54*, 405.
14. Sheehy, E. J., (1948). Agriculture, J. Minist. Agric. Engl., *55*, 189.
15. Groenewald, J. W., and P. J. v. d. H. Schreuder, (1947). Agriculture, J. Minist. Agric. Engl., *53*, 478.
16. Mackintosh, J., (1938). " Calf Rearing." Bull. No. 10, Minist. Agric. Fisheries.
17. Converse, H. T., (1947). " Science in Farming." U. S. Dept. Agric.
18. Robinson, J. F., (1947). Agriculture, J. Minist. Agric. Engl., *54*, 54.
19. Morrison, F. B., (1947). " Feeds and Feeding." 1005.
20. Mitchell, H. H., quoted by Maynard (Ref. 6).
21. Wood, T. B., Quoted by H. E. Woodman, " Rations for Livestock." H. M. Stationery Office, 1948.
22. Blaxter, K. L., and H. A. Price, (1946). J. Agric. Sci., *36*, 301.
23. Hoddell, G. P., (1947). Agriculture, J. Minist. Agric. Engl., *54*, 402.
24. Lloyd, J. L., (1946). Agriculture, J. Minist. Agric. Engl., *53*, 257.
25. Minist. Agric. Bull. No. 13, (1939).
26. Hammond, J., (1946). Agriculture, J. Minist. Agric. Engl., *53*, 34.
27. Howie, A., (1939). Scot. J. Agric., *22*, No. 4.

THE FEEDING OF SHEEP

1. Introduction.
2. Methods of sheep feeding.
    (a) Hill sheep feeding.
    (b) Lowland sheep feeding.
        (i) Upland semi-arable farms.
        (ii) Lowland fertile arable farms.
        (iii) Flying flocks.

(1) Introduction

The lamb, like the calf, begins its life as a non-ruminant and gradually develops the complex digestive system which is so characteristic of the ruminant. On this basis one would expect foods suitable for cattle to be suitable also for sheep and to be utilised with about the same degree of efficiency. Within fairly wide limits this is true.

A second point of resemblance between the two species, this time a functional and not an economic one, is that they both serve a dual purpose, but whereas cattle are kept very largely for meat and milk, sheep are used for the production of meat and wool. There is thus not such emphasis on feeding for milk production for the ewe as there is for the cow. To a degree there are, of course, dual-purpose breeds of both species and, whereas in Britain the emphasis tends to be on the production of mutton, with wool as the secondary product, the reverse is true of Australian practice.

Both species fill an important position in general farming policy. Though they compete with one another to some extent for the same class of nutrients this is not quite so marked as one might expect. The closer-grazing sheep can derive nourishment from pastures which would not support a cow, and the smaller animal can venture into hill regions which are inaccessible to the larger one. Sheep may follow cattle on grassland, so that the feeding of the two species is a complementary rather than a competitive process in a number of instances.

Sheep will do well on grass, which they seem to prefer shorter and finer than do cattle; for this reason they can be used for the close grazing of a ley before it is ploughed. On temporary leys, and especially in the first year, they will do very well, any tendency to scouring being offset, as in the case of cattle, by the provision of coarser foods, such as hay. So far as hay is concerned the leafy legume hays are the best. Silage, if of good quality, and good dried grass are valuable foods.

On lowland arable farms sheep may be folded on to a variety of crops on which they may be fattened. Provided that changes of diet are made gradually, the stock will grow and fatten well. On such crops it seems that sheep are less prolific than under other feeding systems. Possibly both nutritional and hereditary factors operate here, and in a review of fertility in sheep in relation to nutrition, American workers [1] have drawn attention to the fact that it has not yet been shown whether it is better, from the point of view of increased lamb production, to have ewes in uniformly good condition or to keep them relatively thin and then feed them well (" flush " them) just before the breeding season. There is a general agreement, however, that for breeding purposes neither rams nor ewes should be allowed to become too fat, although it is very difficult to define " too fat ". Insufficient protein or vitamin A in the ration will, of course, result in impaired reproduction and so far as the latter is concerned it may be emphasised again that the usual roots given to sheep provide none of this factor, that the concentrates except yellow maize are lacking in it and that hay is an uncertain source.

Protein and mineral requirements are relatively high in the last third of pregnancy and in the early stages of growth. Sheep usually consume freely of the salt licks which are given, but the actual provision of anything more than common salt and perhaps calcium and phosphorus depends very much on local conditions. In all cases a free water supply is desirable, though it is not always an easy matter to ensure this.

Although there are feeding standards in use for sheep under various conditions, they can seldom be applied to the individual animal as is done, for example, for the dairy cow. For this reason feeding is based upon the flock or group and there are two important practical consequences. The first is that where feeding is from troughs, there must be ample feeding space, otherwise the weaker animals may be deprived of their full ration: the second point is that animals of similar age or condition are often fed as a group and distinct from others. As with other classes of livestock so with sheep, successful production depends not only on adherence to known feeding standards but upon careful observation of the condition of the individual beast.

The range of environments in which sheep are kept is greater than that for cattle, with the result that the different breeds are even more highly adapted to a particular altitude, climate, or system of management than are the various breeds of cattle. Breeds which are eminently suited to one country, or even county, are not satisfactory when introduced into another, e.g., Southdowns introduced into certain parts of the Highlands are a failure. In other cases, breeds with certain recognised characteristics in their home counties change noticeably when kept in distant parts; thus, the Border-Leicester is a very different sheep from the English-Leicester from which it originated.

British breeds of sheep, though they may produce less wool than the wool-producing breeds, such as the Merino, are still capable of yielding quite a good weight of satisfactory wool and, moreover, they are notable for their weight of carcase and their depth and quality of flesh. There is a great difference, however, in the mutton produced by various breeds, and by individual sheep of different ages.

TABLE 105

Breed	Carcase wt. (lb.)	Fleece wt. (lb.)	Characteristics of meat
Heavy			
Cotswolds, Lincolns, Leicesters, Devons, Wensleydales	40-90 per quarter	12-20	Tending to be too fat sub-cutaneously if forced, and rather coarse.
Down breeds			
Southdowns, Oxfords, Hampshires, Suffolks	15-25 or more per quarter	6-12	Better quality than the heavier breeds.
Mountain			
Scottish Blackface, Cheviot	10 per quarter	4-6	Best quality, with little subcutaneous fat.

The above table gives a brief summary of the differences between the chief groups; it is not possible here to discuss the details.

One more important factor in sheep feeding which always has to be considered is whether the sheep are to be kept for breeding or for fattening. Certain farms, owing to their situation, nature of the land, or because of the crop rotation, can only carry fattening stock, while poorer, cheaper and lighter land is generally better suited to breeding, and is unsatisfactory for fattening. On many farms a combination is sometimes possible; a green or fodder crop is arranged for the lambs after weaning, the ewes meantime running upon rough pastures, open downs, or drier marsh lands—provided these are reasonably free from infestation with worms or flukes. In such cases, during the suckling period the ewes and lambs run together and share the same food, the ewes often being folded and the lambs running out through a creep-hurdle† into the rest of the field. Lambs under this system can be brought on well if provided with 0.5 lb. per head per day of cake or corn in a trough outside the fold.

Present-day tendencies are all towards the purchase of meat from younger animals, and to meet these requirements the feeder aims to turn out his animals at the age when they have nearly attained adult size, but before added expense has been occasioned by keeping them too long. In other words, he feeds the animals as well as possible, so that the normal growing period coincides to a great extent with the fattening period, and the stock is ready for slaughter at a very much earlier age than was formerly the custom. The advantages to the consumer are that he obtains his meat at a stage where the muscle fibres are fully formed, but before any great amount of fibrous tissue has been laid down, i.e., the meat is tender, the toughness of age being absent. Moreover, when

† A creep-hurdle is so arranged that only lambs can pass through it.

an adult animal is *rapidly* fattening (e.g., a ram, cast ewe, cow or bull) the fat is deposited in layers under the skin, but when a young animal is fattened *slowly but continuously* fat is laid down between the muscle fibre and amongst the muscle bundles rather than under the skin; therefore the younger the animal, the better the appearance of the joint upon the table, and the more palatable it is.

(2) Methods of sheep feeding

There are two main systems of sheep rearing, namely those associated with the hills and with the lowlands. In the case of the former the sheep rely upon the rather sparse vegetation of the highlands for sustenance, one sheep requiring several acres of such land for its upkeep, while in the latter instance the more fertile lowlands are used. The second system may be subdivided into two divisions, associated with grassland and with arable land respectively: in each case one acre of land will provide the nourishment for a number of sheep. The three systems are not necessarily independent of one another, nor are the divisions always quite so clear cut as the above statement suggests. Though sheep are still kept in strength on the hills, the numbers reared on arable land are tending to fall, although they should have a position on such land complementary to cattle and not in competition with them, as so often seems to be thought.

The demand for fat lambs has become such that it now occupies the main place in the programme of the lowland sheep farmer. Besides the quality of the joint, consumers nowadays demand that it should be small in size so as to meet the needs of the small family. Sheep feeders, on the other hand, need thrifty animals which are capable of doing themselves well on the herbage available without much supervision, and with a minimum of expensive supplementing foods. It is for the first reason that there has been such a reduction in the number of the heavy, long wool breeds of sheep, and for the second that the number of Down sheep has been so materially reduced. Their places have largely been taken by the cross between the mountain or hill ewe and a Down ram, so that the progeny have the advantage of a genetic make-up which favours early maturity and the possibility of exploiting this characteristic by the liberal feeding afforded by a generous milking dam.

The earliest fat lambs are put on the market at about 10 weeks old from April to June. They are usually off the better arable land and are the progeny of Down or Down cross breeds. These are followed by selected single lambs from less advanced areas, and by the month of August even some pure-bred mountain lambs are sold fat. All these classes of lambs have come direct from breeding flocks but later their place is taken by lambs which have undergone a period as stores and which have been prepared for the market by feeders on a higher plane of nutrition than was possible in the district in which they were bred. They respond rapidly to the feeding and the best are sold when about 5 months old; others which need still more generous treatment may not be fit for slaughter until October or later, and are grown to not more than about 130 lb., which is considered to be the maximum weight desirable.

(a) Hill sheep feeding.

In the working of a hill sheep farm the land itself does not receive any set system of cultivation and the natural flora are allowed to grow without encouragement or hindrance. The sheep stock are usually the property of the owner of the farm and are rented with it to the occupier, for a settled sheep stock is a very important factor in the successful breeding and feeding of hill sheep.

The sheep on a hill farm are generally divided into groups known as " hirsels ", which number between twenty and thirty score (i.e., 400 to 600) as a rule. Each hirsel is in charge of a shepherd or " herd," and usually remains confined to one particular hill or other natural division of the farm. At the headquarters for each hirsel there is generally a circular stone shelter built upon a lower and level piece of ground. This is known as a " stell ". Hay may be stacked nearby and sometimes a low-roofed shed is provided also.

So far as the actual feeding is concerned, the main flock eats whatever kinds of grasses, heather and other herbage are found on the hill, and in ordinary times these are sufficient for the sheep, though the lower and better areas tend to be reserved for lambing. In some situations, however, the grazing is so poor that the ewe lambs and even some of the breeding ewes have to be wintered, at great expense, on lower lying farms. Hand-feeding, so far as the ewe stock is concerned, does not take place in ordinary years. When the winter is very stormy, however, and especially when falls of snow are heavy and snow lies long on the ground, it becomes necessary to supply hay or a little grain to tide the sheep over the period when the ground is covered. If only a thin layer of snow covers the ground the majority of sheep will manage to scratch or " nose " through it and feed as usual, provided the surface is not frozen hard. Where convenient, turnips are sometimes carried out on sleighs or in panniers on a horse during stormy weather. In the opinion of most sheep-farmers the hay should only be used when absolutely necessary, for sheep that are given a large amount of hay during the winter are inclined to get lazy and cease to forage for themselves so well as when they get none. Grain, however, is used by some farmers at weekly intervals—reckoning at the rate of about half a pound per head per week during the period between tupping and lambing.

In reference to the disastrous winter of 1946-7 in Britain, Phillips and Phillips [2] have suggested that an allowance of 0.5 lb. of hay per ewe per day would be a satisfactory reserve if sufficient were kept by to cover a month of hard weather. They also give details of the effect of

the method of wintering (1937-8) upon the average live weight of lambs
and on the percentage of lambs reared. Their table is reproduced below:

TABLE 106

Method of wintering	Weights (lb.) At birth	May 14	Aug. 31	Lambs reared, %
Improved hill pastures	5.7	18.5	41.8	69.3
1.5 hr./day on timothy	6.0	18.3	40.8	64.5
1.5 hr./day winter foggage ...	6.4	21.2	45.6	72.6
2 feeds/day of dried grass	6.5	18.7	41.8	76.9
2 feeds/day of maize	6.6	22.4	45.7	75.1

The beneficial effects of foggage, dried grass and maize rather suggest
an extra need for total energy, carotene and perhaps protein.

For this system of production the percentage of lambs reared is not
abnormal, but it gives some idea of the wastage involved; it also puts the
problem of the methods which should be adopted to increase the proportion of lambs which can be reared.

In this connection Wallace [3] has studied the needs of ewes during
pregnancy and the effect of the plane of nutrition of the dam on the
well-being of her progeny. His general conclusions will suit all cases,
so that his results may be discussed here and afterwards considered in
the light of the special conditions of hill feeding.

By careful experimental control Wallace was able to show that both
the birth weight of a lamb and the milk yield of the ewe are particularly
affected by the plane of nutrition of the ewe during the last six weeks
of pregnancy. His results provoked the suggestion that the vigour and
weight of a lamb at birth is important, not merely for avoiding losses at
that time, but also for its effect on the ability of the lamb to take the
best advantage of the potential milk supply of the dam—for her milk
yield, as in the case of the cow, depends in part upon the demands which
are made upon it. A good start in lactation means a lamb which is able,
earlier than would otherwise be the case, to take advantage of solid foods.

In his work Wallace did not have among the ill-fed ewes any cases
of " pregnancy disease ", which has been attributed to the undernutrition
of pregnant ewes, especially those carrying twin lambs, and he suggests
that malnutrition as a causative agent may be a matter, not only of the
stage of pregnancy at which it occurs but also of the size of the foetus.
A large foetus, produced by a good level of nutrition, might make too
severe demands on the ewe if a period of semi-starvation followed.

Though Wallace showed the need for adequate feeding during the
last six weeks of pregnancy, it is not possible to separate clearly the
differences in the conditions of the ewes and lambs which were due to
varying intakes of total nutrients from those which were due to differences of protein consumption, for the successively higher planes of
nutrition were increasingly better with respect to protein percentage.
There is, however, no reason for believing that the needs of pregnant

mammals—farm stock, at least—differ fundamentally from one species to another and that sheep are exceptional.

Bearing these facts in mind, the supplementary feeds which are given to hill sheep, during periods of stress, may again be considered. For example, though maize is fairly easy to handle, to store and to feed its low mineral content and its rather poor protein both render it open to suspicion as a supplementary food for a pregnant animal. While the amount of protein needed at a given stage of pregnancy may be subject to quite narrow limits of variation, one cannot assume that in all cases the ratio of digestible protein to total digestible nutrients should be about one to five, for that ratio was determined by experiments where the amount of exercise was limited and where the environmental conditions to which the animals were subjected were not extreme. In the case of hill sheep, however, the amount of energy used in foraging must be relatively very high and in severe climatic conditions the extra heat production required to offset the cold environment is also increased. In the ideal case, the extra energy needed for both purposes can be derived from carbohydrate or fat, but where the total energy supplied in the food is not sufficient for all purposes, then the animal will metabolise protein, either of its food, or of its own tissues, or both. There is not much point in worrying about the nitrogenous ratio of a ration for a pregnant ewe if the total energy supply of the beast is insufficient. Truly enough the diet should provide a good proportion of digestible protein, say 15 - 20 per cent. or more, but both quantity and quality must be provided.

For a ration which is definitely a supplement to the maintenance provided by the hill grazings a protein-rich food is desirable; there is no reason why the usual protein concentrates, such as linseed cake, ground-nut cake, beans, etc., balanced with cereals, should not be fed from troughs at appropriate times.

Wallace's work showed that a ewe which was poorly fed during the early part of pregnancy could make up a good deal of lost ground by better feeding during the last six weeks. Where there is likely to be a shortage of food, either because of an actual lack of it or because climatic conditions render it temporarily inaccessible, it would seem that food reserves are best kept for this critical period.

Mineral deficiencies which are met with in various parts of the country—often they are highly localised—include phosphorus, iodine, cobalt and copper. One group of workers has reported that heather provides the trace elements in relative abundance.[4]

The rise and fall in the nutritive value of natural pasture is well shown by the figures which are provided by monthly chemical analyses of a hill pasture throughout a year, when one may see that lambing occurs when the nutritive value as well as the quantity of the grass is beginning to increase as expressed in the increase in the percentage of protein and silica-free ash with a corresponding decrease in fibre. Weaning occurs naturally at the time when there is a decided reduction in nutritive value, and it is to be noted that tupping takes place when the level is low. The cycle of lambing, weaning and tupping varies with locality, so far as locality influences pasture growth. It is pasture growth—influenced by locality—which is the factor that decides the lambing time.

The figures also illustrate the necessity of supplementary feeding of ewes prior to lambing, and where " flushing " is carried out it also shows why there may be need for the extra food.

It is sometimes said that hill sheep farming cannot afford to pay for the necessary foods which are needed to supplement the natural herbage of the hills. It might be better to put the matter another way and to ask whether the country—and ultimately mankind—can afford to neglect the nutriment provided by the hill regions. As expressed by Fraser[5] this type of sheep farming " has a value and importance not readily calculable on the sole basis of production and profit ".

The products of a hill sheep farm will include (i) ram lambs for breeding, (ii) ewe lambs, (iii) wether lambs, (iv) cast ewes and (v) wool. So far as the feeding of the stock is concerned it is an advantage to discuss the feeding of the lambs first of all and leave the ewes until later.

The nutritional requirements of lambs differ in no fundamental way from those of the young of other mammalian species. In their early life easily digested protein, fat and carbohydrate, together with sufficient calcium, phosphorus, vitamins A and D, plus other trace factors, are needed; the proportion of protein which is desirable has been dealt with elsewhere (Ch. 17). Milk from the ewe is the food par excellence for this purpose. As growth proceeds the rumen develops and the lamb gradually becomes capable of dealing, not only with solid foods such as the easily digested cereal grains and protein concentrates, but also with fibrous foods. The better the start the lamb makes the sooner will it reach this satisfactory stage. If fattening as well as growth is desired an extra intake of food is needed, either of good pasture or of additional concentrates. As in the case of cattle, a store period leads to inefficient utilisation of ingested food because of the high proportion which is used simply for maintenance. Conditions are not always such, however, as to allow the farmer to make the best use of these desirable principles.

Lambing will usually take place on the lower and better parts of the hill grazings; improved hill pasture is suitable for the purpose. Among the mountain flocks, because of the generally low plane of nutrition, twin lambs are relatively rare; such lambs require extra attention if they are to make satisfactory growth.

(i) Ram lambs

Ram lambs, whether for home use, or for sale, get special attention. They are usually bred from specially selected ewes, which have been tupped by well-bred (and often high-priced) rams before these latter are used for the general flock. After weaning, the best are marked, kept in a small field during the day and given special feeding. On some farms, cabbages or other green crops are grown specially for them, and as soon as the turnips or swedes are ready they get these as well.

Hand-feeding is usually rich, and consists in supplying 2 lb. per head per day of a mixture of crushed oats, kibbled old beans or peas, linseed or cotton cake, bran, locust beans and broken, split or flaked maize, along with about 0.5 lb. per head per day of boiled barley and maize, to which cod liver oil, treacle and a little coarse salt may be added. Water must always be kept available. As in other cases, changes of dietary should be gradual.

A certain amount of criticism is often levelled at the system of forcing tup-lambs, because when these latter, perhaps so accustomed to pampering and hand-feeding that they cannot do without it, are put out to the ewes in November and bad weather is experienced, they may fail to withstand the rigours of the weather added to the strain of service. Against judicious hand-feeding and wise attention, however, there can be no objection.

(ii) *Ewe lambs*

The ewe lambs retained for maintaining the numbers of the stock spend their first summer with their dams on the hill grazings, usually receiving nothing but milk and the available herbage. These " hoggs ",* as they are called for their first autumn and winter, are normally wintered at home on better keep. Hay or silage may be supplied, with roots and, if really necessary, small amounts of concentrates, in addition to whatever pasturage is available; if the pasturage is of the improved type, the hoggs will probably do well on it, but conditions vary very greatly with respect to the nature and position of the ground, the season and the beasts themselves. In the following year the hoggs return to the hill pastures and are bred from as " gimmers ", i.e., when they are between one and two years of age, being tupped at about 19 months of age and producing their first lamb at two years.

Depending very much on local conditions there may be a surplus of ewe lambs over and above those required for the maintenance of the flock. If the lower pasturage is good these may be fat enough for sale in the late summer. Others, though not so forward, may be well enough grown to be fit to fatten. They are put on to a good pasture for the first week or until they settle, and then are folded on turnips, swedes (if forward), cabbages or kale, foggage or some other green autumn crop. The change must be made gradually, for a sudden access to turnips may cause scouring. Roots may be carted on to the pastures for a few days The fold should be large enough to allow about 2 square yards per head per day, or more if the crop is poor or if the lambs appear to need more. Iron or wooden hurdles or sheep-netting and stakes are used, and each day a new fold is set ahead of the old one, so that the lambs may lie in the old fold and feed in the new one.

* Hoggs, hoggets or tegs.

Troughs are provided, and very often a hay rack as well. The former are used for feeding the concentrates, and the latter is daily filled with clover, lucerne, rye-grass or meadow hay, or cut straw according to taste and the facilities available, so that 0.25 to 0.5 lb. per 100 lb. live weight is allowed. The concentrates used vary almost with each individual farmer. Some representative mixtures and the amounts used are given below.

TABLE 107

Diet

(1)

Crushed oats   ...   .
Kibbled maize ...   .   equal parts
Undecorticated cotton cake   ...

Lambs are started at 0.5 lb. per head per day, increasing to 1 lb. per head per day after a month or six weeks.

(2)

Winter beans (crushed)   ...
Crushed oats   ...   .   } equal parts
Whole maize   ...   .
Linseed cake   ...   .

Lambs are begun at 0.25 to 0.5 lb., which is increased to a maximum of 1 lb. per head per day.

(3)

To check scouring when first on turnips:
Undecorticated cotton cake   ...   } equal parts
Dried grains   ...   .

0.1 to 0.75 lb. per 100 lb. live weight is given to begin with; later this is gradually changed to the food below.

(4)

Undecorticated cotton cake   ...
Dried grains   ...   .   } equal parts
Flaked maize   ...   .
Linseed cake   ...   .

This diet can be used to finish off the fattening process.

As a rule the tegs of mountain breeds do not well adapt themselves to *winter* fattening on roots, because of the wet nature of the land which soils their fleece, and those not ready for the butcher by Christmas are often wintered over as stores on the pastures of lowland farms, sometimes getting roots and hay carried to them. They are finished off later on early spring green crops.

(iii) *Wether lambs*

Wether lambs are either sold fat or as stores for fattening on the lower-lying arable farms, where, during the winter, they receive such feeding as has been described above for ewe lambs. The production of stores has the same disadvantage with respect to the overall efficiency of food utilisation as in the case of store cattle and for the same reasons.

(iv) *Cast ewes*

Ewes may be discarded for several reasons, such as age, diseased udders or barrenness. Those not fit for further breeding are best sold separately: like the lambs they are sometimes hand-fed for a short time before sale in order to fatten them.

Those draft ewes, which are in a fit condition to breed, i.e., which have sound udders and full but unbroken mouths and which are in fair bodily condition, are usually bought by the arable farmer to form a " flying flock " (p. 370). In view of this practice and the demand there is for good draft ewes, many hill-farmers part with their draft ewes when 4½ years old, whereby they get a bigger price per head, since the ewes are still in good breeding condition and are not too old to be turned into good quality mutton a year afterwards. In most cases, however, draft ewes are sold when 5½ to 6½ years old, and a certain number, which have proved very good breeders, may be kept till 9½ or even 10½ years old.

(b) Lowland sheep feeding.

The object of the lowland sheep farmer may 'be ram-breeding, or tegging, or fattening-off on turnips, or raising fat lambs, or fattening dam and lamb together, according to the farm and locality. Excluding true mountain breeds, the sheep throughout the lower-lying and more fertile parts of Britain can be looked upon as falling into two main groups. Firstly, there are the upland breeding flocks, from whence come store lambs and draft ewes, usually containing from 500 to 1200 ewes or more and kept on the wide-lying hillier and poorer pastures; and secondly, there are the smaller lowland flocks, chiefly kept for fattening on the rich fertile lower arable lands, which are perhaps best typified by Romney Marsh and the pedigree flocks of Down breeds. Few lowland farmers, however, rear all their own lambs, and since sheep food is most abundant on lower richer farms in the winter months, there is an exchange all over the country during the autumn when many upland-bred lambs change hands to be fattened on the winter keep of arable farms. In each of these groups, however, there are almost as many systems as there are counties, for that which suits the flat country of Lincolnshire and East Anglia does not answer when carried out on the Sussex Downs, for example.

(i) *Upland semi-arable farms*.

On upland semi-arable farms the ewe flocks are generally reckoned according to the size of the grazing—one sheep per acre being the usual. In the winter, after the lambs, " culls " (ewes which owing to some bodily disablement are neither fit for keeping nor for placing in the draft) and the regular draft ewes have been sold and after the best of the season's lambs have been added to the breeding stock, the main flock settles down to a period of maintenance only. The sheep, during autumn, roam the pastures practically at will, and in normal years require no hand-feeding whatever unless they are flushed, which is accomplished by improving their nutrition some two to three weeks before they are put to the ram. The stimulating effect of a change from a subsistence diet to a very much more generous one at this season is reflected in the regularity with which individuals of the flock come into œstrus, and the increased ovulation which takes place so that the percentage of twin lambs is greatly increased. It is practised in all British flocks except mountain ones, where, on account of the scanty feed, twin lambs are generally an embarrassment. No food has been proved to contain any special virtue for flushing; the essential is that the total diet should be more generous in quality, quantity and palatability than previously. Rape or fresh young grass, clover layers in the bottom of oat or barley stubbles, late aftermaths, silage, foggage, etc., may be used. Failing supplies of green food, a ration of about 0.5 lb. of crushed oats per ewe per day, either alone or with a little bran or cake added, answers quite well. In such cases, the sheep remain at pasture, and are fed from troughs during the middle of the day. After the rams have been taken out (they are generally allowed to run with the ewes for about 6 weeks, and the " flushing " may continue during the first month of this period) the ewes receive nothing further until perhaps the middle or end of December when they are given a small but gradually increasing root ration. For medium-sized ewes this may reach about 10 lb. per head per day up to the last six weeks of pregnancy. At this stage the ration should be carefully reviewed, bearing in mind the characteristic needs of a pregnant animal. It may then be found that a limit has been reached to the quantity of roots which it is desirable to feed and that concentrates should be now added to the ration. If there is a scarcity of protein concentrates then it may be better to reduce the amount of roots fed, using first-class grass silage in its place. Silage, in fact, is an excellent food at this stage; dried grass is also valuable, for although it is expensive it is not outstandingly so compared with the usual concentrates and it has good qualities which they do not possess. Though roots are succulent, they are essentially sources of carbohydrate and, if they are going to constitute a large proportion of the ration, are better used for fattening (as distinct from growth) than for pregnancy or lactation unless they are balanced with some protein-rich food to give a suitable ratio of starch equivalent to protein. Excessively heavy root feeding just before lambing will bring its own reward in weak and unsatisfactory lambs. As has been pointed out already, the period both before parturition and immediately after it is one in which generous feeding always pays, for there is no cheaper or better food for the lamb than its dam's milk, and only a well-developed lamb can take full advantage of it.

On some farms roots are carted daily on to a convenient pasture; on others, particularly on lighter types of land, the ewes are allowed into a field of roots for a stated period daily.

For 2 or 3 weeks before lambing, a mixture of oats, dried grains, cotton cake, peas, bran and flaked maize, in different proportions, at the rate of 1 lb. per head per day, is often given, and this is continued until the lambs are well forward and the grass starts to grow in the spring, or until autumn sown catch crops are ready to be fed, when it is gradually reduced. The basal nutritive requirements of lowland sheep have been fairly accurately ascertained and are dealt with later. Representative mixtures for ewes before, during and after lambing are:

TABLE 108

Diet.					Amount fed (lb.)/day.
(1)					
Linseed cake ...	...	...	}	equal parts	0.75
Crushed oats ...	...	...			
Bran ...	...	...	...		
(2)					
Linseed cake ...	...	...	}	equal parts	0.75
Peas or beans ...	...	...			
Pea chaff ...	...	...			
(3)					
Decorticated cotton cake	...	}		equal parts	1.0-1.5
Bran	...				
(4)					
Dried grains ...	...	...	}	equal parts	0.5-1.0
Crushed oats ...	...	...			
Linseed cake ...	...	...			

With most flocks, if it is available, up to one half-pound per head per day of seeds hay, meadow hay, or, better still, clover or sainfoin hay, is given in hay racks.

As soon as the lambs will eat from a trough, which may be from 2 to 3 weeks onwards, they may be given some concentrates, such as a mixture of equal parts of ground linseed cake, cracked beans, malt culms and flaked maize. According to their size 0.1 to 0.5 lb./day is allowed for each lamb, the feeding being done inside a hurdle enclosure which the lambs enter by creep hurdles. A hay rack kept filled with clover or rye-grass hay should be available for them as soon as they will eat hay. The whole flock, as soon as lambing is finished and the lambs are strong enough to follow their mothers, is generally changed from pasture to pasture according to the food available.

They are run over young clovers, seeds, and even occasionally over winter wheat or barley early in the spring, if these are very forward. This carries the flock on till weaning time, which, if lambing occurred in January, will be about May, but if lambing was later, e.g., March or early April, may not be much before July. After weaning, the ewes return to the higher, open and poorer land, where they are kept on a low diet, partly for economy and partly to dry up their milk. Later on they are run over stubble, or mustard, or rape, which may carry them up to tupping time again.

Between weaning time and the lamb sales the lambs are kept in good growing condition. They are not usually greatly forced, unless the production of fat lambs, or ram lambs is aimed at, in which case their management follows rather more closely that given in the succeeding account of sheep feeding on lower fertile arable land. Otherwise they are kept upon spring sown tares, rape, or a green mixed crop of oats, tares and peas (or other similar combination), and receive concentrates to the extent of 0.5 to 0.75 lb./day. The exact routine of management varies according to the breed and locality, and also to the time of the year when lambing takes place.

As an example of this system, the following experiments, covering the years 1934-9 may be given.[6] Half-bred ewes were out on pasture until about December, when seeds hay was given from racks, together with 0.25 to 0.5 lb./day of a mixture of whole maize (45 per cent.), rolled oats (45 per cent.) and fish meal (10 per cent.), the higher level of feeding being reached when lambing commenced. After lambing, chopped mangolds were fed to the ewes in the lambing pens, with whole mangolds on the grass. A concentrate mixture, of which the following is a typical example of the several used, was given to the ewes up to 1 lb. per head per day, the amount being gradually reduced towards the end of April and discontinued at the beginning of May.

Decorticated groundnut cake	...	...		1 part
Whole maize	...	...	...	...	3 parts
Rolled oats	...	...	...	...	3 „
Linseed cake	...	...	...	...	1 part
Minerals	...	...	...	...	...	5% of mixture
Dig. protein, %	...	...	...	...	16-18

Lambing usually began in late February and ended a month later, a mixture of decorticated groundnut cake (1 part), linseed cake (1 part), kibbled locust beans (1 part) and flaked maize (3 parts) being fed to the lambs in creeps from mid-March onwards. When the lambs had reached a fasting weight of 70 lb. they were killed. In these trials Border Leicester-Cheviot ewes, with either Hampshire or Suffolk rams were used. The nutritionally significant results are tabulated below (the data have been rounded off).

TABLE 109

Lambs born/ ewe. (Av.)	Lambs reared. %	Birth weights Singles Twins Triplets			Live wt. at sale.	Gain/head/week. (Av.) Singles Twins Triplets		
			(lb.)		(lb.)		(lb.)	
1.97	86	13	11	9	82	6	5	4

About 5 per cent. of the lambs born were singles, 27 per cent. were triplets and the remaining 68 per cent. were twins.

. The above rations are capable of modification by the substitution of alternative protein concentrates, such as cracked or ground beans.

(ii) *Lowland fertile arable farms*

Sheep husbandry on the richest mixed arable lands of the British Isles is a most complicated procedure which can only be considered in relation to the crops of a locality and the crop rotation practised there, and differs greatly from both systems of sheep management already considered.

The average number of a typical lowland flock on a rich arable farm, where the permanent pasture is usually not much more than 20 per cent. to 25 per cent. of the total acreage (and may be less) varies between 80 and 150 or 200. On lighter and poorer arable land, however, as many as 500 to 1000 flock ewes may be kept.

The general management on the lowland farms, where a permanent flock of ewes is maintained all the year round, is the reverse of what occurs in the upland hill farm. In the summer time a smaller head of sheep is carried and the ewes are more or less open-grazed, running behind fattening bullocks and dairy cows, and living on the harsher, drier and less nutritious herbage left by them; while in winter, after the fattening sheep have been brought in, the head of sheep is greatest, the fattening ones and a proportion of ewes being folded on turnips and other crops.

Beginning after weaning and drafting has taken place, the ewes to be kept in the flock are run over poorer pastures, hay aftermath if not too rank, stubbles as they become available, etc., partly from the point of view of economy and partly to dry up the flow of milk. This routine is followed until tupping time approaches, when the ewe flock should get a change to richer keep, to get the ewes into better breeding condition. Some farmers give a little cake about this time, others rely on folding at night on turnips, rape or mustard, the ewes grazing out during the day, while others " flush " more strongly by folding on cabbage, marrow-stem kale and early kohl rabi, or on a late sown mixture of oats, tares and peas—which are still green at tupping time, i.e., from July onwards. Sometimes the tups are put out in the fold, but where this procedure is followed extra care and supervision are needed lest they should fight.

After the tups have been removed, generally in six weeks, the ewes may be grazed on rather poorer keep for the first 2 or 3 months of pregnancy, for the heavy lowland breeds of sheep always show a great tendency to become too fat, and if the ewes are too fat at lambing, parturition may be troublesome. The importance of this over-fatness has, however, been greatly exaggerated by many writers. Heavier feeding should start about six weeks or so before lambing begins, so that the extra nourishment obtained can lead to an increased milk flow for the lambs, rather than that it should produce fat. To effect this, the flock is managed in much the same way as before tupping, being kept on dry pasture during the day and sleeping in a fold of turnips during the night. The fold is moved on each day or every second day according to the rate at which the crop is eaten. If frosts occur the ewes are better kept in the fold each morning until the frost or rime is off the grass, a little hay or good oat straw being given in hay racks in the meantime. Kale is a reliable winter crop which provides excellent food for the ewes throughout the greater part of the winter and spring. The marrow-stem variety should last through to January and the thousand-headed till well into spring.

Lambing usually takes place in a lambing-pen or fold, in which the ewes sleep at night; the ewes are run out during the day on good pasture and return each night to the pen, where for the first few days the ewe and lamb or lambs are made comfortable, the ewe and her progeny thereafter being drafted to the appropriate yard. Yards are generally provided for—(1) single ram lambs; (2) single ewe lambs; (3) twins; (4) mixed or inferior lambs and lambs whose mothers are not up to standard. As soon as the lambs can follow their mothers they are put out of the yard on to white turnips, returning to the yard or other shelter at night. Later on, when strong enough, they are kept out altogether. As in the case of calves and other young stock, there should be careful attention to hygiene. Dirty conditions, leading to scouring in the lambs, will very often more than offset the beneficial effects of good feeding. Lambs should be put out each day whenever they are strong enough, and when the weather is suitable.

For the first few days the ewes are fed on concentrates and rye-grass, clover or lucerne hay, sometimes with the addition of pulped turnips or mangolds, or cabbages or other succulent foods. Clean water must always be available; the ewes should be free to drink if they need to.

For the first month in their lives the lambs do quite well on their mother's milk, and the single ewe lambs will probably need very little, if any, more than this before they are able to fend for themselves. Single ram lambs, intended to become breeding tups, and twins, as well as the mixed lambs, should be offered solid food when they are little more than a week old. It is not until they are four or five weeks old that they will eat an appreciable quantity, but from then the extent to which they augment their milk diet will be reflected in the rate of their growth. At first, when small quantities are being eaten, the more palatable carbo-hydrate foods such as maize, and later a mixture of maize and oats, will be found suitable. As the milk supply declines, some rich protein food is added, such as finely kibbled linseed and decorticated groundnut cake; so that should there be a period between the cessation of the milk diet and grazing on young grass, it is spanned as easily as possible.

It is estimated that a Down ewe of about 160 lb. body weight will yield, on an average, 3 gallons of milk per week, though the range is wide. Her requirements of food for milk production, assessed upon the composition of the milk and assuming a standard of food conversion equal to that of a dairy cow, is 4 lb. S.E. and 1 lb. P.E. per gallon. If this is added to her maintenance requirements (see page 369) the total comes to 24 lb. S.E. with 3.6 lb. P.E. The amount the milking ewe will eat is considerably more than that of a non-lactating sheep and a diet such as the following would be adequate to meet her requirements for a week:

TABLE 110

Food.	Quantity.	Dry Matter.	S.E.	P. E.
	lb.	lb.	lb.	lb.
High quality clover hay ...	10.5	8.76	4.5	0.73
Swedes	150	18.00	10.5	1.05
Total		26.8	15.0	1.8

For each gallon of milk that it is estimated she is secreting, an addition of 4 lb. of the following mixture may be given:

TABLE 111

Dec. groundnut cake ...	1	0.9	0.7	0.42
Flaked maize	1	0.9	0.8	0.08
Oats	2	1.8	1.2	0.15
Total		3.6	2.7	0.65
Total in the whole diet ... (for 3 gallons of milk)		37.6	23.0	3.7

To the single ram lamb section is given a good mixture, fed in a corner to which the lambs only have access (through a lamb-hurdle), such as equal parts of finely ground linseed cake, split white peas, malt culms, and flaked or cracked maize. The amount given may rise to 0.5 lb. per head per day as required.

It has been shown to be economical to feed lambs liberally, at any rate up to 4 months of age, and an early start should be made by offering them appetising food. If they have done well, and this depends to a very large extent on the supervision of the shepherd, each lamb should consume up to 0.5 cwt. of concentrates during the four months.

Folding should be arranged so that the lambs run forward on to a fresh fold through lamb-hurdles, thereby getting the pick of the crop before the ewes, which follow on to clean the land after them. Lambs very soon learn to take advantage of this system, returning to the main fold to suckle and to sleep with their dams over night. It also admits of specially feeding the lambs on lamb mixtures to fatten them as they grow, so that January and February-born lambs may be fit for the butcher in July and August, as they command high prices at that time.

On a well-managed fertile lowland farm a succession of folding crops is arranged so that the lambs are continually getting a change of food right on through the late winter and spring. For example, the flock may sleep on turnip-land, and after a fresh fold has been run over in the forenoon, the sheep are moved on to winter rye, or winter barley, and back again to the roots where they finish the morning's fold and spend the night. When the turnips and swedes are finished, winter rape, winter barley, trifolium, tares, clovers, lucernes and spring rapes, etc., will be ready in succession, and carry the flock on into the summer. At the same time, changes to regular permanent pasture, which are not required for other stock, or to the early-cleared hay-fields, clover aftermath, etc., will in due course become possible, and other regular or catch crops will be available. During this period the lambs will get cake and corn regularly night and morning with one or other of the various lamb-food mixtures, the ewes requiring no hand-feeding since the lambs are no longer dependent upon them for milk. An exception to this will arise in those cases where both ewes and lambs are fattened at the same time. The ewes then generally receive concentrates up to 1 or 1.5 lb. per head per day.

A survey of the rations which are given to sheep has led Halnan and Garner to conclude that usually too little protein is fed.'

After weaning, early lambs are finished off by folding on aftermaths, rape, kale and catch crops, receiving their daily ration of cake and corn, which usually averages about 1 per cent. of their live weight, and when ready for the butcher the heavily forced lowland breeds will give lambs 5 or 6 months old weighing from 80 to 100 lb. live weight, although under the most intensive systems lambs may be ready to kill at little more than 4 months old.

For the winter fattening of lambs bought in the summer and autumn from the upland sheep farms, roots form the main ration. These hoggs feed quite well up till the middle of January when they begin to lose their central temporary incisor teeth, which are changed for the corresponding permanent teeth. When this occurs the roots require to be cut and fed in boxes or troughs lest the lambs begin to lose condition. Changes from grass or forage crops on to turnips, especially when the root ration is not restricted, need to be effected gradually, for if the change is made suddenly scouring and indigestion are almost certain to arise. Most flockmasters usually make the change by folding for only a short period in the middle of the day during the first week or so, and then gradually increasing the time till the sheep are able to sleep in the fold overnight, or they cart a limited quantity of roots on to the sheep pastures for some days previously. If wet weather occurs the sheep are moved back on to the pastures and a quantity of roots is carted there as before.

Under ordinary circumstances the amount of roots required should be calculated as about 15 per cent. to 17 per cent. of the average live weight, taking roots as containing approximately 90 per cent. of water. Along with the roots it is usual to feed hay practically *ad libitum*—the amount consumed being usually small—not much more than about 0.5 lb. per 100 lb. live weight, and the hay racks ("sheep racks") are usually kept filled, one 10 or 12 foot rack being generally enough for every 50 head. The lambs, being still in active growth while fattening, require good hay and a concentrate which has a fairly narrow nitrogenous ratio, so that undecorticated cotton cake, palm kernel cake, groundnut cake, dried brewers' grains, peas, or beans, are suitable foods to add to the concentrated ration. Cotton cake (undecorticated) and dried brewers' grains possess the further advantage that they tend to check the laxative effect of feeding on turnips in the early part of winter. Towards the end of the fattening period materials of higher energy value such as flaked maize, linseed cake, etc., are generally added to the mixture.

As an illustration of this system the following example relating to a flock of Hampshires, may be given.[8] Feeding is begun in April on a fresh ley, to be followed in turn by hop clover, winter tares, spring tares, aftermath clover and rye grass leys. By October kale is ready to carry the flock through the winter. About three weeks before lambing (which takes place in January) 1 lb. of crushed oats and a little linseed cake is given and this concentrate ration is continued for some 8-9 weeks after lambing; a certain amount of hay is also fed and mangolds are included during lambing time and for as long after as they last. The lambs are fed practically *ad libitum,* the object being to turn out the maximum number of ram lambs.

The food requirements of sheep maintained under lowland conditions in Britain were calculated on the lines of Kellner's work on cattle by the late Professor T. B. Wood. His standards have since been substantially confirmed by Woodman and others who showed that the 100 lb. sheep needs 9 lb. S.E. containing 0.38 lb. P.E. per week for maintenance. Wood's estimates of consumption capacity, however, have been shown to be too high and it is generally conceded that his figures must be reduced by about 15 per cent., so that the dry-matter appetite of the 100 lb. sheep, fed on a well-balanced diet of palatable food, is considered to be approximately 20.5 lb. per week, and to vary by about 1.3 lb. for every 10 lb. in body weight.

The revised standards of Woodman, Evans and Eden[9] are given in Table 112:

TABLE 112

Live weight lb.	Maintenance requirement (per week).		Total P.E. required per week, lb.	Production requirement per lb. live weight increase, lb. S. E.
	lb. S. E.	lb. dig. protein.		
60	6.25	0.24	1.50	1.50
70	7.00	0.28	1.50	1.50
80	7.75	0.32	1.75	1.50
90	8.25	0.35	1.75	1.75
100	9.00	0.38	1.75	2.00
110	9.50	0.42	1.75	2.25
120	10.00	0.46	1.75	2.50
130	10.50	0.50	1.75	2.75
140	11.00	0.54	1.75	3.00
150	11.50	0.58	1.75	3.50
160	12.00	0.62	1.75	3.75
170	12.50	0.66	1.75	4.00
180	13.00	0.70	1.75	4.00
190	13.50	0.74	1.75	4.00
200	14.00	0.78	1.75	4.00

There is an important body of opinion which considers that these standards are too high, but taking into consideration the very varied conditions under which sheep are bred and maintained, the higher standard is likely to prove the safer one to follow. It must be pointed out once again that these estimates are for guidance in the feeding of *flocks* of lowland sheep. The individual needs vary very greatly indeed and the feeding standards quoted may well prove to be misleading if applied to small numbers or to individuals.

The theoretical requirements of a teg of 80 lb. fattening at the rate of 2.5 lb. is 11.5 lb. S.E. containing 1.75 lb. P.E. per week and would be met by the following ration:

TABLE 113

	Amount.	Dry matter.	Starch Equivalent.	Protein Equivalent.
	lb.	lb.		
Swedes	80	9.6	5.60	0.56
Hay (Italian Rye) ...	3	2.6	1.30	0.17
Flaked Maize	3	2.6	2.52	0.24
Dried Brewers' Grains ...	1.75	1.6	0.89	0.22
Dec. groundnut cake ...	1.75	1.6	1.24	0.73
		18.0	11.6	1.9

(iii) *Flying flocks*

Since on many lowland arable farms the flying flock is of importance, taking the place of a regular breeding flock, it merits a brief mention here. A draft of good class full-mouthed (but not broken-mouthed, or otherwise unsound) ewes is bought from a regular breeding sheep farm, or through the open market, and is managed on lines similar to the ewes on an arable farm—as already described. A crop of lambs is taken from them in the usual way, but after lambing the ewes are heavily fed so that they are fat at about the same time as the lambs, or very shortly afterwards. In this way there is usually a short period of the year when there are no sheep at all on the farm, and when the newly bought-in draft ewes arrive at the end of harvest they are put on to the stubbles at once. In such cases not more than 80 or 100 ewes are kept. The system suits many lowland farms, and is a very useful adjunct to general farming.

The question of the most suitable stock for this method of sheep production has recently been reviewed.[10] On a Suffolk station the ewes are turned on to good pasture by the beginning of October, so as to be in good condition when mated from the middle of the month onwards. The system provides for most of the lambs to come in March, so that young grass or a run on wheat will stimulate milk production in the ewes and provide a little for the lambs at the age of about a month. Where the chance occurs the ewes are put on to neighbouring leys for a few weeks after tupping. As far as possible, by a system of manuring and resting of the pasture, feeding on grass is practised well into the winter and early on in the spring. Three things which are especially avoided in winter are low meadows, rough, neglected and wiry grazings and too heavy feeding on turnips. The ewes are given a run on sugar beet tops early in winter but no more roots until after lambing, at which time mangolds are fed. Hay of good quality, fed in small amounts in movable racks from Christmas onwards, serves to initiate the ewes into hay feeding, but it needs to be kept dry otherwise the ewes tend to reject it. From a month before lambing until the end of April, the provision of 0.5 lb. per head per day of a mixture of equal parts of rolled oats and cracked beans is advocated, this being given from troughs, which are kept clean and dry by turning them over after each meal.

The foregoing is no more than a very rough outline of some of the commonest methods of sheep feeding employed in Britain. Each particular locality has its own system, i.e., the system which has been found to suit it best; further, each sheep farmer must from time to time vary his methods to keep in line with changes in the season or the weather, with fluctuating market prices of foods, of fat or of store sheep, and also according to the altering conditions of general agriculture.

REFERENCES.

1. Miller, R. F., G. H. Hart & H. H. Cole, (1942). Univ. California Agric. Exp. St. Bull., No. 672.
2. Phillips, R., & Ll. Phillips, (1947). Agriculture, J. Minist. Agric., Engl., 54, 217.
3. Wallace, L. R., (1948). J. Agric. Sci., 38, 93, 243 & 367.
4. Thomas, B., J. R. Escritt & N. Trinder, (1945). Empire J. Exp. Agric., 13, 93.
5. Fraser, A., (1947). " Sheep production."
6. Boaz, T. G., T. L. Bywater & G. C. A. Robertson, (1939). Univ. Leeds & Yorks. Council for Agric. Educ. Bull., No. 210.
7. Halnan, E. T., & F. H. Garner, (1947). " The Principles and Practice of Feeding Farm Animals."
8. Private communication from Dr. W. S. Gordon, Director, Agric. Res. Council Field Station, Compton, Berkshire.
9. Woodman, H. E., R. Evans and A. Eden, (1937). J. Agric. Sci., 27, 205.
10. Steward, W. R., (1946). Agriculture, J. Minist. Agric. Engl., 53, 344.

GOATS

1. Introduction
2. General nutritional characteristics of goats
3. The feeding of goats

(1) Introduction

Although many millions of goats are kept in various parts of the world for their meat, milk, or hair, very few studies have been made of their efficiency as converters of vegetable matter into animal food suitable for human consumption. In Europe, where they have received attention as milk producers, study has been directed chiefly to volume of milk produced rather than to efficiency of production. There are many different breeds in existence, kept under very diverse conditions with respect to feeding and management, but precise information about them is meagre.

(2) General nutritional characteristics of goats

Goats are ruminants, whose general feeding habits are rather like those of sheep, but they are closer-grazing than sheep and will contrive to find nourishment in circumstances where even the latter would not.

Although comparatively few digestibility trials have been made with goats, such data as are available suggest that there is little difference between goats and sheep. The following table has been compiled from the data of Schneider[1]:

TABLE 114

Species	Foodstuff	Organic matter	Digestibility coefficients (%)			
			Protein	Fibre	N. Free Ext.	Ether Ext.
Sheep	Lucerne hay ...	61	72	45	69	31
Goats	Lucerne hay ...	59	74	41	69	19
Sheep	Clover hay (red) ...	56	67	45	61	47
Goats	Clover hay (red) ...	59	68	44	66	39
Sheep	Grass, mixed ...	71	74	69	71	60
Goats	Grass, mixed ...	73	70	66	79	64
Sheep	Hay, meadow ...	63	60	62	64	52
Goats	Hay, meadow ...	60	53	62	60	52
Sheep	Maize	94	78	30	99	87
Goats	Maize	91	67	—	94	80
Sheep	Cottonseed meal ...	90	82	—	95	97
Goats	Cottonseed meal ...	80	91	41	63	92
Sheep	Soya-bean meal ...	94	94	101	96	52
Goats	Soya-bean meal ...	91	91	101	89	47

Table 114—*continued.*

Species	Foodstuff	Organic matter	Digestibility coefficients (%)			
			Protein	Fibre	N. Free Ext.	Ether Ext.
Goats	Beet pulp, dried ...	72	34	63	79	72
„	Maize meal	81	46	44	89	84
„	Potato peelings ...	81	40	14	93	39
„	Soya silage ... :..	64	79	55	52	72
„	Vetch, mixed, pre-bloom, fed green	71	74	68	73	57

The lack of experimental investigation of the food requirements of goats is shown by the fact that Schneider gives less than 40 foods for which digestibility data have determined for this species, as compared with about 1,500 for sheep. For this reason alone it will be easy to understand that there is very little knowledge of the precise food requirements of goats.

Although one group of workers[2] reported that the basal metabolic rate of goats was appreciably lower than that of sheep of a corresponding size, the data accumulated by Brody[3] for different species of a great range of bodyweights suggest that, pending the acquisition of fresh data, the feeding standards to be adopted for goats may be taken as being the same as for sheep. This, of course, applies only to mature animals.

The same kinds of foods may be fed as to sheep. In particular goats make good use of coarse foods, but this does not mean that food which is unsuitable for sheep may be fed profitably to goats, for there are no indications that goats differ from other ruminants in their needs for protein for growth, or for vitamin A or other factors which are needed by cattle and sheep.

Some figures have been provided by Plimpton[4] for the weights of goats at birth and at various ages almost up to maturity; they are reproduced in Table 115.

TABLE 115

Age (mth.)	Birth	1	2	4	6	12	18	21
Wt. (lb.) ... ... :..	8	21	32	57	73	108	136	144

(3) The feeding of goats

The kids are usually allowed to suckle their dams up to the age of 3 to 4 months, or even a little longer, weaning on to solid foods, such as hay and mixed concentrates, taking place gradually. In some cases the goat milk may be needed, when the question of the curtailment of the supply for the kid and its substitution by other foods then arises. Because they are so similar in composition, cow's milk may be substituted for that of the goat with little apparent harm, provided that the substitute milk is sound and clean, is fed at the right temperature and is given regularly—initially about 1 lb. of milk for each of three daily feeds has been suggested.[5] After the age of 6 weeks or so, whole milk may be gradually replaced by skim milk if the loss of the fat is made good by the feeding of suitable concentrates. The procedure is similar to that concerning the calf; it must not be forgotten that the removal of fat from milk also means the loss of vitamins A and D, a loss of which should be made good by the feeding of a teaspoonful of cod liver oil.

As in the case of calves, good legume hay should be provided for the kids at an early age. The kind of concentrate mixture to be provided will be that which is suitable for lambs, e.g., crushed oats or maize, wheat bran, linseed or groundnut meals, together with dried grass, bean-meal, etc. In the early stages of growth the protein content of the mixture should be about 20 per cent. It has been suggested that the amount to be fed should be about as much as the kids will clean up at each feed, when they are fed twice daily. Small amounts (2—3 per cent.) of bone meal and of animal protein may be included in the rations of the youngest animals. Later the needs for calcium and phosphorus, and for protein will diminish (Ch. 17 [3]).

So far as the adult animals are concerned they may be left to browse such vegetation as is available at the particular season, but, although goats are efficient utilizers of coarse grazing, the latter will need to be supplemented at times. Good quality hay, or silage, or roots, or dried grass, may be used, and there is no reason why crops such as kale should not be utilized. In spring and summer the goats will normally find their nutritional requirements supplied by grazing, but in autumn and winter the replacements suggested will be needed. About 4 lb. of hay or its equivalent, plus 0.25 to 0.5 lb. of a concentrate mixture such as will be provided by crushed oats (2 parts), bran (1 part) and cracked beans (1 part), or even simple linseed, groundnut- or cottonseed-cake meals, will meet the normal needs of the adult animal. In the absence of feeding standards the quantities of food to be given and its nature must depend on the condition of the individual beast and on the general principles which have been outlined in Section III.

Although there are many parts of the world where the milk yield of the milk-goat is very small, there is no doubt that with suitable feeding and attention, the animal is a good milk producer. In studies made on milk goats of the ages 2, 3 and 4 years respectively, Knowles and Watkin showed that the milk yield rose from 2,200 lb. to 2,850 lb. for a 300 day lactation, the fat content of the milk remaining at about 4.4 per cent.[6] While the average milk-goat will produce more milk in proportion to her body-weight than will a cow, the maintenance energy requirements of the smaller animal are proportionately higher, so that the efficiency of milk production, as measured by milk energy produced per pound of total digestible nutrients consumed, is about the same in both cases (about 35 per cent. on an energy basis).[7] Goat milk is very similar in composition to that of the cow and feeding for production may be on the same basis. In summer, with good pasturage, there may be little need for the feeding of any appreciable amounts of concentrates, but as the pasturage deteriorates and also in winter, supplementary foods will need to be given. About 4 lb. of such a concentrate mixture as is suitable for dairy cows (Ch. 20) may be given for each gallon of milk produced. A suitable ration for the winter feeding of a milk goat is given in Table 116.

TABLE 116

	lb./day
Good legume hay, or dried grass	2
Roots or silage	1–2
Concentrate mixture, such as:	
(a) Maize, 8 parts; oats, 8; bran, 2; linseed meal, 1; or	
(b) Oats, 3; bran, 2; linseed meal, 2; cracked beans, 1	
depending on the milk yield	2–6

Of the concentrate mixtures given above (a) would be best used in conjunction with good silage and (b) when roots were being fed. Production ration (a) is not good enough without the basal ration being satisfactory in protein content; it would be improved by the inclusion of more linseed meal or groundnut meal.

REFERENCES

1. Schneider, B.H., (1947). "Feeds of the world; their digestibility and composition."
2. Ritzman, E. G., E. L. Washburn, and F. G. Benedict, (1936). New Hampshire Agr. Exp. Sta. Tech. Bul. 66.
3. Brody, S., (1945). "Bioenergetics and growth."
4. Plimpton, A. A., (1941). Animal Breeding Abs., 9, 30.
5. Spencer, D. A., (1939). U.S. Dept. Agric. Yearbook, 758.
6. Knowles, F., and J. E. Watkin, (1938). J. Dairy Res., 9, 153.
7. Brody, S., (1939). J. Nutrition, 17, 235.

THE FEEDING OF HORSES

(1) Introduction.
(2) Management in relation to nutrition.
    (a) General.
    (b) Watering.
    (c) Choice of foods.
    (d) Horses at pasture.
(3) Feeding standards and their application.
    (a) Introduction.
    (b) Feeding for maintenance.
    (c) Feeding for production.

(1) Introduction

Though the horse is a herbivorous animal, it differs very much from the ruminants in the anatomy of its digestive system and in the mechanisms of the digestion and absorption of food. In the adult horse mastication is usually relatively slow and very thorough. The masticated food passes into a simple type of stomach, quite unlike the complicated system of the mature ruminant, where food is acted upon by acid secretions. Food tends to be retained in the stomach for a rather long period after feeding, but during feeding it passes through the stomach both rapidly and in the order in which the foodstuffs have been ingested.[1] Whilst active feeding is going on, the organ remains about two thirds full.

The absence of a rumen and of that enormous microbial population, which is found therein in the ruminant, means that the horse is unable to utilize bacteria to assist in the breaking down of foods *before* the food passes on to what is, in mammals, the main site of absorption, namely, the small intestine. From this point of view the horse would seem to be less well fitted for dealing with fibrous foods than cattle and sheep, and this has been experimentally confirmed by digestion trials with various foodstuffs, as described elsewhere in this book (p. 15).

The horse, however, has a very large cæcum, which can retain food for some twenty-four hours. Here there is certainly a very large bacterial population, which may assist in the breakdown of some cellulose in the food and synthesize some of the water-soluble vitamins, but what chances there are for the absorption of the latter products is not fully known. Recent work tends to confirm what the general behaviour of horses under different systems has suggested, namely, that the horse may not be as fully independent of dietary sources of members of the vitamin B complex as is the ruminant: this is a matter of some practical importance.

The needs of foals, during the suckling period and in the following rapid phase of early growth, do not differ materially in any fundamental way from those of the young of other species; ample supplies of good quality protein, with sufficient mineral and vitamins, are needed, together with a total energy supply sufficient for the size and condition of the animal. Likewise, the last third of the gestation period is one when mares should receive an abundant amount of those same nutrients. Because of the relatively simple digestive system, even when the animal is beyond the suckling stage, too high a proportion of fibre must not occur in the rations of horses.

In Europe and America the ruminant species are used primarily for producing meat, milk or wool: in each case the product demands good attention to the protein supply of the ration. Horses, however, except in the cases of breeding establishments, are used for work, and there is no experimental evidence to suggest that the performance of muscular work requires any appreciable amount of protein. Although some of the products of protein breakdown can be used for work, carbohydrate is a cheaper and more efficient source of the necessary glucose. The additional food necessary for productive purposes in working horses is therefore of the carbohydrate type. To feed pure carbohydrates would not only be expensive but it would bring in a host of complications from the point of view of practical feeding; and so, as stated above, the carbonaceous foods, which contain a certain amount of protein along with their predominance of carbohydrate, are the ones for work. The coarser foods, which might otherwise provide carbohydrate, are rather bulky for the digestive system of the horse and they have to give place more and more to cereal grains as more or harder work is required from the animal. This, however, means that the ration given to the horse tends to deviate in type more and more from the natural food of the species, which is herbage. Digestive upsets in hard-working horses therefore tend to be rather common. Under natural conditions the horse derives from herbage, not only such protein as it needs, but sufficient carbohydrate, carotene and—perhaps aided by the bacterial population of its own digestive tract—enough of the members of the vitamin B complex. The breakdown of carbohydrate in the body for the purposes of providing energy involves enzyme systems with which several members of the vitamin B family are directly concerned. Recent evidence [2] points to the dependence of the horse upon its food for some of its intake of these vitamins. It may be perhaps that severe work and the rapid production of muscular energy, increase substantially the need for aneurin, etc. If that is so, then the beneficial effects of bran, given *with* cereal foods, receive a rational explanation. Furthermore, the improvement in condition, which has been reported to follow the inclusion of small amounts of dried yeast in rations, has a similar basis.

On the whole town horses are probably poorly fed. Their fertility is low [3] and their liver reserves of vitamin A seem to be inadequate, so far as the few analyses reveal (Ch. 6). Horses in towns are often given very poor hay, high in fibre and low in protein and carotene, with little green food. Oats provide ample carbohydrate but they contain no carotene.

Bran is better used by its daily inclusion in the ration than by being given in one or two large bran mashes at the week-end. Country horses, which usually have some grazing available to them regularly, are probably much better off. The foods which are of particular application to horses are dealt with in a subsequent paragraph.

Rations should be balanced for the particular purpose they are intended to serve and, so far as horses especially are concerned, one should not be content merely to satisfy the energy and protein requirements which their condition and the nature of their work suggest. An attempt should be made to see that the ration is complete in all possible respects, which is most unlikely to be the case if the range of foods is very small and the ration is seldom or never varied.

Finally, it should be made clear that the use of starch equivalents for the feeding of horses is not so simple a matter as in the case of cattle and sheep. It will be remembered that the starch equivalents of the various foods were measured for cattle, and, although there may not be much difference between the two species with regard to their use of concentrates, it is still true that the horse is much less capable than the cow of handling the very fibrous foods. This reservation applies with some force to the coarser straws, from which cattle may derive some little nourishment but which will be a liability to the horse.

(2) Management in relation to nutrition

(a) General.

In any stud it should be the duty of some responsible individual to assess the general condition and fitness for work of each horse, to see that the food purchased and the rations fed are of the right kind and quality, and to modify the feeding standards to suit the requirements of the various horses.

All horses should be watered and fed an hour and a half before the first horse is due to leave the stable for the commencement of the day's work: it is most important that this feeding time is not shortened, for no horse should be called upon to start a heavy day's work after a hurried morning meal. If the animals are out all day each carter should be given a supply of thoroughly mixed feed, chopped hay and grain, sufficient to satisfy the requirements of his horse during the day. Horses when away from the stable all day should be fed from the nose-bag at regular intervals and time must be found for this purpose, for, unlike the ruminant, the horse requires feeding on the principle of little and often. An almost unfailing cause of intestinal trouble among horses is the practice, now fortunately becoming less common, of working horses for many hours without food and then expecting them to digest and assimilate a big feed when they return home in the evening in an exhausted condition.

As with other species, sound feeding practice and careful hygiene should go together; food utensils must be scrupulously clean.

Purchased, ready prepared " chop " may or may not be good, depending on the quality of the ingredients which have been used. Under a

recent order (Feeding Stuffs [Regulation of Manufacture] Order, 1947),
definite limits are set for the proportions of concentrates, cereal
by-products, chopped hay and chopped straw in the " National " preparations (See Appendix 2). It is a matter for the purchaser to see that such
a product is fresh and of good quality; the surest way, of course, is for
him to prepare his own product from good quality ingredients, making it
in fairly small batches so that the crushed concentrates have no chance to
deteriorate.

(b) Watering.

Horses should be watered as often as possible so as to make certain
that they get what they need; they should not be kept short of water for
a prolonged period and then be allowed to drink very large quantities at
a time. All horses not supplied with a constant supply in a water pot at
the head of their stalls should be given the opportunity to drink the last
thing at night, particularly during the summer months. When a horse
returns home very hot and thirsty he should be allowed to drink a
moderate quantity of cold water. When the first pressing thirst has been
quenched more water may be offered.

As to the much debated question whether horses should be watered
before, during or after feeding, the rational and most satisfactory method
is to let them have water whenever they want it, in which case they will
not need to take very large quantities at a time. It is generally supposed
that if a horse is allowed to drink immediately after feeding, the water
entering the full stomach washes the food out and carries it away to the
large bowel undigested. From experiments carried out by the author it
was found that when the stomach was full, a large drink of water did not
mix with the stomach contents at all but passed directly out along the
lesser curvature of the stomach leaving the stomach contents intact. On
the other hand, if only a small feed was given and then the horse was
allowed to drink a large quantity of water, it did mix with the food and
carried a small amount into the small intestine. Other tests have shown
that, provided that the animal has become used to the system, watering
may be done before, after or during a meal without interfering with the
digestion or absorption of the food eaten.[45]

A horse returning home tired and thirsty will not eat his food well
until he has had a drink and one which has eaten a lot of dry food often
feels thirsty and therefore should be allowed a drink if he wants one.
Nevertheless, as stressed many times in this book, feeding and watering
routines should be regular; where changes have to be made they must be
as gradual as possible. Where an animal has been used to one particular
system, such as watering before meals, a sudden change to watering after
feeding may produce a digestive upset, although this is usually temporary.
If horses are given water liberally and often, however, it has never been
proved that watering after feeding does any harm, and where digestive
disturbances do follow, then the system of management as a whole should

be investigated; dried sugar beet pulp, for example, needs to be moistened before it is fed, otherwise it may swell in the stomach.

(c) Choice of foods.

With certain exceptions, foods that are generally suitable for other grass-feeding animals are suitable for the horse, provided that the diet is balanced so as to supply the proper amounts of energy, protein, fat, starchy foods, dry matter and minerals. The foods must also be palatable and of such physical character that it is possible for the horse to eat them without difficulty.

The cereal grains.

There is a belief common in some quarters that oats are the only suitable cereal grain for horses, but it is quite a mistake to imagine that even the bulk of the concentrate allowance must necessarily consist of oats, for, provided that the mixture is balanced, many combinations of concentrates may be used in their place. However, if the price of oats compares favourably with that of other foods they may with advantage form the greater part of the diet. The quantity given naturally depends upon the work the animal does; half a bushel, about 20 lb., is a common daily allowance for hunters in work.

Other ripe grains may be used to replace oats, provided that one bears in mind the variations between them in starch equivalent, in fibre, mineral and vitamin contents, and in the nature and amounts of protein they contain. It is the nature of the final, complete ration which is important, not so much the characteristics of a single constituent. If a ration is so dominated by one foodstuff that one is afraid to change it, then it is probably a poor dietary. Though oats have come to be regarded as the " natural " food for horses in Britain, other grains are used in other lands throughout the world.

Where the ration for a horse consists almost entirely of oats and hay, the question of the replacement of one cereal by another may become important, but so unvaried a diet has little to commend it from the nutritional point of view. In the case of such simple rations, then, on an energy basis, approximately 0.8 lb. of cracked, dent maize, or slightly larger amounts of crushed barley or crushed wheat, may replace 1 lb. of oats. Because, however, of the differing physical consistencies of the various cereals in the mouth or in the gut, some fibrous foods need to be mixed with wheat and maize, or else digestive disturbances may follow: barley, with its 5 per cent. of fibre, is less troublesome. It is usually recommended, in such rations, that the intakes of maize, barley, or wheat, should be limited to about 10 lb. per day. The inclusion of bran with these foods will improve the physical and nutritional qualities of the ration.

Cereal by-products.

For physical reasons medium or broad bran is the most suitable of the wheat offals to feed to horses. It should be used less for the replacement of oats or other grain in a ration than for the supplementing of the cereals. When it is given dry, mixed with other concentrates, its physical properties are useful in opening up the starchy masses and it helps to prevent the bolting of food. It is a most useful food to give with cereal concentrates. Its laxative action may well be as much associated with its mineral or vitamin contents as with its fibrous nature.

Protein concentrates.

Some of the samples of hay which are fed to horses are found on analysis to be little better than straw; they are very high in fibre and low in protein. It is possible, therefore, that horses which are given rations consisting of poor hay and oats may receive insufficient protein. Beans, preferably of the species Faba, about a year old, and cracked or coarsely ground, may be used with some advantage to replace 1 or 2 lb. of oats in a ration. Peas, split or coarsely ground, gram, or even small amounts of soyabean, similarly treated, can be used.

Oil-seed cakes, used with the same discretion and fed to provide the comparatively small amount of protein which is needed in the ration, are very useful foods. Linseed, decorticated groundnut or cottonseed, palm kernel or other cakes, broken and mixed well in a ration, are all of value when used in amounts of 0.5 to 1 lb./day, depending on their protein contents.

Compound horse foods are also available. The "National Horse Foods" (see Appendix 2) must contain between 3 and 5 per cent. of oil, 13-16 per cent. of protein and not more than 10 per cent. of fibre. Maximum and minimum limits are fixed for the various constituents.

Succulent foods.

Apart from such animals as have regular access to pasture, succulent foods are probably insufficiently used for horses. A ration consisting of poor hay and oats is likely to be deficient in a number of factors, for example carotene, besides being comparatively unpalatable.

Horses welcome an occasional allowance of succulent foods. Of roots, carrots, mangolds, swedes and turnips (up to 20-30 lb./day) are most commonly used, and carrots supply the vitamin A precursor, carotene. For stabled horses, grass or other green fodder should always be supplied as soon as it is available. Clover and vetches may also be given and are particularly valuable owing to the amount of calcium they contain, but they require to be fed with greater care than is the case with grass owing to their liability to ferment in the stomach. All green foods of this class should be fresh.

Conserved crops.

Good quality hay is needed for horses: too often one sees a product which is stemmy, coarse and fibrous. Like any other food to be used for livestock it should be sound, and not dusty or mouldy. Though the legume hays tend to be rejected in Britain for horse feeding because their leafiness is liable to make them dusty, lucerne hay, for example, is widely used in America and with good results. Such a variety of hays has been fed with success that one may say that most failures with particular kinds are either due to the use of poor quality material or to bad management. The chopping of hay is a matter concerned more especially with the prevention of the bolting of the grain with which it is fed, than with economy of utilisation, for tests have shown [6] that the saving achieved does not amount to 10 per cent. of the grain ration. Dustiness in hay, where it is certain that it is not due to the action of moulds, may be countered by slightly damping it at the time it is fed; surplus damped material should not be saved.

Silage is a good food for horses if it is of good quality and is carefully fed. Watson [7] quotes examples of its use in many parts of the world. It requires gradual introduction into the ration, as with many other foods, and extreme care must be taken to see that it is not mouldy or decomposed. Both oat-and-vetch silage in this country and maize silage in the United States have been fed in amounts up to some 14 lb./day. Silage is thus a supplement to the ration and not a replacement for hay.

The use of good quality dried grass for horses is also to be recommended. A relatively small quantity would improve the usual ration of the town horse quite considerably and even country horses might benefit from its use during the winter scarcity of fresh green foods or silage. Dried grass for this purpose should preferably be the long type, and certainly not the finely divided, rather dusty material. Miller and Muir [8] have suggested its considerable use to replace hay and oats in the conventional rations.

Dried sugar beet pulp.

This foodstuff is being given increasingly to working horses. Its virtues are that it contains a high proportion of soluble carbohydrate, with some 7 per cent. of digestible protein; on the other hand it must be remembered that the factory extraction process has removed water soluble carbohydrates, vitamins and salts. Its deficiencies in this respect should be offset by the feeding of suitable green foods, either fresh or conserved. Lastly, because of its pronounced swelling power after water absorption, it should be well soaked before it is fed.

(d) Horses at pasture.

Horses turned out to pasture usually derive much benefit from the change; the improvement in town horses is often such as to constitute an indictment of their normal feeding regime. For this species the grazing should be good, the sward not too hard and the pasture must not be too heavily stocked with horses year after year, otherwise parasitic infestation may be serious. During the greater part of the year horses on average pasture will not only maintain condition but put on weight, but as the year advances and the grass begins to decline in quality a supplement must be given. For this purpose good hay and possibly concentrates are necessary. As with milch cows, it is very important to supply this supplement before there is any loss of condition rather than when the loss has become obvious.

When working horses are turned out to graze during the summer nights some additional food is required beyond the amount of grass the animals would graze. Such food is best supplied in the form of oats mixed with a little cut hay and given in the morning before work and again at mid-day. No hard and fast rule can be laid down as to the amount necessary, as this depends upon the condition of the pasture and the nature of the work done by the horse. Farm horses which are at grass during the summer should be brought into good hard condition before harvest operations begin, and it is therefore a mistake to restrict the corn allowance too much during the period of comparative slackness preceding harvest.

(3) Feeding standards and their application

(a) Introduction.

In the formulation of the production ration for a dairy cow one may assess, with reasonable accuracy, the quantities of nutrients needed to yield one gallon of milk of known composition. The chief " product " of horses, however, is work, and, though their needs for energy for maintenance may be gauged fairly well, the problem of feeding standards for work is a very different matter.

On farm land the nature of the soil differs from field to field and from day to day. The soil may be stiff and heavy, or light and friable; it may be wet or dry. The gradient and therefore the pull exerted by a horse for a given load differs from field to field and in different parts of the same field. Weather conditions, the character of the road surface, the speed at which the work is done and the nature of the animal itself all have an effect on the total energy expended by a horse in a day. Furthermore, one man doing the same work will tire a horse much more easily than will a more careful driver.

Although in any particular case it might be possible, using proper scientific equipment, to measure in calories the energy expenditure associated with the given task, the results would be only of very general value, for the conditions under which work is done and the nature of the work itself vary so considerably that the energy required for the performance of the work is equally variable. One uses the suggested feeding standards simply as guides and, as in the case of other species, modifies them to suit the particular individual. The feeding standards themselves have been framed, partly on the basis of limited experimental work [*] and partly as the result of long experience of the practical feeding of horses under a variety of conditions.

(b) Feeding for maintenance.

The nutritional requirements for the maintenance of a horse have been studied by many workers interested in animal nutrition and various estimates have been made as to the minimum amount of food required.

Linton has suggested [10] that a total of 13,000 kilo-calories of metabolisable energy would meet the demands of a 1,000 lb. horse, i.e., a horse kept under average conditions, provided that the rations yielding this energy contain sufficient protein and a proper amount of bulk. This quantity of metabolisable energy would be obtained from about 5 lb. of starch equivalent, that is, from 16 lb. of average meadow hay, which is about as much as an idle light draught horse would eat in a day. It would contain about 0.72 lb. of protein equivalent and 13.75 lb., or slightly less than 1.5 per cent. of the animal's live weight, of dry matter.

One may suggest, then, that the maintenance requirements of a 1,000 lb. horse are 5 lb. starch equivalent containing 0.5 lb. protein equivalent, while calculations based on Rubner's Surface Law indicate that requirements of horses of other weights can be met approximately by an addition or subtraction of 0.3 lb. starch equivalent, containing 0.05 lb. protein equivalent, for each 100 lb. body weight difference. Thus the requirements for a horse weighing 1,400 lb. are 6.2 starch equivalent, 0.7 protein equivalent. Assuming the meadow hay to have a S.E. value of 31 and a P.E. of 4.5 per cent., 16 lb. of this hay will provide 4.96 lb. S.E. and 0.72 lb. P.E.

This estimate of the maintenance requirements of horses is sufficiently accurate for all practical purposes, and forms a useful basis on which to build rations for work.

During periods of idleness the rational and commonsense method of feeding horses is to restrict the diets to little more than maintenance requirements. It is an error to imagine that because a horse is idle the time is opportune to fatten him up and improve his condition. If a horse is in poor condition (provided that he is not diseased) it may be taken for granted that either he has been overworked or has been under or badly fed, for a healthy horse can be maintained in good condition even during long periods of reasonably strenuous work. If for any reason a horse has to cease work suddenly owing to lameness, advent of hard frosts, etc., his allowance of concentrates should immediately be cut down and for the first day or two laxative foods should be given. As will be seen later, the total energy needs of a 1,500 lb. horse doing 6 hours of hard work daily will be about equal to that provided by 15.5 lb. of starch equivalent. Of this 9 lb. is being fed for the work done. Since concentrates have more than twice the energy value of hay, the reduction in the ration of the horse must come largely from the concentrates. Where the horse is working for only half a day on Saturday, there should be a proportionate reduction of the allowance, while the food for the idle day on Sunday should be reduced to about maintenance needs and should consist mainly of good hay with some bran but very little in the way of concentrates.

The emphasis which is put on the feeding of hunters, as distinct from draught horses, is more an indictment of the poor average feeding of the latter class than an expression of new and fundamentally different physiological processes brought into operation by the periodically severe exercise of the former. In the case of working horses, the daily routine may be roughly the same for long periods, so that the food intake may not require much adjustment in quantity, whereas the much more variable programme of the hunter demands a close observation of the physical condition of the animal from day to day and a dietary based on such observation. It is not within the province of this book to survey the general physiological problems involved in the performance of muscular work and those who require further information will find Brody's summary* a useful one; nevertheless, one or two points of broad application may be touched upon. There is evidence to show that the percentage of energy obtained as actual muscular work from the breakdown of the sources (glycogen, glucose, etc.) used for the contraction of muscle, falls off rapidly at high speeds of movement, although at walking speeds the fall may not be readily apparent. The needs of a fast moving horse may thus be out of all proportion to the load (its own weight) involved: there is evidence in the case of both horses and men which suggests that for a peak effort of muscular exertion, the energy expenditure may be something like a hundred times the basal metabolic rate, as compared with about twice basal metabolism for simple maintenance. Performance at such a level implies highly efficient blood supply, pulmonary ventilation, etc., in addition to the provision of adequate nutrients. For the effective performance of muscular work at such high rates, the ready availability of the various enzymes and co-enzymes—involving members of the vitamin B complex, for example— would seem to be essential. The fact that the horse is unable to do without some dietary source of such trace factors probably means that greater care needs to be taken to ensure their presence in the diet of the animal working at a high rate, even though the total amount of work done may be less than in the case of the slower moving one. There are many problems in this field which have as yet no answer.

(c) Feeding for production.

(i) *Pregnancy*

In regard to breeding mares it should be remembered that if a mare is working while pregnant the food that formerly supplied her needs may not be adequate as the foetus grows, either in quantity or quality. Judging from the large number of " washy " foals that are born there is room for improvement on many farms in this respect. The needs for a pregnant mare are, as for other pregnant animals, for sufficient energy, protein, calcium, phosphorus and vitamins, particularly in the last phase of pregnancy. The leguminous green crops, such as tares, lucerne, clover, etc., should be given if available before foaling; if the foals are born early, e.g., in March or April, naturally these crops are hardly ready in the majority of districts. Calcium phosphate may be conveniently supplied by including in the diet approximately 0.25 lb. of sterilised meat-and-bone meal, steamed bone flour or fish meal, which should be given throughout the whole period of pregnancy. The diet of in-foal mares should not be too bulky, so that the straws should be excluded from the diet. The food should not be too fattening, i.e., it must not contain a marked preponderance of starchy foods but must contain sufficient protein to allow for the proper growth of the fœtus. Good hay, and a balanced, cereal grain-protein concentrate mixture, such as is used for cattle, together with a supply of one of the above-mentioned mineral-rich commodities, with green food in season will supply all that is necessary. Though maize and cereal by-products such as bran are given to brood mares by breeders, in large proportions they are not ideal foods for breeding stock owing to their fattening nature and unbalanced mineral composition. The object to be aimed at in feeding breeding mares is to keep them in good condition, neither too fat nor too lean, and to see that they get sufficient exercise to keep them healthy. At the time of foaling, and for two or three days after foaling, rich food should be withheld and during this period the diet should consist of light, slightly laxative foods, good hay, and an unstinted amount of clean fresh water.

(ii) *Lactation and growth*

After parturition the mare should be fed generously, but not lavishly, particular attention being paid to the protein, mineral and vitamin fractions of the diet. Milk yields are seldom measured so that success depends entirely upon adherence to the principles laid down in Chap. 17(5) and upon observation of the condition of mare and foal.

Foals are weaned at from 4 to 6 months of age, depending upon the need of the farmer to work the mare, but for as long as possible the mare should be left with her foal and kept from work; in any case she should be given at least one month's rest with the foal, and weaning should not be done until the foal is at least 4 months old. The mare should never be kept away for longer than three hours during the period she is suckling, and should be given nothing more than light work. If by mischance she returns from work hot and excited she should be allowed to cool off before being taken to the foal, and the udder should be partly milked out, because milk kept under pressure in the udder is not normal. The udder should be wiped over with a clean cloth and warm water. Initially, weather permitting, both mare and foal should be kept at grass during the day, and later it is better to leave them out altogether, but some shelter should be provided in the field. The foal will begin to nibble at dry food when about a month old. After weaning, provided that it has been well nourished and the pasture is good, no other food will be necessary than good grass. If, however, the foal has been badly nourished by the mare, or if it is desired to bring the foal into good condition early or if the pasturage is poor, then some concentrated food must be allowed. As a first food the following mixture has proved very successful: oatmeal 3 parts, maize meal 1 part, linseed cake meal 1 part, and white fish meal or meat and bone meal 0.5 part, the exact quantity depending on the foal's condition, bearing in mind the great potentialities for growth of young stock. Separated cow's milk, provided that it has been pasteurised to kill tubercle bacilli, is a valuable source of protein and may be given in almost unlimited quantities. During the winter, when no pasture is available, the foal should be well fed with first quality hay and suitable concentrates so as to provide sufficient energy and protein: every effort should be made to include a daily portion of fresh green food. A very common mistake is to undernourish yearlings and two-year-olds at this critical stage of life by giving them large quantities of inferior fibrous roughages supplemented with roots. A mixture of freshly crushed oats 4 parts, bran 2 parts, linseed meal or good quality compound cake meal 0.5 part, with chaffed meadow or clover hay and an addition of from 5 to 10 per cent. of fish meal will give good results. The quantity to be allowed depends upon the size of the animal—from 4 to 6 lb. of concentrates a day will be suitable for the average yearling. Pulped roots may also be given mixed with the concentrates and chaff and a suitable quantity of bean meal, lentil meal, maize gluten feed or other nitrogenous food of this nature may be sprinkled over the roots. The animal should be fed twice daily, allowed access to an unlimited amount of clean fresh water and have good quality hay within reach.

The hand-rearing of the foal that has lost its mother at or soon after birth has always been a difficult problem. The easiest, and certainly the most satisfactory, method is to obtain a foster mother and induce her to suckle the foal. In artificial feeding the main difficulty is to obtain a food similar to mare's milk, and even though the chemical nature of the food may simulate in close degree the milk it is desired to copy, yet the biological value of the natural and artificial products may be considerably different. This is probably the explanation of the many failures that follow attempts to rear foals on cow's milk, which usually forms the basis of the orphaned foal's food. Cow's milk differs from mare's milk in that it contains more total solids, more protein (casein and albumin), more ash and less sugar, (Chap. 17).

To make cow's milk* approximate to that of the mare as nearly as possible water must be added to dilute it and sugar (preferably lactose) added to make good the deficiency of carbohydrate. Owing to the fact that the casein of cow's milk curdles or clots in the stomach in large lumps whereas the casein of mare's milk after clotting is of a more flocculent nature, lime water is added to prevent the formation of large clots. Morrison[11] gives the following instruction for rearing foals:— "Choose milk from a cow in the first part of the lactation period and one giving milk low in fat, if possible. Put 4 tablespoonfuls of lime water and 2 teaspoonfuls of ordinary cane sugar in a pint jar and then fill it with fresh milk. Feed about one-fourth pint about every hour for the first day or so, warming the milk to 100°F. and using an ordinary nursing bottle with a large nipple. This must be carefully cleansed and sterilised.

"If the foal is doing well, the amount of milk may be gradually increased and the period between feedings lengthened, until the animal is fed only 4 times a day. After a few days unmodified whole milk may be substituted and the foal taught to drink from a pail. In 5 to 6 weeks sweet skim milk may gradually replace the whole milk and after 3 months the foal may be given all it will drink 3 times a day. As soon as possible, the foal should be fed solid food, such as crushed or ground oats, bran, a little linseed meal, and legume hay, and it should have the run of a paddock where there is good grazing."

Because artificially reared foals are usually kept indoors during their earliest life, the mixture should be improved by the inclusion of some high grade cod liver oil, about one half-teaspoonful to the pint. This, however, must be done with caution for, as has been pointed out,[12] foals do not thrive on milk rich in fat. Lactose is the best kind of sugar to add to the milk; failing this, glucose is the next most suitable. The feeding must be done with meticulous regularity, the temperature of the milk must always be at blood heat, and the utensils must be kept scrupulously clean. The foal should be encouraged to nibble at concentrates as soon as it shows any inclination to do so. It is perhaps not generally recognised what a large amount of milk a mare can secrete; for example, a Clydesdale mare, when milked by hand for the purpose of hand-rearing a foal (owing to the dam's fractious nature), yielded as much as 5 gallons daily.

(iii) *Work*.

Of the many standards suggested for work requirements the following is probably as simple and as satisfactory as any: for every hour of hard work allow 1 lb. of starch equivalent and 0.15 lb. of protein equivalent per 1,000 lb. live weight. Thus if a horse weighing 1,400 lb. is doing 6 hours hard work a day he requires, in addition to maintenance food, 8.4 lb. starch equivalent and 1.26 lb. protein equivalent.

* Heated to destroy tubercle bacilli.

The total food requirement for the day for this horse is therefore:

TABLE 117

	Starch Equivalent	Protein Equivalent
	lb.	lb.
For Maintenance	6.2	0.70
For Work	8.4	1.26
	14.6	2.0

In recommending this standard, " per hour of work " is intended to mean actual work performed.

Much confusion exists regarding the interpretation of the terms light, medium and hard work. It is almost impossible to define the terms satisfactorily and the best method is to feed in the manner suggested in the following pages, increasing the amount of food fed if the horse fails to maintain condition or decreasing it where the animal shows signs of becoming fat. No two horses will perform the same amount of work with an equal expenditure of energy and no two horsemen will get the same amount of work out of the same horse.

From the general point of view the question of " bulk " has been dealt with already and it remains to re-emphasise its importance in the feeding of hard-working horses. One has to reconcile the need for concentrates, which heavy work entails, with the limited capacity of the digestive system of the horse and with the animal's requirements for a certain amount of fibre in the ration to facilitate the processes of digestion. For each particular animal there is an optimum capacity for food and, within reasonable limits, a favourable proportion of fibre in the ration. To require the animal to work more severely than the above conditions will allow must entail either the usage of body substance, with loss of condition, or digestive upsets, or both. The working horse is compelled to combine, to a greater or lesser degree, muscular work with the work of digestion, whereas in Europe and the United States at least, other species of livestock have time to rest following the ingestion of food.

One is not likely to go far wrong if the diet of working horses is so constructed that the total dry matter in it ranges from 1.5 to 2 per cent. of the animal's live weight and for idle horses from 1 to 1.25 per cent. of the live weight. Balancing the ration so that it contains just enough dry matter and no more than is necessary is one of the most important details in the dieting of horses. For example, a stud of heavy trotting vanners requires for maintenance and work, starch equivalent and protein equivalent as follows:

TABLE 118

	Starch Equivalent	Protein Equivalent
	lb.	lb.
Requirements for Maintenance ...	6.5	0.75
Requirements for Work	9.0	1.35
Total	15.5	2.1

The total dry matter in the diet should be approximately 1.75 per cent. of the live weight; assuming the average live weight of the horses in the stud to be 1,500 lb., then the total dry matter should be about 27 lb. A diet in accordance with these requirements may be constructed as follows, making use of meadow hay, oats, maize and beans:

TABLE 119

Food		Protein Equivalent	Starch Equivalent	Dry Matter
	lb.	lb.	lb.	lb.
Hay (meadow) ...	16	4.96	0.72	13.76
Oats	10	6.10	0.75	8.70
Maize	4	3.28	0.27	3.48
Beans	2	1.32	0.39	1.74
	32	15.7	2.1	27.7

The dry matter is 1.8 per cent. of the live weight, and the ration therefore agrees with the standards laid down. In practice it proved satisfactory.

Suppose now that oat straw were to be substituted for the hay. The 16 lb. of meadow hay (S.E. 31) supplies 5 lb. of starch equivalent, a quantity which might be furnished by 29 lb. of oat straw (S.E. 17). The word "might" is used because—discounting for the moment variations in the quality of different samples of straw—the horse is less efficient in deriving nourishment from fibrous foods than is the bullock; actually the horse would probably need more than 29 lb. of oat straw to provide it with as much energy as 16 lb. of good hay. However, even the use of 29 lb. of oat straw would increase the total dry matter of the ration to some 39 lb. or 2.6 per cent. of the live weight of the horse: this percentage is much too high. Moreover, by substituting oat straw for hay the ration is completely altered in other very important respects, as a study of the analysis of the altered diet will show:

TABLE 120

Food		Starch Equivalent	Protein Equivalent	Dry Matter
		lb.	lb.	lb.	lb.
Oat Straw	...	29	4.93	0.29	24.94
Oats ...	...	10	6.10	0.75	8.70
Maize ...	...	4	3.28	0.27	3.48
Beans ...	...	2	1.32	0.39	1.74
		45	15.6	1.7	38.9

If this altered ration is now compared with the standard requirements, it will be seen that whereas the starch equivalent may be sufficient, there is a deficiency of nearly half a pound of protein equivalent.

The complete substitution of oat straw for the hay is not therefore an economical proposition and is clearly wrong. This does not mean, however, that no oat straw should be given to horses; on the contrary good oat straw is better than bad hay, and good quality oat straw can sometimes be used *in moderation* to replace part of the hay allowance,* provided that the horses are not doing hard work. In many cases, oat straw instead of hay is given to horses on the assumption that because it is cheaper per ton it is necessarily more economical to use, whereas the reverse is often the case.

Wheat straw is not suitable for working horses and should never be used. For ruminants, in proper combination with other foods, it supplies approximately 11 lb. of starch equivalent per 100 lb., but horses expend more energy in digesting the straw than they obtain nutriment from it.

The above arguments show that, to a certain extent, the proper proportion of dry matter in a diet automatically controls the supply of concentrates and therefore it should be given due consideration when formulating rations for horses.

Pea and bean straws may be used for horses in small quantities but they vary greatly in nutritive value, depending upon the proportion of nutritive leaf to fibrous stalks. As leguminous straws of this nature are more difficult to dry than cereal straws they are sometimes mouldy in patches, and when in this condition should not be used. A sudden change of diet to include a large proportion of either pea or bean straw is almost certain to cause digestive disturbances.

* This is not a practice to be recommended, especially in the case of town horses, without some reservations. If the horses have access to grazing occasionally—say once a week or once a fortnight—or if the hay fed is always of first-class quality and contains moderate amounts of carotene, or if dried grass or fresh green foods are regularly available, then the substitution may be made. No one should imagine, however, that good hay and straw are foods so much alike that they may be interchanged at random.

As to the manner in which the coarse fodder should be given, this depends upon the class of horse and the kind of work it is doing. In large commercial stables it has clearly been shown that chaffing or cutting all the hay, and straw if it is used, effects a great monetary saving, for when horses are given long hay from racks there is always a certain amount of wastage in scattering, which in big commercial studs represents a considerable sum per annum. There is a further advantage in cutting all the hay inasmuch as it affords a certain method of controlling the amount of bulky food consumed by the animals. At the same time the practice of chaffing all the coarse fodder is open to abuse, for when wheat straw or inferior oat straw is mixed with the grain and cut hay the horses are compelled to eat it. In stables where the horses are not at work every day, or are out for only part of the day, it is advisable to give the greater part of the hay uncut; then the horses can occupy their time picking hay from the racks. With hard-working horses the object should be to get them to finish their evening meal in reasonable time so that they can lie down and rest as long as possible.

(iv) *Work: rations for work horses.*

The four rations in Table 121 have been used in practice, the first two being due to Mr. J. W. M'Intosh, M.R.C.V.S. Below is given an example of the way in which the required amounts of starch and protein equivalents, appropriate to the work done, have been calculated from the feeding standards already given: it relates to ration 1.

Starch equivalent for maintenance of 1,700 lb. horse ... ... 7.1 lb.
Starch equivalent for 1,700 lb. horse doing 6 hours hard work ... 10.2 lb.

∴Total requirements for S.E. ... ... 17.3 lb.
Protein equivalent for maintenance of 1,700 lb. horse ... ... 0.85 lb.
Protein equivalent for 6 hours work by 1,700 lb. horse ... ... 1.53 lb.

∴Total requirements for P.E. ... ... 2.4 lb.

In the case of the third ration it will be noticed that the amount of food fed is less than is needed for hard work. Here, although the work was only of medium degree, the physical condition of the horses suggested that insufficient food was actually being given.

As another present-day example of 1,500 lb. horses doing medium work in London, it has been found that a ration of 20 lb. of hay, 11 lb. of oats and 1 lb. of bran per day is barely sufficient for 6-7 hours of work.

In Table 122 are given some suggested rations for different classes of horses. From many points of view they represent a considerable improvement on some of the other rations which have been quoted, not so much in starch and protein equivalents as in the many minor factors which help to ensure efficient physiological performance.

TABLE 121

Ration No.	Horses' wt. lb.	Nature of work done	Food		Starch Equiv. lb.	Protein Equiv. lb.	Dry Matter lb.	Starch Equiv. (lb.)			Protein Equiv. (lb.)		
				lb.	lb.	lb.	lb.	Ration	Stand.	Diff.	Ration	Stand.	Diff.
1	1,700	6 hours heavy transport at walking pace.	Maize	7.25	5.95	0.48	6.31						
			Oats	9	5.49	0.68	7.83						
			Dried Grains	2	1.02	0.25	1.80						
			Hay	17.5	5.43	0.79	15.00						
				36	17.9	2.2	30.9	17.9	17.3	+0.6	2.2	2.4	—0.2
								Dry matter content 1.8 per cent. of live wt.					
2	1,500	8 hours very heavy, mostly at the trot.	Maize	10	8.2	0.67	8.7						
			Dried Grains	6.3	3.2	0.78	5.7						
			Beans	0.7	0.46	0.14	0.6						
			Hay	14	4.34	0.63	12.0						
				31	16.2	2.2	27.0	16.2	15.5	+0.7	2.2	2.1	+0.1
								Dry matter content 1.8 per cent. of live wt.					
3	1,500	7 hours of medium work. Horses not in good condition.	Oats	12	7.3	0.90	10.44						
			Bran	3	1.26	0.30	2.64						
			Hay (Italian Rye)	12	4.32	0.72	10.32						
			Oat Straw	8	1.36	0.08	6.88						
				35	14.2	2.00	30.3	14.2	17.0	—2.8	2.0	2.3	—0.3
								Dry matter content 1.8 per cent. of live wt.					
4	1,500	Farm horses doing 8 hours hard work.	Hay	14	5.04	0.84	12.04						
			Maize	10	8.20	0.67	8.70						
			Oats	5	3.05	0.37	4.35						
			Bran	2	0.84	0.20	1.76						
			Beans	2	1.32	0.39	1.74						
				33	18.5	2.5	28.6	18.5	18.4	+0.1	2.5	2.5	0.0
								Dry matter content 2 per cent. of live wt.					

TABLE 122

Type of horse	Amounts to be fed in lb.					S.E.	P.E.	Daily wt of food
	Oats	Hay	Dried grass Best	Med.	Super hay			
Heavy draught	15	15	—	—	—	14.5	1.8	30
	12	9	6	—	—	14.2	2.0	27
	12	9	—	7	—	14.4	1.9	28
	12	8	—	—	8	14.2	1.7	28
Medium	10	10	—	—	—	9.7	1.2	20
(Heavy	6	8	5	—	—	9.6	1.4	19
chargers over	7	7	—	5	—	9.5	1.3	19
15 h.h.)	8	6	—	—	6	9.8	1.2	20
Light	8	10	—	—	—	8.5	1.1	18
(Cavalry under	6	8	3	—	—	8.4	1.2	17
15 h.h.)	6	7	—	4	—	8.4	1.1	17
	6	9	—	—	5	9.1	1.1	20

These are a number of suggested alternatives; the original paper should be consulted for still further examples.

(v) *The feeding of mine animals.*

The feeding of animals employed underground is complicated by many and varied factors. Working conditions differ not only in every mine, but in different sections of the same mine. Some of the variations may be cited, e.g., differences in the height of roadway, gradients, presence or absence of water either in the form of " droppers " from the roof or an admixture of water and mud on the roads, weight of load, length of working shift and periods of rest between the shifts. When one adds to these factors the statement that all breeds, ages and sizes of animals from 9.0 h.h. to 17.0 h.h. are employed underground it will be realised that to obtain the best results from feeding is a complicated problem.

A mixture fed to the animals in one group of pits is made up in the following proportions: hay, 288; straw, 140; oats, 216; maize, 240; beans, 76 parts.

When straw is omitted it is replaced by additional hay. The hay and straw are chopped, while the grains and beans are crushed, the whole ration being afterwards well mixed. Bran, linseed and rock salt are available as separate issues as and when required. This ration and the following one would be improved by the inclusion of a small proportion of dried grass (first quality).

The scale of rations is based on the sizes of the various animals and ranges from 12 to 30 lb./day.

The following ration (Table 123) has been used with success for small ponies in a colliery, the average weight of feed, including hay and mixed corn, being 12 lb. per head, although it varies from time to time according to the work the animals do.

TABLE 123

Food.		Starch Equivalent.	Protein Equivalent.	Dry Matter.
	lb.	lb.	lb.	lb.
Meadow Hay ...	2.34	0.72	0.10	2.10
Seed Hay ...	2.34	0.84	0.14	2.10
Oats	4.32	2.63	0.32	3.75
Maize	2.40	1.97	0.16	2.10
Beans	0.60	0.40	0.12	0.52
	12	6.6	0.8	10.6

Pit ponies are fed liberally, and particular care is taken to see that the food supplied is of good quality. They are usually fed and watered three times in twenty-four hours when in the stables. In accordance with the Coal Mines Act, 1911, Third Schedule, water and food are also provided in the working places. On returning to their stables after completing their shift of 6 to 7 hours the feed is provided in the mangers ready for them.

REFERENCES.

1. Marshall, F. H. A. & E. T. Halnan, (1946). "Physiology of Farm Animals."
2. Carroll, F. D., H. Goss & C. E. Howell, (1949). J. Animal Sci., 8, 290.
3. Marshall, F. H. A. & J. Hammond, (1947). Min. Agric. Fisheries Bull., No. 39.
4. Tangl, F., (1902), quoted by Morrison, "Feeds and Feeding", 1947.
5. Scheunert, A., (1913). Arch. Physiol., 151, 396.
6. Bohstedt, G., B. Roche, I. Rupel & J. Fuller, (1930). Wiscon. Agric. Exp. Sta. Bull., No. 102.
7. Watson, S. J., (1939). "The Science and Practice of Conservation."
8. Miller, W. C. & W. B. Muir, (1940). J. Roy. Army Vet. Corps, 12, No. 1.
9. Brody, S., (1945). "Bioenergetics and Growth."
10. Linton, R. G., (1917). Vet. Journal.
11. Morrison, F. B., (1947). "Feeds and Feeding."
12. Linton, R. G., (1937). J. Dairy Res., 8, 143.

CHAPTER 24

RABBITS

1. **Introduction**
2. **The digestion of food constituents by rabbits**
3. **Feeding standards and practical feeding**
    (a) Maintenance.
    (b) Reproduction and lactation.
    (c) Growth.
    (d) Rations.

(1) Introduction

The domestic rabbit is maintained for two purposes, namely meat and fur production and, having been selectively bred with the object of exploiting these two sources of profit, it differs quite markedly from its original wild ancestor. On the one hand the ability to grow quickly and to a great size has been cultivated and on the other, the production of fine quality pelts of fur of a distinctive character. While the success of both of these activities depends primarily upon an adequate supply of suitable food, commercial considerations make it imperative that the supply be furnished in the most economical manner possible.

Under natural conditions the rabbit seems to be an herbivorous animal. It is a non-ruminant and, with its relatively large caeca, generally resembles the horse in the anatomy of its digestive tract. The mouth of the animal is better fitted for cutting and gnawing foodstuffs than for grinding them.

(2) The digestion of food constituents by rabbits

Due to the fact that a few of the early results of digestibility trials carried out on rabbits produced data comparable with those for sheep, it was at first assumed that the powers of digestion of the two species were about equal. Later work, however, has shown that this is not so. In the table below are set out data relating to a number of common foodstuffs for sheep, rabbits and horses.

There is surprisingly little difference between the three species so far as protein digestibility is concerned and relatively little for nitrogen-free extractives. In the utilisation of fibre the order of diminishing efficiency is sheep, horse, rabbit, but it will be observed that lucerne fibre is better used by the rabbit than by the two other species. This efficient use of fibre in foods when the fibre content is not high nor too lignified is typical of the animal.

TABLE 124

Foodstuff	Animal species	Organic matter	Protein	N.F. Extract	Fibre	Fat
			Dietary constituent, dig. %			
Oats	Sheep	77	78	83	37	82
	Rabbit	64	79	72	18	90
	Horse	75	79	79	44	30
Lucerne	Sheep	58	73	68	39	47
	Rabbit	81	89	88	66	71
	Horse	57	71	69	44	—
Meadow hay	Sheep	63	60	64	62	52
	Rabbit	47	60	64	18	43
	Horse	51	54	56	44	21
Lucerne hay	Sheep	61	72	69	45	31
	Rabbit	61	76	73	39	16
	Horse	58	74	68	39	6
Grass	Sheep	76	77	77	78	46
	Rabbit	64	77	67	50	41
	Horse	51	66	62	33	—

Literature ref. [123]

The most comprehensive work which has appeared on the digestibility of foodstuffs by rabbits is summarised below, the figures representing average data for the different groups.[4]

TABLE 125

Class of food	Energy	Protein	Fat	Nitrogen-free Ext.	Fibre	Total dig. nutrients %
	Average digestibility, % of					
Hay, non-legume	40	55	48	58	17	40
Hay, legume	55	75	48	58	17	60
Green roughages and roots	95	85	80	95	85	8*
Concentrates	85	85	95	90	50	75-80

(*. Cooked potatoes, 16)

Although the above figures have been rounded off for purposes of tabulation and although there are variations within each group, the data show fairly clearly the efficiency of rabbits with the different classes of food. They make somewhat better use of protein, slightly less of nitrogen-free extractive and fat, and much less of fibre than sheep; they may in fact be more fittingly compared with the horse.

The rabbit is an example of a species which practises coprophagy (which has also been described as " pseudo-rumination "[5]), since it excretes two types of fæcal pellets; the soft kind, excreted chiefly during the night, it immediately swallows. The differences between the two kinds of fæces are shown in Table 126.

TABLE 126

	Firm fæces	Soft fæces
Crude protein %	10.92	34.97
Ether extract %	4.10	3.55
Crude fibre %	35.53	13.89
N-free Extractives % ...	41.10	36.59
Ash %	8.35	11.00

(On dry matter basis)

In an earlier chapter it was pointed out that the horse is unable to make as efficient use of the products of the microbial population of the cæcum as the sheep, goat or cow may do of their rumen products. Apparently the rabbit represents an intermediate stage in efficiency between true ruminants and the equine family. By re-consuming the soft pellets the rabbit can take in an increased amount of " vitamin B," together with protein which has been synthesised by bacteria. The rabbit is less dependent upon dietary sources of vitamin B than is the horse, while its protein intake is improved.

So far as the practical feeding of rabbits is concerned, this evidence serves to show that it can use coarse foods with reasonable efficiency, provided that they are not too mature and highly lignified. The full range of foods, except for those which are very fibrous and lignified is thus available; economic considerations are usually the deciding factor in deciding which are actually to be used. Hay is a common food for rabbits, but, from what has been said earlier concerning the nutritive value of this material, one should be sure that the hay is a good, leafy type. Even so, its employment is limited.

One result of the effective use of the protein of foods by rabbits as compared with their limited powers to digest fibre is that the average food has a slightly narrower nutritive ratio for this species than for ruminants, although the effect is less marked where the foods used are immature green crops, or where the fibre content is low.

(3) Feeding standards and practical feeding

(a) Maintenance.

The different breeds of rabbit range in bodyweight from about 2 lb. to as much as 20 lb.,[5] although the more commonly kept varieties weigh about 8 lb. when mature.

Despite this several-fold variation in bodyweight, there appears to be no change of conformation and Lee[7] has shown that the basal metabolic rate of rabbits is covered by Brody's suggested equation (p. 248). The values obtained by Lee are given in Table 127.

In Wilson's monograph on rabbit feeding,[8] various diets which have been used for maintenance purposes have been analysed; the results support Brody's contention that the needs for maintenance are approximately twice those for basal metabolism. For this reason, in Table 127

TABLE 127

Bodyweight { Kg.	1	2	3	4	5
lb.	2.2	4.4	6.6	8.8	11.0
B.M., Cal./day	62	101	141	180	219
Maintenance, Cal./day ...	124	202	282	360	438
Weight of dig. nutr. for maintenance, oz./day ...	1.1	1.8	2.5	3.2	4.0

the requirements given by Lee for basal metabolism have been doubled and converted into the equivalent quantity of digestible nutrients.

Maintenance protein needs for mature animals are as for other species, about 10 per cent. of the total digestible nutrients being required in the form of protein of average biological value.

Rabbits which receive rations including good proportions of fresh green foods and some hay, will require little supplementation of the diet with the fat-soluble vitamins, although 0.5-1.0 per cent. of cod-liver oil may be necessary during the winter months to provide vitamins A and D. Unless too large quantities of potatoes (cooked) and household waste are included in the diet, the animals should not lack members of the vitamin B-complex.

Maintenance rations for rabbits can be made up entirely of green foods and hay,[8] with small amounts of roots. Suitable green foods include grass and clover mixtures in the spring and summer and kale during the rest of the year, eked out with cabbage, lettuce and weeds such as dandelion. The hay can be supplemented by dried grass. Since animals which are being kept for wool or fur production do not provide true examples of simple maintenance, the standards which have been suggested may be increased slightly to suit the particular circumstances. Suggested rations are given in Table 129.

(b) Reproduction and lactation.

Like other mammals the breeding doe has appreciable need of additional nutrients during the last third only (10 days) of the period of gestation, provided that, at other times, she is maintained in good condition. The increase in the total amount of food then necessary follows the general lines indicated in Chap. 17, [4], the intake of food being increased by some 25 per cent., while the protein need is enhanced 100-150 per cent. This change in the basic nature of the diet involves a diminution in the amount of hay and green food which may be fed, cereal and oil-seed concentrates being used instead, together with wheat offals and small amounts of food of animal origin. Less emphasis need be placed upon the nature of the protein given than in the case of carnivorous species. Of the cereal foods oats, wheat, barley and maize have all been found suitable, while the various grades of bran may be used. Among the oil-seed meals (decorticated types) groundnut, linseed, soya-bean, sunflower and sesame are useful. Cottonseed cake is not suitable.[8] Animal proteins such as fish meal, or dried milk, are of value for the calcium and phosphorus they provide, quite apart from their protein contents.

As the data in Table 66 show, rabbit milk is rich in protein; it also contains about 15 per cent. of fat. Since the volume secreted by a lactating doe may be as much as 35 g./Kg. bodyweight, feeding must make allowance for this relatively large energy production. One gramme of the milk will have a food energy content of approximately 2 Cal., so that, for a partial efficiency of milk production of 50-60 per cent., the additional allowance of energy per Kg. of bodyweight for a doe in lactation will need to be about 1.25 to 1.5 oz. of digestible nutrients per day. Compared with the maintenance allowances given in Table 127, the total requirements for milk production are thus two to three times as great. At the height of lactation, therefore, the doe may need three times as much food as for simple maintenance. Such a large intake necessarily limits the amounts of succulents which may be consumed.

The high protein content of the milk necessitates the use of protein concentrates in the ration to bring the percentage of digestible protein up to 20-25 per cent. Legumes will provide calcium, but the ration would probably be improved by the addition of 1-2 per cent. of steamed bone flour, since rabbit milk is rich in mineral matter. A salt lick will also need to be provided.

(c) Growth.

The data given below illustrate the rapidity of growth which may occur in young rabbits under favourable conditions.[9]

TABLE 128

Age, days	0	14	30	45	60	75	90	105	120	135	150
Weight, g. ...	60	225	400	700	1050	1400	1750	2000	2200	2350	2500
Gain/day, g. ...	—	11	15	21	23	23	20	15	12	10	10
Gain %, on previous weight....	—	275	77	75	50	33	25	14	10	7	6
Wt., multiple of birth wt. ...	—	3.7	6.7	12	17	23	29	33	37	39	41

The actual size attained by individual animals varies inversely with the number in the litter, while as in the case of other species the amount of milk produced by the doe probably depends on the demands made upon her. The two contrasting requirements seem to produce the best results, on the basis of the *litter* and not just on individual weights, when there are about six animals in it.

Little precise experimental work has been done on the way in which the energy requirements of growing rabbits vary with age. The daily gain in weight of an animal of 1 Kg. bodyweight is such that its equivalent energy would be about 25-30 Cal., which is one fourth the maintenance requirement for a mature animal of the same weight. It would seem, therefore, that the early needs of the young of this species for growth and maintenance are probably twice the maintenance needs of the mature animal of the same weight; towards maturity the ratio falls to unity; this trend is suggested by the much slower increase in weight after the age of about 105 days. One authority* has reported that beneficial results were obtained by giving to young growing stock higher initial and lower subsequent intakes of food than is commonly the practice. This ability of young stock to take advantage of a high plane of nutrition has been observed in other species. (Ch. 17 [3].)

A correspondingly high percentage of protein in the ration is needed for early growth. Milk provides a high initial level of protein which may be implemented just before the weaning period by the feeding of fresh green foods and concentrate mixtures rich in protein.

(d) Rations.

(i) Maintenance.

Using Table 127 for the energy needs of mature animals and American data for the total digestible nutrients for various foods when they are given to rabbits, the table below shows the approximate amounts (oz.) of the various foods which would provide the maintenance energy of animals of different weights.

TABLE 129

| Bodyweight | Kg. | 1 | 2 | 3 | 4 | 5 |
	lb.	2.2	4.4	6.6	8.8	11.0
Greens (fresh), roots		14	22	30	40	50
Young lucerne, grass, clover, or potatoes, cooked ...		7	11	15	20	25
Legume hay, good		2	3	4.5	6	7
Cereal grains, oil-seed meals		1.3	2.2	3	4	6
Bran, brewer's grains (dry) ...		1.8	3	4	5	5

Examples of rations which have been recommended are numbers 1, 2 and 3, below, the amounts referring to oz./day.

TABLE 130

No.	Lit. ref.	Greens or roots.	Cereals.	Hay.	Mash (or pellets).	Dig. nutr.	Weight of rabbit.
						oz.	lb.
1.	(8)	Greens, ad lib.	—	Ad lib.	—	—	5
2.	(6)	1	1	1	(Cereals, plus 10% fish-meal) 1	2	5
3.	(9)	Fodder-beet, 4-5	1.5	3	—	3	6.5

A variety of foods is better than one or two, while the protein content of the ration must be kept in mind. Some hay, or dried grass, or green food should always be included.

(ii) Reproduction and lactation.

Here the basic rations must be modified. The large intakes of energy needed for the last stage of pregnancy (about 1.5 times maintenance needs) and for full lactation (up to four times maintenance) usually cause the intakes of succulent foods to be reduced. Concentrates, including the protein rich foods, have to be increased. If no fish meal is given, then bone-meal may be required to furnish calcium and phosphorus.

Rations 1, 2 and 3 of Table 131 have been used for the pregnant doe, the rest of them being used during lactation. The mashes should contain about 10 per cent. of animal protein, such as fish meal.

TABLE 131

No.	Lit. ref.	Greens or roots.	Cereals.	Hay.	Mash.	Dig. nutr. oz.	Weight of rabbit. lb.
1.	(11)	20 rising to 27 (wilted).	—	—	—	1.6-2.2	6
2.	—	1	1.5-2	ad lib.	1	>2.5	5
3.	(11)	10	—	5	2.5	5	5
4.	(11)	25	—	10	3-4	10	5
5.	(8)	ad lib.	4, to 12th day, reduced to 1 by 18th (mixture of two kinds) ad lib.	ad lib.	—	—	5
6.	(10)	Little		ad lib.	Pellets ad lib.	—	Average

(iii) Growth and fattening.

Rations which have been used successfully are of the type given in the following table; No. 4 is a fattening ration.

TABLE 132

No.	Lit. ref.	Greens or roots.	Cereals.	Hay.	Mash or pellets.
1.	(8)	ad lib. from 48th day.	From the 88th day to 188th 1	ad lib.	—
2.	(12)	11, @ 9 weeks rising to 17, @ 28 weeks.	—	—	app. 1.5
3.	(12)	10-11	—	—	Fresh kitchen scraps 1.5 rising to 6
4.	—	—	1	3	Potatoes, cooked, 3; plus 2 of mash*
5.	(10)	Small amt.	—	Small amt.	As much as can be consumed in 30 mins. of mixture of cereals (4 pt.) and protein concentrate (1 pt.)

* Bran 1; ground oats 1; middlings 1; flaked maize 4; meat meal 1. To a mixture of this kind 1% of salt, 2.5% limestone flour and 1.5-2% of cod-liver oil were added.

(iv) General routine of feeding.

The use of large amounts of green food is often troublesome; it tends to produce damp hutches. Difficulties may be experienced in obtaining regular supplies, while such food does not keep well and its nutritive value tends to vary. American practice makes less use of it than British, although good breeding performance has been claimed for the following mixture; bran 15, barley meal 20, groundnut meal 15, linseed cake 10, meat and bone meal 8, dried grass meal 30, chalk 1, and common salt 1.[13]

In actual feeding, water should always be provided. Where the animals have a high proportion of succulent foods in the ration, their water consumption will be small, but a diet containing hay and concentrates may be expected to cause a need for water up to 150 ml. per day.[2]

Rabbits are usually fed twice a day, the bulk of the concentrates being given in the morning, and the remainder along with the roughages at night, although perfectly satisfactory results can be obtained by feeding once only in the evening. Very young rabbits should be fed in small quantities three or four times a day, as they are apt to foul their food if it is given in large quantities at one time.

REFERENCES

1. Schneider, B. H., (1947). " Feeds of the world; their digestibility and composition."
2. Brüggemann, H., (1937). Biedermanns Zentralbl. (B) Tierenährung, 9, 374.
3. Watson, S. J., and E. A. Horton, (1936). Emp. J. Exp. Agric., 4, 25.
4. Voris, L., L. F. Marcy, E. J. Thacker, and W. W. Wainio, (1940). J. Agric. Res., 61, 673.
5. Taylor, E. L., (1940). Vet. Rec., 52, 259.
6. Wilson, W. King, and W. McCartney, (1940). Imp. Bur. Animal Nutrition, Tech. Comm. No. 12.
7. Lee, R. C., (1939). J. Nutrition, 18, 473.
8. Page, D., (1942). Emp. J. Exp. Agric., 10, 103.
9. Hagelin, K. F., (1935), quoted in ref. 6, above.
10. Kellogg, C. E., (1939). U.S. Dept. Agric., Yearbook, 891.
11. Legendre, G., (1934). Rev. Zootech, 13, 223, and 14, 357.
12. Wilson, W. King, (1947). Harper Adams Utility Poultry J., 32, 52.
13. Bruce, H. M., (1947). J. Hyg., 45, 169.

PIGS

(1) Introduction

The pig differs considerably from the herbivorous species which have hitherto been considered both in the type of food which it can digest and in its general management.

It is usually described as an omnivorous animal, a description which refers to the range of foods that may be given to it rather than to its powers of dealing easily with any class of foodstuff. Its digestive system is simpler than that of the ruminants or of the horse, for it has neither rumen nor capacious cæcum; in consequence it has less power of digesting fibre, especially lignified fibre, than the herbivorous species, and it is much more dependent on dietary sources of the water soluble vitamins. Under the conditions of management which usually pertain, this inability of the pig to deal with fibre has led it to compete with man for supplies of cereal grains for food. In the past it was also thought that rather high intakes of animal protein were needed by the species.

Unlike those other animals, the pig may produce litters of eight or more young ones; this brings in a new feature, namely, that of anæmia due to a nutritional deficiency of iron. It is a deficiency sufficiently common to require definite steps being taken to prevent its occurrence in young pigs.

The starch equivalent system applied so commonly to cattle, sheep and, with some reservations, to horses, cannot be used with any confidence for pigs except for a limited range of foods, low in fibre and therefore consisting largely of cereal and protein concentrates. Because the range of foods is, in fact, so very limited and because most of the different foods are very much alike in the fibre contents and starch equivalents, in practice one often refers to the nutritional needs of pigs in terms of pounds of " mixed meals".

With regard to management there is also a big difference between pigs and the herbivorous species. Although fat lambs are produced in quite large numbers and although baby beef may also be raised, pigs, apart from breeding sows, are fed for simultaneous growth and fattening but with two quite clear-cut objects in mind, in the one case the production of pork and in the other of bacon. The fact that a sow has a large number of piglets and that feeding is for growth and fattening means that every effort must be made to avoid checks. This, in turn, puts great emphasis on the feeding of the breeding sow throughout pregnancy—and especially during the last third of it—on adequate supplies of water, on the right kind of food during lactation, and on smooth transitions for the young pigs from one type of food to another, e.g., milk to solid foods. As will be seen later definite principles must be followed if a suitable kind of animal is to be produced during a given time at such a level of food consumption as will be economic.

Pigs are usually fattened to a much higher degree than is the case with cattle or sheep and, because of this, considerable care has to be exercised with regard to the quantity and kinds of dietary fat which may be ingested at various stages of development.

There are no fundamental differences between pigs and other species of farm mammals with respect to general requirements for growth, reproduction, lactation and fattening.

(2) Foods for pigs

Here there are two problems, namely, how to feed breeding stock and young pigs for pork and bacon. Although, broadly speaking, the same classes of food are available for both purposes, there are some differences which must be remembered. Feeding for pregnancy requires attention to the provision of adequate amounts of energy, protein, vitamins and minerals at different stages, the maximum demand coming during the last third of the gestation period, when protein requirements particularly are enhanced.[1] On the other hand the growing animal begins with large needs for protein, mineral elements and vitamins, but, where fattening is concerned, requires more carbohydrate than protein. The effects of foods on the flavour of the body fat of the sow are not of very great concern, whereas they are most important where bacon and pork are being produced. Similarly, provided that it satisfies her needs, the sow may receive reasonable amounts of coarser foods, but the nutritional requirements for rapid growth and fattening limit their use quite considerably in the other cases.

Barley and the finer grades of wheat bran, both of which contain some 5 per cent. of fibre, have always been looked upon as the cereal foods most suitable for pig feeding. Provided that they are finely ground, however, oats may be fed at high levels—up to 50 per cent. or more of the ration for pigs above 50 lb. bodyweight. About 1.2 lb. of farm-ground oats are needed to replace 1 lb. of barley. Ground wheat is rather unsatisfactory from the points of view of its lack of palatability and its sogginess when moist, while maize, which might otherwise have been used in conjunction with the rather coarser grades of bran to give a ration of the desired fibre content, contains too much rather highly unsaturated fat for it to be used to a greater extent than about 25 per cent. of rations. In the United States, however, maize is used as the main source of carbohydrate for pig feeding and germ only is regarded as being a troublesome cause of soft carcase fat. As substitutes for cereal foods, potatoes are good, provided that they are cooked, but it takes about 4 lb. to replace one pound of barley; dried potato slices and flakes are equally useful. Where rather large amounts of potatoes are fed, however, attention must be paid to the protein, mineral and vitamin contents of the ration. It is noteworthy that the fibre of potatoes, which is not lignified, is quite well digested by pigs, while Woodman[2] has shown that fodder cellulose, made by the de-lignification of straw, is about 80 per cent. digested provided that the amount fed does not exceed about 2 lb. per day. Beet pulp is rather too fibrous to enable much use to be made of it, but if it is moistened, the ration may include 10 - 15 per cent. at the fattening stage.

Of the protein concentrates beans and peas do not lead to the production of soft body fat, nor does palm-kernel cake, but linseed, soya-bean and groundnut cakes or meals do: in this respect the solvent extracted products, with their lower fat contents, are better. Poor quality fish meal is also unsuitable. Animal muscle proteins, unless accompanied by large amounts of fat, are very useful, but, like the milk proteins of whole or skim milk, they should be fed with the idea of physiological economy in mind, that is, with the object of supplementing vegetable proteins. Dried yeast supplies good protein in addition to the richness of its vitamin B content, for which chiefly it is fed, but its very high phosphorus content (5 per cent. P_2O_5) necessitates a compensating intake of calcium and vitamin D. A useful review of the food values of dried yeast, dried clostridium residue and dried penicillin felt has been made by Braude.[3] Woodman[4] has recently determined the protein contents and digestibilities for pigs of a number of protein concentrates. His data are given in the table below, where they are adjusted to the nearest integer and where the contents of total and digestible crude protein refer to the materials as fed. It should be observed how rich a protein source is whalemeat meal [of the grade low in ash (2 per cent.)—there is a second which contains some 15 per cent. of mineral elements].

TABLE 133

Constituent	Whale-meat meal	White-fish meal	Feeding meat meal	Feeding meat meal (extr.)	Extrd. decort. ground-nut	Bean meal	Dried yeast
Crude protein, total %	88	58	66	67	54	28	42
Crude protein, dig. %	88	95	94	88	93	80	89
Digestible crude protein content, on wet basis	77	55	62	58	50	22	37

The pig is one of the species which give full opportunity for the exploitation of the supplementary relationships between different dietary proteins. Maize and meat offals have long been a favourite combination in many regions of the United States, while in Britain white-fish meal and cereals are very commonly used. When there is a good supply of skim milk it may be used to good effect in association with oats. There is no doubt that many more combinations of this kind remain to be tested, especially those of the more readily digested protein concentrates; many of the rations in frequent use appear to be much more rich in protein than one would expect to be necessary, especially where late growth and fattening are concerned.

Kitchen waste and processed swill are both used to a large extent in the feeding of pigs. Provided that one has a fairly good idea of the composition of such foods they are very useful, but they tend to be deficient in three factors, namely fat-soluble vitamins, members of the vitamin B-complex and some mineral elements. Where they are used to any extent, care should be taken to provide suitable supplements, such as cod-liver oil, yeast and mineral mixes.

Dried grass meal, if it is of good quality and is given in the form a thick slop, can be used with good results both for growing and fattening pigs.

(3) The feeding of breeding stock

In feeding sows and boars the aim is to keep them in good breeding condition, neither too fat nor too lean, for if sows are to produce two litters in twelve months, as is commonly done, and to rear them successfully, they require careful feeding. Before the sow is mated she should have recovered completely from the effects of rearing her last litter and be in a thriving condition. Thereafter she should be fed so that she continues to thrive right up to the time of farrowing, for a strong litter of pigs will make heavy demands on their mother, particularly during the first fortnight of their life. For this last period the dam's appetite may be somewhat capricious no matter how well she is fed, so that she is liable to lose weight during the few weeks when the litter relies entirely upon her for food.

If two litters are born in a year it should be arranged that the first is farrowed in March so that the second can be produced in September before the cold weather sets in. Many breeders mate their sows with the boar in October and April so that the piglings are born in February and August, thus possibly giving them a better chance to avoid the cold weather when they are very young.

In-pig sows should be kept out of doors as much as possible so that they can get plenty of fresh air, sunlight and exercise. When possible, breeding stock from the earliest age should be given the opportunity to roam at will in fields or woodlands, where they can eat grass, acorns or beech-mast, and root up worms, insects and grubs.

The amount of grass which a sow may consume when on good grazing may easily be over-estimated. A quantity of about 14 lb./day seems to be a good intake and this quantity is equal in energy value to no more than 2 to 3 lb. of meal.

To sows and boars kept in confinement, grass and other green crops should be given freely; the leguminous soiling crops are valuable on account of their richness in calcium. A supply of foods rich in minerals, or the addition of mineral mixtures to foods, is necessary if healthy litters are to be expected.

At first it is neither necessary nor desirable to give sows such concentrated foods as are given to fattening pigs; roots and other succulent foods, such as potatoes, swedes, turnips, carrots, artichokes and parsnips may be allowed fairly freely, but as the period of pregnancy advances very bulky foods must be reduced and their place taken by more concentrated materials, so as to reduce bulk. Too often a sow is left to find most of her own food by foraging, not only during the early days of pregnancy, but almost to the time of farrowing. By foraging on good pasture she may do well enough during the first half of pregnancy, but over the later part, and especially in the last quarter, she cannot accommodate any great amount of bulky food.

Mitchell [1] and his associates have shown that the average requirement of extra energy for foetus and dam throughout the period is about 6 per cent. During the early part of gestation little additional food is indeed required, but in the last third of pregnancy the growth of the young becomes rapid and substantial demands for extra nutrition arise. It is very important to see that the pregnant sow is then supplied with sufficient food of the right kind so that the foetuses are not developed at the expense of the dam. Insufficient food, particularly if it is deficient in protein, means that the sow will be in poor condition after farrowing and may not be able to produce the large quantity of milk required for her numerous progeny.

Although the nature of the carbohydrates and fats which are fed to brood sows is not of prime importance, it is essential that high quality protein be given. Moreover, when gilts are mated from 6 to 8 months of age, which is quite a common custom, they are still growing, and food of the right kind has to be supplied for the needs of the growing body as well as for the piglings in utero. The strain thrown on a young gilt when she is required to produce and nourish a big litter of pigs is very great, and it is therefore a sounder practice to wait until she is 10 to 12 months old. Where, however, gilts are mated at the earlier ages there will be a need for nutrients over and above those which are described in the following paragraphs for the more mature beasts.

The diet as a whole ought to provide about 17 per cent. of crude protein during the last six weeks of pregnancy. Suitable rations are given in Table 134 opposite.

TABLE 134

Ingredient			Ration 1	Ration 2	Ration 3 (Supplement)
Lucerne meal	...	...	—	—	25
Crushed oats	...	...	30	15	—
Bran	...	...	—	37	—
Middlings	...	...	25	—	—
Maize meal	...	...	30	—	—
Barley meal	...	...	—	35	—
Fish meal	...	...	—	10	50
Whale-meat meal	...	...	5	—	—
Ext. soya-bean meal		...	7	—	25
*Mineral mixture	...	...	3	3	—
Protein content, per cent.	...		17	17	44
Fibre content, per cent.	...		5	7	—

* (40 per cent. ground chalk, 40 per cent. steamed bone meal, 20 per cent. salt.)

With the above rations about 0.5 oz. of cod-liver oil per day may be given. Rations 1 and 2 can be fed at the rate of about 1 lb. of mixture to each 25 lb. of bodyweight. Ration 3 is a suitable one for sows which have some grazing, plus cereal mixes or swill; it is essentially a protein *supplement* and may be fed at the rate of 3 - 5 lb./day, the precise amount depending on the condition of the sow and the nature of the rest of the ration.

There are plenty of opportunities for variation in the above rations, for other oil-seed meals, of low fibre content, can be used. In the second ration the amount of oats used may be increased and that of the bran diminished, using dried yeast or penicillin felt to keep up the total protein and vitamin B.

The sow should be introduced to the farrowing pen at least ten days before she is due to farrow and be given the opportunity to make her bed where and as she wants it. This she will do about 24 hours before farrowing, without that restlessness and anxiety which would otherwise occur, and she will then farrow down with the minimum loss of energy.

Once the sow has been penned, constipating foods must be avoided. She should be allowed out for exercise each day, and for a day or two before farrowing the ordinary meal can with advantage be replaced by hot wet mashes of bran with some crushed oats. For a short time after parturition it is good to continue the mash, adding milk or a milk by-product to it if possible, until the appetite has fully returned, when the sow may be fairly rapidly brought on to the quantity of meal that she was getting before.

According to the size and vigour of her litter, the sow's needs for food will continue to increase for a fortnight and then be maintained until the fourth or fifth week, when the young have begun to take appreciable quantities of solid food. She should be allowed out of her pen, and encouraged to go out to grass or exercise.

As much as 8 lb. of mixed meal containing at least 20 per cent. of crude protein, of which approximately one-third is preferably of animal origin, is needed for milk production (p. 270). A simple and fairly satisfactory guide which has been recommended for estimating daily food needs is to feed to condition or to allow 1 lb. of meal for each piglet, and 2 lb. for the sow.[5] Twelve lb. of high-quality meal are generally sufficient for a sow with a litter of 8 to 10 pigs, but there will be exceptional cases where more may be needed. The following mixtures supply these requirements:

TABLE 135

Ingredient	Ration 1	Ration 2	Ration 3	Ration 4 (Supplement)
Maize meal	—	—	22	—
Barley meal	10	32	10	—
Sussex ground oats ...	30	—	30	—
Fine middlings ...	35	35	10	—
Linseed cake or Groundnut - cake meal	7	10	8	—
Soya-bean meal ...	7	—	8	50
Bean meal	—	10	—	—
Fish meal	5	5	5	25
Lucerne meal ...	3	—	—	25
Dried yeast	—	5	4	—
Mineral mixture* ...	3	3	3	—
Protein, per cent. ...	20	22	20	42
Fibre, per cent. ...	5	4	5	7

(* As in Table 134.)

It is better for the sow to have access to grazing or to other fresh green food if this is possible. With rations such as 2 and 3 above, a cod-liver oil supplement will be needed. Ration 4 is a protein supplement which is suitable for feeding with cereal mixtures to raise the total protein of the ration to about 20 per cent. It is common American practice to put the grain and protein fractions of the diet into separate feeding compartments and allow the sows to select freely.[6]

At no time should the sow be short of water, and the best arrangement is to have it always available so that she can help herself as she requires it.

(4) The feeding of growing pigs

(a) General feeding up to 100 lb. liveweight.

The dam's milk is not only the most suitable food, but also the cheapest and, as nothing can compensate for an inadequate supply from birth to weaning, this should be the breeder's first concern. If the dam is milking badly and the young are undernourished it is reflected in ill health, slow development and in an unsatisfactory financial return, for the pig's life is too short to allow it to recover from an initial setback.

No matter how well fed the dam may be, however, there is one factor which it is difficult to regulate—that is the supply of iron. Young animals are born with a reserve of iron in their liver, kidneys and spleen which is generally sufficient to carry them over the period in which they rely solely on milk for their sustenance; but the supply in the young is sometimes inadequate. The amount of iron excreted in milk is very small and cannot be increased by feeding iron supplements to the dam. In the same way it appears that the body reserves of the fœtus remain unaffected by dosing the dam during pregnancy.[7] It is necessary, therefore, for the young animal to ingest sufficient iron at a very early age if anæmia is to be avoided. Herbivorous animals begin to eat green food at a much earlier stage than young pigs do, but if the latter are given liberty to roam in the open, they pick up the very small quantity of iron which supplies their needs, either by eating fresh vegetation or small quantities of earth containing iron. Where the diet is deficient signs of anæmia may be observed as early as two weeks old, though they are often delayed until the fourth to the sixth week of life. The little pigs must be given an adequate supply of iron or iron-containing food not later than the second week either by allowing the sow and her litter to have freedom in a paddock soon after farrowing, or by administering an iron supplement as part of the diet.[8] The latter alternative presents practical difficulties in the way of expenditure of time and labour which can ill be spared. A good way of giving iron is that recommended by Schofield and Lloyd Jones[9] in Canada, who found that anæmia can be prevented by giving a massive dose of 300 mg. of "reduced iron", an inert powder so fine that when placed in the mouth it cannot be rejected. This is given when the pigs are a few days old. Another precaution which is often advocated but which is not always successful is to place suitable clods of earth for young pigs to root in the sty.

Young pigs will start to nose dry meal at about 3 weeks and a week to ten days later they will be consuming an appreciable amount. They will not take to wet food so readily, but if their own supply of meal, which must be fed through a "creep", is not completely to their liking, or is deficient in quantity, they will eat the sow's ration, which is seldom suitable for them, and is often the cause of indigestion and diarrhœa. There is no basic reason why young pigs should be fed wet rather than dry food, as the one is as well digested as the other. Cow's milk and its by-products are very useful foods for young pigs and if they are introduced in sufficient quantities at an early date will go a long way to smooth out the depression of growth rate which often occurs at weaning. Milk in any form can with advantage be added to the meal as soon as the pigs show that they can deal with wet food.

After the fourth week the sow's milk supply begins to fall and the pigling relies more and more for its nourishment upon solid food. So quickly may the transition be made that it is possible to wean a litter when six weeks old, but this is not advisable because early weaning often results in a pronounced post-weaning check, the effects of which are obvious throughout life. Where a sow is to have two litters each year no longer than eight weeks can conveniently be allowed to the sow for lactation and thus weaning is most often carried out at that age. If it is delayed until later the change over is hardly felt at all and the extra time given may benefit the sow as well as the young pigs.

Skilled attention is required in the management of pigs at weaning if ill effects are to be avoided—the time and trouble expended then is well spent and the more gradually the change is made the better. The sow should be allowed out without the litter for longer and longer periods each day and when it is seen that the flow of milk is decreasing naturally and that there is no undue tension or signs of inflammation of the udder, the separation may be completed.

Rations which have been found suitable for young pigs of different ages are given in the table below.

TABLE 136

Ingredients	Class of pig					
	Sucklings, fed through creeps		Weaning to 50 lb.		50 to 100 lb.	
	Ration 1	Ration 2	Ration 3	Ration 4	Ration 5	Ration 6
Barley meal ...	25	—	22	15	57	7
Flaked maize ...	25	—	22	20	—	7
Oatmeal	—	15	—	—	—	—
Fine middlings ..	30	10	43.5	53	32	47
Ground linseed ...	—	4.5	—	4.5	—	—
Skim milk	—	70	—	—	—	—
Fish meal	15	—	10	7	7	7
Lucerne meal ...	4.5	—	2	—	—	2
Dried grass meal	—	—	—	—	3	—
Potato flakes ...	—	—	—	—	—	30
Mineral supplement	—	—	—	—	1	—
Cod-liver oil ...	0.5	0.5	0.5	0.5	—	—
Protein content, %	20	19†	18	18	16	15
Fibre content, %	3	5†	3	4	5	4

(† Dry-matter basis)

The treatments of pigs reared for pork or for bacon will not need to differ radically from one another in the early stages of growth (See also Ch. 17 [3]). Both groups may be allowed unrestricted food intake up to a bodyweight of about 100 lb., when the pigs reared for pork will be almost ready for slaughter. Their consumption of mixed meals may be expected to be of the order of 1 lb. for each 25 lb. liveweight. Some care is needed near the end of the respective feeding periods for both pork and bacon pigs, so that foods which may be liable to cause undesirable qualities in the flesh, as, for example, fat of low melting-point, may be avoided.

The examples given in the above table illustrate the way in which the rations may be varied as the pigs grow. More fibre and less protein are found in the rations, while cod-liver oil, used for the growth of the piglets, may be discontinued when once the animals have acquired a reserve, especially when grass or lucerne meals are being fed or when there is access to fresh green crops. Examples 5 and 6 incorporate the recent finding of Woodman and Evans, namely, that the amount of animal protein (fish meal) in the rations of bacon pigs of reasonable weight need not be more than about 7 per cent.[10] and that potato slices or flakes may constitute 30 per cent. of the ration, provided that the protein content is satisfactory.[11]

Considerable energy is expended by young pigs in fighting for trough space, so it is to the owner's advantage to provide a trough of sufficient size to allow all the pigs to feed comfortably at the same time. The trough for little pigs should be shallow, so that they can eat from it without difficulty, and placed behind a creep so that the sow cannot get to it. On no account must the food in the trough he allowed to become sour or stale; small quantities should be given at a time and the trough should be scalded frequently. At first it is advisable to feed the piglets several times a day, but three times daily will be quite satisfactory by the time they are 50 lb. in weight. Although feeding twice a day may be sufficient when the pigs are bigger, if carried out with young pigs it results in gorging, over-distension of the stomach and indigestion. Whatever quantity of food is needed should be eaten up readily at each meal and only that amount should be given at one time which can be cleared up in about 20 minutes.

In cold weather especially, or if the accommodation is damp or draughty, warm food is definitely beneficial for young pigs, sick animals, and farrowing sows, though it is not necessary for fattening pigs kept under reasonably warm conditions. The food for the young pig, if it is to be fed wet, should have the minimum amount of hot water added to it to bring it to body temperature.

(b) Feeding for pork.

The object here is to produce a relatively small carcase of good quality. Good proportions, texture of flesh, and amount and distribution of fat are found in pigs which have been brought on rapidly without check. A fairly lean type of carcase, obtained from young pigs whose liveweight is around 100 lb., is desirable.

The general plan of feeding does not necessarily differ from that of the feeding of bacon pigs, save in one or two minor respects. In the first place it may be easier to rear the pigs indoors, so that their feeding may be under complete control, and, secondly, as already indicated, it is necessary to omit from the diet foods which may produce unwanted qualities of the flesh after the pigs have attained weights of about 50 lb. For this latter reason foods rich in low melting fats should be replaced by equivalent ones which do not suffer from the disadvantage. There is also a tendency to reduce in amount or omit fish meal from the ration, using in its place milk products and other foods of high protein content.

Weights (3 lb. at birth) of 20-30 lb. may be expected to be achieved at weaning, of 50 lb. at about 12 weeks, of 100 lb. in 18 weeks and

130 lb. in 20 to 22 weeks. The amounts of food given should be on the basis previously indicated.

(c) Feeding for bacon production.

The carcase required at the bacon factory is one that is long, deep and well fleshed and comparatively small boned, with a rather thick belly and a moderate amount of fat evenly distributed throughout the body and lightly laid over the back.

The investigations of McMeekan and Hammond have clearly shown how management affects carcase quality.[12] The older method of feeding a pig to capacity from weaning to the time it was butchered as a fat animal is now known to be inimical to the production of first-class bacon, i.e., with a desirable proportion of lean meat to fat and bone. In normal growth, development is first most rapid in bone, then in flesh, and lastly—when the body is well grown—in fat formation. During early stages of growth, head, neck and legs are big in proportion to the size of the body; as the animal matures there is an increase in body length, including that of the more valuable part, the loin; then later the trunk grows in depth and thickness. If management during the early stages has been bad, for example where steady growth has been interrupted by a store period, and fattening is then hastened, a carcase is produced which though fat is badly proportioned, with the better cuts ill developed. To get a carcase suitable for bacon purposes the animal must be well fed throughout the earlier stages of its life, and never stinted but at the same time not overfed when approaching maturity. While it is true that restricted feeding in the later stages results in a slightly longer period of keep than would be the case if the animal were fed to capacity throughout, this disadvantage is definitely offset by an actual saving of food, for under such a system a smaller total supply of food is required to produce the same weight of carcase.

Up to a weight of about 100 lb. the bacon pig may be fed in the general way which has been described for young pigs. Because there is less emphasis on the quality of the carcase at that weight and age, there is more freedom of choice of food and of management than with the animal which is bred for pork.

Soon after the above weight has been attained, the high demands for mineral elements, protein and the fat-soluble vitamins tends to fall; the emphasis now is more and more on fattening and not on simple growth. To correspond with these changes unrestricted food consumption gives place to controlled food intake, the protein content of the ration is reduced by degrees and increasing quantities of carbohydrate are given. There is need for care with respect to the fat-forming constituents of the diet during the last stages of fattening.

Swill, dried grass and potatoes are foods which may constitute quite large proportions of the diet. The many studies of Woodman and Evans on the nutrition of the bacon pig have shown the variety of foods which can be used and have indicated standards for feeding.

Suitable rations are given in the tables below, the first of which is for pigs of 100 to 150 lb. bodyweight and the second for 150 lb. upwards.

TABLE 137

Ingredients	Ration 1	Ration 2	Ration 3	Ration 4 (Supplement)	Ration 5 (Supplement)
			Pigs of 100 - 150 lb.		
Barley meal	65	—	42	50	50
Ground wheat	—	—	—	—	25
Maize meal	—	—	—	—	20
Middlings	23	28	15	30	—
Extr. oil-seed meal	10	—	—	5	—
Fish meal	5	10	10	10	2
Lucerne meal	—	2	—	5	3
Dried grass meal	—	—	33	—	—
Potato slices	—	60	—	—	—
Mineral mixture	2	—	—	—	—
Protein, %	17	16	18	19	11

TABLE 138

Ingredients	Ration 6	Ration 7	Ration 8 (Supplement)	Ration 9	Ration 10 (Supplement)
			Pigs over 150 lb.		
Ground oats	—	—	—	—	25
Barley meal	—	4	50	50	—
Maize meal	—	6	—	—	70
Middlings	28	4	30	13	—
Extr. oil-seed meal	10	—	—	7	—
Fish meal	—	—	15	—	5
Lucerne meal	2	—	5	—	—
Dried grass meal	—	—	—	28	—
Dried yeast	—	5	—	—	—
Potato slices	57.5	—	—	—	—
Swill, conc.	—	80	—	—	—
Mineral mixture	2.5	1	—	2	—
Protein, %	14	20	20	15	13

Of the foodstuffs listed in the tables, suitable extracted oil-seed meals include groundnut, soya-bean or others of low fat and fibre contents. Fish meal can be replaced wholly or in part by meat meal, or by some of the vegetable protein concentrates, where conditions will allow. Bean meal is a useful protein source.

Ration 1 is of a simple type, capable of much modification by the replacement of one of the ingredients by an equivalent, as for example a *partial* substitution of ground maize and oats for barley. Ration 2 is derived from experiments of Woodman and Evans[11] on the use of potato slices and flakes. It is of interest to quote their words regarding these foods:

" (These) forms of dried potatoes, when forming part of pig rations containing additional supplies of protein and minerals, are superior to barley meal in feeding value and markedly superior to ground oats. The potato slices compare closely with maize meal, while the potato flakes have a value not far short of that of flaked maize."

The third ration, also due to these workers, illustrates the use of dried grass meal [11]; it should be remembered that the grass meal needs to be fed as a slop, if the best results are to be derived from its use.

American practice, for the feeding of pigs which have access to pasturage, is indicated by rations 5 and 10, which are intended to supplement grass, while ration 4 is one which could be used in conjunction with the feeding of cooked potatoes or swill. Of the other rations, 6 is another example of the use of potato slices at even higher levels for the final fattening stages, 9 shows a ration employing a high proportion of grass meal while containing no animal protein; in this respect it conforms to the recent recommendations of Woodman and Evans regarding the omission of white-fish meal from the rations of bacon pigs when their weights are above 100 to 150 lb.[10] Ration 7 is one in which processed concentrated swill is used; its nature would vary with the quality of the swill.

Where facilities are available, young pigs intended for bacon can with advantage be reared out of doors until they are about 50 lb. in weight, for such treatment goes a long way to ensure the production of vigorous, healthy animals. From this stage the pigs may be put into fattening pens, the aim being to control the amount of exercise the animal enjoys and the amount of food consumed. At 100 lb. bodyweight the intake of mixed meals, or its equivalent of other foodstuffs, will be 4 - 5 lb. per day, but from that time onwards food consumption is restricted, the quantity increasing by 0.5 lb. for every 20 lb. rise of bodyweight.

Advantage is taken of the increasing power of pigs to deal with coarse foods as they increase in age by a·practice which was evolved in Germany and is now universally associated with the name of Lehmann. When first consuming solid food, young pigs can deal only with material which is of the nature of a concentrate and so, under the *Lehmann system of feeding*, they are given a ration composed of 70 per cent. cereal meal and 30 per cent. of a protein-rich food which is fed to appetite until their capacity reaches approximately 2.5 lb./day, when they should be about 50 lb. in weight. From then on their increase in appetite is met by allowing them as much of any easily procurable, cheap, coarse food as they can consume, but the basic ration remains fixed at 2.5 lb. throughout life. In this way the pig's increasing power of dealing with roughage is exploited to the full and results in a considerable saving of expensive cereals.

Particularly under the stress of war-time conditions of feeding, the scheme has met with a good deal of modification. The high level of protein originally used has been scaled down to 10 per cent. of white-fish meal or of its protein equivalent. This means that the type of ration which is used for pigs up to 50 lb. can be continued afterwards, the only change in dietary regime being the gradual increase in the proportion of coarse foods. Apart from other factors the gradual change is itself an example of good management. In Table 138, ration 8 is one which has a somewhat higher content of animal protein than the one suggested above and which is capable of being used in the way described.

Although potatoes form by far the best supplementary ration, mixtures of potatoes with mangolds, kale or cabbage, and forage crops such as fresh grass, rape and silage, or milk and whey have been used with equal success.

A common method of feeding is to give the bulk of the supplementary food in the morning and the rest, together with the basal ration, for the evening feed. A modification of a continental practice is now officially advocated here to deal with surplus whey. Potatoes are fed to appetite and 1 to 1.5 gal. of whey per head are given daily throughout the fattening period. In addition a basic ration of 1.5 lb. of cereal meal with 3.5 oz. of fish meal is supplied each day up to the time the pigs reach a weight of 120 lb., when the protein supplement may be discontinued.[14]

When modified Lehmann feeding systems are in use, care should be taken concerning the nature of the basal ration, particularly where cooked potatoes are being fed, for Nasr and Baker[15] have shown that whereas pigs may survive on *raw* potato–B deficient diets, because of microbial vitamin syntheses, they die on *boiled* potato–B deficient rations. This constitutes another interesting case of the inter-relationships between the nature of the diet, the intestinal flora and the health of livestock.

REFERENCES

1. Mitchell, H. W., W. E. Carroil, T. S. Hamilton, and G. E. Hunt, (1931). Ill. Agr. Exp. Sta. Bul. No. 375.
2. Woodman, H. E., and R. E. Evans, (1947). J. Agric. Sci., *37*, 202 and 211.
3. Braude, R., (1948). Chem. Ind., 259.
4. Woodman, H. E., and R. E. Evans, (1948). J. Agric. Sci., *38*, 200.
5. Woodman, H. E., (1948). Min. Agric. Fisheries Bul. No. 48. H.M. Stationery Office.
6. Zeller, J. H., and N. R. Ellis, (1939). U.S. Dept. Agric. Yearbook, 723.
7. Hart, E. B., C. A. Elvehjem, and H. Steenbock, (1930). J. Nutrition, *2*, 277.
8. Foot, A. S., and S. Y. Thompson, (1947). Agriculture, J. Min. Agric. Engl., *54*, 308.
9. Schofield, F. A., and T. Lloyd Jones, (1939). Canad. J. Comp. Med., *3*, 63.
10. Woodman, H. E., and R. E. Evans, (1948). J. Agric. Sci., *38*, 354.
11. Woodman, H. E., and R. E. Evans, (1943). J. Agric. Sci., *33*, 1.
12. McMeekan, C. P., (1940-1). J. Agric. Sci., *30*, 276, 387 and 511, and *31*, 1.
13. Woodman, T. E., and R. E. Evans, (1948). J. Agric. Sci., *38*, 51.
14. Braude, R., (1941). Agriculture, J. Min. Agric. Engl., *48*, 10.
15. Baker, F., and H. Nasr, (1950). " The advancement of science," VI.

SMALL DOMESTICATED
CARNIVORA

(1) Introduction

With respect to the purpose for which they are kept, the animals which are to be considered under the above heading may be conveniently divided into the following groups, (a) animals, such as dogs and cats, which are maintained as pets, (b) those, like the fox and mink, which are bred for their fur production, and (c) working animals, such as sheep-dogs, police-dogs and racing greyhounds.

All of these animals are carnivorous. In them the mouth is best adapted for tearing flesh and not for the grinding of food, while the stomach is relatively large, with the intestine small and ill-suited for dealing with very bulky foods. In the natural state, the food of this group of animals is meat—the flesh of such smaller animals as they can catch—and on this account there is a popular belief that dogs and cats must have large amounts of meat in their diet, if they are to remain in good health. Because such ideas can cause a good deal of dietary mis-management, the problem deserves further examination here.

The wild animal does not rely solely on the muscular tissue of its prey; on the contrary it will consume in addition such parts as the liver and bones. Under these circumstances the creature enjoys a good intake of fat and, quite apart from its consumption of protein, makes reasonably sure of its supplies of vitamin A and those other factors which are present in fairly high concentration in liver. Where the animals are kept in captivity, however, they have to compete with human beings for supplies of animal protein, with the result that the "meat" they are given tends to be different from their natural food. For one thing, the residual meat available for animals often includes the poorer, less easily digested material; it seldom consists of the highly nutritious liver and other organs. Secondly, the food is usually deficient in fat, while small bones, which such small animals could manage fairly easily, are often replaced by those of the large domestic species. It follows, therefore, that the class of material which is available for the dog, etc., is of a much more restricted type than the natural diet provides. There is, however, a further difference in that the second source of meat for these species is food which is not fit for human consumption and which needs to be cooked before it may safely be given to animals. In the cooking, some loss of nutritive qualities is inevitable. On the whole, then, there is little comparison between the meat of the wild animal and that which is given to the captive one. Another point which is quite often forgotten is that the free carnivore does not eat twice daily with unfailing regularity, but seeks its prey chiefly when moved by actual hunger. To be successful in its search it has to be in good condition, not overfed and lethargic. Far too many domestic pets are mere caricatures of the natural animal.

There are other characteristics which the members of this class of creatures share in common, a very important one being that they produce litters of several young, which means that a high level of feeding is necessary for successful reproduction and lactation. Another factor is the poor capacity of carnivores for dealing with fibrous foods.

(2) General nutritional requirements

(a) Quantitative.

(i) *Total nutrients.*

Although the available data concerning the energy needs of the smaller carnivorous species are relatively few, those which have been obtained experimentally support the statements made in Section III with respect to the relationship between bodyweight and basal metabolic requirements.

Despite the wide variations in bodyweights between the different breeds of dogs and the contrast between the weights of dogs and minks, it seems that maintenance energy needs, to a first approximation, can be taken as twice those of basal metabolism. The data of Dechambre[1] for dogs can be regarded as applying fairly well to the other species. Dechambre's figures are given in Table 139, both in calories and in terms of the *approximate* amount of a suitable ration (p. 426) which might be fed daily to the animals. Additional data from Brody[2] have been included.

TABLE 139

| Bodyweight | | Maintenance needs | | | Bodyweight | | Maintenance needs | | |
| | | | Food | | | | | Food | |
Kg.	lb.	Cal.	Kg.	lb.	Kg.	lb.	Cal.	Kg.	lb.
1	2.2	140	0.07	0.15	30	66	1,690	0.84	1.8
2	4.4	234	0.11	0.24	40	88	2,020	1.00	2.2
4	8.8	388	0.19	0.42	50	110	2,330	1.17	2.6
5	11	520	0.26	0.57	60	132	2,640	1.32	2.9
10	22	855	0.43	0.95	80	176	3,250	1.62	3.6
15	33	1,080	0.54	1.2	100	220	3,630	1.81	4.0
20	44	1,265	0.63	1.4					

Once again the large needs of small animals, in proportion to their bodyweights must be stressed.

Although complete data are lacking there are no reasons for believing that the needs of the carnivorous species for growth, reproduction and lactation represent departures from the general principles which have been laid down elsewhere. The young, growing animal will require two or three times as much food as a mature one of the same weight, which is being fed simply for maintenance. As in the case of working horses, energy needs for work depend upon the amount of work done. Dechambre has suggested that the performance of light work by the mature beast will involve an increase in energy supply of about 30 per cent. above maintenance levels, while hard exercise may necessitate a 70 per cent. increase in the dietary energy which must be supplied. (It is of interest to note that a hard working horse also needs an increase of 50-100 per cent.) Such figures are no more than guides, the final adjustment of food intake depending upon the condition of the animal. Here it should be said that the carnivorous animal in good condition is lean rather than fat; physical well-being should be reflected in the sleek appearance of the animal rather than in excessive weight.

(ii) *Protein.*

As in the case of other domestic species, the protein needs of dogs, foxes and other carnivorous animals are determined by the age, weight and condition of the individual beast. There is no reason for putting the maintenance requirements for protein at any higher level than some 10 per cent. of the total calories supplied; the chief difficulty is to make sure that all of the other factors accompany the protein in adequate amounts. A related phenomenon is the limited capacity of carnivora for dealing with fibrous foods, a matter which will need further consideration in connection with practical feeding. It suffices here to say that diets containing 10 per cent. or less of suitable proteins have been found adequate for the maintenance of dogs,[3] while foxes[4] and minks do not seem to show material departures from this standard, provided that the quality of the protein is good. In practice some latitude is usually allowed for safety.

So far as growing animals are concerned it has been shown that puppies flourish on a ration, the dry matter of which contains 20 per cent. of protein of average quality,[5] while earlier workers came to the conclusion that about 25 per cent. would be quite a suitable level.[6][7] In careful examination of the growths of fox pups on diets containing, on a dry matter basis, 13, 16, 19, 22, 25, 28, 34 and 40 per cent. of protein, respectively, American workers[8] found that, between weaning at 50 days and the end of the fastest growing period (161 days), the minimum needs lie between 22 and 25 per cent., while from 161 to 259 days the requirements fall to 19-22 per cent. In feeding practice 25-34 per cent. and 19-25 per cent., respectively, are recommended. A consideration of the rations fed to minks suggests that the same proportions are needed at corresponding ages, namely, 50-60 days and about 100 days.

Comparatively little work has been done on protein needs for reproduction and lactation in carnivorous species, but the general nature of development during pregnancy must require diets containing some 25 per cent. protein towards the end of that period. The milk of the bitch[9] is high in protein (8-9 per cent.) and in fat (11-12 per cent.) and, volume for volume, contains more than twice as much energy in the form of digestible nutrients as cow's milk. Feeding should thus be generous during the lactation period. Cow's milk is a weak substitute for the dam's milk when orphan pups are to be reared.

(iii) *Fat.*

There is a great variety of opinion as to the amounts of fat which should be included in the diets of carnivora. Quality is perhaps as important as quantity. Under natural feeding conditions, quite apart from the glyceride fraction of fats, this constituent of food is the vehicle for the necessary vitamin A. Dogs can thrive on diets containing as much as 40 per cent. of fat, provided that the large amount of fat in the ration does not lead to other necessary factors being present at too low a level. There is evidence that pups need about 10 per cent. after weaning; in this connection the high fat content of the milk of the bitch may be re-emphasised. The fat secreted in the milk is also more highly unsaturated than butter fat.[10] On the whole there seems to be sufficient reason for fixing the required fat intake for the growing dog at about 10 per cent. by weight of the ration: satisfactory diets for foxes have also contained about this proportion.

(iv) *Carbohydrate, mineral elements and vitamins.*

When once the intakes of protein, fat and total energy have been fixed, that of carbohydrate is also settled. The chief matter for consideration is, therefore, the nature of the carbohydrate to be fed; this is discussed later.

There is a good deal of evidence to suggest that the ratio of calcium to phosphorus in the diets of carnivores is extremely important. Perhaps because of the way in which the species have developed in the course of time, dogs and foxes seem to be very susceptible to rather slight changes in the Ca/P ratio. For example, in the heavier breeds of dogs a large intake (250 I.U./day) of vitamin D was found to be insufficient to prevent rickets when the Ca/P ratio was 1.7/1.[11] In the case of Great Danes 12 I.U./day sufficed for a ratio of 1.2 but there was very poor bone formation when the ratio was increased to 2/1.[12] Suitable limits for the Ca/P figure are about 1.2 to 1.4. Heavier animals seem to be more sensitive to imbalance than the light breeds. The nature of the carbohydrate fraction of the diet is also important, especially in very young animals (p. 15). Troubles have been encountered in fox-breeding very similar to those described above for dogs.

From a general aspect vitamin requirements have been dealt with in Section I and the following table merely adds greater detail. For convenience the data have all been referred to needs/Kg. bodyweight; the upper or even higher limits should be chosen for productive animals.

TABLE 140

Vitamin	Daily needs	Element		Daily needs
A	20-30 I.U.*	Calcium		127 mg.
D	10-20 I.U.	Phosphorus		67 mg.
Aneurin	15-25 μg.	Chlorine ⎫	as	
Riboflavin	25-50 μg.	Sodium ⎭	salt	149 mg.
Niacin	200-400 μg.			

*Twice as much carotene

The figures have been adapted from the suggestions of Michaud and Elvehjem." Data relating to mineral requirements have also been included. Although the lists are not complete, diets which can meet the figures quoted will probably be fairly satisfactory in respect of the remaining factors.

(b) Qualitative.

There is plenty of evidence to suggest that the needs of dogs—and hence, most probably, of foxes and minks—are very much the same as those of the rat. So far as the protein fraction of meat is concerned, there is thus no reason why meat should be an essential constituent of the diet. Other proteins, of vegetable origin, should be satisfactory, provided that they supply the necessary amino-acids in the desired amounts, and in fact dogs " and foxes " have been raised on rations devoid of animal protein.

When domestic animals such as the dog forgo their natural food, then, as previously explained, the meat they receive is not usually identical with what they themselves would catch and eat. Even when some meat is included in their rations there are good reasons for not leaving to chance their intakes of (a) vitamin A, (b) calcium and phosphorus and (c) members of the vitamin B-complex. For this reason it is advisable that the diet should always be supplemented with suitable sources of vitamin A, e.g., cod-liver oil, of calcium and phosphorus, e.g., good bone meal, and of members of the B-complex, e.g., dried yeast, or wheat germ, or a liver preparation. Where raw meat of good quality is to be had, then the need for the last item is less urgent, but no chances should be taken with the others, especially in the feeding of pups.

If meat is in short supply fish can be used quite well as a protein source; when it can be obtained dried milk is also very useful, especially for growing stock. Failing these substances—and it is seldom possible or even desirable that the whole of the protein in the ration should come from animal sources—protein of vegetable origin can be used. Provided that such foods are well chosen with respect to amino-acid composition, then dietary levels of protein very slightly, if any, higher than those which have been described in the previous paragraphs, should suffice. The proteins of cereals, oil-seeds and similar foods are all suitable, provided that certain precautions are taken. For dogs, rations of (a) 1 qt. of milk and 160 g. of bread per day, or (b) 1 qt. of milk plus (up to) 2,500 g. of potatoes and carrots per day have both proved satisfactory for periods of a year. It is not suggested that so simple a diet as this should be adopted; it merely illustrates the fact that meat is not always necessary.

Where the difficulty does occur is in the somewhat low digestibility of the carbohydrate fraction of the diet when foods of vegetable origin are used. Lössl [14] showed that for dogs the digestibility of the fibre of wheat meal or of boiled potatoes is very variable and that one cannot safely assume that this species will deal well with rations containing more than about 2 per cent. of fibre. In a similar manner Maynard and Loosli [15] showed that the mink has a limited capacity for digesting the fibre of cereals. Starch is fairly well absorbed (about 90 per cent. when it has been cooked but only 50-70 per cent. when raw) but a ration which contained 10 per cent. of wheat bran adversely affected general digestibility for minks, though not for foxes.[16] Cereals may thus be used, provided they are not too fibrous. Oil-seed cakes may also be fed if they satisfy these requirements, e.g., soya-bean meal has been used quite satisfactorily and likewise decorticated groundnut-cake meal. Some of these meals are also useful in providing reasonable proportions of fat. For preference, mixtures of vegetable proteins designed to exploit supplementary amino-acid relationships, should be used (p. 53).

(3) Practical feeding

(a) Introduction.

Dogs may not reach their mature bodyweights for many months, whereas the fox is mature in some 7 months, by which time the male may weigh 12-15 lb. and the vixen 10-12 lb. Mature weight, about 2.5 lb. in the male and 2.0 lb. in the female, is reached in five months in the mink. Despite these disparities of size the general systems of practical feeding for the several species are very much the same. As in the case of other animals, food and food utensils must be absolutely clean; vessels should not be left with food remains in them. Feeding should be regular and ample water should be allowed. When food is being mixed it should not be made in large batches and then left for long periods of time; where that has happened and certain kinds of fish have been included in the ration, the results have on occasion proved disastrous ("Chastek paralysis" through avitaminosis. B_1 in foxes). If some meat can be given raw, so much the better, provided its quality is assured;

where it has to be cooked, any liquor in which it is cooked should be included in the ration. When complex rations are being fed the food should be well ground, very thoroughly mixed and, if it is dry, made moist enough to be crumbly; it should not be possible for the animal to pick out particular fractions. Provided there is discretion in the selection of the ingredients, complex rations are likely to prove more suitable than very simple ones.

(b) The feeding of mature animals for maintenance and work.

Commercial breeders of foxes and minks usually feed the animals once daily, namely, in the evening; there is much to be said for the same system applied to dogs. The working dog in fact is generally fed in this manner.

Despite the fact that the teeth of carnivorous species are adapted for tearing flesh, present-day scarcity usually requires that meat should be minced thoroughly and mixed in well with the rest of the ration, which it will help to flavour.

Minks.

It has been the custom to provide a large proportion of the ration of mature minks in the form of meat. Of the daily ration of 4 to 5 oz. of food more than a half has taken this form, but economic considerations have caused less expensive diets to be sought.

Examples of diets which have been tried for minks, the first an American one using a considerable amount of meat [17] and the second a European one in which fish is extensively employed,[18] are given below.

TABLE 141

Ration 1		Ration 2	
	(Wt.)		(Wt.)
Fresh lean meat	10 parts	Fish waste	app. 80 parts
Fresh lamb liver	3 ,,	Slaughter-house offal ...	5 ,,
Canned fish	2 ,,	Vegetable feed	10 ,,
Lettuce	1 ,,	Bonemeal	1 ,,
Cooked cereal mixture * ...	5 ,,	Dried yeast	0.5 ,,

* Composition: Oatmeal 30, Yellow maize meal 22, Wheat middlings 25, Dried skim milk 10, D. yeast 5, Dried blood 5, Bonemeal 1, Gd. limestone 1.5, Iodised salt 0.5, Cod-liver oil 0.3.
(A mixture as complex as this is by no means essential.)

The meat usually given is horse flesh and the fish consists of the cheaper grades, while the cereal mixture of Ration 1, or a similar product, may often be purchased commercially. Ration 2 is reported to have been in satisfactory use during the period 1939-1945, at a farm where about 300 minks were kept and some 6,500 animals were reared.

American breeders have also substituted ground, fresh fish in place of half of the fresh meat allowance with quite good results. Dried meat is less successful than the fresh food, probably due to loss of digestibility through the drying process, or destruction of an essential amino-acid, or loss of a necessary non-protein fraction, or a combination of these causes. The cereal mixture in the ration can be a simple one of equal parts of oatmeal, maize meal and bread crumbs.

Foxes.

Mature foxes will need about 1 lb. per day of a mixed ration, which includes meat, fish and cereals. Smith[4] has stated that the amount of protein required is about 0.08 to 0.14 lb., depending on the size of the animal; too high a level is undesirable.

Meat and fish, either raw or dried, constitute a big proportion of the ration, often as much as one half to three quarters of the required protein. Fish has been used very widely; the precautions to be adopted in such cases to prevent a deficiency of aneurin have already been discussed. The rest of the protein may be derived from vegetable sources, soya-bean meal being a good one. Attention needs to be paid to the vitamin and mineral intakes.

A suggested ration is given in Table 142.

TABLE 142

Ingredient	%	Ingredient	%
Meat meal	4.8	Soya-bean meal (hydraulic) ...	4.8
Liver meal	2.4	Ground fresh vegetable ...	5.0
Bread crumbs	7.5	Oatmeal	7.5
Lucerne meal	2.5	Wheat germ	2.5
Fish meal	5.0	Ground green bone	5.0
Water	53.0		

Dogs.

These may be either pets or working animals; usually one finds a tendency to overfeed the former.

Commercially prepared foods are available, often in biscuit form. The value of these preparations depends very much on the nature and quality of the ingredients used in their manufacture.* They are customarily intended to be supplemented with other foods. In the following table are given four rations which have been found satisfactory, two of them involving the use of fresh meat, one requiring a certain amount of meat and fish scrap and the fourth deriving almost the whole of the protein from vegetable sources.

* When biscuits are purchased, information should be sought as to their composition. Neither the food value of the material, nor the way in which it can be incorporated in rations, can be gauged without such evidence.

TABLE 143

Ration 1	Ration 2	Ration 3		Ration 4	
g.	g.		%		%
Horse flesh,	Meat & Veg.	Maize, ground,		Maize	35
fresh ... 200	broth ... —	yellow ...	46	Bran	30
Biscuits,	Milk 400	Bran, fine,		Meat scrap ...	10
commercial 450	Bread 300	wheat ...	20	Fish	10
		Groundnut		Dried milk ...	10
		meal ...	29	Salt	1
		Cod-liver oil...	1	Bone meal ...	2
		Salt	1	Lucerne meal	2
		Bone meal ...	2-3		

Notes:—
(a). Ration 1, which was used at the Royal (Dick) Veterinary College, was satisfactory for moderate activity for dogs of about 27 Kg.; it provided 111 g. of protein and 23 g. of fat.
(b). The second ration was in use at a greyhound racing kennel. Of the 129 g. of protein it provided, 85 g. came from the meat and vegetable broth used.
(c). On a dry matter basis both rations 3 and 4 [19] provide more than 20% of total protein.

For the dog owner who wishes to make up rations, it is perhaps easiest to divide the foods to be given into three sections, one to provide protein mainly, a second one to give carbohydrate and the last to ensure good intake of minerals and vitamins. The following table shows how a variety of foods might be employed to this end.

TABLE 144

Supplying:	Foods	Weights
		Parts
Carbohydrate	Cooked potatoes, including carrots, beet, etc., from time to time.	3
	Breadcrumbs, or biscuit, or oatmeal, or ground maize.	4
Protein	Cooked, boned fish,* or Raw or cooked, minced meat,* or Soya meal, or Groundnut (dec.) meal.	2
Minerals and vitamins	Low-temperature blood meal.	0.25
	Wheat germ.	0.25
	Dried yeast or dried liver.	0.25
	Steamed bone flour or dried skim milk.	0.25
	Cod-liver oil (small daily dose).	
	Salt.	

* 1 Part of fish or meat meal may replace 3 parts of fresh or frozen food.

On a dry matter basis a ration of the above kind contains about 20 per cent. of dig. protein. One pound of this ration should provide

800-900 Cal. of digestible energy. The food is best mixed well and then made crumbly by the addition of gravy or other flavouring material. Bones may be supplied but they should not be of the kind which splinter easily. Variety should be aimed at with respect to the three different components, so far as circumstances will allow.

(c) Feeding for reproduction and lactation.

It is in feeding for reproduction and lactation that most skill and care is required. More attention has to be directed to the satisfaction of protein requirements and to ensuring that the supply of vitamins and minerals is adequate.

Whereas dogs, foxes and minks may only be fed once daily under ordinary routine conditions, it is usual to give pregnant and nursing animals two or three feeds. Animals to be used for breeding need to be well managed right throughout their lives; misguided economies in their youth may subsequently cause serious losses in breeding performance.

A ration which is evidently suitable for mink breeding has already been given in Table 141; feeding at higher levels of intake will be needed during lactation and the last third of pregnancy. In the case of foxes it does not seem to be essential to have more than about 20 per cent. of raw meat in the average ration; dried meat, and fish can usefully be employed, in conjunction with good, relatively non-fibrous, vegetable sources of protein such as groundnut, soya bean and linseed meals. Small amounts of wheat-germ meal, lucerne meal, blood meal, dried yeast and, where it can be obtained, milk, either raw or dried, are valuable additions, which are beneficial out of all proportion to the amounts involved. Small quantities of vegetables may be fed, but their fibre content and relatively low digestibility must be remembered. Bread and mixed cereals can be used. Cod-liver oil should also be given regularly; it is suggestive, though not conclusive, evidence of insufficiently high levels of vitamin A in the rations of foxes on breeding stations, that the amounts of vitamin A found in their livers have in some cases [20] been only about one-fiftieth of that in wild foxes. The ration given in Table 145 has been suggested as being suitable for feeding to foxes just before mating and during the reproductive period. [21]

TABLE 145

Ingredients	%	Dry mixture ingredients	%
Raw meat (muscle 7 pts., glandular 3 pts.)	40.0	Bread meal	16
Dry mixture given opposite ...	25.0	Oatmeal	16
Vegetables, finely grd., carrots,		Wheat-germ meal	16
lettuce leaf, tomatoes ...	10.0	Fish meal	16
Green bone, ground	5.0	Lucerne meal	8
Water	19.7	Dried skim milk	8
Cod-liver oil	0.3	Soya bean meal	8
		Linseed meal	4
		Wheat bran	4
		Brewers' yeast	4

Fish may replace one-quarter of the meat, while good quality dried meat can be used in equal amount (dry matter basis).

For dogs, modifications of the rations given in Table 144 will yield diets suitable for pregnant and lactating animals. The proportions of potatoes and bread may be reduced to 2 and 3 respectively and that of the protein supply, at least half of which should preferably be meat or fish, increased to 3 parts. During the last third of pregnancy the amount fed to the pregnant bitch will need to be increased to one and a half to twice as much as its maintenance allowance, while the quantity needed for lactation, though depending upon the number and sizes of the pups in the litter, may be expected to be about twice maintenance needs. In both pregnancy and lactation consideration of the needs of the individual animal is essential, for both under- and over-feeding are to be avoided. Apart from food, a supply of clean water must always be accessible.

In the case of these species there may be need for somewhat lighter feeding during the few days around the time of parturition.

(d) Feeding growing animals.

As in the case of other species, pups are best allowed to begin to eat small amounts of solid food before they are weaned, so that weaning may be a gradual process.

As the needs of growing animals are relatively high, dogs are usually given three feeds daily and foxes and minks in commercial breeding establishments two feeds a day. Towards maturity the number of feeds per day is reduced gradually to that given to grown animals.

Where the amount of food given to a mature non-breeding fox may be just under a pound a day, the pups are given 25 per cent. more than this during the active period of growth. It is customary to give just as much food as can be cleaned up at a single feed; in this way the demands of the growing animal are given full play. Feeding may be based on the diet of Table 145, lowering the intake of vegetable foods by half in the early stages of growth. Cod-liver oil, for its vitamin A and D content, must be given to speed up growth and to ensure good bone formation.

Another ration which has been found satisfactory for foxes is one in which fish (canned type), wheat-germ meal and ground wheat provided 71 per cent. of the total, potatoes 23 per cent., green vegetables 5 per cent. and dried yeast 1 per cent. This was suitable for feeding from weaning to slaughtering."

Diets which are suitable for raising minks have been given in Table 141; the modifications which may be suggested for the very young animals are simply those of cutting down the proportions of vegetables in the ration slightly during the early growth period.

In the case of the dog, weaning may take place at about 6 weeks of age, but before then the pups should have been offered cow's milk (where possible), with which a little minced meat, or fish, and bread or biscuit have been mixed. Gradually the nature of the diet may be changed. For this purpose the general diet of Table 144 may be taken as the basis. In early growth the vegetable and cereal fraction may be cut by about a half, meat and fish providing most of the animal protein. As the animal progresses towards maturity the amount of vegetable material can be increased and the proportion of animal protein decreased. Because of breed differences in size, it is not possible to give a time-table for this; instead it should be remembered that the period of rapid growth in most young animals is the first third of the time between weaning and maturity. American workers have proved that the protein requirements for growth when expressed as a fraction of the ration, are not different as between the large and small breeds.[5] Feeding should be done regularly, preferably from individual dishes or troughs; the animals are best allowed ten or fifteen minutes in which to clean up their quota, the vessel then being taken away. In early life the overall maintenance requirements of a pup may be twice that of a mature animal; half way to maturity they are likely to be one and a half times, but these figures are only rough guides.

(e) Probable dietary deficiencies.

The carnivora seem to depend upon dietary supplies of all of the vitamins, except perhaps vitamin C. Deficiencies of vitamin A and D, of members of the B-complex as a whole and of calcium and phosphorus are not uncommon. It should be remembered that in the development of nutritional science, the dog has been the animal which has been used to determine some of the undesirable consequences of deficiencies of vitamin A, vitamin D and niacin. More skill is needed in feeding carnivorous animals, especially in times of shortages of animal protein, than other types. Too low a protein intake may well produce deficiencies of other factors.

REFERENCES

1. Dechambre, P., (1919). Receuil Med. Vet., *95*, 220.
2. Brody, S., (1945). "Bioenergetics and Growth."
3. Melnick, D., and G. R. Cowgill, (1937). J. Nutrition, *13*, 401.
4. Smith, G. Ennis, (1935). Rept. Supt. Canad. Exp. Fox Ranch.
5. Heiman, V., (1947). J. Amer. Vet. Med. Ass., *111*, 304.
6. Lössl, H., (1932). Zeitschr. Hundeforschung, *2*, 95.
7. Morgan, A. F., (1935). Vet. J., *91*, 204.
8. Harris, L. E., C. F. Bassett, L. M. Llewellyn, and J. K. Loosli, (1947). J. Animal Sci., *6*, 486.
9. Daggs, R. G., (1931). J. Nutrition, *4*, 443.
10. Campbell, D. M., (1938). Vet. Med., *33*, 470.
11. Morgan, A. F., (1940). N. Amer. Vet., *21*, 476.
12. Michaud, L., and C. A. Elvehjem, (1944). Nutrition Abs. Rev., *13*, 323.
13. Koehn, C. J., (1942). Alabama Polytech. Inst., Agric. Exp. Sta. Bull., No. 251.
14. Lössl, H., (1934), quoted by E. Mangold. Nutrition Abs. Rev., *3*, 647.
15. Loosli, J. K., and L. A. Maynard, (1939). Proc. Amer. Soc. Animal Prod., 400.

16. Bernard, R., S. E. Smith, and L. A. Maynard, (1942). Cornell Vet., *32,* 29.
17. Hodson, A. Z., and L. A. Maynard, (1938). Amer. Fur. Breeder, *10,* 38.
18. Nordfeldt, S., (1947). Nutrition Abs. Rev., *18, 453.*
19. Michaud, L. M., and C. A. Hoppert, (1947). J. Amer. Vet. Med. Ass., *111,* 390.
20. Holmes, A. D., F. Tripp, F. G. Ashbrook and C. E. Kellogg, (1941). U.S. Dept. Int. Wildlife Res. Bull., No. 3., 15.
21. Kellogg, C. E., (1939). U.S. Dept. Agric. Yearbook, 871.
22. Lunde, G., and E. Mathiesen, (1939). Nutrition Abs. Rev. *9,* 496.

POULTRY

(1) Introduction

In Section III of this book some comparison was made between the anatomy of birds and that of mammals from the nutritional point of view. It was pointed out that in birds the mouth is far better adapted for picking up small particles than for dealing with finely divided foods, that grinding of ingested food by the gizzard replaces mastication, that the digestive tract is of a relatively simple type, incapable of dealing with large proportions of fibrous food, and that the taste and smell of food appear to be less important as measures of palatability than colour and brightness.

Poultry are kept for two main purposes, either as producers of eggs or as birds for the table. To some extent the two purposes are quite distinct, there being nothing very closely resembling, for example, the dual-purpose breeds among mammals. The best table bird is a young one, the flesh of a fowl which has had two seasons as a laying bird being generally of a lower quality. These two purposes naturally influence the feeding systems which may be used.

Under natural conditions birds will consume grass and other green foods, seeds and berries, and insects, but man's selection of heavier birds, or those with high egg production, for breeding purposes, has altered the position somewhat. More intensive systems of production have involved demands for increased intakes of food which natural conditions cannot often meet. More concentrated supplies of foods have been sought for poultry feeding. A policy of this kind creates new problems since it requires two fundamental questions to be answered;

first of all the specific needs of birds under various conditions must be examined and, secondly, very full knowledge of the chemical composition of foods is necessary. Partly for economic reasons and partly because birds are very convenient creatures easily handled in fairly large groups, with relatively small food requirements and rapid growth rates, a vast amount of research has been carried out on them during the last three decades or so.

From the point of view of broad nutritional principles the feeding of birds does not differ from that of mammals, but there are differences of detail which are interesting scientifically and important economically.

So far as present knowledge goes the order of increasing difficulty in feeding is roughly adult ruminants, herbivorous species of mammals, omnivorous animals like the pig and, finally, carnivorous animals and birds in intensive production. Not all of the known nutritional factors need be supplied preformed in the ration of a cow, whereas the list for poultry is of formidable length. The practical feeding of birds requires considerable care if the best results are to be obtained. It is of interest to note that leg troubles of three kinds and involving three different groups of factors, namely vitamin D, riboflavin, and the manganese-choline-biotin group, can arise in birds as the result of faulty feeding. Furthermore, birds require vitamin D_3 and not calciferol, which is relatively ineffective for them.

Compared with mammals, young birds seem to have generally higher growth rates, so that suboptimal feeding has worse effects in the case of chicks than in, say, calves.

Among birds there are distinct species differences with respect to growth; for example, the optimal growth rate of the turkey poult is distinctly higher than that of the chick and it is correspondingly easier to fail to meet the greater nutritional requirements involved.

In many ways the intense laying bird demonstrates new aspects of feeding principles. Whereas the feeding of mammals usually involves a consideration of calcium and phosphorus intakes together, the fact that egg-shell consists largely of calcium carbonate necessitates special attention being given to calcium. Although the disastrous results of poor feeding at critical reproductive stages in the life of mammals has been discussed on many occasions in preceding chapters, the fact that the mammalian egg is small, rather difficult to handle and is so soon embedded in the uterine wall, hinders close observation of the precise effects of dietary changes upon its development. On the other hand the avian egg lends itself to the study of such phenomena as the effects of diet upon the hatchability of eggs or upon the early growth of the chicks.

(2) The general feeding of birds

At appropriate stages the separate nutritional requirements for growth and egg production will be considered; in this section the general nature of the foods and feeding systems which are suitable are briefly surveyed.

(a) Suitable foods.

Birds require protein, fat, carbohydrate (very small amounts of fibre), vitamins A, D, E and K, almost the whole range of the B-complex, together with the usual inorganic elements. Further attention will need to be paid later to these requirements; here they are mentioned because they tend to limit the foods which may be fed to birds for intensive production, to the following chief classes:

(i) Grass and other green foods, in limited amounts.

(ii) Cereal grains and cereal by-products of low fibre content.

(iii) Oil-seed meals, of limited fibre content.

(iv) Animal proteins, such as fish meal, which are used most efficiently when they supplement vegetable sources.

(v) Cod-liver oil, or other source of vitamins A and D_3.

(vi) Potent sources of the vitamin B-complex, such as dried yeast and the several grades of bran.

(vii) Mineral supplements, especially of calcium carbonate and common salt.

(viii) Insoluble grit for increasing the efficiency of digestion.

These requirements are fairly exacting.

(b) Feeding systems.

Where the birds have free range of pasturage of good quality, the feeding problem is simplified, since grass supplies so many necessary dietary factors. In such cases a supplement of suitable concentrates may be fed.

The form in which concentrates are given, either as part of the ration of birds on free range or almost the whole of the ration on battery systems, is important. There are the possible alternatives of feeding mixtures of cereal grains, etc., more or less as they are purchased, of grinding the ingredients fairly coarsely and giving the mixture dry (dry mash), of giving the mixture after sufficient water has been added to it to make it just crumbly (wet mash), or of mixing the ingredients very well and then pelleting them.

The first method has the disadvantage that the birds may select portions of the food, e.g., whole grains, the appearance of which attracts them, while perhaps neglecting the finely divided materials, e.g., bran, which are necessary to balance the ration.

By the second method of feeding the matter of selection is disposed of. If, however, some of the ingredients to be used are rather powdery, there may be difficulties for the birds in picking up and swallowing such material. Furthermore, the rate of deterioration of vitamin A supplements, when mixed in such dry mashes, is rather high. Nevertheless, dry mashes have been and still are in extensive use.

Wet mashes are an improvement on dry ones in so far as birds may consume more food in a given time and with less difficulty. Furthermore, there tends to be less food scattered, but more attention is needed in seeing that no food remains to become sour.

The commercial pelleting of foods has greatly increased during recent years. By pelleting the ingredients, the possibility of the preferential selection of any one of them is removed. The size of the pellets may be suited to the age of the birds, the rate of food intake is increased, the food is easily handled and is not so easily scattered, and vitamin concentrates are rather more stable. The disadvantages of this method of feeding are that the breeder has no control of the composition of the pellets (it would not be economic to buy pelleting machinery except for a very large output). However, reputable firms find that it pays to produce as efficient a product as possible, while the general composition of pelleted poultry foods in Britain is now controlled by law (Appendix 2).

In practice all of the systems described, and combinations of some of them, are in use and, provided that the possible drawbacks of each (questions of labour as well as nutritional principles are involved) are realised and steps are taken to meet them, they work well. From time. to time research papers appear giving the results of comparative trials made to determine which is the best method. Such trials seldom reveal outstanding differences between the methods, as for example the feeding of pellets as opposed to mash,[1][2] but one should not forget that the trials are carried out by skilled personnel who are fully aware of the possible difficulties. It by no means follows that the same results will be obtained by unskilled or careless hands.

It is not easy to feed laying birds on the individual basis which can be used for dairy cows. Usually the feeding standards, which have been determined for various circumstances, have to be used for the feeding of groups of birds rather than for individuals. This does not mean, however, that records of food intake and of egg production should not be kept; it is only by the use of records that the poorly productive birds can be culled.

(3) The feeding of chickens

(a) Maintenance requirements.

A number of workers have reported data for the maintenance needs of chickens. In the following table, estimates for total nutrients, made by Halnan for British breeds of poultry,[3] and by Brody[4] and Titus[5] in America, are given. Halnan's figures were given in terms of starch equivalent which, for comparison with the other results, have been converted into the approximately corresponding weight of a basic layer's mash.

TABLE 146

Weight of bird. lb.	Maintenance needs (g.)				
	Halnan		Brody	Titus	Halnan Dig. protein
	S.E.	Feed			
3	47.5	76	63	‥	1.9
3.6	50*	80*	67	64	—
4	51.8	82	72	—	2.5
5	56.0	88	85	—	3.1
6	60.2	95	96	—.	3.7
	* Calculated				

Considering the nature of the assumptions made for the purposes of calculation, the agreement is very good. The data of Halnan are based on several years' trials and it will be noticed that he suggests the use of a more liberal allowance than Brody. Present evidence points to Halnan's data being the more useful, since Brody himself has obtained results which indicate that his standards are too low for the smaller birds.

The important point, as in the case of mammals, is that the maintenance needs of small birds are higher in proportion to their body weights than those of large fowls.

Halnan's estimates of the quantities of digestible protein required per day, when calculated as a percentage of the total calories required for maintenance, lie approximately in the range 4-6 per cent., which is somewhat lower than the general level of 10 per cent. suggested in Section III. The difference is not a significant one, however, when it is remembered that the estimated 10 per cent. assumes the intake of proteins of rather low biological values, whereas fowls are usually fed well-balanced protein rations.

(b) Feeding for egg production.

(i) *Efficiencies of conversion of organic nutrients.*

The additional food which is necessary for egg production depends upon the number of eggs produced in a given time, the quantity of nutrients present in the average egg and the efficiency with which the fowl is able to convert the substance of the ingested food into that of eggs.

Although the composition of an egg is by no means invariable,[6] the following data, which are given by Halnan,[3] suffice for the purposes of making an estimate of the food needed for egg production. Fat, concentrated almost exclusively in the yolk, accounts for about 10.5 per cent. of the weight, protein, which is distributed between both white and yolk, constitutes 10.9 per cent., the shell 9.1 per cent., water 68.6 per cent. and the ash, apart from that of the shell, 0.9 per cent. The main variations are not usually to be found in these major components of the egg, but in the amounts of trace factors which help to determine hatchability, etc.

An average egg weighs about 2 oz., or, in more conveniently rounded figures, 50 g. With regard to protein, therefore, the formation of an egg means the production of 5-6 g. of egg protein. If the efficiency of conversion of digested food protein to egg protein were 50 per cent., the production of one egg per day would involve a protein intake of 10-12 g. of digestible protein, while an efficiency of only 33 per cent. would increase the requirements to 15-18 g. When these figures are compared with the amount of maintenance protein for a bird of 6 lb. weight, one may see that requirements for egg production are indeed high.

The total digestible nutrients of an average egg are about 17-20 g. Here again efficiencies of conversion of absorbed food into egg nutrients of 100, 50 and 33 per cent. would require corresponding intakes of about 18, 36 and 54 g. respectively, compared with maintenance needs of the order given in Table 146.

Various workers have shown ' that this net efficiency of energy conversion is usually about 50%, the corresponding value for protein being about half as great again (68%). Practical poultry breeders, however, are more interested in gross efficiencies, which take into account both (a) the food used for the maintenance of the bird and (b) the number of eggs produced in a given period. Naturally the allowance under (a) depends upon the size of the bird, but for birds of about 4 to 5 lb. weight, as for example, White Leghorns or Leghorn-Rhode Island crosses, the efficiencies are approximately those given in the following table.

TABLE 147

Eggs produced per year.	Gross efficiencies, %		
	Energy.	Protein.	Fat.
100	8	15	2
200	13	30	5
300	17	40	6
400	20	45	7

These represent the efficiencies which may be attained by good general poultry husbandry; much lower ones are likely to result from poor feeding. Halnan ' quotes percentages, over two year periods, as follows: energy, 22%, and protein, 33%.

(ii) Practical feeding

The fundamental requirements remain the same no matter what system of feeding is adopted. Halnan suggests that the needs for the production of a 2 oz. egg are generally satisfied when 12.5 g. of dietary protein and 38 g. of starch equivalent (about 50 to 60 g. of ordinary concentrate mixtures) are provided. If one has a knowledge of the anticipated egg production the daily needs for maintenance and egg production may easily be calculated. Where pullets are concerned the food given must cover maintenance needs, egg production and, in addition, the final growth which the bird has still to make. The demands made by the moult are dealt with separately in this chapter. There are various slight difficulties in the application of these nutritional principles caused by the different feeding systems which are in use, so that the following examples are general ones capable of being modified to some extent.

All-mash feeding.

In the case of all-mash feeding, whether the mash is wet or dry, the food must contain protein and total digestible nutrients in the right proportions for combined maintenance and production. For example, a 4 lb. bird would need 52 g. of starch equivalent for maintenance and 38 g. for the production of one egg per day, the total being 90 g. Corresponding figures for digestible protein would be 2.5 g. and 12.5 g., a total of 15 g. The mash, therefore, must provide protein and starch equivalent in the ratio of 15 : 90, or 1 : 6. Now most cereal grains have a corresponding ratio of about 1 : 8 and the protein concentrates one of 1 : 1 or 1 : 2. Mixtures of cereals and protein concentrates may be mixed to give the desired ratio by the use of the method described elsewhere (Ch. 19). In the course of many years of research, however, it has been found that there are certain combinations of foods which are best suited for the purpose and, in Table 148 below, this experience is summarised [8] in a general ration for feeding with grain.

TABLE 148

Ingredients	%
Ground cereal grains and their by-products	56–68
Minimum animal protein supplements	7–9
Additional protein supplements	12–14
Riboflavin supplements (potency 20 μg./g.)	5–7
Lucerne meal, dehydrated	4–10
Bone meal or rock phosphate (defluorinated). app.	1
Ground limestone. app.	2

In this general type of ration, all of the needs of the laying hen are considered except the extra supply of vitamins A and D it is desirable to include (as cod-liver oil, or a similar concentrated source) and grit, the flint type about once a month and limestone when laying is established.

As examples of the useful supplementary relationships it is advantageous to exploit in rations for poultry one may mention (a) the excellent properties of soya-bean meal when combined with maize meal and maize gluten or with maize meal and wheat middlings, (b) maize gluten when combined with blood meal, and (c) sesame meal and soya-bean.

Rations of this general kind can be pelleted, of course, and the same feeding principles apply. The amount which it would be necessary to feed per day would be about 150 g. or 5-6 oz., for a bird of average weight, since such rations furnish about 60 g. of starch equivalent per 100 g. of food. In the case of birds which are to be used for breeding, extra care must be taken to include in the rations all those factors which are concerned in good hatchability and in a high survival rate of the hatched chicks. This usually involves particular attention to the vitamin and mineral elements of the food.

In Table 149 are given four suggested rations, each of which contains about 12 per cent. of digestible protein and a starch equivalent of 60-70. They are thus balanced for a high rate of egg production.

TABLE 149

Ingredients	Ration 1	Ration 2	Ration 3	Ration 4
Ground yellow maize ...	37.2	41.0	44.0	23.5
Sussex ground oats	10.0	10.0	10.0	10.0
Wheat bran	6.0	10.0	—	15.0
Middlings	20.0	10.0	16.0	35.0
Dried milk	5.0	5.0	5.0	5.0
Meat meal	2.0	4.0	2.0	—
Fish meal	2.0	—	2.0	3.0
Lucerne meal	7.0	7.0	7.0	5.0
Soya-bean meal	2.5	4.5	5.0	—
Linseed meal (hydr. process)	2.0	2.0	2.0	—
Salt	0.6	0.6	0.6	0.5
Cod-liver oil	1.4	1.4	1.4	1.5
Ground limestone	3.3	3.0	2.5	—
Steamed bone meal	1.0	1.5	2.5	—
Dried yeast	—	—	—	2.5
Literature reference ...	(9)	(9)	(9)	(3)

The American author stipulates the inclusion of about 2 per cent. of manganese sulphate in the salt to be used.

Mash-and-grain feeding.

In the mash-and-grain system, a mash is fed together with one or more of the suitable cereals, such as wheat, clipped oats, kibbled maize, barley (screened to remove the awns), or dari. Since the cereal grains have a relatively low ratio of digestible protein to total nutrients, they need to be balanced with a mash containing a high proportion of protein. The cereal fraction of the diet may be used to provide maintenance (a little more than maintenance in the case of the protein) leaving the mash to be fed in proportion to the egg production of the birds. The system is flexible, therefore, but needs some skill in its execution. If the birds have no access to grass, then kale or other green food should be supplied, or else good grass or lucerne meal should be included in the mash. As a source of calcium some limestone grit, in addition to flint grit, may be provided. Cod-liver oil will furnish vitamins A and D. In this type of management, 1.5 to 2.0 oz. of the grain is given to each bird, most of it being fed at the end of the day, with the mash given at midday. Naturally the composition of the mash will depend upon the weight of the birds concerned (since this determines maintenance needs), their egg production and the quantity and kind of cereal grains available. For cases where one-third to half of the total food is to take the form of cereals, suitable mashes could be framed on the basis of the proportions of the various ingredients of the four rations of Table 149; the proportions of the various ingredients to be used would be those in the table, but excluding the oats, maize and, in Ration 4, some of the middlings.

Birds on free range.

Where the birds have access to fresh grass it is more difficult to assess the amount of supplementary food to give them. One authority believes that the amount of food saved by grass is only about 5 per cent.; nevertheless it enables some of the ingredients such as lucerne meal, which are included for the sake of their vitamin content, to be reduced or even omitted from the ration. A suitable ration would be, ground maize, 20; fine ground oats, 10; bran, 20; middlings, 40; fish meal, 10.

So far as the fibre contents of rations are concerned, the best guide is chemical analysis; a fibre content of 10 per cent. is probably the acceptable upper limit. Apart from analyses, a rough guide to the dietary suitability of a dry, mealy ration is the volume 1 oz. of it occupies when it has been placed in a 100 ml. measuring cylinder and gently tapped once. A volume of more than 70 ml. indicates too bulky a food.

Feeding on kitchen scraps and balancer meal.

One of the most difficult cases of all now has to be considered, that of the small, " backyard " poultry keeper, who, in Britain, has to manage with household scraps, supplemented by " balancer meal." The latter is a protein concentrate, consisting of wheat offals, maize or maize by-products, oil-seed meals, some animal protein, barley, and brewers' by-products, together with bone flour. It is assumed that the household waste, consisting largely of potatoes, bread, meat scraps, etc., will supply rather more than the maintenance quota for a laying bird, provided that the food is not a mixture of fibrous vegetable materials. Balancer meal, given at the rate of about 2 oz. per bird each day, supplies the rest of the food for production. Cod-liver oil (1-2 per cent. of the dry matter, or in the proportion of 1-2 oz. for 10 days rations), flint and limestone grits, and a little fresh green food, such as cabbage, need to be fed. The total feed per bird should not amount to more than about 12 oz. per day.

The final matter to be considered in this section is the way in which the diet influences the number of eggs which are produced for breeding and the proportion of these which ultimately yield healthy chicks. A useful review of this field has been made by Cruickshank.[*]

(iii) *Diet in relation to breeding.*

The quantities of nutrients which are needed for the production of eggs, a high proportion of which will give healthy chicks, ready to utilize efficiently the food they are offered soon after hatching, are greater than those needed for egg production for human food.

As in the case of milk production in dairy cattle, it is true to a first approximation that the results of underfeeding of laying birds, so far as the amounts of total energy and protein supplied are concerned, are mainly loss of production; fewer eggs are produced under such circumstances. Besides total energy and protein, calcium must be regarded as a major component of the diet of a laying bird, since the average egg contains about 2 g. of calcium, mainly as calcium carbonate, in the shell. Such an amount of calcium is equivalent to about 5 g. of chalk or limestone. If one assumes that a good laying bird will receive some 150 g. of food per day and that the efficiency of utilization of the calcium carbonate of the ration is about 66 per cent., then the diet will need to include about 5 per cent. of calcium carbonate for the formation of good egg-shell. The need for including in the ration of laying birds a good supply of chalk, bone meal and limestone grit, is thus apparent; in the absence of adequate calcium, soft-shelled eggs will be produced and, apart from their susceptibility to damage, their hatchability is low. A detailed review of calcium and phosphorus metabolism in poultry has been made by Tyler.[10]

From what has been said in Section I, concerning the functions of the vitamins, and because the chick embryo has to depend for its development on the supplies of nutrients present in the egg, one may judge that there are many dietary factors concerned in the proportion of fertilised eggs which ultimately produce healthy chicks.

Of the fat-soluble vitamins A and D are needed, while, in the absence of vitamin E, the chick embryos may die as soon as the second day of incubation. In the absence of vitamin K the resulting chicks may die of hæmorrhage following trivial injuries, such as wing-banding.

Fairly high levels of intake of riboflavin, pyridoxine and pantothenic acid are essential for satisfactory growth of the embryo chick. Although the effects of simple deficiencies of single vitamins have been described in Section I, it is foolish to treat the feeding of breeding poultry simply as a matter of supplying so much of each of the vitamins. Foods which are known to be potent sources of all the members of the B-complex should find their place in the ration.

Of the inorganic elements, manganese has received some attention. In laying and breeding birds, a dietary deficiency of manganese leads to lowered production and poor hatchability. It may be necessary to increase the manganese content of a ration not because the element is usually lacking in foods but because the large amounts of calcium given to laying birds tends to have an adverse effect on manganese absorption.

The sequence of events in the formation of an egg has a nutritional significance. Yolk formation is rather slow and begins several days before the egg is laid, while the production of the white and of the shell are events which occupy only about the last day. The yolk is rich in protein and fat, the latter containing the fat soluble vitamins. It follows that dietary changes can have relatively little influence upon the nature of the egg produced until a number of days after they have been made; conversely the results of faulty feeding are liable to persist for some time after this has been corrected.

The colour of egg yolk is no certain indication of its vitamin A potency, since the yellow is due, not to carotene or vitamin A, but to xanthophyll. Since most foods which are rich in xanthophyll are also good sources of cryptoxanthin and carotene, a deeply coloured yolk usually indicates a high level of vitamin A. On the other hand, laying birds which have received little green food or maize, but have had supplies of cod-liver oil, may lay eggs with pale yolks of high vitamin A potency.

(c) Feeding for growth.

(i) Fundamental bases.

In the early stages birds grow very rapidly, as the following table reveals. For the satisfactory development of chicks two things are necessary, (a) good feeding of the hen, so that the newly emerged chick is well fitted to take advantage of the food which is offered to it and (b) a correspondingly high level of intake of nutrients at the times after emergence when it is most needed. Because birds depend upon ingested food for almost the whole range of vitamins, it is essential that the diet offered should be well-balanced and complete. The data of Table 150 are based upon results reported by Halnan,[3] for White Leghorn and Light Sussex breeds.

TABLE 150

Age of chicks (weeks) ...	2	4	6	8	10	12	14	16	20	24	28
Total energy of body substance (100 cal.) ...	1.1	1.9	3.0	4.0	5.4	7.4	9.6	12.4	20	24	32
Increase (per cent.) over previous figure	—	70	60	33	35	36	30	29	—	20	33
Protein content of body (g.)...	11	24	37	54	75	98	128	160	280	340	380
Increase (per cent.) over previous figure	—	120	50	45	40	30	30	25	—	22	13
Ash content of body (g.) ...	1.5	4.0	7.0	11	16	21	29	38	65	90	95
Increase (per cent.) over previous figure	—	170	75	60	50	30	40	30	—	40	6

Halnan declares that the data show the great need for both protein and inorganic elements in the early phase of growth; he has constructed rations for growing birds which are designed to meet these needs (Table 151).

Quite apart from the weights of nutrients which must be supplied for chicks, the rates of increase of the body constituents, when calculated as a percentage of those existing at the beginning of short successive periods of time, are also of interest. Increases of 70 per cent. of the total energy of the body, of 120 per cent. of its protein content and of 170 per cent. of its mineral matter between the second and fourth weeks of the life of the chick, illustrate the high metabolic rates which must be involved and the need for the provision of a ration complete in all respects. They also show how, as in the case of mammals, the requirements of the organism are for the development of the bones, the muscles and for fat formation in that order.

The problem which arises is how these needs are best met. As the capacity of chicks for digesting fibrous foods is quite limited they must be given concentrated foods of low fibre content. Even at the age of six months, a substantial proportion of the energy stored in the body substance is protein. The precise fraction of the dietary energy which should take the form of digestible protein depends upon the biological value of the latter, and several groups of workers have carried out feeding tests to obtain information on the matter.

American workers showed that as the protein content of chick rations increased from 13 to 21 per cent. of the feed, it was used with increasing efficiency for growth, whereas a continued increase to 25 per cent. then produced a sharp fall in percentage utilization.[11] They found, too, that so long as the percentage did not fall below 13 per cent., it made little difference to the magnitude of the final live weight, although that weight was attained in increasingly long times as the protein content of the ration fell. Other workers have made similar observations. The practice to be followed depends on the purpose for which the bird is required. If it is a table bird, then quick growth and fattening are desired, but where the bird is to be used for egg production, all that is necessary is to have it in good condition by the time it comes into lay.

As protein concentrates are relatively expensive foods, they should be used efficiently. In the chapter on proteins (p. 53) some account was given of the supplementary values of proteins. It was pointed out that cereal proteins tend to be deficient in lysine, while groundnut, soya, yeast and legume seed proteins are relatively poor in methionine. Combinations of these proteins can produce mixtures which are of higher biological value than the individual constituents.

For growing chicks a mixture of ground maize, maize gluten and soya-bean meal, such that the separate ingredients contribute 25 per cent., 33 per cent. and 42 per cent. respectively of the protein of a ration (the level of protein in the ration being 16 per cent.) was shown to have a high biological value, while a mixture deriving its protein from ground maize, wheat middlings and soya-bean meal in the proportions of 25 per cent., 33 per cent. and 42 per cent., was even slightly better.[12] Earlier work[13] had revealed good supplementation between maize gluten and soya-bean meal, between meat scraps and soya-bean meal and between maize gluten and fish meal, but the good effects of mixtures using fish meal depend on its method of preparation, which should be a low temperature process.

Sunflower-seed meal,[14] rape-seed meal[15] and groundnut meal[16] for growing chicks may be used successfully when they are included in balanced rations. It is to be expected that more extensive use of oil-seed proteins will become common as knowledge of their value for supplementing animal and vegetable proteins increases.

More recently work has been carried out to determine whether combinations of vegetable proteins are sufficient for optimum growth or not. On the whole they seem to be less efficient than mixtures containing animal proteins, but part of the effect seems to be due, not to proteins, but to other factors, probably members of the vitamin B-complex which are present in the animal proteins."

(ii) *The practical feeding of chicks.*

It being assumed that housing is good, with plenty of room for the birds, and that water is freely available at all times, the chief points connected with the feeding of chicks are (a) whether the birds are intended for table use or for egg production, (b) the nature of the diet in relation to the age of the chick, (c) what physical form the diet should take and, (d) how often the feeds should be given.

Birds which are for early table use may be fed at a higher level than others, as already explained. It is the usual practice to feed a diet containing 16-20 per cent. of protein until the chicks are about six weeks old, following which, over a period of a month, the ration is changed gradually to one containing 14-16 per cent. of protein. The next change, to a layer's ration, may be more rapidly brought about and will be made when the birds are about six months old.

Some suggested all-mash rations are given in the following table:

TABLE 151

Ingredient	To 8 weeks			12 weeks on			Layer's basic ration
	1	2	3	1	2	3	
Maize, grd. yell.	19	33	30	32.5	45	39	45
Fine grd. oats ...	10	5	10	10	14	10	10
Bran, wheat ...	25	14	10	20	10	—	10
Middlings ...	24	23	10	18	20	16	26
Dry skim milk ...	10	7	10	6	—	10	—
Fish meal ...	—	7	—	7.5	6.5	5	7.5
Meat meal ...	—	—	10	—	—	5	—
Soya-bean meal	—	—	10	—	—	—	—
Linseed meal ...	—	3	1	—	3	—	—
Lucerne meal ...	5	—	8	—	—	5	—
Dried yeast ...	3	3	—	2.5	—	—	—
Cod-liver oil ...	1.5	2	0.5	1.5	1	0.5	1
Minerals* ...	2.5	3	1.5	2	0.5	0.5	0.5
Cottonseed meal†	—	—	—	—	—	8	—
Protein content, %	16	18	24	18	16	22	16
Literature ref. ...	(18)	(3)	(9)	(18)	(3)	(9)	(3)

* Containing 0.5% common salt, based on the ration.
† See Ch. 13 (4b).

Two of the rations quoted in the above table are American.

If the ration is given in the form of a wet mash, then, after the first 24 hours when only water and warmth will be needed, five feeds per day may be given until the chicks are about three weeks old. At that time the number may be reduced to four and then, at the age of five weeks or so, further reduced to three. From the age of three months onwards, two feeds per day are usually given.

When grain and mash are being fed, a small amount of pinhead oatmeal, maize grits, or cut wheat may be given to begin with. Subsequently increased amounts of whole wheat and kibbled maize may be fed and the nature of the mash changed. Since the grain contains rather a low proportion of protein for growth, the mash with which it is to be fed must contain rather more protein than the type given to birds on all mash rations. Such mashes might be as follows:

TABLE 152

Ingredient	Mash 1	Mash 2	Ingredient	Mash 1	Mash 2
Ground yellow maize	25	—	Dried yeast ...	2.5	—
Fine ground oats ...	15	19	Soya-bean meal ...	—	5
Bran...	20	10	Cod-liver oil ...	1	2.8
Middlings	15	15	Limestone or chalk	0.8	5.6
Lucerne meal ...	5	15	Steamed bone meal	0.8	2.4
Dried skim milk ...	5	10	Salt	0.4	1.2
Fish or meat meal	7.5	10			
Linseed meal ...	2	4	Protein, % ...	18	21

The second ration contains 1 per cent. more protein than is now permitted in Britain in commercial baby chick foods; its content of dried milk is also too high. Substitution of some of the dried milk and/or fish meal by increased amounts of middlings or small amounts of potato flakes, would bring it into line. It contains all the limestone which is needed until egg production begins. The permissible upper limit for the protein content of a grower's mashes is 18 per cent. The second ration would need still further substitution in the manner indicated to make it conform.

Where there is access to grass still further changes, as suggested previously (p. 439), may be carried out in order to reduce the cost of feeding.

The amount of grain fed may be increased gradually to about half of the total amount of the ration by the time the birds are about three to four months old, the total quantity then fed being of the order of 3-4 oz. per day.

In the case of growing birds it is important that the ratio of the total amount of calcium ingested to the quantity of phosphorus in the diet should lie within the limits 1.5 : 1 to 2 : 1. An increase in the amount of calcium is not desirable until laying begins. Where a ration is being given which is well balanced with respect to calcium and phosphorus, no good would be done by giving limestone grit in addition to chicks.

(d) Fattening.

As soon as the cockerels can be distinguished from the pullets they should be separated and kept by themselves. They are generally reared under brooders in the same manner as pullets until 8 or 9 weeks old, but are then gradually hardened off and, if conditions are favourable, are transferred to folds or night arks in the fields; they may be caponised beforehand. There they remain until about 17 weeks old, when they are removed to fattening batteries, where they undergo a fortnight's special feeding, to be sold eventually at about 4 to 4.5 lb. If, however, they are to meet the demand for a smaller carcase, say 2.5 to 3 lb., the special fattening process is undertaken about 3 weeks earlier. In some cases ordinary crate feeding is supplemented by a process of cramming for a week or ten days.

When the birds reach 2 lb. in weight they can be put on a fattening diet and fed three times daily on a mixture composed of barley meal, middlings, and Sussex ground oats, mixed with milk to a proper consistency, when they will rapidly put on weight. Feeding is carried out in the crates three times daily.

The ration shown in Table 153 is said to give very good results:

TABLE 153

Ingredients			%	Ingredients			%
Ground maize	...	...	25	Middlings	...	...	20
Sussex ground oats ...		...	15	Meat and bone meal		...	5
Barley meal ...	...	...	10	Soya-bean meal	...	...	5
Bran ...	...	...	15	Dec. groundnut cake meal ...			4.5
				Salt ...	...	...	0.5

Where the birds are to be fed forcibly, i.e., crammed, the following mixture has been recommended by Halnan:[3]

TABLE 154

Ingredients			Parts	Ingredients			Parts
Fine ground oats	...	...	13	Melted mutton fat, or palm oil*			1
Dried skim milk	...	...	1	Water	...	...	20

* Other fats are suitable, if not of too low melting point.

The fat of fowls, like that of cattle, has a colour which is characteristic of the breed, that is, some have deeply pigmented fat while in others it is white. If the pigmented foods are withheld for a reasonable length of time from those whose fat is normally yellow, then the colour becomes greatly reduced and approximates to that of the other breeds.

Green vegetables as well as grass, clover and such like meal, yellow maize and carrots should be avoided when one is fattening fowls of breeds in which there is a tendency to store the xanthophyll pigments, and their place should be taken by such relatively pigment-free foods as buckwheat, oats, potatoes and skim milk.

(e) The effect of diet upon the moult.

This can best be understood when it is realised that feathers represent about 26 per cent. of the total weight of a bird [2] and that at least once a year all the feathers must be renewed; during the first year of life there may even be four partial or complete moults. The feathers of the adult bird contain nitrogen equivalent to about 94 per cent. of protein, together with 1 per cent. of ash. Of the protein, the amino-acid, cystine, constitutes a large fraction, for which reason it is advisable during the moult to feed good supplies of protein rich foods and grain, so that the process may be hastened. Protein concentrates, which are rich in the sulphur-containing amino-acids, such as blood meal, meat meal, dried yeast, soya-bean meal and similar vegetable sources, should be fed. Sunflower, groundnut and sesame meals (dec.) appear to have useful amino-acid compositions from this point of view. If this supply is forthcoming and the bird is in sound health, the normal moulting period of 20 weeks can be reduced to some 8 or 9 weeks, not by a greatly increased rate of growth of the individual feathers but by the casting of considerable quantities of them at one time and their prompt replacement instead of the slow loss of a few feathers over a prolonged period.

If the need of food for feather production is embarrassed by a simultaneous demand for some other activity, such as egg-laying in the adult or growth and egg production in the pullet, then none of these processes can be carried on at maximum rate and moulting is slowed down. If the dietary protein supplied is sufficient for only one activity, moulting has preference, egg-laying ceases, and even growth may be suspended. When the extra needs of young birds coming into their first laying season are not met, a neck moult commences and the promising start in egg laying is brought to an abrupt end. Nevertheless the modern high producing adult hen can lay eggs and moult at the same time provided her nutritional needs are met.

When there is an economic advantage in so doing, the moult may be induced earlier than would otherwise be the case by a sudden, temporary restriction of the diet. When the moult has then begun it is hastened to completion by generous feeding, as described above. Good feeding will produce a resumption of laying or will increase egg production to its pre-moult level. Changes of management are liable to hasten the onset of moulting, but the likelihood is diminished if the plane of nutrition is made rather better than the previous one.

(4) The feeding of turkeys

Although the general feeding of turkeys does not differ in principle from the feeding of fowls, there are one or two points of detail which need consideration. Turkeys are bred for meat and, except for the increase of stock, not for egg production, so that, in the feeding of these birds, the emphasis is largely on growth.

(a) The food requirements of poults.

Under conditions of intensive production one of the factors which has made difficult the rearing of turkeys is the very high growth rate of the poult, a rate appreciably greater than that of the chick. A day old poult weighs about 2 oz., but, by the time it is six weeks old it may weigh as much as 2 lb., a sixteen-fold increase. At eight weeks of age the weight may be as great as 4 lb. Increases of this magnitude reveal the great potentialities of the poult for growth and, since the young bird depends upon its food for almost all of the vitamins, as well as minerals and proteins, it is not difficult to understand why there have been failures in producing these birds.

Although it is usual to give chicks no food during the first day after their emergence from the shell, it is inadvisable to do so with poults; there is experimental evidence to show that leaving this species without food for 24-48 hours increases the mortality rate in the young birds.[19]

The general feeding methods are the same as for chicks. For example, where there is intensive production the poults may be put on a wet mash until they are about 8 weeks old, when the ration is gradually changed to that of a grower's mash. Either all mash or a mash-and-grain method may be adopted; in the latter case it has been recommended that oats should constitute 70 per cent. of the grain which is fed. One difficulty which is encountered is that of inducing the poults to eat their first rations. This phenomenon has been encountered in research experiments, as well as in poult production for profit and there is possibly a palatability factor involved.[20] Usually chopped greens, or chopped carrots, sprinkled on the top of the mash, assists in the overcoming of this difficulty. A small amount of flint grit should also be scattered about for the birds to pick up. Ample room and an abundance of fresh water are necessary, while cleanliness of food troughs and good lighting in the houses are important.

Until the poults are five or six weeks old they need about five feeds per day; if a dry mash is used the troughs can be left open all day. Where a mash and grain system is being introduced the first and last feeds of the day may be of grain (or pellets). When the birds are six weeks old, the morning feed of grain is omitted, followed by one of the feeds of mash a few days later.

The general types of ration which are suitable at various stages of growth are rather like those given to chicks, except that more energy, and higher proportions of protein and vitamins are essential for optimum growth.

The protein needs of poults have received much attention and it has been suggested that they are about one quarter to one third as high again as those of chicks, when expressed as percentages of suitable rations.[9] Because of the shortage of animal proteins, attempts have been made (not always on the most logical basis) to use rations containing only vegetable proteins. For example, the first two rations of Table 155 contain only small amounts of vegetable protein and produce poults weighing about 3 lb. at eight weeks of age. On the other hand the next four rations show clearly that optimal growth had by no means been achieved in the first examples quoted. The workers [20] who presented the second group of rations conclude that " early poult growth can be markedly increased by raising the energy, protein and unidentified vitamin content of the ration ". They also came to the conclusion that the requirements of the poult for some of the unidentified factors, like those which have been isolated already, are higher for the poult than the chick. The remaining rations are specimens of those in use in Britain where, at present, it is difficult or impossible to meet the protein needs laid down by the American workers. Stress must be put on the fact that increase of protein alone will not necessarily improve growth.

TABLE 155

Ingredient	Ration number								
	1	2	3	4	5	6	7	8	9
Maize, ground ...	25.5	17	12.3	12.6	14.4	24.4	20	25	20
Sussex grd. oats	10	10	10	10	10	10	10	10	10
Crushed wheat ...	—	—	15	18	20	12	—	—	—
Bran, wheat ...	10	10	—	—	—	—	14	10	10
Middlings ...	10	15	—	—	—	—	35	17	36
Fish meal ...	—	—	6.5	3	—	—	—	9	11
Meat meal ...	4.5	4.5	—	—	—	—	3	—	—
Soya meal ...	30	29.5	36	36	36	36	5	—	—
Dried yeast ...	—	—	4	4	4	4	—	—	—
Lucerne meal ...	5	5	—	—	—	—	5	5	3
Dried milk ...	—	—	—	—	—	—	5	17	6
Buttermilk ...	—	—	7	7	7	7	—	—	—
Liver meal ...	2	1.5	3	3	2	—	—	—	—
Whey, dried ...	—	4.5	2	2	2	2	—	—	—
Bone meal ...	—	—	1.2	1.4	1.6	1.6	—	2	—
Limestone ...	2	2	1.5	1.5	1.5	1.5	—	—	3
Salt ...	1	1	0.5	0.5	0.5	0.5	1	1	1
Cod-liver oil ...	—	—	1	1	1	1	2	2	—
Literature ref. ...	(21)	(21)	(20)	(20)	(20)	(20)	(22)	(22)	(22)
Total protein, %	24	23	30	28	26	25	18	19	19
Veg. protein, % ...	20	20	23	24	23	24	14	9	11
Poults weight at 8 weeks (g.) ...	1366	1279	1748	1623	1183	953	—	—	—

Notes.
1. In rations 1 and 2, not actual liver meal but a liver and glandular concentrate was used.
2. The salt used in rations 1 to 6 was iodized.
3. In rations 3 to 6 dicalcium phosphate was used; bone meal could be employed quite well.
4. Rations 3 to 6 contained 250 p.p.m. of manganous sulphate; rations 1 and 2 were also enriched in manganese.

In rations 3 to 6 there are no wheat offals, foods less rich in fibre taking their place. Although research of this type shows the possible growth rates which can be achieved, it does not follow that it would necessarily be cheaper than rations producing slower rates of growth; such diets could be useful for meat production but probably not for breeding.

Finely ground oats only should be used for rations for poults. Where a mash-and-grain system is in use, Titus [9] suggests that oats (pinhead) should constitute 50 - 75 per cent. of the grain allowance, although English practice tends towards the employment of more cut-wheat and kibbled maize.

If the poults have access to grass. the rations need to be modified accordingly. Lucerne meal may be diminished in proportion or omitted altogether; the quantities of cereals may be increased slightly and the amounts of dried milk cut down. No hard and fast rules can be made to cover all such cases.

Diets must be balanced for the intense growth which is described by the American workers, who found, contrary to the reports of other experimenters [23]—who had probably failed to achieve balanced rations— that their birds showed good feathering, displayed no tendency to feather picking or cannibalism or to abnormal leg disorders.

With the high growth rates of turkeys are high requirements for vitamins, as the following table reveals; the data refer to 1 lb. of food.

TABLE 156

Species and condition	Requirements for					
	A I.U.	D I.U.	B₁ I.U.	B₂ μg.	Niacin mg.	Pantothenate μg.
Chick, growing ...	1500	180	180	1500	5	4300
Poult, growing ...	3600	360	180	1700	50	—
Chicken breeding ...	4700	540	180	1250	—	2500
Turkey, breeding ...	4700	540	180	1250	—	—

As previously indicated with reference to other species, calcium and phosphorus intakes are needed at higher levels when there are increased proportions of protein in the ration. For a level of 26% of protein in the diet, 2-2.5% of calcium and 1% of phosphorus are required.

Up to the age of eight weeks between 2.5 and 3 lb. of feed will be needed for each increase of 1 lb. of bodyweight; between two and six months the quantity required will increase to 4-6 lb., while in the last stages of growth and fattening, some 8-10 lb. are necessary. For growth after 2-3 months a ration such as that of No. 9 in Table 155 can be employed. In such circumstances the system in use might be to give a morning feed of 0.5 to 1.0 oz. of grain, to allow the dry mash *ad lib.* or to feed 3-4 oz. of the mash wet (or pelleted) during the middle of the day and to end with 1.5 to 2.0 oz. of grain in the evening. The allowance will need to be increased steadily as described above.

For breeding stock a ration containing ground maize 30, finely ground oats or barley 20, middlings 22, bran 5, dried skim milk 5, meat meal 4, fish meal 3, lucerne meal 5, ground limestone 4, salt 0.5, and cod-liver oil 1.5%, is suitable when given as a mash. Flint grit would be needed. Where the birds have access to fresh green food, or are receiving grain supplements, the ration is modified in accordance with principles already described.

(5) The feeding of ducks

The feeding of ducks is determined partly by their being used for meat and, though to a lesser extent, for egg production and partly by their nature, for though the rest of the digestive system is very like that of the fowl, the beak is adapted to dealing with a different, moister type of food. According to Titus,[*] both ducks and turkeys require less food than chickens to attain any given bodyweight up to 5 lb.

The various mixtures of grains and meals supplied to hens are equally suitable for ducks, but the method of feeding should be modified to suit the requirements and general habits of the latter. While the hen employs feet as well as beak in her search for food, the duck is dependent solely on her blunt shovel-like bill, as her webbed feet are not adapted for scratching. A duck's bill is admirably fitted for tearing herbage and for sifting mud and water in which is found the animal food that forms such a large part of the bird's diet. Under artificial conditions her food consists largely of grain and mash, but the " sifting " instinct still remains. In order to satisfy this instinct, the grain may be given in the drinking dishes, so that the ducks have to seek for it. Mash on the other hand should not be given near water, as much of it will be wasted in the " sifting " process; it should always be fed wet, not sloppy, but mixed to the same consistency as for hens. A good plan is to give the ducks their mash in their house after they have been shut up for the night. They should be kept shut in till about ten o'clock in the morning as they usually lay early in the day.

If ducks have their liberty they will find a great deal of their own food, particularly if they have access to a stream or a pond. All that they require in the way of additional food is a light feed of grain in the morning and wet mash when they come home at night. Ducks greedily devour small animals such as slugs, tadpoles, etc., and where these are not available a liberal allowance of meat or fish meal should be given. Fresh green stuff, such as grass or kale, and oyster shell must also be provided in good quantity.

Young ducklings grow very fast and recent researches support the idea that the vitamin requirements of ducklings are of the same order as those of turkey poults.[21] Ducklings that are to be fattened for the table must be heavily fed so that they may be brought to a marketable condition as quickly as possible. For the first few weeks they may receive a chick mash mixed with boiling water to the proper consistency, and given five or six times a day. By the end of a month the number of meals may be gradually reduced to three, and the ducklings put on a more fattening diet. Boiled rice, boiled potatoes, Sussex ground oats and barley meal, mixed with buttermilk or skim milk, are amongst the best foods for fattening purposes; fish or meat meal should also be included. Although the birds will use household waste quite well, they should not be given such quantities of it as will produce an unbalanced diet. As growing birds they need good protein, much of which they may find for themselves by foraging, but if there is any doubt about the amount of food they are picking up on free range, then the mash given to them should be modified accordingly. With liberal feeding, the birds should be ready for killing at 10 or 12 weeks old.

Ducklings which are to be reared for stock should be given less fattening food and should be allowed as much liberty as possible on clean grassland; if it is to remain in a fresh unworn state, each duck must be allowed about 250 square feet of ground. They eat a large amount of green stuff, and when grass is scarce, kale, chickweed, etc., must be supplied.

Ducks have a natural tendency to become fat, so that in feeding stock birds foods such as maize must be given in moderation. Their appetite capacity is considerably greater than that of hens, for an average duck in full lay will eat up to 7 oz. (dry weight) of wet mash per day if it is given in three feeds. About a half of this can be provided in the form of grain if necessary. Where there is good free range, a reduction of one third to one half of this quantity may be possible. As in the case of chickens it is advisable to have both types of grit available.

(6) The feeding of geese

The staple food of the goose is grass. The bird possesses a short powerful bill, curiously ridged in the inside, which enables her to crop the grass very closely; in fact geese will graze a field closer than almost any other animal.

Geese thrive best when they can roam over fields and waste places preferably within reach of a pond or stream. If water is supplied in a container it should be deep enough to allow the birds to submerge their heads. One feed in the day is usually sufficient, and this may take the form of wet mash given at night when the birds are brought home; boiled grain may be given occasionally. Failing grass, succulent food such as lettuce, cabbage or swedes must be supplied.

The goslings are very independent, and will soon learn to find a large amount of their own food, but mash should be given two or three times a day when the birds are very young. This may be composed of such foods as scalded biscuit meal and Sussex ground oats.

Geese are impatient of confinement, and it is not advisable to pen them up closely with the idea of fattening them. A few weeks before they are to be marketed, they may be placed in large grass runs and fed liberally on boiled potatoes and boiled rice, dried off with barley meal to which a little meat or fish meal may be added. Grit and green food should also be supplied.

(7) The feeding of other birds

Comparatively little systematic work has been done on the feeding of other birds than those already described, although a useful review of the needs of game birds has been provided by Nestler.[25] Such data as are available for pheasants, partridges and quail, show that the young birds are rather more like the poult in their requirements than the chick.

More recent work on pheasant chicks suggest that the type of diet suited to their needs is, for example, ground yellow maize 18, middlings 14, finely ground oats 10, soya-bean meal (expeller type) 30, fish meal 10, liver meal 3, dried skim milk 5, dried whey 2, dried brewer's yeast 4, dicalcium phosphate 1, limestone 1.5, high potency cod-liver oil 1.5 and salt, 0.5 per cent., with the addition of 250 p.p.m. of manganous sulphate. Such a ration provides nutrients at the following levels; protein 29, glycine 1.7, fat 5.2, fibre 4.2, calcium 1.74, phosphorus 1.10 and salt (added) 0.5 per cent., together with 80 p.p.m. of manganese and, on the basis of 1 lb. of food, 9,500 I.U. of vitamin A, 1,800 I.U. of vitamin D and 3, 26 and 930 mg. respectively of riboflavin, niacin and choline.

REFERENCES

1. Morgan, R. B., and B. W. Heywang, (1941). Poultry Sci., 20, 62.
2. Morris, L., (1947). Poultry Sci., 26, 122.
3. Halnan, E. T., (1948). " Scientific Principles of Poultry Feeding." Min. Agric. Fisheries Bul. No. 7.
4. Brody, S., (1945). " Bioenergetics and Growth," 479–483.
5. Titus, H. W., (1929). Poultry Sci., 8, 80.
6. Cruickshank, E. M., (1941). Nutrition Abs. Rev., 10, 645.
7. Leitch, I., and W. Godden, (1941). Imp. Bureau of Animal Nutrition, Tech. Comm., No. 14.
8. Cravens, W. W., H. J. Almquist, L. C. Norris, R. M. Bethke, and H. W. Titus, (1944). U.S. Nat. Res. Council Rept. No. 1., Recommended nutrient allowances for poultry.
9. Titus, H. W., (1939). U.S. Dept. Agric. Yearbook.
10. Tyler, C., (1948). Nutrition Abs. Rev., 18, 261 and 473.
11. Hammond, J. C., W. A. Hendricks, and H. W. Titus, (1938). J. Agric. Res., 56, 791.
12. Van Landingham, A. H., T. B. Clark, and B. H. Schneider, (1945). Poultry Sci., 24, 105.
13. Van Landingham, A. H., T. B. Clark, and B. H. Schneider, (1942). Poultry Sci., 21, 346.
14. McGinnis, J., P. T. Hsu, and J. S. Carver, (1948). Poultry Sci., 27, 389.
15. Kondra, P. A., and G. C. Hodgson, (1948). Sci. Agric., 28, 264.
16. Altschul, A. M., G. W. Irving, W. F. Guilbeau, and H. C. Schaefer, (1948). Poultry Sci., 27, 402.
17. Emerson, R., J. Houston, R. H. Thayer, and R. MacVicar, (1949). Poultry Sci., 28, 431.
18. Fermor, C. E., (1947). " Good Poultry Keeping."
19. Chilson, W. T., and H. Patrick, (1946). Poultry Sci., 25, 86.
20. Scott, M. L., G. F. Heuser, and L. C. Norris, (1948). Poultry Sci., 27, 773.
21. Fritz, J. C., J. L. Halpin, and J. H. Hooper, (1947). Poultry Sci., 26, 78.
22. Halnan, E. T., and F. H. Garner, (1947). " The Principles and Practice of Feeding Farm Animals."
23. Lloyd, M. D., C. A. Reed, and J. C. Fritz, (1949). Poultry Sci., 28, 69.
24. Hegsted, D. M., and R. L. Perry, (1948). J. Nutrition, 35, 411.
25. Nestler, R. B., (1939). U.S. Dept. Agric. Yearbook.

LABORATORY ANIMALS

1. Introduction.
2. Rats.
3. Mice.
4. Guinea-pigs.
5. Golden hamsters.
6. Ferrets.

(1) Introduction

The feeding of laboratory animals does not differ in principle from the rules which have been elaborated in Section III of this book, in fact much of the study of the fundamental bases of nutrition has been made with such small animals, mainly because they have short life and reproductive periods and, being small, their food intake is correspondingly small, enabling numbers of them to be used at not too great a cost.

In this chapter it is intended to give no more than a general account of the feeding of the different species from the point of view of the maintenance of colonies, together with a few of the diets which represent the nearest approach that has yet been made to synthetic, i.e., perfectly controlled, diets. A more full account may be found in one of the reference works quoted.[1][2][3][4][5] Of the animals here considered, five are rodents and one is a carnivore.

(2) Rats

The domesticated varieties of the rat, particularly the albino and hooded ones, have been used to a very great extent for nutritional research during this century, for much of the investigation of vitamins, mineral elements and amino-acids was first carried out with these animals, the results then being applied to trials with other species. Quite apart from studies of the values of particular nutrients, much fundamental work on the differences of dietary requirements of a given species under varying physiological conditions, e.g., growth and lactation, has been made possible by these useful animals.

Because of the additional cleanliness and economy which it makes possible, the practice is growing of giving pelleted or cubed food to rats. Large cubes may be left on the floors of the cages but a cleaner and simpler method is to put the pelleted food into hoppers, which are filled from outside the cage. A baby-chick size of pellet is useful and, apart from the wastage of the first day or two after the introduction of such a system, the method is economical.

In some colonies the same type of ration is given to stock of all ages, chiefly because comparatively few of the animals are kept for maintenance purposes, most of them being in the stages of growth, pregnancy or lactation; in other cases different foods are used for the different conditions and this is the better practice.

The rat has a simple type of digestive system. Although it will consume a large variety of foods, it is able to make very little use of fibrous ones; this is especially true of the young rat. Usually the diet is compounded of ground cereals, oil-seed meals, small amounts of fish and meat meals, dried yeast, skim milk powder, grass meal, and mineral and vitamin supplements. Where a complex mixture of this kind is not used the basal diet commonly consists of cereal grains or bread, supplemented with small amounts of fresh green food or of meat. This method is more troublesome, less hygienic and no better than the use of balanced pelleted mixtures. In the following table are given some of the diets which have been in use successfully, often for many years, in the laboratories of commercial organisations and research centres.

TABLE 157

Ingredients	Diet 1	Diet 2	Diet 3
	%	%	%
Cereals			
Ground wheat ...	19.2	—	—
Ground oats ...	19.2	18	—
Ground barley ...	9.5	12 (Malted)	—
Ground maize ...	9.5	24	11
Wheat offals			
Coarse bran ...	—	—	8
Fine middlings ...	19.2	26.8	34
Oil-seed meals	—	—	21 (Coconut 16, groundnut 5)
Animal proteins			
Fish meal ...	4.7	—	2.5
Meat-and-bone meal ...	9.5	—	—
Blood meal ...	—	2.4 (Soluble)	—
Dried liver ...	—	—	2.5
Dried skim milk	7.0	15.6	6.5
Adjuncts			
Wheat germ ...	—	—	2.0
Dried yeast ...	1.2	—	5.0
Mineral mixture	0.5 (NaC1)	1.2	2.5
Vitamins ...	0.5 (Cod L.O.)	—	See below
Molasses ...	—	—	5.0
Supplements	5 g. green food. (10 ml. skim milk for growth)	See below	Small fresh-milk ration for lactating rats
Protein, % ...	20	17	22
Fat, % ...	5	3	4
Fibre, % ...	4	4	3

The first ration is one which has been used successfully at a British research institute, the weaning weights of the young rats being 42 - 3 g. at 23 days; the allowance of green food is regarded as essential. Ration 2 is one used in the United States; the reported weight at 21 days is 52 g., but in this case a paste food is fed to nursing dams and the young up to 6 weeks of age. The paste consists of casein 25, whole milk powder 25, wheat germ 20, and lard 30 per cent.[7] Other rats receive 1 g. of yeast per day and 3 g. of wheat germ weekly. For the last system the average weight of the bucks at 100 days is very high, namely 358 g.

Ration 3 is in use in a large industrial breeding colony, where it is considered undesirable to have too large an intake of vitamins A and D, the levels in the ration being 8 and 1 I.U./g. respectively. The food is given in pelleted form.[8]

In a very thorough review of the requirements of laboratory animals, Russell[2] concludes that 20 per cent. of mixed protein, or 20 per cent. of casein supplemented with 0.2 per cent. cystine, or 25 per cent. of casein, is needed for reproduction and lactation in rats. For maintenance, about 10 per cent. seems to be enough.

Although the evidence is not conclusive, it would seem that 10 - 20 per cent. of fat in the diet of does produces better performance than lower levels.

Although the rat is normally dependent upon dietary sources for its supplies of vitamin B, there may be conditions when this is not so. The phenomenon was first observed by Fridericia,[9] in feeding to young rats a diet lacking in vitamin B, one of the ingredients of the ration being raw rice starch. Some of the animals began to excrete large amounts of undigested starch and, very surprisingly, to grow at normal rates. This effect, which has been called " refection " provides an example of a rodent depending for its supplies of vitamin B upon bacterial agents which under specific conditions become established in the digestive tract.[10]

Food consumption naturally varies with the size of the animals; the requirement per day of a concentrated type of ration, such as those just described, is about 15 g. for adult does and 20 g. for bucks. The average period of gestation is 21 days, during which time the food intake of the pregnant doe may increase to 33 per cent. above maintenance levels.

Newly born albino rats weigh 4 - 5 g., a weight which can rise to 40 - 50 g. by the end of the suckling period of some 21 - 23 days. It is not surprising, therefore, with an average number of seven young in a litter, that the food intake of the dam is high. The average additional food requirement of the doe for each of the young is 3 - 4 g./day (13 Cal.) over the period of lactation. The dam's food needs for maintenance and lactation may thus range from 25 to 40 g., depending on the size of the litter. [8]

Although rats have been so intensively studied there are still surprising variations in experimental results between different laboratories, even when diets are being compounded to the same formula. Apart from any possible differences due to breed, one cause of variation is almost certainly that due to variations of composition in what are nominally the same foods. Hinton[11] has shown how some of the vitamin B of wheat offals is very localised, so that differences of milling technique might quite well produce two foods of different potency. Only those workers who have tried to maintain the constancy of composition of a basal diet will realise how difficult a task it can be. The solution to the problem, so far as the experimental worker is concerned, would seem to be the use, not of ordinary foods, but of chemically pure constituents. A good deal of progress has been made towards the formulation of such diets. The big test of them is whether they will allow satisfactory reproduction and lactation when used as the sole food for several generations, for it is by no means so difficult to devise diets for maintenance purposes. A young rat, for example, may receive from its dam almost enough iron to last it for its full life, provided that haemorrhage does not occur, or the production of young is not expected from it; in such a case a diet could contain much less iron than would be satisfactory for reproduction and lactation and yet be quite good enough for maintenance. These results are not only interesting in themselves but they indicate that *long range* research on the feeding of the larger animal species upon which man depends for food is very necessary. The laboratory animals serve as the pilot animals for such research, so that the more obvious factors may be determined with speed and economy. In this connection the words of Sica and Cerecedo with reference to rats,[12] which are quoted below, find a close parallel to those of Wallace[13] on lambs, quoted in Chap. 17.

" Survival of new born rats is dependent largely on their weights at birth."

The most systematic and exhausting trials of synthetic diets yet carried out—and there have been many extremely careful and well planned ones—seem to be those of Folley, Henry and Kon[14] and of Nelson and Evans,[15] the former workers carrying on their tests for a longer period (5 generations). Both groups used very similar diets, in which 20-24 per cent. of casein supplied the protein, 60-64 per cent. of sucrose provided the carbohydrate, the fat content varied from 8-15 per cent., and the mixture of salts from 4-5 per cent. In addition there were supplements of fat-soluble vitamins A, D, E and K, and of thiamin, riboflavin, pyridoxine, nicotinic acid, choline, calcium pantothenate, p-aminobenzoic acid, inositol, biotin and folic acid. In the experiments of the English workers reproduction and lactation deteriorated with each succeeding generation; fresh liver contained factors which led to approximately normal physiological processes.

(3) Mice

Although the nutritional needs of mice seem to be very similar to those of rats, far less study has been made of the details.

For stock colonies the same kind of diet as for rats, compounded in cubes or pellets, is satisfactory. Mixed meals may be given in food pots, but there is usually much contamination of food by the excreta when this practice is followed, although special cages have been designed to overcome the difficulty.[16]

Most of the research on synthetic diets for this species is of very recent origin.[17] [18] [19] Apart from a higher proportion of casein and the use of dextrose or dextrin, the most successful rations have closely resembled those given above for rats. Though there has been successful breeding through as many as four generations, the performance has not been as good as on normal stock foods. Some factor or factors may still remain to be identified. Different strains of mice, as with rats and other species, vary in their quantitative needs for nutrients [20]; it seems probable that the variations relate to the vitamin and mineral fractions of the diet rather than the major ones.

There are some workers who believe that a diet which is suitable for reproduction will be good for lactation, too.[12] The matter is still the subject of enquiry, but one would have thought that the higher plane of nutrition needed for lactation than for pregnancy might result in more searching requirements for nutrients. Where reproduction is concerned it is possible, of course, that a slightly faulty diet might appear to be sound, simply through the female drawing on her own bodily stores to provide for the foetuses; her reserves might be inadequate, however, for the greater demands of lactation. That it is not due to innate deficiencies of the young seems to be proved by the fact that they are capable of being reared by foster mothers on stock diets. It is certain that a diet which is excellent for the growth of the weaned young may be a failure for lactation.[17]

Again it is of interest to make comparisons between the results obtained with laboratory animals and the larger species. In this instance the failure of a diet to promote satisfactory reproduction in sows, although it gave good growth of young pigs, may be quoted.[21]

Mice weigh about 1 g. at birth and reach a weight of 9 - 10 g. by the time they are weaned at about 3 weeks; the mature animals range in weight from about 25 - 35 g. Mature mice consume about 4 g. per day of the pelleted type of ration described above.

(4) Guinea-pigs

Guinea-pigs are of interest nutritionally because they are one of the few species which require constant dietary supplies of vitamin C to maintain health.

The basis of most of the diets which are used for the species is green food, plus a concentrate mixture. At one laboratory, for example, each mature animal receives a ration of 1.5 to 2 oz. of a mixture of equal parts of rat cubes, oats and bran, together with 2.5 to 3.5 oz. of green food.[22] The latter must be fresh, otherwise some of the food factors present in the material are destroyed.

Bruce and Parkes [23] attempted to produce a pelleted diet for guinea-pigs which would be sufficient in itself, but they found that the added vitamin C (either the synthetic substance or that present in lucerne meal) was destroyed during manufacture or storage. The animals were reared successfully on pellets plus either vitamin C, or green food, or good quality dried cabbage.

Guinea pigs appear to need all the dietary factors which are required by rats, together with ascorbic acid—and maybe additional ones. Although much work has been done on the requirements of this species, too great a proportion of it has been in connection with vitamin C, so that it is not yet possible to produce a synthetic diet which will give even normal growth. Recent work [24] showed that a purified basal ration containing all the known nutrients except vitamin B12 would not produce anything like normal growth until 25 per cent. of lucerne meal was used to replace an equal percentage of sucrose; it was suggested that the good results then might be due to bulk, for a similar effect was obtained from the ash of the lucerne meal added to 15 per cent. of gum arabic. The basal ration plus 30 per cent. of dried sugar beet pulp was also effective. This last discovery and the way in which the species thrives on green foods may both be connected with the anatomy of the animal, which has a large caecum.

(5) Golden hamsters

As a laboratory animal the golden hamster is of more recent introduction than the species already considered in this section, the use of the animal going back to about 1930. Knowledge of its nutritional requirements is thus less detailed than for the rat.

A survey of the diets which have been used successfully for these animals suggests that one which is adequate for the rat will suffice for them, too. Synthetic diets which permitted good growth of the young, but which were inadequate for reproduction, have been reported; these diets, however, were lacking in folic acid at least.[25] As might be assumed, the diets were very similar to those which have been used for the rat.

(6) Ferrets

Little is known of the specific nutritional needs of this carnivorous species,[26] but there are no grounds for the belief that they differ radically from those which have been described for the dog, fox and mink in Chapter 26. It is worth while to repeat here the statement that the "raw meat" which is commonly given to carnivorous animals differs in many ways from the food that the animal would consume under natural conditions. It is liable to be deficient in vitamins A and D and in calcium. Care must be taken to see that there is a certain supply of these factors for the animals which have the greatest need of them, namely, growing, pregnant or lactating animals.

Where raw meat is given the amount needed is of the order of 4 oz. per adult per day, to be supplemented by cereal foods and by milk. The diets which have been found satisfactory for the other carnivores should be adequate here also.

REFERENCES

1. Worden, A. N., (Ed.) (1947). "The UFAW handbook on the care and management of laboratory animals."
2. Russell, F. C., (1948). Commonwealth Bur. Animal Nutrition, Tech. Comm. No. 16.
3. Loosli, J. K., (1945). New York Acad. Sci., *46*, 45.
4. Griffith, J. Q., and E. J. Farris, (1942). "The rat in laboratory investigations."
5. Snell, G. D., (Ed.) (1941). "Biology of the laboratory mouse."
6. Thomson, W., (1936). J. Hyg., *36*, 24.
7. Mendel, L. B., and R. B. Hubbell, (1935). J. Nutrition, *10*, 557.
8. Tainsh, P., (1944). Private comm. quoted in (1) above.
9. Fridericia, L. S., (1926). Skand. Arch. Physiol., *49*, 55.
10. Kon, S. K., (1945). Proc. Nutrition Soc., *3*, 217.
11. Hinton, J. J., (1944). Biochem. J., *38*, 214.
12. Sica, A. J., and L. R. Cerecedo, (1947). Science, *107*, 222.
13. Wallace, L. R., (1948). J. Agric. Sci., *38*, 93.
14. Folley, S. J., K. M. Henry, and S. K. Kon, (1947). Brit. J. Nutrition, *1*, 39.
15. Nelson, M. M., and H. M. Evans, (1947). Arch. Biochem., *13*, 265.
16. Brownlee, G., (1947). Quoted in (1) above.
17. Fenton, P. F., and G. R. Cowgill, (1947). J. Nutrition, *33*, 703.
18. Foster, C., J. H. Jones, F. Dorman, and R. S. Kobler, (1943). J. Nutrition, *25*, 161.
19. Ball, Z. B., and R. H. Barnes, (1941). Proc. Soc. Exp. Biol. Med., *48*, 692.
20. Cerecedo, L. R., and L. J. Vinson, (1944). Arch. Biochem., *5*, 147.
21. Russell, W. C., A. E. Teeri, and K. Unna, (1948). J. Nutrition, *35*, 321.
22. Gordon, W. S., (1948). Private comm. Director, Agr. Res. Coun., Field St., Compton, Berks.
23. Bruce, H. M., and A. S. Parkes, (1947). J. Hygiene, *45*, 70.
24. Booth, A. N., C. A. Elvehjem, and E. B. Hart, (1949). J. Nutrition, *37*, 263.
25. Hamilton, J. W., and A. G. Hogan, (1944). J. Nutrition, *27*, 213.
26. Pyle, N. L., (1940). Amer. J. Pub. Health, *30*, 787.

THE EFFICIENCY FACTOR IN NUTRITION

1. **The purchase of foodstuffs.**
   (a) Purchase on the basis of overall nutritive value.
   (b) Purchase on the basis of protein content.
2. **The efficiency factor in nutrition.**
   (a) Introduction.
   (b) The efficiencies of different species and systems.

(1) The purchase of foodstuffs

(a) Purchase on the basis of overall nutritive value.

From time to time the owner of livestock usually has to purchase foodstuffs in order to supplement those which he himself produces. For such occasions some standards of comparison between foods are essential so that the best food for the purpose may be obtained at the lowest cost. It is with economic considerations of this kind that this brief section is concerned.

It must be made quite clear at the outset that there is no general solution to the problem, for the guiding principles upon which the purchase will be made are variable and depend not only on the foods to be bought but also on the ration which they are to supplement and the purpose for which the livestock are being fed. If, for example, the animals are fully grown and are being fattened for market, then there is no urgent need for protein-rich foods; those containing a high proportion of carbohydrate will serve the purpose and may be much cheaper. In such a case the standards of comparison between the different foods for sale may well be those of the amounts of energy which could be obtained for the same monetary expenditure. Where ruminants are involved it is advantageous to buy foods on a starch equivalent basis, for, as previously explained (Ch. 18), the starch equivalents of foodstuffs are actually indices of their *net* energies for the fattening of bullocks. If oats, having a starch equivalent of 61, can be bought for £20 per ton, this means that the price of 100 lb. is £20 ÷ 22.4, the cost of one pound of S.E. thus being

$$\frac{£20}{22.4 \times 61} = £0.0147$$

Should barley, of starch equivalent 71, be available at £19 per ton, then the price of one pound of S.E. would be £0.0119. It would thus be cheaper to buy the barley.

As indicated in Chapter 18, however, starch equivalents are not necessarily additive. Two foods may have the same starch equivalent but yet have very different effects when they are added in equal amounts (on a S.E. basis) to the same basal ration of the same animals, for one of them may help to balance the basal diet by providing factors in which it is lacking, while the other may be quite unable to do so. It is perhaps unlikely that two foods so similar as oats and barley would have widely different effects, but it does mean that very ·definite limits should be put to this kind of attempt at reducing the complexities of nutrition to simple slide-rule operations.

Where non-ruminants are involved, or where rations are being constructed for purposes other than fattening, the starch equivalent system becomes of still less use. Møllgaard and Lund in 1929, for example, showed that the values which foods have for fattening mature cattle are not those which they possess for other purposes. An extreme example may be chosen to illustrate this point. For fattening purposes, a pure carbohydrate and a pure protein could be almost equally good, whereas the former would be useless for growth or for milk production.

Although the above criticisms have been applied to the starch equivalent method of comparing the nutritive values of foods, they may also be used for the net energy system. It is not suggested that the two methods are useless but that the arithmetical data which they provide are not in themselves adequate. The livestock owner must consider the starch equivalent or net energy of the food he is about to buy in relation to his background knowledge of the general principles of nutrition.

The two systems which have been discussed above both aim at relating the foodstuff to its actual productive effect, e.g., gain in weight of fattening cattle, whereas a third method which is used does not go so far. Foods may be compared on the basis of the number of pounds of digestible nutrients which may be purchased for a given sum of money. In this instance the concept of net energy is not introduced and even the intervening stage of metabolisable energy is avoided. Apart from the conversion of the pounds of digestible fat into the corresponding weight of digestible starch, the method has few complications. Although the use of starch equivalents and net energies may be advantageous for particular foods and for special classes of livestock, where there is a long history of experimental trials and of practical feeding, the buying of food on the basis of total digestible nutrients has much to commend it. It is not a perfect method but it is relatively simple and fairly free from assumptions which may not be justifiable in all cases.

Whichever method is employed, however, one must remember that the tables showing the compositions and nutritive values of foods are composed of average data. A particular sample of food may have a chemical composition differing quite markedly from the average figures quoted in the tables. Wherever it is possible, it is best to have analytical data relating to the sample of food in question. To avoid trouble and expense this may mean buying foods in bulk on the basis of an analytical report or else purchasing the goods under guarantee from the supplier.

Some foods are less variable in composition than others, but hay, dried grass and swill require careful consideration. Finally, the inadequacies of chemical analysis and the innate ambiguities of terms such as " crude fibre " ought to be remembered.

(b) Purchase on the basis of protein content.

It happens quite often that it is necessary to buy foods rich in protein so that quantities of grain, or beet pulp, or potatoes, or similar food-stuffs, which a farmer may have in hand, may be used to provide rations suitable for growth, reproduction or lactation.

In this case the amount of digestible protein which can be bought for a given outlay of money is the broadest basis upon which calculations can be made. Here also it is very desirable to have an actual analysis of the food, showing both its protein and fibre contents. The cost of one pound of digestible protein should be worked out in a manner similar to that described for purchase on the basis of starch equivalents.

Quite apart from the possible errors which are introduced into calcu-lations by the limitations of chemical analyses, other mistakes may be made when protein-rich foods are bought without taking into account the quality of the protein in the materials as well as its quantity. Where rations are being constructed for fully developed ruminants, protein quality is relatively unimportant in most cases because of the inter-vention of the rumen bacteria. Nevertheless this factor cannot be ignored where highly productive animals, such as cows in heavy lactation, are involved, since there is undoubtedly a better response to the feeding of some food proteins than others. Non-ruminants are greatly affected by the biological values of their dietary proteins.

Consideration of the quality of bought protein, without an examina-tion of the nature of that of the basal diet, would be valueless. The best opportunities for using the supplementary relationships between the different dietary proteins are provided by the food proteins of relatively low biological values. There would be little point, for example, in pur-chasing an expensive protein-rich food to *supplement* a basal ration the biological value of the protein of which was equal, or very nearly equal, to 100. Apart from the cases which have been quoted in Chapter 4, there must be many opportunities for practical trials of different com-binations of food proteins, using as a basis for the construction of the rations the information that is already in existence as to the amino-acid composition of the proteins.

Before concluding this brief section, stress must again be put on the need for examining rations in their entirety. Useful though the concepts of net energy, starch equivalent and digestible protein have been in the past, there is little doubt that they have helped to put too much reliance on the ability of very simple calculations to express a concept so complex as the " nutritive value " of rations. An extreme example may again be quoted to illustrate this point. Consider the case of a basal ration which is low in protein and devoid of carotene or vitamin A, and which is to be supplemented by either dried grass meal or an oil-seed meal. Although, on the basis of protein content alone, the former food might be 10-20 per cent. dearer than the latter, livestock would remain in good appetite longer and would utilise their dietary protein more efficiently, when kept on a ration which included the grass meal rather than the oil-seed meal. Whether it would be economic to buy the grass meal would depend on how long the animals were to be kept on the ration, how they had been fed previously and other factors. It might well be advisable to buy both grass meal and oil-seed meal, but in any case the decision is not one which could be arrived at on the simple basis of the cost of the respective meals and the contents of digestible protein.

(2) The efficiency factor in nutrition

(a) Introduction.

In various chapters of this book there have been discussions of the efficiency with which the food given to livestock is converted into some desirable product, such as milk. It is inevitable, in this period, that the final chapter of a book on animal nutrition should be concerned with nutritional efficiencies generally. During the last century in particular, one discovery after another has helped to reduce the human death rate due to disease, with the result that the world's population increases more and more rapidly. With the increasing population comes an enhanced need for food, food which, by the use of present techniques, must be derived from a fixed land surface. To say that there is at present a great deal of undeveloped land, which could be put to the growing of food, is not to solve the problem but merely to concern ourselves with the penultimate step; the final problem remains.

Apart from various factors which eventually may operate so as to reduce the rate of increase of the world's population, there are several ways of increasing the amount of food which can be produced. These include the development of new land (or water) for the production of crops, the use of better methods of crop husbandry in order to increase the weight of food produced per unit area of land, and increased efficiency in the conversion of crops into animal foods suitable for human consumption. This book can be concerned only with the last of these methods. Excluding for the moment beasts of burden, the numbers of which may be expected to decline in face of the competition of machines, and the relatively few animals which are kept as pets or for the entertainment of man, the rest of the domestic animals are maintained purely for food production. It seems necessary, therefore, to enquire into the efficiency with which the operation is carried out.

(b) The efficiencies of different species and systems.

Before proceeding further, the word " efficiency " requires to be defined rather carefully. Economic efficiency, in the sense of balancing food against gold or credit notes, is not concerned, for no amount of money will satisfy the hunger of a man or give well-being and growth to a child. Nor is it the efficiency of isolated physiological processes, such as that of conversion of the protein of the production ration of a cow into milk protein, which is the issue. Rather is it the efficiency of a complete cycle of operations, taking into account all the nutrients which have been put into the system and all the products which are suitable for human food. In the case of a chicken, therefore, we are concerned on the one hand with the quantity of nutrients required for the formation of the egg from which the bird was produced plus the total amount of food consumed by the bird during its life, and, on the other hand, with nutrients of its entire egg production and the edible portion of the fowl. Where a dairy cow is concerned, the balance is between the nutrients needed by the animal from gestation to the time of its death and the nutritive value of the milk produced, of the edible portion of the carcase and of the calves obtained.

The examination is thus an enquiry into the efficiency of different systems of feeding during the whole productive life of livestock. It also entails a comparison between the efficiencies of the different species for converting feeding stuffs into animal food for human consumption. One particular system of animal management may be more suitable for one region than for another and, if that is the conclusion obtained after an impartial investigation, it must be accepted. There is, of course, always a good deal of opposition to change. One meets students, who, being told of some system of animal feeding which is not widely used in their particular district, will subsequently describe the system quite carefully, adding, however, " it is not economic ". To them and to livestock owners of a similar kind " uneconomic " has no deeper meaning than " unfamiliar "; both groups are heedless or ignorant of the way in which animal feeding systems have changed in the past and may have to change yet again. It is but two centuries since the cultivation of roots on a large scale enabled reasonable numbers of cattle to be maintained throughout the winter in Britain without many of them having to be slaughtered for lack of winter food; the extensive use of oil-seed cakes and the move towards intensive milk production are even more recent.

Having decided upon the operations the efficiencies of which are to be investigated, the next step is to select the method of examination. This is a subject which has been discussed in previous chapters but which will lose nothing by brief repetition. Full information is required of the amount of food consumed during the periods in question, of the chemical composition of the food, of the weight and composition of fæces excreted, and of the weight and composition of the products. These are very severe requirements and, apart from some outstanding, rather isolated examples with the different species, the work has never been done on the scale that is required. Brody [1] and Leitch and Godden,[2] however, have provided excellent summaries of the information that is available; it is largely from their accounts that the subsequent figures have been drawn.

Since the composition of the digestible dry matter of food and that of the products may differ widely, it is useless to try to express the efficiency of a particular feeding system as the percentage of digestible dry matter which appears in the products. As in previous instances, the problem has to be split up into convenient sections. The best attempt to gain a single picture of overall efficiency is to work in terms of the digestible energy consumed and the energy of the products obtained; this method, however, is far from perfect. Additional useful information is provided if the protein of diet and products is considered in a similar way.

An example of this method of approach [2] is given in Table 158 below, which represents the balance sheet for a dairy cow for a whole year.

TABLE 158

	(Weights in lb.)					
	Dry matter	Protein equiv.	Fat	Carbo-hydrate	Gross Dig. energy	Starch equiv.
Feed consumption						
Winter ration						
Maint., 213 days	2,918	157.6	34.1	1,384	1,661	1,257
Prodn., 520 gal.	1,499	311.5	74.3	821	1,382	1,277
Grass, good, *91 days	2,339	482.3	91.9	1,156	1,993	1,720
Grass, poor, 61 days	953	83.4	7.1	500	619	543
Pregnancy allowance						
61 days	83	17.1	3.1	41	71	61
Total	7,792	1,051.9	200.5	3,902	5,726	4,858
Products					*Total calories*	
Milk, 600 gal.	744	204.0	210.0	288	1,800,900	
Calf, birth value	7	6.3	1.1	—	16,358	
Total	751	210.3	211.1	288	1,817,258	
Efficiency	9.6%	20.0%	4.8%	—	*Energy* 17.1%	

* This covers residual milk production to a total of 600 gal. and 30 days' pregnancy allowance.

This animal, which was fed in conformity with the standards of the Ministry of Agriculture, thus gave back 17 per cent. of the total energy of her ration in the form of food for human consumption; the protein return, at 20 per cent. was rather better than this.

In a very similar way balance sheets may be drawn up for the different species and the varying systems of management, so that comparisons of efficiency may be made. One may contrast the efficiency of the milk-producing animal—usually the cow—with that of the meat producers, such as beef cattle, sheep and pigs, or with the egg-producing fowl. In the following sub-sections data of this kind are set out; *it must be remembered that they represent efficiencies of present-day systems and do not constitute the results of exhaustive trials of all possible methods.*

(i) Milk production.

The figures of Table 159 show the efficiencies of milk production. Comparisons may be made between the efficiencies at different levels of milk production, or between winter and summer feeding, or between a full year and a " whole life " in which 1800 gal. of milk, 3 calves and the carcase of the cow are the products.

TABLE 159

				Efficiency %		
			Dry matter	Energy	Protein	Fat
Winter feeding:						
6 gallons daily ...	...	...	24.0	40.9	47.0	11.4
4 gallons daily ...	...	...	19.7	35.1	43.5	9.7
2 gallons daily ...	...	...	12.7	24.6	35.1	6.5
Summer feeding: grazing only.						
4 gallons daily ...	...	...	19.3	29.5	25.7	9.5
Complete year:						
600 gallons } Spring calving	...		10.7	19.5	23.6	5.5
1 calf* } Autumn calving	...		9.6	17.1	20.0	4.8
Whole life:						
1,800 gallons } Average of						
3 calves* } Spring and	...	...	7.5	13.9	18.1	4.1
Cow beef } Autumn						
*Birth value						

Despite the many references cited by Leitch and Godden, there seems to be no doubt that the problem of productive efficiency has not been exhaustively studied. Many of the researches have been of very short duration, or with very few animals; only in a few instances have the trials continued throughout whole lactations. Extremely few experiments have been carried on for a second or subsequent lactation. There is an urgent need for much research in this field. The high yielding animal, on the basis of existing data, appears to have an advantage over the lower yielding one. Investigation is needed of the efficiencies of cows over the whole life period under different systems of feeding; food intakes should not be kept to those levels which are now the accepted standards. There is also a need for research on the relative capacities of different breeds for utilising coarse foods. Such programmes of research require to be planned at least on a national—and preferably on an international—basis, for they are beyond the resources of individual livestock owners. Apart from the authorities already quoted, Yates, Boyd and Pettit [3] have produced a survey of work done on level of food intake in relation to milk production.

(ii) Meat production.

Some of the problems of this type have already received mention in connection with the production of baby beef. The data calculated by Leitch and Godden are given in Table 160 below: the weights quoted are liveweights.

TABLE 160

| | Efficiency % | | |
	Energy	Protein	Fat
Beef			
Baby beef, birth to 7 cwt.	8.6	15.5	3.5
Baby beef, birth to 9 cwt.	11.1	11.1	5.1
Fat bullock, birth to 10.7 cwt. (grass fattened) ...	8.2	8.9	3.7
Fat bullock, birth to 12.5 cwt. (stall fattened) ...	7.9	8.7	3.5
Lamb			
Fattening period, 70 to 100 lb. in 12 weeks	17.2	13.2	8.4
Bacon and pork			
Bacon, 40 to 220 lb. with restricted feeding	28.2	15.2	14.5
The same, but with unrestricted feeding	22.3	13.3	11.3
Pork, 40 to 160 lb., restricted feeding	27.4	19.0	13.6
The same, but with unrestricted feeding	22.1	15.3	11.0

In this instance, also, far less work has been done than is needed.

(iii) Egg production.

The efficiency of egg production has been computed to be as follows:

TABLE 161

| | Efficiency % | | |
	Energy	Protein	Fat
Medium light bird (4 lb.)			
1 egg per day	19.6	43.6	7.0
200 eggs per year	13.3	29.8	4.7
120 eggs per year	9.0	20.2	3.2

For heavier birds the corresponding efficiencies are somewhat less.

(iv) Species differences.

On the basis of the above figures, the high yielding cow is the most efficient food producer, both from the energy and protein aspects. The better laying birds approach the high yielding cow in protein conversion efficiencies, but fall well behind in energy. Pigs, though more efficient than beef cattle or sheep, occupy third place in the list.

(v) Conclusion.

The efficiencies which have been quoted for the various species and systems are those which pertain under present conditions of feeding. Other methods or combinations of methods might give very different results—one has but to remember the relatively poor use which pigs make of high proportions of fibre—but there is no doubt that the time has come for the carrying out of larger, better planned and better controlled animal feeding experiments than have ever been done in the past.

This is not to belittle the achievements of past workers, whose resources were much smaller than those which are now necessary; in any event, much of the work will have to be based upon their results.

Long term investigations of productive efficiency by animals of different species and different breeds, under varying feeding systems appear to be essential. Such matters as reproductive efficiency also require examination. Many types of worker are needed for such work. Possibly a good deal of useful pilot research could be done with some of the smaller laboratory animals. Certainly wide vision is necessary if, under the pressure of the need for food for human beings, the creation of a zoological counterpart to the agricultural " dust-bowl " is to be avoided.

REFERENCES

1. Brody, S., (1945). " Bioenergetics and Growth."
2. Leitch, I., and W. Godden, (1941). Imp. Bureau of Animal Nutrition, Tech. Comm. No. 14.
3. Yates, F., D. A. Boyd, and G. H. N. Pettit, (1942). J. Agric. Sci., 32, 428.

COMPOSITION AND NUTRITIVE VALUE OF FEEDING STUFFS*

	Average composition per cent, as shown by chemical analysis						Digestible nutrients per cent					Calculated from digestible nutrients		Per 100 lb.	
	(1) Dry Matter	(2) Crude Protein	(3) Oil (Ether Extract)	(4) Carbohydrate (Nitrogen-free Extractives)	(5) Crude Fibre	(6) Ash	(7) Dig. Crude Protein	(8) Dig. True Protein	(9) Dig. Oil (Ether Extract)	(10) Dig. Carbohydrate (Nitrogen-free Extractives)	(11) Dig. Fibre	(12) Nutritive Ratio (approx.)	(13) V.	(14) Starch Equivalent	(15) Total Digestible Nutrients
1. Roots															
Artichoke, Jerusalem	20·4	1·5	0·2	16·9	0·7	1·1	1·0	0·4	—	15·8	0·2	1:16	92	16·4	—
Carrots	13·0	1·2	0·2	9·3	1·4	0·9	0·8	0·4	0·1	8·9	0·7	1:12	87	8·8	—
Kohl Rabi	12·7	2·0	0·1	8·2	1·4	1·0	0·7	0·3	—	7·4	0·6	1:11	90	8·3	—
Mangolds, white-fleshed globe	10·7	1·0	0·1	8·2	0·7	0·7	0·7	0·1	—	7·5	0·3	1:11	70	5·5	—
,, intermediate	12·0	1·0	0·1	9·4	0·7	0·8	0·7	0·1	—	8·5	0·3	1:13	70	6·2	—
,, yellow-fleshed globe or tankard	13·2	1·2	0·1	10·2	0·8	0·9	0·7	0·1	—	9·4	0·3	1:14	70	6·8	—
,, long red	13·1	1·0	0·1	10·3	0·8	0·9	0·7	0·1	—	9·5	0·3	1:14	70	6·8	—
Parsnips	15·0	1·3	0·3	11·3	1·2	1·0	1·0	0·6	0·1	10·9	0·7	1:12	86	10·6	—
Potatoes	23·8	2·1	0·1	19·7	0·9	0·7	1·1	0·6	—	17·7	—	1:16	100	18·5	—
Sugar-beet	23·4	1·1	0·1	20·4	1·1	0·7	1·1	0·6	—	19·3	0·4	1:25	75	15·0	—
Swede Turnip	11·5	1·3	0·2	8·1	1·2	0·7	0·8	0·3	—	7·5	0·8	1:11	85	7·3	—
Tulip Bulbs (pigs)	48·0	5·2	0·7	37·4	2·0	2·7	3·5	2·0	0·5	35·0	1·0	1:11	—	—	40·6
Turnip	8·5	1·0	0·2	5·7	0·9	0·7	0·6	0·2	—	5·2	0·3	1:9	77	4·4	—
2. Leaves of Roots															
Artichoke tops	32·3	3·4	1·1	17·4	5·4	5·0	2·0	1·7	0·5	13·1	2·2	1:8	91	16·2	—
Carrot leaves	18·2	3·4	0·9	7·1	2·5	4·3	2·2	1·5	0·5	4·7	1·4	1:3	91	7·7	—
Kohl Rabi leaves	13·5	2·8	0·4	7·1	1·6	1·6	1·9	0·4	0·2	5·7	0·9	1:4	93	6·8	—
Mangold leaves	11·0	2·4	0·4	4·6	1·6	2·0	1·6	0·6	0·2	3·5	0·9	1:3	92	5·3	—
Potato haulm	23·0	2·5	1·0	10·2	6·2	3·1	1·1	0·9	0·2	6·1	2·2	1:8	78	7·2	—
Sugar-beet tops	16·2	2·0	0·5	8·7	1·6	3·4	1·4	0·4	0·3	7·2	1·1	1:6	84	8·6	—
Swede Turnip leaves / Turnip leaves	11·6	2·2	0·4	5·3	1·5	2·1	1·5	0·9	0·2	4·2	0·8	1:4	93	5·3	—

* Reproduced from the Ministry of Agriculture's Bulletin, No. 48, by permission of Dr. Woodman and the Controller, H.M. Stationery Office.

COMPOSITION AND NUTRITIVE VALUE OF FEEDING STUFFS—continued

	Average composition per cent. as shown by chemical analysis						Digestible nutrients per cent.						Calculated from digestible nutrients		Per 100 lb.
	(1) Dry Matter	(2) Crude Protein	(3) Oil (Ether Extract)	(4) Carbohydrate (Nitrogen-free Extractives)	(5) Crude Fibre	(6) Ash	(7) Dig. Crude Protein	(8) Dig. True Protein	(9) Dig. Oil (Ether Extract)	(10) Dig. Carbohydrate (Nitrogen-free Extractives)	(11) Dig. Fibre	(12) Nutritive Ratio (approx.)	(13) V.	(14) Starch Equivalent	(15) Total Digestible Nutrients
3. Other Green Foods															
Cabbage, drumhead	11·0	1·5	0·4	5·9	2·0	1·2	1·1	0·7	0·2	4·6	1·4	1:6	94	6·6	—
,, open-leaved	15·3	2·5	0·7	8·1	2·4	1·6	1·8	1·2	0·4	6·5	1·7	5	94	9·5	—
Chickweed	9·2	1·7	0·2	2·9	1·1	3·3	1·7	1·2	0·17	7·5	1·8	5·7	92	10·3	—
Kale, Thousand head	15·8	2·2	0·4	8·4	3·1	1·7	1·7	1·1	0·3	6·1	1·6	4·9	93	9·1	—
,, Marrow-stem (unthinned)	14·0	2·2	0·5	6·9	2·5	1·9	1·4	—	0·15	5·8	1·0	5	—	—	8·5
,, Marrow-stem (minced) (pigs)	14·0	2·2	0·5	6·9	2·5	1·9	1·6	1·0	0·18	6·4	1·5	5·2	93	9·0	—
,, Marrow-stem (singled-out)	13·9	2·1	0·3	7·2	2·5	1·2	1·4	0·7	0·2	4·9	1·1	5	94	7·5	—
Purple sprouting Broccoli	12·3	1·9	0·4	7·4	1·5	1·4	1·9	1·3	0·2	4·9	1·1	4	90	7·2	—
Mustard	14·9	2·9	0·4	7·3	2·9	1·3	2·0	1·3	0·5	3·9	1·9	3	87	6·9	—
Rape	14·1	2·8	0·8	5·7	3·5	1·3	2·0	1·3	0·5	3·9	1·9	3	87	6·9	—
4. Cereals															
Barley in flower	31·4	2·2	0·5	16·8	9·9	2·0	1·5	1·3	0·3	12·1	6·4	12	79	16·1	—
Maize	19·4	1·7	0·5	10·4	5·6	1·2	1·0	0·6	0·3	6·7	3·1	10	83	9·1	—
Millet	13·0	1·3	0·2	6·2	4·1	1·2	0·7	0·4	0·1	3·8	2·2	9	82	5·4	—
Oats in flower	23·2	1·9	0·6	10·4	8·5	1·8	1·4	1·2	0·4	6·5	4·9	9·6	75	10·0	—
Rye	23·4	3·0	0·9	10·3	7·5	1·7	2·1	1·4	0·5	7·0	4·9	6	80	11·3	—
5. Grasses															
Pasture Grass, close-grazing:															
Non-rotational	20·0	5·3	1·1	8·9	2·6	2·1	4·5	3·8	0·7	7·8	2·1	2·5	95	14·7	—
Rotational, with 3-weekly intervals *	20·0	4·5	1·3	9·3	3·1	1·8	3·7	3·2	0·8	8·0	2·5	3·3	94	14·6	—
Rotational, with monthly intervals *	20·0	3·5	1·0	9·2	4·5	1·8	2·6	2·3	0·5	7·6	3·7	4·8	91	13·4	—

* Data for fore-flush period should be taken as for non-rotational close-grazing.

Pasture Grass, extensive grazing.

Spring value, running off during summer	—	11·2	91	4	2·6	7·3	0·4	1·7	2·5	2·0	4·0	9·7	0·8	3·5	20·0
Winter pasturage (after close-grazing allowing free growth from end of July to December)	11·8	11·4	90	5·5	2·6	7·9	0·15	1·5	2·0	1·6	4·4	10·3	0·6	3·1	20·0
Pasture Grass, closely-grazed (pigs)	11·3	—	—	2·4	1·9	6·4	—	2·8	3·5	1·7	3·4	8·9	0·8	5·2	20·0
Pasture Grass, rotational grazing (pigs)	—	—	—	5	2·1	7·3	0·25	1·2	1·9	1·6	3·9	10·5	0·6	3·4	20·0
Rice Grass	—	8·6	85	7	3·3	5·1	0·3	0·9	1·3	2·4	5·0	11·2	0·6	2·9	22·1
Ryegrass, perennial	—	10·6	81	7	4·0	7·4	0·5	1·3	1·8	2·6	7·1	11·5	0·7	2·9	24·8
„ Italian	—	11·4	85	6	3·6	7·7	0·2	1·3	2·1	2·8	6·2	11·6	1·0	3·4	25·0
Sorghum	—	8·0	79	8·1	3·3	5·8	0·5	0·7	1·2	1·4	6·2	9·6	0·6	2·1	19·9
Timothy	—	14·0	79	11	4·8	11·1	—	1·0	1·6	2·2	9·2	17·6	1·0	3·1	33·1
6. Green Legumes															
Alsike	—	6·3	79	3	2·2	3·6	0·4	1·5	2·1	1·5	4·5	5·1	0·6	3·3	15·0
Crimson Clover	—	8·9	81	5	3·5	5·2	0·5	1·5	2·1	1·9	6·2	6·9	0·7	2·8	18·5
Red Clover, beginning to flower	—	10·2	86	4	3·0	6·3	0·5	1·7	2·5	1·6	5·2	8·1	0·7	3·4	19·0
Trifolium (see Crimson Clover)															
White Clover, beginning to flower	—	8·8	88	3	2·6	4·7	0·5	1·9	2·8	2·1	4·3	6·9	0·8	4·4	18·5
Beans, beginning to flower	—	7·1	88	3	1·6	4·1	0·3	1·5	2·3	2·0	3·3	5·7	0·8	3·2	15·0
Kidney Vetch	—	7·9	83	7	2·7	5·7	0·1	0·6	1·4	1·3	5·1	8·6	0·6	4·1	18·0
Lucerne (in early flower)	—	10·3	80	3·2	3·2	6·6	0·13	2·4	3·1	2·4	7·2	9·9	0·4	4·5	24·0
„ (in bud)	—	11·3	84	2·8	3·1	6·8	0·3	2·1	3·6	1·8	6·2	9·0	0·5	3·8	22·0
„ (before bud)	—	9·0	91	2·2	2·1	4·6	0·3	1·6	3·2	1·8	3·3	5·7	0·6	3·5	15·0
Peas, beginning to flower	—	6·8	77	3	3·0	3·7	0·3	1·6	2·4	1·2	5·9	7·8	0·6	3·5	16·8
Sainfoin, in flower	—	7·6	76	4	3·2	4·8	0·4	1·4	2·3	1·5	6·9	7·2	0·5	3·2	20·0
Tares, in flower	—	7·5	83	4	2·3	4·9	—	1·6	2·2	1·6	5·1	8·4	0·8	3·5	17·5
Trefoil	—	9·1	83	4	2·8	5·9		1·6	2·4		5·1		0·8		20·0
Vetches (see Tares)															
7. Miscellaneous															
Bracken (dried)	—	14·8	49	14	6·7	20·2	0·8	1·6	2·1	5·3	24·4	46·9	3·0	13·8	93·4
Brushwood	—	8·1	87	5	2·5	5·2	0·3	1·1	1·6	1·5	26·7	40·3	1·9	4·6	75·0
Buckwheat	—	5·2	91	3	0·8	3·7	0·2	0·9	1·5	1·1	4·3	7·8	0·6	2·5	16·3
Comfrey	—								2·2	2·0	1·7	7·5	0·3	2·5	11·5
Dandelion	—								1·4	2·0			0·7	2·8	14·5
Gorse	—	8·9	39	10	9·6	10·9	0·5	1·5		2·8	24·0	18·1	1·1	5·3	51·3
Heather	—	6·0	31	14	7·0	8·6	1·5	0·7		2·9	22·7	16·6	4·3	3·5	50·0
Heather (dried-tips)	—									3·4	34·3	44·6	5·2	5·2	92·7

COMPOSITION AND NUTRITIVE VALUE OF FEEDING STUFFS—continued

	Average composition per cent. as shown by chemical analysis						Digestible nutrients per cent.						Calculated from digestible nutrients		Per 100 lb.
	Dry Matter (1)	Crude Protein (2)	Oil (Ether Extract) (3)	Carbohydrate (Nitrogen-free Extractives) (4)	Crude Fibre (5)	Ash (6)	Dig. Crude Protein (7)	Dig. True Protein (8)	Dig. Oil (Dig. Ether Extract) (9)	Dig. Carbohydrate (Dig. Nitrogen-free Extractives) (10)	Dig. Fibre (11)	Nutritive Ratio (approx.) (12)	V. (13)	Starch Equivalent (14)	Total Digestible Nutrients (15)
7. Miscellaneous—contd.															
Artichoke tops (dried)	87·5	12·7	2·2	48·1	14·2	10·3	7·6	6·1	1·1	33·6	4·1	1 : 5	82	37·3	—
Ash leaves (dried)	88·0	10·1	2·3	59·0	8·9	7·7									
Beech leaves (dried)	84·6	5·6	3·1	47·0	25·2	3·8									
Elm leaves (dried)	88·0	15·9	2·9	49·9	8·6	10·7	11·6	8·5	0·7	40·7	4·9	4	91	50·0	—
Hop leaves and bine (dried)	89·4	12·5	3·5	38·1	24·5	10·8	8·0	6·1	2·5	27·1	7·6	5	69	31·1	—
Horse chestnut leaves (dried)	85·9	14·7	2·0	48·5	14·9	7·8									
Leaves of Trees in July (dried)	84·0	10·5	3·0	49·3	14·2	7·0	6·2	3·7	2·4	32·5	5·3	7	82	37·6	—
Nettles (dried)	88·6	18·3	7·7	38·0	10·6	14·0	12·8	9·3	4·9	30·0	6·0	4	89	46·5	—
Oak leaves (dried)	85·2	14·8	3·8	41·9	20·6	4·1									
Poplar leaves in Oct. (dried)	84·0	10·8	8·7	39·6	17·4	7·5	6·0	3·4	6·9	26·2	5·6	8	73	33·9	—
Willow leaves (dried)	89·9	15·3	5·4	40·4	19·5	8·9									
8. Silage															
Alsike	24·6	3·3	1·8	10·7	6·7	2·1	2·0	1·4	1·2	6·1	3·3	6	81	10·5	—
Bracken (early growth)	25·2	3·8	0·6	11·2	7·9	1·7	0·2	—	0·4	4·9	2·0	—	61	4·8	—
Clover, red	21·7	4·4	1·2	7·1	6·5	2·5	2·9	1·7	0·6	5·1	3·5	3	81	9·2	—
Grass (first quality)	21·0	3·8	1·0	9·8	4·3	2·1	2·7	1·0	0·6	7·3	3·1	4·3	91	12·8	—
Grass (second quality)	24·5	3·5	0·9	11·3	6·6	2·2	2·4	0·9	0·5	7·4	3·1	5·4	84	12·6	—
Grass (hay maturity)	25·0	2·6	1·0	10·5	8·4	2·5	1·8	1·0	0·5	6·1	4·9	7	75	10·2	—
Lucerne	25·0	4·2	2·1	8·8	7·4	2·5	2·8	1·7	1·0	6·2	3·1	4	81	11·1	—
Maize	18·5	1·6	0·8	9·0	5·7	1·4	0·8	0·4	0·4	7·9	3·2	13	82	8·6	—
Maize, Jaune Gros, English grown	21·0	2·3	1·2	11·3	4·9	1·3	1·5	0·6	1·1	5·4	3·4	9	82	12·1	—
Mangold leaves	22·4	3·0	1·1	10·0	3·3	5·0	2·0	0·7	0·5	6·1	1·8	4	87	7·9	—
Marrow-stem Kale	15·9	2·0	0·5	7·2	3·7	2·5	1·5	1·0	—		2·8	6	89	9·2	—

Mustard	8.0	90	5	1.9	5.2	0.4	1.1	1.6	2.3	3.8	6.1	0.4	2.5	15.1
Oats, green	8.9	72	11	5.1	5.9	0.4	0.6	1.1	1.8	8.5	10.7	0.8	1.9	23.7
Pea haulms and pods	11.6	85	6	3.4	5.9	1.3	0.2	2.0	4.1	6.0	8.6	1.4	3.5	23.6
,, pods	15.9	83	7.5	5.5	9.8	0.9	0.4	2.3	1.8	8.4	12.8	1.0	3.5	27.5
Potatoes	18.6	95	17	1.7	18.4	0.1	0.2	1.2	1.4	0.7	21.7	0.5	2.2	26.5
Potato haulms	8.0	86	8	2.6	5.0	1.2	0.3	0.9	5.6	4.4	9.1	2.7	3.2	25.0
Rye	5.5	81	7	3.4	3.4	0.2	1.8	3.0	2.0	4.4	8.2	0.5	1.6	13.1
Sainfoin	10.2	77	4	1.2	5.5	0.8	0.3	0.5	0.9	8.0	7.2	1.5	4.3	24.0
Sugar-beet pulp, Wet	6.5	90	14	2.5	5.4	0.1	0.2	1.5	7.4	2.3	9.1	0.2	1.0	11.6
,, tops	9.5	91	7	1.7	7.2	0.3		1.6	2.0	3.4	8.8	0.7	2.4	23.0
,, tops plus Wet Sugar-beet pulp	10.3	90	6	3.3	7.5	0.4	0.7	1.1	2.3	2.1	6.2	0.6	2.4	15.9
Sunflowers	9.8	80	10	5.2	6.6	0.7		1.5	5.7	6.8	12.5	0.6	2.1	22.2
Turnip tops	8.6	90	5	4.6	5.2	0.5	0.5	2.2	2.2	2.8	12.9	0.6	2.1	17.4
Vetch and oats, green fruity	12.8	76	7	5.5	8.7	0.9	1.1	3.8	3.2	8.0	11.6	1.2	3.4	27.3
,, ,, acid brown	13.0	76	4		6.4	1.2	1.9		2.3	11.4	12.9	1.5	5.6	34.6
Sweet Silage														
Clover, red	11.6	77	4	3.8	7.8	1.0	1.9	3.9	2.3	8.5	11.6	2.0	5.6	30.0
Grass	13.0	74	9	5.9	7.5	1.3	0.7	3.0	2.7	9.9	12.9	2.7	3.8	32.0
Lucerne	7.7	61	4	4.3	4.2	1.6	1.2	3.0	3.5	10.7	6.1	3.2	4.0	27.5
Stack Silage, Ryegrass and Clover	10.5	70	29	5.6	7.6	0.8	0.5	0.5	2.9	10.3	13.6	1.1	4.3	32.2
9. Hay														
Barley (just past milk stage)	42.7	85	10	15.4	28.9	0.8	—	4.6	6.4	24.9	45.8	1.9	7.0	86.0
Clover, crimson	33	77	4	12.3	23.1	1.0	5.5	8.3	7.2	26.2	35.5	2.4	12.0	83.3
,, red, poor	30	72	7	11.6	24.6	1.0	4.0	5.7	5.1	28.9	37.8	2.1	11.1	85.0
,, ,, good	38	84	5	11.3	26.0	1.7	5.5	8.5	6.0	24.0	37.1	2.9	13.5	83.5
,, ,, very good	43	89	4	11.0	26.8	2.1	5.5	10.7	7.0	22.2	35.8	3.2	15.3	83.5
,, ,, damaged	22	59	5	13.2	18.3	0.7	4.8	6.1	5.0	33.1	30.5	1.5	11.9	84.0
Couch Grass											62.0		8.3	93.0
Lucerne, before flowering	32	76	3	11.3	21.1	1.1	8.1	12.1	7.3	16.5	31.1	2.4	16.2	84.0
,, in full flower	27	68	4	13.2	18.1	1.2	6.2	9.7	8.0	27.5	29.2	2.6	14.2	83.5
,, in half flower (very good quality)	37	81	2.4	12.2	20.4	—	9.8	13.9	8.0	25.4	30.6	1.1	18.9	84.0
Meadow Hay, poor	22	59	11	15.6	19.3	0.5	2.5	3.4	5.0	33.5	38.2	1.5	7.5	85.0
,, ,, medium	32	73	11	17.9	21.8	0.8	3.8	3.6	6.2	26.3	39.4	1.6	8.6	85.7
,, ,, good	37	80	8	15.0	25.7	1.0	6.5	5.4	7.7	19.3	41.0	2.5	9.7	85.7
,, ,, very good	48	93	6	12.7	30.1	1.6	6.9	9.2	8.5	22.5	40.5	3.0	13.5	84.0
,, ,, aftermath, good	43	88	5	14.0	26.1	1.6	5.0	6.9	7.7	19.7	39.3	3.4	11.5	85.2
,, from wet meadows	45	92	6	12.2	27.2	2.1	6.0	7.4	7.4	28.4	40.6	4.6	12.4	85.0
,, from salt meadows	36	77	10	16.4	24.6	1.4	3.0	4.3			41.7	2.7	8.1	88.3

COMPOSITION AND NUTRITIVE VALUE OF FEEDING STUFFS—continued

	Average composition per cent. as shown by chemical analysis						Digestible nutrients per cent.					Nutritive Ratio (approx.) (12)	Calculated from digestible nutrients		Per 100 lb.
	Dry Matter (1)	Crude Protein (2)	Oil (Ether Extract) (3)	Carbohydrate (Nitrogen-free Extractives) (4)	Crude Fibre (5)	Ash (6)	Dig. Crude Protein (7)	Dig. True Protein (8)	Dig. Oil (Dig. Ether Extract) (9)	Dig. Carbohydrate (Dig. Nitrogen-free Extractives) (10)	Dig. Fibre (11)		V. (13)	Starch Equivalent (14)	Total Digestible Nutrients (15)
9. Hay—contd.															
Millet hay	86.6	10.8	2.2	38.5	29.4	5.7	6.1	4.8	0.9	23.4	17.6	1:7	76	36	—
Mineral-deficient hay (mainly purple molinia and brown bent)	86.0	11.1	1.9	40.4	29.5	3.1	5.5	5.3	0.2	15.7	16.4	6	65	24.6	—
Oats (milk stage)	86.0	8.1	2.6	40.7	27.8	6.8	4.4	—	1.6	22.9	14.5	9	76	34.0	—
Reed hay	90.0	8.6	1.2	43.2	29.0	8.0	2.5	2.3	0.5	19.7	15.6	15	75	29	—
Rice Grass, poor	81.3	6.4	1.3	40.6	24.9	8.1									—
Rye, before flowering	85.7	10.4	2.5	39.0	28.5	5.3	7.3	6.2	1.5	27.3	17.1	7	83	44	—
" in flower	86.0	6.3	2.0	38.6	34.4	4.7									—
Ryegrass, perennial	86.0	10.4	2.6	41.1	25.4	6.5	6.4	5.1	1.1	26.3	13.2	6	82	38	—
" Italian	84.2	11.2	3.5	41.6	22.1	7.6	6.9	5.5	1.7	27.9	12.8	4	89	44	—
Sainfoin, before flowering	83.5	15.4	3.2	32.5	24.9	6.7	10.9	7.8	2.1	25.2	10.7	4	84	40	—
" in flower	83.3	13.2	2.5	28.0	28.0	7.3	9.6	7.5	1.6	25.3	11.8	2	79	37	—
Tares, beginning to flower	83.3	19.8	2.3	28.5	23.4	9.3	15.1	10.8	1.4	18.5	12.6	4	82	36	—
" in full flower	84.0	14.2	2.5	32.8	25.5	8.3	9.4	6.6	1.5	19.7	12.8	6	78	32	—
Tares, and Oats (Tares in flower)	85.7	11.6	3.3	36.3	24.2	8.6	6.5	4.2	1.7	23.3	12.3	3	80	34	—
Timothy	84.0	8.5	2.4	41.1	28.5	5.2	4.0	3.2	1.0	25.5	15.1	6	77	35	—
Trefoil	86.0	15.4	3.4	33.2	24.5	7.5	11.8	8.6	1.6	23.2	10.8	5	82	37	—
Vetches (see Tares)															
Seeds hay (Ryegrass and Clover)	86.0	12.0	2.8	37.4	27.5	6.3	6.2	3.6	1.2	22.0	13.2	6	73	30	—
" good quality	85.0	13.0	2.3	37.8	23.1	8.8	7.8	6.3	1.3	25.5	13.0	5	85	40	—
Wheat (milk stage)	86.0	5.7	1.6	47.3	25.2	6.2	3.1	—	0.9	29.3	14.7	15	83	40.6	—
10. Straws															
Barley straw, spring	86.0	3.3	1.8	42.4	33.9	4.6	0.8	0.6	0.6	22.5	18.3	52	54	23	—

Barley awns	86.0	4.8	1.8	46.1	21.9	11.4	2.2	1.3	0.5	22.0	18.7	19	43	19	—
„ cavings	86.0	4.4	1.9	41.3	33.1	5.3	2.2	1.7	0.5	18.0	17.2	16	42	17	—
Bean straw (including pods)	86.0	4.5	0.8	33.0	43.1	4.6	4.0	3.1	0.6	11.1	16.4	7	22	7	—
„ stems and leaves	86.0	7.6	1.1	34.8	42.4	3.4	1.4	1.0	1.7	13.0	12.2	18	60	21	—
„ cavings	86.0	7.7	0.9	34.8	36.2	6.3	1.7	1.2	0.7	13.6	15.1	20	63	19	—
„ pods	86.0	4.8	1.2	42.6	28.5	6.3	1.0	0.8	0.6	19.4	18.3	20	50	39	—
Buckwheat straw	84.0	4.6	1.1	32.6	38.2	5.2	2.2	1.7	1.0	21.9	10.2	29	81	16	—
„ husks	86.8	9.1	1.8	35.3	43.5	5.7	0.6	0.4	0.5	19.8	19.7	21	51	67	—
Clover straw (red)	84.0	2.3	0.6	21.4	44.6	1.3									
Flax stems minus leaves	88.4	18.4	1.8	37.4	62.8	7.9									
Lentil pods	85.0	3.5	3.4	35.0	19.5	5.8									
Linseed chaff (see also Flax by-products)	88.4	9.0	0.7	42.4	40.7	6.0									
Lupin pods	87.3	2.9	0.8	45.3	29.2	11.2									
Maize, stripped stalks	87.8	4.8	2.2	29.0	36.9	4.9									
Millet, chaff and husks	88.0	2.9	1.9	42.4	40.8	10.3									
Oat straw, spring	86.0	6.0	2.1	44.8	33.9	6.5									
„ chaff (glumes), spring	86.0	4.4	2.2	42.0	22.8	4.9									
„ cavings	86.0	1.9	1.5	43.1	30.9	8.8									
„ straw winter	86.0	4.9	1.9	46.3	34.6	5.9									
„ chaff (glumes) „	86.0	3.2	2.3	45.3	24.1	5.6									
„ cavings „	85.0	3.8	2.3	40.7	29.3	5.7									
„ straw chaff „	83.6	6.0	3.4	39.0	32.6	5.8									
„ „ „ fermented	86.0	9.2	1.6	36.0	32.4	8.1									
Pea, haulm	86.0	11.7	2.4	35.8	33.4	6.6									
„ cavings	86.4	9.0	1.2	38.7	28.0	3.8									
„ straw	84.0	2.5	1.4	32.9	35.5	14.1	4.3	3.4	0.7	18.5	13.7	17	45	8	—
Rape straw	90.2	3.8	1.6	41.7	37.8	2.6	1.8	0.7	0.5	20.4	14.0	15	41	20	—
Rice husks	86.0	3.1	1.4	37.6	38.0	3.9	0.4	0.1	0.9	11.5	0.4	3	22	35	—
Rye straw, spring	86.0	3.5	1.3	29.1	36.9	7.7	0.6	0.4	0.8	17.0	17.3	15	41	60	—
„ straw, winter	85.7	6.0	1.5	43.0	40.0	8.3	0.6	0.4	0.7	15.3	20.4	14	37	62	—
„ chaff	89.2	7.4	2.0	38.3	44.1	10.2	1.1	0.7	0.4	11.3	22.0	22	63	31	—
Soya bean pods	84.0	9.0	1.7	29.8	30.4	5.3									
„ „ straw	86.7	10.4	1.7	32.9	26.1	8.8									
Tare or Vetch straw	85.7	2.9	1.3	35.9	40.9	6.1	4.1	3.2	0.8	15.4	16.4	13	35	8	—
„ „ pods	86.0	8.6	1.1	42.7	31.9	10.9									
Wheat straw, spring	86.0	2.1	1.3	40.7	35.9	5.3	0.1	—	0.4	14.7	18.0	13	39	336	—
„ cavings, spring	86.0				22.7										
„ straw, winter	86.0	3.8	1.8	39.8	36.6	8.6	0.1	—	0.4	15.0	18.3	13	38	342	—
„ cavings, „	86.0				32.0										
„ chaff (glumes) „	86.0	3.7	1.2	42.6	27.7	10.8									

COMPOSITION AND NUTRITIVE VALUE OF FEEDING STUFFS—continued

	Average composition per cent, as shown by chemical analysis						Digestible nutrients per cent					Calculated from digestible nutrients		Per 100 lb.	
	Dry Matter (1)	Crude Protein (2)	Oil (Ether Extract) (3)	Carbohydrate (Nitrogen-free Extractives) (4)	Crude Fibre (5)	Ash (6)	Dig. Crude Protein (7)	Dig. True Protein (8)	Dig. Oil (Dig. Ether Extract) (9)	Dig. Carbohydrate (Dig. Nitrogen-free Extractives) (10)	Dig. Fibre (11)	Nutritive Ratio (approx.) (12)	V. (13)	Starch Equivalent (14)	Total Digestible Nutrients (15)
II. Grains and Seeds															
Cereals															
Barley	85·1	10·0	1·5	66·5	4·5	2·6	7·6	7·0	1·2	60·9	2·5	1:9	98	71·4	—
Dari	88·9	9·6	3·8	71·2	1·9	2·4	7·7	6·7	3·0	60·5	1·0	1:9	100	74·1	—
Maize	87·0	9·9	4·4	69·2	2·2	1·3	7·9	7·4	2·7	63·7	0·8	1:9	100	77·6	—
Millet	87·5	10·6	3·9	61·1	8·1	3·8	8·0	7·4	3·1	45·8	2·7	1:7	95	58·9	—
Oats	86·7	10·3	4·8	58·2	10·3	3·1	8·0	7·2	4·0	44·8	2·6	1:7	95	59·5	—
Rice	88·6	8·3	1·8	64·7	8·8	5·0	—	—	—	—	—	—	—	—	—
Rice, polished	87·6	6·7	0·4	78·0	1·5	0·8	5·8	5·5	0·2	75·8	0·7	1:13	100	82·1	—
Rye	86·6	11·5	1·7	69·5	1·9	2·0	9·6	8·7	1·1	63·9	1·0	1:7	95	71·6	—
Wheat	86·6	12·1	1·9	69·0	1·9	1·7	10·2	9·0	1·2	63·5	0·9	1:7	95	71·6	—
Cereals (pig digestion trials)															
Barley Meal	86·0	10·5	1·5	66·6	4·8	2·6	8·6	—	1·2	59·1	0·5	—	—	—	70·9
Maize Meal (dry-fed)	87·0	9·6	4·4	69·4	2·0	1·6	7·5	—	2·8	63·5	0·5	—	—	—	77·8
,, ,, (soaked)	87·0	9·6	4·4	69·4	2·0	1·6	8·1	—	2·7	63·8	0·7	—	—	—	78·3
,, ,, (cooked)	87·0	9·4	4·5	69·7	1·6	1·8	8·1	—	2·9	64·4	0·4	—	—	—	79·4
Maize (flaked)	89·0	10·4	5·6	71·6	1·5	1·1	9·9	—	2·7	69·5	0·5	—	—	—	86·0
Oats (Sussex ground)	87·0	11·6	4·6	54·8	11·4	3·6	8·7	—	4·7	44·5	5·4	—	—	—	69·2
,, (farm-ground)	87·0	11·2	4·7	58·2	10·0	2·9	9·6	—	4·1	43·2	—	—	—	—	62·0
,, (crushed)	87·0	9·7	4·8	58·2	11·1	3·2	6·7	—	3·1	38·3	—	—	—	—	52·0
Legumes															
Beans	85·7	25·4	1·5	48·5	7·1	3·2	20·1	19·3	1·2	44·1	4·1	1:2	96	65·8	—
Butter ...	89·2	23·6	1·1	56·4	3·7	4·4	15·6	14·8	0·7	52·4	2·3	1:4	97	68·4	—

Gram	89·0	23·4	1·1	54·3	5·1	5·1	15·5	14·7	0·7	50·5	2·9	3	97	66·6	—
Lentils	86·0	25·5	1·9	52·2	3·4	3·0	21·9	19·1	1·2	48·5	1·8	3	99	70·0	—
Lupins, Sweet (yellow)	87·7	42·1	5·6	25·0	10·5	4·5	38·1	35·0	4·6	19·0	9·6	1	96	71·1	—
" " (blue)	87·3	33·9	5·9	37·0	7·2	3·3	30·3	28·4	4·8	28·6	7·0	1·5	97	72·1	—
Mutter	89·5	22·1	1·5	58·5	4·1	3·3									
Peas	86·0	22·5	1·6	53·7	5·4	2·8	19·4	16·9	1·0	49·9	2·5	3	98	69·0	—
Vetches	86·7	26·0	1·7	49·8	6·0	3·2	22·9	20·0	1·5	45·8	3·9	2	97	69·5	—
Oil Seeds															
Beech Mast	88·9	13·3	27·4	25·5	18·5	4·2	10·7	10·1	24·1	16·8	7·4	7	94	86·2	—
Brazil Nuts	95·0	16·5	68·0	4·0	2·8	3·7									
Coconut	85·0	5·5	59·0	15·0	4·0	1·5									
Cotton Seed, Egyptian	91·2	19·6	23·9	21·5	21·2	5·0	13·4	12·0	20·7	10·7	16·1	6	94	80·6	—
" " Bombay	91·5	17·9	19·4	29·9	20·0	4·3	12·3	11·0	16·8	15·0	15·2	6	94	74·3	—
" " Brazilian	90·6	21·1	23·2	25·0	17·0	4·3	14·4	12·9	20·1	12·5	12·9	5	94	83·7	—
Ground-Nuts, Earth or Pea-Nuts ...	94·0	26·8	44·9	17·5	2·6	2·2	24·1	22·2	40·3	14·7	0·2	4	99	131·4	—
Hemp Seed	91·1	18·2	32·6	21·1	15·0	4·2	13·7	12·8	29·3	16·8	9·0	7	96	103·7	—
Kapok Seed	89·5	23·0	22·0	18·5	20·0	6·0									
Linseed	92·9	24·2	36·5	22·9	5·5	3·8	19·4	18·1	34·7	18·3	1·8	5	99	119·2	—
Niger Seed'	95·0	23·0	38·0	13·0	16·0	5·0									
Palm Nut Kernels	91·6	8·4	48·8	26·8	5·8	1·8	8·0	7·8	46·5	22·5	3·5	16	99	143·6	—
Poppy Seed	92·8	20·9	32·5	23·3	8·6	7·5									
Rape Seed	92·7	19·6	45·0	18·0	5·9	4·2	15·9	13·8	42·8	14·4	1·5	8	99	130·5	—
Sesame Seed	94·5	20·5	47·2	15·0	6·3	5·5	18·4	16·8	44·8	8·4	1·4	6	99	133·2	—
Shea Nuts	94·5	7·5	49·0	32·0	2·9	3·1									
Soya Bean	90·0	33·2	17·5	30·5	4·1	4·7	29·5	26·2	15·8	20·8	1·7	2	98	78·9	—
Sunflower Seed	92·5	14·2	32·3	14·5	28·1	3·4	12·8	11·1	30·7	10·3	9·4	8	92	103·8	—
Miscellaneous Seeds															
Acorns, fresh	50·0	3·3	2·4	36·3	6·8	1·2	2·7	2·2	1·9	32·6	4·1	15	95	41·2	—
" dried	85·0	5·7	4·1	61·6	11·6	2·0	4·6	3·8	3·3	55·5	7·0	16	95	70·2	—
Buckwheat	85·9	11·3	2·6	54·8	14·4	2·8	8·5	7·5	1·9	42·3	3·5	6	93	53·4	—
Chestnuts, Sweet (kernel)	60·0	7·0	7·0	43·0	1·5	1·5									
Cleaver or Goose Grass seed ...	87·1	11·2	1·9	54·4	16·2	3·4									
Corn Cockle	88·2	15·2	5·0	58·1	6·2	3·7									
Corozo Nut (Vegetable Ivory) ...	89·5	4·6	0·9	76·0	6·9	1·1	1·9	—	0·3	70·6	4·5	40	97	75·5	—
Grape Seeds	91·0	8·5	11·5	21·6	47·1	2·3									
Hop Seeds	89·0	30·5	18·5	16·0	16·5	7·5									
Horse Chestnut, fresh...	50·8	4·3	1·5	40·9	2·5	1·6	2·6	1·5	1·2	33·3	0·8	14	99	38·0	—
" " dry	81·2	6·9	2·4	65·2	4·1	2·6	4·1	2·4	2·0	48·4	1·2	13	99	56·2	—
Locust Beans (pods plus seeds) ...	85·0	5·8	1·3	69·0	6·4	2·5	4·0	3·2	0·7	65·5	3·7	18	97	71·4	—
" " (pods)	87·0	4·0	1·0	70·0	9·0	3·0									

COMPOSITION AND NUTRITIVE VALUE OF FEEDING STUFFS—continued

	Average composition per cent. as shown by chemical analysis						Digestible nutrients per cent.					Calculated from digestible nutrients		Per 100 lb.	
	(1) Dry Matter	(2) Crude Protein	(3) Oil (Ether Extract)	(4) Carbohydrate (Nitrogen-free Extractives)	(5) Crude Fibre	(6) Ash	(7) Dig. Crude Protein	(8) Dig. True Protein	(9) Dig. Oil (Dig. Ether Extract)	(10) Dig. Carbohydrate (Dig. Nitrogen-free Extractives)	(11) Dig. Fibre	(12) Nutritive Ratio (approx.) 1:	(13) V.	(14) Starch Equivalent	(15) Total Digestible Nutrients
11. Grains and Seeds, Misc.—contd.															
Locust Beans (seeds)	88.0	16.0	3.0	59.0	7.0	3.0									—
Lucerne Seed Meal	88.0	33.1	10.5	31.9	8.1	4.4	27.8	23.9	9.0	27.7	5.0	2	97	75.6	—
Mangold Seed	86.1	11.9	5.3	28.8	33.2	6.9	7.2	4.6	3.2	17.8	11.6	5	76	30.3	—
Plantain Seed	88.8	16.2	8.0	38.6	22.5	3.5	27.5	23.8	6.8	26.9	7.5	1.8	96.4	72.0	—
Red Clover Seed Meal	87.5	32.6	7.8	31.2	9.2	6.7									—
Rye Grass Seed Meal (perennial plus Italian)	87.5	9.5	1.9	62.9	9.1	4.1	6.4	5.7	1.6	52.0	1.9	9	96	60.7	—
Sainfoin Seed Meal (unmilled seed)	88.0	26.4	6.0	33.7	17.9	4.0	22.8	19.3	5.3	25.2	7.3	2	92	60.0	—
„ „ (milled)	88.0	35.4	7.0	33.0	9.1	3.5									—
Spurrey Seed	89.0	13.7	10.7	54.6	6.8	3.2									—
Sugar-beet Seed	90.0	12.3	5.5	36.0	40.6	6.6	7.4	4.8	3.3	15.0	14.0	5	71	28.1	—
Old Trefoil Seed	90.0	33.5	5.5	36.0	11.0	4.0									—
Yorkshire Fog Seed (unshelled)	88.5	13.1	14.5	42.5	11.9	6.5									—
„ „ (shelled)	87.3	17.2	18.0	41.1	6.4	4.6									—
12. Oil Cakes and Meals															
Beech Mast Cake, shelled	89.4	36.3	8.4	30.2	6.7	7.8	32.0	31.0	7.6	22.9	1.6	1	97	69.7	—
„ „ unshelled	84.0	18.2	8.5	27.5	25.1	4.7	13.6	13.1	7.7	14.0	4.0	3	88	42.8	—
Castor Bean Meal, unshelled	89.9	29.2	1.4	15.9	37.0	6.4	23.6	22.0	1.3	6.9	3.3	0.6	70	24.9	—
„ „ „ (de-toxicated)	88.6	21.2		42.4	12.4	5.5									—
Coconut Cake	88.7	19.5	8.0	42.5	13.6	6.4	16.6	16.2	7.8	35.1	7.3	4	100	76.8	—
Cocoa Bean Cake	89.2	23.8	9.2	40.4	10.0	5.8	15.3	14.9	6.5	35.4	8.6	4	100	73.6	—
„ „ Meal (extracted)	87.1	24.9	6.7	42.1	19.0	6.1									—
Cotton Cake, Bombay	87.7	20.2	4.8	35.2	21.7	5.8	15.6	14.8	4.5	18.9	4.4	2	84	40.0	—
„ „ Brazilian	89.0	27.1	5.4	27.1	24.9	4.5	20.8	19.7	5.0	14.7	5.2	2	84	42.0	—

Feedstuff	1	2	3	4	5	6	7	8	9	10	11	12	13	14	15
Cotton Cake, Egyptian	87.9	5.0	23.2	32.6	21.3	5.8	17.8	16.8	4.6	17.7	4.5	2	84	41.6	—
,, decorticated	90.2	8.0	41.2	26.5	7.8	6.7	35.4	33.9	7.5	17.7	2.2	1	97	68.4	—
,, semi-decorticated	89.0	10.8	34.8	26.3	11.0	6.2	37.6	36.0	7.6	17.4	2.1	1	97	70.1	—
Cotton Seed Meal	91.3	8.0	43.6	25.8	7.7	6.2	42.0	40.6	6.8	19.7	0.5	1	98	73.0	—
Grape Seed Cake	88.5	7.5	12.0	25.5	36.4	4.6	27.7	26.8	8.2	18.4	2.6	1	86	56.8	—
Ground-Nut Cake, decorticated	89.7	9.1	46.8	23.2	22.9	5.8	29.2	28.3	1.5	20.0	2.9	1	84	44.4	—
,, ,, undecorticated	89.7		30.2	21.8	25.3	5.7	50.0	21.8	0.3	19.1	3.6	1	89	46.0	—
Ground-Nut Meal, undecorticated extracted	92.4	1.9	31.8	29.1	5.2	4.3	22.8	24.2	7.7	10.5	1.9	1	86	31.5	—
Ground-Nut Meal, decorticated extracted (pigs)	88.0	0.6	53.8	22.5	23.9	5.9	26.2	18.0	1.3	8.9	2.1	2	84	39.2	73.4
Hemp Seed Cake	89.3	8.6	30.8	18.3	25.7	7.7	20.0	23.9	6.4	10.1	5.1	1	97	74.0	—
Kapok Cake	88.7	1.7	34.8	16.8	25.8	9.3	25.3	26.3	8.7	28.5	4.3	1	97	74.5	—
,, Meal	86.4	7.1	27.0	20.2	9.1	6.3	27.8	30.0	9.1	25.8	4.5	1	96	63.7	—
Linseed Cake, English made	88.8	9.5	29.5	35.5	8.7	5.2	30.8	20.2	2.8	27.2	4.1	7	86	46.3	—
,, ,, foreign	89.0	9.9	32.3	32.2	9.0	5.9	22.2	10.2	8.3	11.1	2.5	8	97	84.3	—
Linseed Meal, extracted	88.2	3.1	35.7	33.9	20.9	6.5	10.4	9.0	11.5	47.0	0.5	9	100	84.0	—
Madia Cake	89.3	10.4	31.9	18.5	4.1	7.6	9.4	8.5	2.0	70.4	1.2		100	86.5	—
Maize Germ Meal	89.2	12.5	13.0	56.0	1.5	3.6	8.7	23.4	1.3	74.5	4.9		89	51.6	—
,, ,, flaked	89.0	4.3	9.8	72.5	1.3	0.8	26.0	3.5	4.7	19.8	9.9		85	62.2	—
,, Meal, degermed, cooked	88.0	1.5	9.2	75.2	17.5	0.8	6.1	16.4	17.0	20.5	5.1		100	73.2	—
Mustard Seed Cake	88.0	7.5	18.0	40.0	16.0	5.0	17.5	16.0	5.3	39.4	8.0		100	71.3	—
,, ,, Meal (extracted)	88.0	2.0	22.8	40.6	18.2	6.6	17.1	27.5	1.9	43.5	5.8		95		—
Niger Cake	22.8	5.8	32.5	23.5	30.0	9.4	11.4	24.7	0.5	37.6	4.1		95	62.3	—
Olive Cake	89.4	17.9	6.3	29.3	13.4	5.4	29.2	25.9	9.0	13.9	0.7		94	59.5	—
Palm Kernel Cake, English made	88.9	6.0	19.2	46.5	16.0	3.9	29.4	38.4	7.6	20.5	1.0		97	53.9	—
,, ,, Meal, extracted	89.0	2.0	19.0	49.0	16.0	4.0	30.7	32.3	2.4	26.2	1.4		97	73.0	—
,, ,, ,, extracted (pigs)	90.0	2.0	19.0	49.0	16.0	4.0	40.0	39.9	10.7	11.7	5.3		96	67.0	55.9
Poppy Seed Cake	90.0	9.8	36.9	21.7	8.3	13.8	34.0	35.0	10.0	9.4	2.4		97	57.7	—
Pumpkin Seed Cake	90.5	24.2	45.2	8.3	8.2	8.5	41.8	36.3	2.2	14.9	3.7		97	68.9	—
Rape Cake	94.4	9.6	35.5	25.6	8.3	12.4	38.8	30.7	5.1	20.4	3.6		95	64.0	—
,, Meal, extracted	91.4	3.1	36.9	32.7	9.3	7.3	40.3	15.7	1.4	24.7	5.3		88	72.5	—
Safflower Cake, decorticated	89.3	7.7	47.9	19.7	6.2	6.9	33.6		12.2	14.6				49.5	—
,, ,, undecorticated	88.4	9.7	20.2	25.1	33.0	3.4	17.2		6.5	20.6					—
Sesame Cake, English	91.4	11.9	44.5	20.9	4.5	8.8									—
,, ,, French	90.7	11.1	37.7	16.8	17.1	8.8									—
,, Meal, extracted	91.5	2.4	46.4	26.7	7.7	10.8									—
Shea Nut Cake	94.0	6.5	12.1	60.7	4.8	5.9									—
Soya-Bean Cake	90.0	5.6	43.1	26.3	5.1	5.4									—
Sunflower Cake, decorticated	85.5	1.5	44.7	31.9	12.1	5.5									—
,, ,, Meal, extracted	88.7	13.8	37.4	20.4		6.7									—
,, ,, undecorticated	90.4	7.4	19.1	28.9	30.0	7.5									—

COMPOSITION AND NUTRITIVE VALUE OF FEEDING STUFFS—continued

	Average composition per cent. as shown by chemical analysis						Digestible nutrients per cent.					Calculated from digestible nutrients			
	Dry Matter (1)	Crude Protein (2)	Oil (Ether Extract) (3)	Carbohydrate Nitrogen-free Extractives (4)	Crude Fibre (5)	Ash (6)	Dig. Crude Protein (7)	Dig. True Protein (8)	Dig. Oil (Dig. Ether Extract) (9)	Dig. Carbohydrate Nitrogen-free (Extractives) (10)	Dig. Fibre (11)	Nutritive Ratio (approx.) (12)	V. (13)	Starch Equivalent (14)	Total Digestible Nutrients (15)
12. Oil Cakes and Meals—*contd.*															
Walnut Cake	86·6	35·0	12·2	27·6	6·7	5·1	31·5	29·0	11·6	23·5	1·7	1:1·7	98	78·5	—
13. By-Products															
Apple Pomace, fresh ...	25·8	1·5	1·1	17·1	4·7	1·4	0·7	0·5	0·5	11·9	—	18	92	12·4	—
" " dried ...	88·3	4·0	3·5	51·8	27·2	1·8	1·6	1·2	1·7	36·3	1·7	26	78	32·3	—
Pear Pomace, dried ...	95·3	5·6	4·2	53·9	30·1	1·5									
Ash Fruits, dried ...	85·0	11·1	10·3	42·3	17·2	4·1									
Banana Flour	87·0	2·9	0·5	79·0	2·4	2·2									
From preparation of pearl barley :															
Barley Bran (with husks) ...	91·8	5·9	1·3	51·8	26·4	6·4	8·8	8·3	2·0	60·1	1·1	7	99	72·3	—
Medium Barley Dust ...	86·0	12·0	6·0	49·0	13·0	6·0									
Fine Barley Dust ...	87·4	11·9	2·2	65·5	4·6	3·2									
Barley Feed	89·0	13·0	2·8	59·9	6·1	4·2									
Brewers' Grains, fresh ...	32·4	7·5	3·4	14·6	6·1	1·4	5·5	5·2	2·4	9·1	2·4	3	86	18·4	—
" " dried ...	89·7	18·3	6·4	45·9	15·2	3·9	13·0	12·1	5·6	27·6	7·3	4	84	48·3	—
Distillers' " fresh ...	26·2	8·4	3·0	10·4	3·6	0·8	6·2	5·8	2·6	6·4	1·7	2	86	16·2	—
" " dried ...	92·0	27·7	11·6	40·8	10·1	1·8	19·6	18·7	10·2	25·3	4·8	3	84	57·2	—
Ale and Porter Grains, fresh ...	27·0	6·5	2·1	11·5	5·7	1·2	4·8	4·5	1·8	7·1	2·2	3	86	14·8	—
" " " dried	90·7	19·9	6·8	43·2	17·6	3·2	14·0	13·1	6·0	25·8	8·5	3	84	49·2	—
Malt Bran	91·2	7·8	2·4	57·2	19·2	4·6									
" " Coombs ...	90·0	24·4	2·0	42·4	14·0	7·2	19·9	12·0	1·5	30·9	12·7	3	75	43·4	—
Bean Husks (chaff or hulls) ...	88·0	3·5	0·2	37·1	42·9	4·3	—	—	0·2	21·3	37·8	—	83	48·5	—
Blood Meal	86·0	81·0	0·8	1·5	—	2·7	72·7	63·6	0·8	—	—	—	100	62·9	—

Bracken Roots ...	22·8	2·4	0·2	12·8	5·4	2·0									
,, ,, (dried)	90·0	9·5	1·2	51·0	20·0	8·3									
Bread (stale) ...	66·2	8·0	0·7	55·5	0·6	1·4									
,, Meal ...	90·7	13·0	0·9	73·0	0·8	3·0									
Broad Bean-Pod Meal	90·0	15·0	1·0	51·4	16·0	6·6	10·1	6·0	0·6	40·4	9·3	5	92	53·6	—
Burdock Roots ...	23·0	2·2	0·1	18·1	1·6	1·0									
Cabbage Meal (dried)	95·0	22·9	5·4	47·7	7·1	11·9									
Cacao Shells ...	89·1	14·5	3·1	46·5	18·3	6·7									
Carrot Slices (dried)	86·2	7·9	2·1	56·7	10·7	8·8									
Cashew Kernel Husks	90·8	12·4	11·3	53·9	11·3	1·9									
Celery Waste (leaves and stalks)	13·6	2·0	0·2	6·7	1·8	2·9									
Cellulose (commercial)	94·0	0·1	0·8	12·5	80·0	0·6									
Fodder Cellulose (from wheat straw by paper process)	90·0	0·3	0·5	14·6	71·8	2·8				5·6	65·1		94	66·8	—
Fodder Cellulose (from wheat straw by paper process) (pigs)	90·0	0·3	0·5	14·6	71·8	2·8				9·8	61·1				70·9
Chicory Roots ...	23·0	1·2	0·2	19·2	1·4	1·0									
Cider Sludge ...	13·5	3·7	0·2	8·3	0·7	0·6									
,, ,, (centrifuged)	36·9	10·3	0·3	23·6	0·9	1·8									
Clover Cobs (husks)	87·6	14·2	1·9	40·0	24·2	7·3									
Coffee Bran ...	90·6	2·4	0·8	24·8	61·7	0·9									
,, Grounds (dried)	89·0	11·5	12·0	38·5	25·0	2·0									
,, Silver Skin	92·7	13·2	1·2	32·5	33·2	7·4									
Cottonseed Bran	91·6	3·4	6·4	49·7	34·8	2·5									
,, Husks	90·6	3·9	0·9	36·7	46·6	3·1									
Couch Grass Roots (dried)	85·0	5·0	0·6	56·5	20·7	12·8									
Elm Fruits (dried)	88·4	24·6	15·3	15·0	6·4	2·3									
Figs, dried ...	70·8	3·3	0·4	58·4	—										
Fish Meal, white	87·0	61·0	3·5	1·5	—	21·0	55·0	51·0	3·3	1·2			100	58·9	—
Flax By-Products :															
Feeding Linseed (residue from dressing of seed) ...	90·0	23·5	26·0	26·3	9·6	4·6	4·8		3·7	11·1	14·7	7·2	76	29·8	—
Flax Bolls (capsules with seed)	88·5	17·0	24·0	25·0	17·0	5·5									
Flax Chaff (whole of seed removed)	87·9	7·0	2·4	33·5	38·3	6·7									
Flax Chaff (containing about 10 per cent. seed)...	87·3	8·0	5·0	35·1	32·2	7·0									
Flax Shives (dam-retted flax)	90·1	2·6	1·1	24·4	57·5	4·5									
,, ,, (green scutching)	90·8	8·7	7·6	25·2	42·9	6·4									
Grass, dried (frequently cut)	90·0	20·3	5·8	41·9	14·0	8·0	16·7	14·4	3·6	36·0	11·3	3·3	94	65·7	
,, ,, (cut less frequently)	90·0	15·8	4·5	41·4	44·4	8·0	11·7	10·4	2·3	34·2	16·7	4·8	91	60·3	
Greaves ...	90·5	58·6	25·5	—	—	6·4	55·7	21·0	23·5	—	—	1	100	106·1	
Ground Nut Husks	85·0	6·0	1·3	20·0	54·6	3·1									

V.D.

31

COMPOSITION AND NUTRITIVE VALUE OF FEEDING STUFFS—continued

	Average composition per cent as shown by chemical analysis						Digestible nutrients per cent					Calculated from digestible nutrients		Per 100 lb.	
	Dry Matter (1)	Crude Protein (2)	Oil (Ether Extract) (3)	Carbohydrate (Nitrogen-free Extractives) (4)	Crude Fibre (5)	Ash (6)	Dig. Crude Protein (7)	Dig. True Protein (8)	Dig. Oil (Dig. Ether Extract) (9)	Dig. Carbohydrate (Dig. Nitrogen-free Extractives) (10)	Dig. Fibre (11)	Nutritive Ratio (approx.) (12)	V. (13)	Starch Equivalent (14)	Total Digestible Nutrients (15)
13. By-Products—contd.												1 :			
Ground Nut Skins	93.5	15.9	22.4	41.9	10.6	2.7	—	—	—	—	—	—	—	—	—
Hatchery Waste (dried)	93.7	45.7	30.8	4.8	—	12.4	—	—	—	—	—	—	—	—	—
Hawthorn Berries	30.0	1.4	0.8	19.4	7.5	0.9	—	—	—	—	—	—	—	—	—
Hominy Chop, High Grade	89.9	10.6	8.0	64.3	4.4	2.6	7.0	6.1	7.3	58.0	3.3	12	95	78.2	—
„ „ Low Grade	90.9	9.5	6.2	64.0	8.5	2.7	6.3	5.5	5.6	57.7	6.4	12	95	76.9	—
Hops, spent, fresh	25.0	4.3	1.9	11.4	5.9	1.5	1.3	0.8	1.2	5.4	1.0	7	83	8.4	—
„ „ dried	89.1	15.3	6.8	39.6	21.0	6.4	4.7	3.0	4.4	19.0	3.6	7	83	29.8	—
Hop Meal	93.0	27.5	9.9	32.0	17.0	6.6	—	—	—	—	—	—	95	55.8	—
Horse-Chestnut Meal (alcohol-extracted)	90.0	6.6	6.7	67.1	7.2	2.4	—	—	4.0	48.2	1.3	—	—	—	58.2
„ „ (alcohol-extracted) (pigs)	90.0	7.0	7.0	66.2	7.6	2.4	1.3	—	2.9	49.1	—	—	96	55.0	—
Horse-Chestnut Meal (water-extracted)	90.0	6.6	6.7	67.1	7.6	2.2	—	—	4.6	46.2	—	—	—	—	59.2
„ „ (water-extracted) (pigs)	90.0	7.0	7.0	66.2	—	2.2	1.3	—	3.6	48.3	1.2	—	—	—	—
Lentil Husks (chaff or hulls)	90.0	7.0	0.7	47.5	25.6	3.1	1.3	—	0.7	33.4	17.2	40	89	46.7	—
Lime Fruits	88.0	11.1	3.0	9.7	13.5	2.1	—	—	—	—	—	—	—	—	—
Linseed Bran	31.9	3.6	18.8	35.7	2.3	11.8	—	—	7.4	—	—	—	—	—	—
Locust Bean Germ Meal	91.1	55.3	5.2	21.5	18.0	6.7	15.9	11.2	1.3	28.4	9.5	2.5	91	50.1	—
Lucerne Meal, English (from crop just coming into flower bud)	91.0	22.3	2.9	36.4	24.5	11.4	11.6	9.3	0.7	27.8	11.2	3.5	86	44.1	—
Lucerne Meal, English (from crop in early flower)	91.0	16.2	2.4	37.7	16.0	10.2	16.3	14.7	—	31.5	7.9	2.4	92	50.2	—
Lucerne Leaf Meal, American	91.0	21.4	1.9	40.6	22.7	11.1	11.7	9.9	7.4	24.5	7.4	—	—	46.8	46.8

	1	2	3	4	5	6	7	8	9	10	11	12	13	14	15
Maize, bran	88.2	8.4	4.2	62.0	11.7	1.9	5.5	4.8	3.6	53.4	3.9	12	95	67.0	—
,, gluten feed	89.6	23.5	3.4	56.7	3.5	2.5	20.0	18.4	2.7	49.3	2.5	3	100	75.6	—
,, meal	90.9	35.5	4.7	47.5	2.1	1.1	30.6	30.3	4.4	42.6	—	2	100	81.5	—
,, malt coombs	86.5	30.7	14.5	39.6	5.8	5.9	17.4	10.6	12.4	34.9	4.5	4	75	59.4	—
,, feeding meal from corn-flour	89.8	20.4	1.0	59.0	1.1	1.0	17.0	15.5	3.5	51.3	3.3	4	100	77.6	—
,, sprouted	22.4	3.1	6.9	16.7		0.5									—
,, starch feed	90.9	22.8	3.1	52.7	7.6	0.9	19.2	18.4	6.2	44.8	5.5	3	100	81.8	—
Malt, dry	93.4	13.8	15.0	64.9	9.0	2.6	11.0	8.8	2.4	56.4	4.5	6	96	71.5	—
Meat and Bone Meal*	90.3	50.3	13.2	1.0		24.0	39.2	29.2	14.3	—		1	100	67.8	—
Pure Meat Meal	89.2	72.2	11.0	—		3.8	67.2	63.6	12.5	0.5			100	91.0	—
Feeding Meat Meal (high fat)	90.5	60.0	2.9	0.5		19.0	56.4	42.4	9.8	3.9			100	72.3	—
,, ,, (low fat)	93.0	66.7	17.4	4.0		19.4	58.6	43.4	2.4	—			—	59.6	—
Crude Carcass Meal (pigs)	90.5	44.5	—	4.6		24.0	37.2	—	15.6	4.1			100	—	72.3
Milk, buttermilk	9.2	3.4	0.8	4.1		0.7	3.4			4.8		2	100	9.2	
,, cow's, whole	12.8	3.4	3.9	4.8		0.7	3.2			5.0		4	100	17.1	
,, separated	9.4	3.5	0.1	5.0		0.8	3.3			5.0		2	100	8.3	
,, skimmed, deep set	9.7	3.5	0.4	5.0		0.8	3.3			5.0		2	100	9.1	
,, skimmed, shallow set	10.0	3.5	0.7	5.0		0.8	3.3			5.0		2	100	9.8	
,, whey	6.6	0.7	0.2	5.0		0.7	0.6					9		6.1	
Colostrum (first-drawn)	25.5	17.6	4.2	2.7		1.0									
Dried whole milk	95.8	25.5	26.5	37.4		6.4									
,, separated milk	89.7	32.8	1.5	47.9		7.5									
Condensed whole milk (unsweetened)	38.6	11.2	11.4	14.0		2.0									
,, separated milk (unsweetened)	31.4	12.4	0.3	15.7		3.0									
Dried buttermilk	90.0	35.3	7.0	40.0		7.7									
Semi-solid buttermilk	29.9	11.8	2.4	13.2		2.5									
Whey paste	46.0	6.2	0.8	35.0		4.0									
Dried whey	92.2	12.6	1.4	70.5		7.7									
From preparation of lactose: No. 1 Extract from whey	57.0	15.0		30.0†		12.0	4.0	3.6	2.0	35.6	8.1	12	88	45.5	—
No. 2 ,, ,,	49.0	13.0		27.0†		9.0	12.0	10.5	5.4	48.0	0.8	5	99	71.1	—
Mussels (dried)	98.3	10.6	1.1	2.7		83.9									—
Oat Bran (from preparation of oatmeal)	90.5	8.0	3.6	51.0	21.9	6.0									
,, Meal	91.8	16.0	6.7	65.5	1.6	2.0									
,, Clippings	90.0	7.3	1.7	45.3	27.2	8.5									
,, Husks	94.0	16.2	1.0	54.0	33.0	4.0									
,, Kernels	91.7	5.0	6.4	65.3	1.9	1.9		0.4		19.4	10.9		66	20.6	
,, "Meal Seeds" (coarse)	90.9	10.1	2.0	51.0	30.0	3.0									
,, ,, (fine)	90.9	5.2	5.2	57.8	14.5	3.3									
,, Feed (ordinary)	92.0	5.5	2.4	52.5	27.6	4.0									

* Brands of meat and bone and of feeding meat meal containing no more than 4 per cent. of oil, are now available.

† Including 5 per cent. of lactic acid.

‡ Including 10 per cent. of lactic acid.

COMPOSITION AND NUTRITIVE VALUE OF FEEDING STUFFS—continued

	Average composition per cent. as shown by chemical analysis						Digestible nutrients per cent.						Calculated from digestible nutrients		
	Dry Matter (1)	Crude Protein (2)	Oil (Ether Extract) (3)	Carbohydrate (Nitrogen-free Extractives) (4)	Crude Fibre (5)	Ash (6)	Dig. Crude Protein (7)	Dig. True Protein (8)	Dig. Oil (Dig. Ether Extract) (9)	Dig. Carbohydrate (Dig. Nitrogen-free Extractives) (10)	Dig. Fibre (11)	Nutritive Ratio (approx.) 1: (12)	V. (13)	Starch Equivalent — Per 100 lb. (14)	Total Digestible Nutrients — Per 100 lb. (15)
13. By-Products—contd.															
Oat Feed (high grade)	91·0	10·3	5·0	53·7	17·5	4·5									
Cockle	87·7	13·0	5·8	62·7	3·6	2·6									
„ Dust	93·0	10·0	11·0	55·0	13·0	4·0									
Parsnip Seed Meal	93·2	18·0	22·7	28·1	17·5	6·9									
Pea Germ Meal	92·5	32·0	2·9	48·9	2·2	6·5									
„ Husks (chaff or hulls)	87·8	5·3	0·7	31·1	47·9	2·8	3·6	3·2	0·5	27·9	45·0	21	83	64·2	
„ Pod Meal (from canning industry)	90·0	13·5	1·2	54·1	15·5	5·7	9·7	4·4	0·8	41·5	9·6	5·5	92	54·8	
Penicillin Felts (dried)	95·2	42·3	4·0	27·9	9·8	11·2	31·3	20·1	2·0	22·8	8·6	1·1	95·6	62·2	
„ „ (dried) (pigs)	95·2	42·3	4·0	27·9	9·8	11·2	28·0		1·1	18·3	8·0				56·8
Plantain Meal	86·2	2·2	0·7	80·6	0·7	2·0				52·5	1·1		95	51·0	
Potato Sludge	86·0	3·4	0·1	68·2	8·8	5·5									
„ Slump	90·0	24·3	3·7	40·8	9·5	11·7	12·2	9·4	1·8	20·4	2·0	2	90	31·8	
„ Pulp (dry)	86·0	3·4	0·1	68·2	8·8	5·5	4·7	0·7		56·6	2·1	14	95	55·8	
„ Cossettes (Meal)	88·0	8·6	0·5	73·4	2·0	3·5	3·4		0·15	63·4	1·0	21	100	68·8	
„ Meal (pigs)	88·0	8·6	0·5	73·4	2·1	3·5	3·8	2·1		70·7	1·3	19			75·7
„ Flakes	90·0	8·2	0·3	75·6	2·1	3·8	6·7			70·8	1·6	12	100	75·2	
„ Flakes (pigs)	90·0	8·2	0·3	75·6	1·6	3·8	4·0	2·2		75·6	1·6	17			83·9
„ Slices	89·0	9·3	0·2	74·0	1·6	3·9	7·0			68·6	0·8	10	100	73·2	
„ Slices (pigs)	89·0	9·3	0·2	74·0	1·9	3·9				72·5	0·5				80·0
„ Peelings (machine)	11·0	1·0	0·8	6·6	0·7	0·7									
„ Peelings (hand) (pigs)	21·2	2·1	0·1	17·0	2·6	1·3	1·6	1·0		16·4	0·5				18·5
„ Dust	94·9	9·3	0·1	76·6		6·2									
Rice meal	91·1	12·9	13·7	49·5	6·4	8·1	7·5	6·6	11·6	39·0	1·6	9	100	72·3	
„ sludge, dried	86·0	26·2	2·1	55·2	1·1	1·4	21·5	16·3	1·0	50·3	0·7	3	90	61·7	

Rye Bran	87·5	16·7	3·1	58·0	5·2	4·5	12·5	10·8	2·4	1·7	4	79	46·9	66·7
Sago Pith Meal (pigs)	87·0	1·7	0·4	77·2	4·3	3·4	0·0	0·0	0·3	—	—	—	—	—
Seaweed Meal (dried):														
Laminaria	83·7	11·4	1·1	45·8	8·6	16·8	6·1	4·4	0·9	39·8	7	82	38·7	28·6
" (pigs)	83·7	11·4	1·1	45·8	8·6	16·8	1·3	0·0	0·8	25·5			37·0	
Fucus	88·7	5·2	4·2	53·6	9·4	16·3	0·0	0·0	4·0	41·8		75		34·4
" (pigs)	88·5	5·2	3·7	53·6	9·4	16·3	0·0	0·0	3·4	26·7				
Soya Bean Husks				32·6	39·3	5·0	0·6	1·0			38			
Straw Pulp (alkaline treatment)*														
From Barley Straw	16·9	0·8	0·3	6·8	7·8	1·2	1·0		0·1	5·7	12	77·7	11·7	
" Oat Straw	18·3	0·5	0·3	7·0	9·3	1·2	5·3		0·2	6·8	13	76·7	60·6	
" Wheat Straw	19·4	0·4	0·2	7·7	9·9	1·2	3·1		0·1	7·5	22	75·9		23·2
Sugar Beet Grated (pigs)	26·2	1·6	1·2	22·2	1·1	1·1	6·3			1·0	11		58·3	
" Frozen (dried)	92·5	5·5	0·1	72·7	8·7	4·4	2·6				25	94	51·6	
" Pulp, wet	15·0	1·6	0·6	9·6	3·1	0·6	1·2			2·8		80·5		
" " dried	90·0	8·9	0·6	59·1	18·3	3·1		5·0		16·3			50·6	70·0
" " dried (pigs)	90·0	8·9	0·6	59·1	18·3	3·1				15·4		80·5		67·2
" " molassed	90·0	10·8	0·4	58·2	15·1	5·5		3·0		13·5				
" " molassed (pigs)	90·0	10·8	0·4	58·2	15·1	5·5				12·7				
" Molasses	74·7	3·5		66·0		3·0						87		
" Tailings	14·3	1·0	0·1	8·5	1·7	6·4								
" Cane Molasses	74·2	3·1		64·7		2·6						87		
Sultanas (dried)	76·7	1·4	0·7	70·9	1·1		1·1							
Swill (pigs):														
Urban Swill, Winter	25·0	3·7	3·0	14·5	1·8	2·4	2·3	1·6	2·3	0·8	8·7			
" " (processed)	31·9	4·7	3·0	18·5	1·8	3·1	2·9	2·0	2·9	1·0	8·7			
" Summer	25·0	4·1	3·1	12·4	2·4	3·0	2·7	2·4	2·5	0·9	6·5			
" " (processed)	30·1	4·9	3·7	15·0	2·9	3·6	3·3		3·0	1·1	6·5			
" Summer (dried & balanced)	89·7	24·8	10·9	29·8	7·8	16·4	18·7	13·2	8·9	3·6	2·3			
Military Camp Swill (meat-rich)	31·4	6·4	8·9	13·7	0·5	1·9	5·8	4·9	8·5	0·3	6			
" " (ordinary quality)	25·0	4·2	4·2	12·3	1·5	2·8	2·6	1·9	3·2	0·8	7·7			
Swill (ruminants):														
Urban Swill (processed)	29·7	3·9	2·3	17·6	1·5	4·4	2·4	?	1·9	0·7	8·7			22·2
Tapioca Flour	88·0	1·8	0·5	81·1	2·5	2·1	1·2		0·1	1·9	69			28·1
" Ampas	87·3	0·9	0·3	80·5	4·9	0·8								20·1
" Roots	87·1	1·9	0·3	81·6	1·9	1·4								24·4
Trefoil " Cosh " (pods)	85·7	14·0	2·0	40·0	23·0	6·7								61·5
Tomato Flour (skins and seeds)	93·3	23·1	20·5	17·8	25·7	6·2								38·7
Walnut Shells	92·3	1·7	0·7	31·9	56·6	1·4						98	22·3	22·4
Whale Meat Flakes	88·0	60·0	12·0		16·0	16·0						100	83·5	

* Means of trials at the Jealott's Hill Research Station.

COMPOSITION AND NUTRITIVE VALUE OF FEEDING STUFFS—continued

	Average composition per cent. as shown by chemical analysis						Digestible nutrients per cent.						Calculated from digestible nutrients		Per 100 lb.
	(1) Dry Matter	(2) Crude Protein	(3) Oil (Ether Extract)	(4) Carbohydrate (Nitrogen-free Extractives)	(5) Crude Fibre	(6) Ash	(7) Dig. Crude Protein	(8) Dig. True Protein	(9) Dig. Oil (Dig. Ether Extract)	(10) Dig. Carbohydrate (Dig. Nitrogen-free Extractives)	(11) Dig. Fibre	(12) Nutritive Ratio (approx.)	(13) V.	(14) Starch Equivalent	(15) Total Digestible Nutrients
13. By-Products—contd.															
Whale Meat Meal	92·0	60·0	16·0	—	—	16·0									
" " (high protein, low ash) (pigs)	94·4	87·7	3·4	1·2	—	2·1	76·9	71·7	3·3	1·1	—	1 :	—	—	85·4
Wheat Germ Meal (vacuum heated)	89·8	32·0	9·2	41·9	2·0	4·7									
Malt Bran	90·6	12·9	3·3	61·1	10·2	3·1									
Wood Sugar Syrup	71·6	0·6	—	66·5	—	4·5									
Wheat Feeds:															
Pure Grades															
Finest grade, fine middlings	86·7	17·0	4·2	60·8	2·3	2·4	12·6	11·6	3·7	51·1	—	5	97	69·0	—
Second grade, coarse middlings or sharps (fine wheatfeed)*	86·0	15·9	4·5	55·9	6·0	3·7	11·6	10·1	3·9	45·9	1·4	5	86	56·5	—
Fourth grade, bran	87·0	15·1	3·8	52·8	9·5	5·8	10·9	8·9	2·6	37·4	2·2	4	77	42·6	—
Broad bran	87·0	14·7	4·0	52·1	10·3	5·9	11·0	9·0	2·8	36·9	2·2	4	77	42·6	—
War-time Grades															
Fine Wheatfeed (75% extraction)	87·0	16·3	5·1	54·1	7·5	4·0	12·2	—	3·1	41·2	2·0	4·1	80	49·0	—
" " (75% extraction) (pigs)	87·0	16·3	5·1	54·1	7·5	4·0	12·7	—	3·5	41·2	1·6	4·4	—	—	63·4
Fine Bran (85% extraction)	87·0	15·2	4·5	53·5	9·4	4·4	10·8	—	2·6	39·6	1·9	4·4	77	44·0	—
" " (85% extraction) (pigs)	87·0	15·2	4·5	53·5	9·4	4·4	11·9	—	3·0	39·7	1·6	—	—	—	60·0
Coarse Bran (85% extraction)	87·0	15·0	4·3	52·3	10·3	5·1	11·0	—	0·9	37·5	2·8	3·9	77	40·4	—
" " (85% extraction) (pigs)	87·0	15·0	4·3	52·3	10·3	5·1	10·3	—	1·5	33·3	1·2	—	—	—	48·2
Fine Millers' Offals (85% extraction)†	87·0	14·1	4·3	53·4	10·3	4·9	9·9	—	2·4	38·7	3·3	4·8	77	43·4	—

* Home-produced middlings were marketed before the war under the names of Weatings (with a guarantee of not more than 5·75 per cent. of fibre) and Superfine Weatings (with a guarantee of not more than 4·5 per cent. of fibre).

Fine Millers' Offals (85% extraction) (pigs)*	87·0	14·1	4·3	53·4	10·3	4·9	9·0	—	2·7	34·7	1·6				51·4
Coarse Millers' Offals (85% extraction)*	87·0	12·3	3·9	51·4	13·4	6·0	7·6	—	0·1	34·8	4·4	5·2	75	34·9	—
Coarse Millers' Offals (85% extraction) (pigs)*	87·0	12·3	3·9	51·4	13·4	6·0	6·7	—	1·8	28·7	1·7				
Yeast, dried	93·7	41·5	1·0	41·4	0·2	9·6	35·6	29·4	0·4	34·1	—	1	100	68·3	41·2
,, ,, (pigs)	93·7	41·5	1·0	41·4	0·2	9·6	37·1	30·8	—	38·6	—	1	100	61·2	—
,, Wood Sugar (dried)	90·0	47·1	1·3	34·3	—	7·3	42·4	32·3	0·3	30·2	—				75·7

* Wheat diluted with 10 per cent. barley before milling.

MINERAL COMPOSITION OF SOME COMMON FEEDING STUFFS

—	Total Ash per cent.	Lime (CaO) per cent.	Phosphoric Acid(P$_2$O$_5$) per cent.	Potash (K$_2$O) per cent.	Chlorine (Cl$_2$) per cent.
Mangolds	0·9	0·02	0·09	0·45	0·16
Potatoes	1·0	0·03	0·18	0·60	0·04
Potatoes (dried)	3·5	0·08	0·39	2·19	0·30
Potato peelings (hand)	1·3	0·04	0·10	?	0·07
Swedes	0·7	0·08	0·08	0·30	0·04
Cabbage	1·2	0·20	0·15	0·40	0·02
Kale, thousand head	1·7	0·39	0·13	0·52	0·16
Kale, marrow stem	1·9	0·43	0·12	0·55	0·21
Sugar-beet tops	3·4	0·34	0·11	0·58	?
Tulip bulbs	2·7	0·08	0·38	?	0·04
Pasture grass (rotational close-grazing)	2·0	0·28	0·16	0·60	0·19
Grass meal (18 per cent. protein) ...	8·8	1·20	0·75	2·70	0·80
Vetches, in flower	1·5	0·50	0·15	0·50	?
Clover, red, flowering	1·6	0·40	0·15	0·50	0·05
Lucerne (before bud)	1·8	0·45	0·13	0·48	0·05
Lucerne (in bud)	1·8	0·77	0·14	0·56	0·05
Lucerne (early flower)	2·4	0·96	0·12	0·43	0·08
Lucerne meal	9·2	2·73	0·78	1·82	0·55
Pea-pod meal	5·7	1·37	0·54	1·32	0·32
Broad-bean-pod meal	6·6	0·83	0·54	2·34	0·47
Pea-pod silage	1·8	0·50	0·14	?	0·05
Pea-haulm-plus-pod silage	4·1	0·54	0·16	?	0·11
Meadow hay, good	6·2	1·00	0·43	1·60	0·37
Red clover hay	7·0	1·60	0·39	2·20	0·24
Seeds hay	6·3	2·00	0·60	1·80	0·30
Lucerne hay (half flower)	8·0	2·74	0·51	1·52	0·34
Oat straw	4·9	0·36	0·18	1·50	0·30
Wheat straw	5·3	0·29	0·13	0·80	0·20
Bean straw (including Pods)	4·6	1·20	0·30	1·90	?
Pea straw	6·6	1·60	0·40	1·00	?
Barley	2·6	0·07	0·84	0·57	0·12
Maize	1·3	0·02	0·82	0·40	0·07
Oats	3·1	0·14	0·81	0·55	0·07
Wheat	1·7	0·05	0·86	0·60	0·08
Beans	3·2	0·18	0·88	1·28	0·03
Peas	2·8	0·10	0·90	1·00	0·04
Lucerne Seed Meal	4·4	0·29	1·34	?	0·13
Red Clover Seed Meal	6·7	0·32	1·33	?	0·13
Rye Grass Seed Meal	4·1	0·29	0·69	?	0·11
Sainfoin Seed Meal (unmilled seed) ...	4·0	1·02	0·91	?	0·11
Sainfoin Seed Meal (milled seed) ...	3·5	0·23	1·11	?	0·11
Bran	5·8	0·20	2·80	1·50	0·09
Middlings (weatings)	3·7	0·13	1·50	1·40	0·07
Castor bean meal (de-toxicated) ...	6·4	1·02	1·70	?	0·10
Coconut cake	5·4	0·50	1·50	2·00	?
Cotton cake, undec.	5·8	0·30	2·50	1·60	0·05
Cotton-seed meal	6·0	0·36	2·70	1·60	0·04
Ground-nut cake, undec.	5·7	0·20	1·00	1·10	?
Ground-nut cake, dec.	5·8	0·20	1·30	1·50	0·03
Horse-chestnut meal (alcohol-extracted)	2·4	0·31	0·25	?	0·08
Horse-chestnut meal (water-extracted)	2·2	0·52	0·36	?	0·06
Linseed cake	5·2	0·51	1·70	1·30	0·09
Palm-kernel cake	3·8	0·30	1·10	0·50	0·16
Soya-bean cake	5·4	0·30	2·00	1·80	0·03
Soya-bean meal, extr.	5·5	0·30	2·10	1·90	0·03
Fish meal, white	22·0	10·00	9·00	1·20	1·00
Meat meal, pure	3·8	0·40	0·70	0·10	0·27
Meat meal	19·0	8·00	7·20	0·70	1·20
Meat and bone meal	24·0	10·50	9·30	0·80	1·40

MINERAL COMPOSITION OF SOME COMMON FEEDING STUFFS
—continued

—	Total Ash per cent.	Lime (CaO) per cent.	Phosphoric Acid(P₂O₅) per cent.	Potash (K₂O) per cent.	Chlorine (Cl₂) per cent.
Blood meal	2·7	0·05	0·22	0·31	0·85
Yeast, dried	9·6	0·30	5·50	2·00	0·03
Penicillin felts (dried)	11·2	0·81	5·59	?	0·28
Milk, whole	0·8	0·17	0·20	0·20	0·10
Milk, separated	0·8	0·15	0·20	0·20	0·10
Whey	0·7	0·10	0·10	0·15	0·07
Brewers' grains, dried	3·9	0·40	1·60	0·20	0·06
Distillers' grains, dried	1·8	0·40	0·68	0·20	0·06
Locust bean meal	4·0	0·85	0·26	0·70	0·20
Maize, meal, degermed...	0·9	0·02	0·39	0·33	0·03
Maize, flaked	0·9	Trace	0·60	0·25	Trace
Maize germ meal	3·6	0·10	0·90	1·30	?
Maize gluten meal	1·1	0·05	0·30	0·05	?
Maize gluten feed	2·5	0·10	0·70	0·20	?
Rice meal	8·6	0·10	2·50	0·70	0·14
Sago pith meal	3·4	0·33	0·11	0·54	0·56
Seaweed meal (dried) :					
Laminaria	16·8	4·62	0·21	1·25	0·69
Fucus	16·3	1·60	0·11	1·80	1·32
Sugar-beet pulp, dried	3·1	1·20	0·18	0·59	0·05
Sugar-beet pulp, molassed	5·5	1·20	0·17	1·34	0·48
Swill, Urban	2·4	0·23	0·18	?	0·19
„ „ processed...	3·1	0·29	0·23	?	0·24
„ „ dried and balanced ...	16·4	4·80	3·45	?	0·75
„ military camp (meat rich) ...	1·9	0·17	0·25	?	0·28
„ „ (ordinary quality) ...	2·8	0·34	0·14	?	0·24
Tapioca flour	2·2	0·22	0·25	1·04	0·02
Steamed bone flour (dry matter) ...	88·7	45·80	31·10	?	?
Whale meat meal (high-protein, low-ash)	2·1	0·05	0·90	?	0·03

Note.—The above data are compiled, as far as possible, from recent British analyses. Inevitably, however, some of the data have been taken from the results of old, and in some cases, foreign analyses. The table has been revised and enlarged in the light of new analyses since its first appearance in the 1932 edition of *Rations for Livestock*, but the compiler (Dr. H. E. Woodman) would welcome suggestions from readers who may be able to supply reliable data for the purpose of further revision and extension. The sign ? indicates absence of data.

Appendix 2*

THE SECOND SCHEDULE

CONDITIONS AS TO CONTENT

PART A.—COMPOUNDS

1. NATIONAL CATTLE FOOD No. 1 (DAIRY RATION)

The compound shall—	Percentage by Weight Minimum	Maximum
(a) conform to the following analysis:—		
Oil	3	6
Albuminoids (protein)	16	21
Fibre	—	10
Calcium expressed as calcium carbonate ...	2	3½
Chlorine expressed as sodium chloride ...	1	1½
(b) contain the following:—		
Wheat by-products	10	—
Cereals	10	—
Low protein oilseed cake	5	20
High and medium protein oilseed cake ...	15	—
Undecorticated oilseed cake and undecorticated oilseed cake meal (or any one or more of them)	—	15
Ground chalk and limestone flour (or either of them)	1½	2

2. NATIONAL CATTLE FOOD No. 2 (DAIRY RATION)

The compound shall—	Percentage by Weight Minimum	Maximum
(a) conform to the following analysis:—		
Oil	3	6
Albuminoids (protein)	17	21
Fibre	—	10
Calcium expressed as calcium carbonate ...	2	3½
Chlorine expressed as sodium chloride ...	1	1½
(b) contain the following:—		
Wheat by-products	10	—
Cereals	10	—
High and medium protein oilseed cake ...	20	—
Undecorticated oilseed cake and undecorticated oilseed cake meal (or any one or more of them)	5	15
Low protein oilseed cake	5	15
Ground chalk and limestone flour (or either of them)	1½	2

3. NATIONAL CATTLE FOOD No. 3 (RATION FOR REARING YOUNG STOCK)

(1) the compound shall—	Percentage by Weight Minimum	Maximum
(a) conform to the following analysis:—		
Oil	3	6
Albuminoids (protein)	18	23
Fibre	—	8½
Calcium expressed as calcium carbonate ...	2	3½
Chlorine expressed as sodium chloride ...	1	1½

*Reproduced from "The Feeding Stuffs (Regulation of Manufacture) Order, 1947," by permission of the Controller, H.M. Stationery Office.

3. NATIONAL CATTLE FOOD No. 3—*cont.*

	Percentage by Weight	
	Minimum	Maximum
(b) contain the following:—		
Wheat by-products	10	—
Cereals	10	—
Low protein oilseed cake	—	15
Linseed cake	10	—
High protein oilseed cake	10	—
Undecorticated groundnut cake and undecorticated groundnut meal (or either of them) ...	—	5
Ground chalk and limestone flour (or either of them)	1½	2

(2) The compound shall not contain any undecorticated cottonseed cake or undecorticated cottonseed cake meal.

4. NATIONAL HORSE FOOD (FOR TOWN AND OTHER WORKING HORSES)

	Percentage by Weight	
	Minimum	Maximum
(1) The compound shall—		
(a) conform to the following analysis:—		
Oil	3	5
Albuminoids (protein)	13	16
Fibre	—	10
Calcium expressed as calcium carbonate ...	1	1½
Chlorine expressed as sodium chloride ...	—	1
(b) contain the following:—		
Wheat by-products	10	30
Oats	15	30
Barley	10	20
Beans	—	15
Linseed cake	7½	10
Low protein oilseed cake	15	20
Molasses	5	7½

(2) Brewer's dried grains may be substituted for wheat by-products up to a maximum of 15 per cent. by weight of the completed compound.

5. NATIONAL PIG FOOD No. 1 (SOW AND WEANER RATION)

	Percentage by Weight	
	Minimum	Maximum
(1) The compound shall—		
(a) conform to the following analysis:—		
Oil	—	4½
Albuminoids (protein)	16	19
Fibre	—	8¾
Calcium expressed as calcium carbonate ...	1½	2¾
Chlorine expressed as sodium chloride ...	—	¾
(b) contain the following:—		
Wheat by-products	10	—
Total cereals	10	—
Wheat	—	10
Oats	—	15
Low protein oilseed cake	—	15
Any animal protein rich substances	5	10
Molasses	—	5

(2) Any of the compound manufactured during the months of October to April inclusive shall contain cod-liver oil equivalent to either:—

(a) not less than one per cent. of cod-liver oil containing 500 international units of Vitamin A and 50 B.S.I. units of Vitamin D per gramme, or

(b) not less than one half of one per cent. of cod-liver oil containing 800 international units of Vitamin A and 100 B.S.I. units of Vitamin D per gramme.

(3) The compound shall not contain any cottonseed cake or cottonseed meal (decorticated or undecorticated).

6. NATIONAL PIG FOOD No. 2 (FOR FATTENING PIGS)

	Percentage by Weight	
	Minimum	*Maximum*
(1) The compound shall—		
(a) conform to the following analysis:—		
Oil	—	4½
Albuminoids (protein)	13	16
Fibre	—	9
Calcium expressed as calcium carbonate	1	2¾
Chlorine expressed as sodium chloride	—	¾
(b) Contain the following:—		
Wheat by-products	10	—
Total cereals	10	—
Wheat	—	15
Oats	—	15
Low protein oilseed cake	—	15
Any animal protein rich substances	5	10
Molasses	—	5

(2) The compound shall not contain any cottonseed cake or cottonseed meal (decorticated or undecorticated).

7. NATIONAL POULTRY FOOD No. 1 (LAYING MASH OR PELLETS FOR SUMMER FEEDING)

	Percentage by Weight	
	Minimum	*Maximum*
(1) The compound shall—		
(a) conform to the following analysis:—		
Oil	2½	—
Albuminoids (protein)	16	19
Fibre	—	9
Calcium expressed as calcium carbonate	2½	6
Chlorine expressed as sodium chloride	¼	1
(b) contain the following:—		
Wheat by-products	10	—
Cereals	10	—
Low protein oilseed cake	—	15
Any animal protein rich substances	5	10
Molasses	—	5

(2) The compound shall not contain any cottonseed cake or cottonseed meal (decorticated or undecorticated).

8. NATIONAL POULTRY FOOD No. 1A (LAYING MASH OR PELLETS FOR WINTER FEEDING AND FOR BATTERY KEPT BIRDS)

	Percentage by Weight	
	Minimum	*Maximum*
(1) The compound shall—		
(a) conform to the following analysis:—		
Oil	2½	—
Albuminoids (protein)	16	19
Fibre	—	9
Calcium expressed as calcium carbonate	2½	6
Chlorine expressed as sodium chloride	¼	1
(b) contain the following:—		
Wheat by-products	10	—
Cereals	10	—
Low protein oilseed cake	—	15
Any animal protein rich substances	5	10
Molasses	—	5

(2) The compound shall contain cod-liver oil equivalent to either:—

(a) not less than one per cent. of cod-liver oil containing 500 international units of Vitamin A and 50 B.S.I. units of Vitamin D per gramme, or

(b) not less than one half of one per cent. of cod-liver oil containing 800 international units of Vitamin A and 100 B.S.I. units of Vitamin D per gramme.

8. NATIONAL POULTRY FOOD No. 1A—*cont.*

(3) The compound shall not contain any cottonseed
cake or cottonseed meal (decorticated or undecorticated).

9. NATIONAL POULTRY FOOD No. 2 (GROWERS' MASH OR PELLETS FOR
SUMMER FEEDING)

	Percentage by Weight	
(1) The compound shall—	Minimum	Maximum
(*a*) conform to the following analysis:—		
Oil	2½	—
Albuminoids (protein)	15	18
Fibre	—	9
Calcium expressed as calcium carbonate ...	2½	3½
Chlorine expressed as sodium chloride ...	¼	1
(*b*) contain the following:—		
Wheat by-products	10	—
Cereals	10	—
Low protein oilseed cake	—	15
Any animal protein rich substances	5	10
Molasses	—	5

(2) The compound shall not contain any cottonseed
cake or cottonseed meal (decorticated or undecorticated).

10. NATIONAL POULTRY FOOD No. 2A (GROWERS' MASH OR PELLETS FOR
WINTER FEEDING)

	Percentage by Weight	
(1) The compound shall—	Minimum	Maximum
(*a*) conform to the following analysis:—		
Oil	2½	—
Albuminoids (protein)	15	18
Fibre	—	8½
Calcium expressed as calcium carbonate ...	2½	3½
Chlorine expressed as sodium chloride ...	¼	1
(*b*) contain the following:—		
Wheat by-products	10	—
Cereals	10	—
Low protein oilseed cake	—	15
Any animal protein rich substances	5	10
Molasses	—	5

(2) The compound shall contain cod-liver oil equivalent to either—

(*a*) not less than one per cent. of cod-liver oil
containing 500 international units of Vitamin
A and 50 B.S.I. units of Vitamin D per
gramme, or

(*b*) not less than one half of one per cent. of cod-
liver oil containing 800 international units of
Vitamin A and 100 B.S.I. units of Vitamin D
per gramme.

(3) The compound shall not contain any cottonseed
cake or cottonseed meal (decorticated or undecorticated).

11. NATIONAL BABY CHICK FOOD (BABY CHICK MASH OR PELLETS)

	Percentage by Weight	
(1) The compound shall—	Minimum	Maximum
(*a*) conform to the following analysis:—		
Oil	2½	—
Albuminoids (protein)	16	20
Fibre	—	6
Calcium expressed as calcium carbonate ...	2½	4
Chlorine expressed as sodium chloride ...	¼	¾

11. NATIONAL BABY CHICK FOOD—*cont.*

	Percentage by Weight	
	Minimum	*Maximum*

(1) The compound shall—
   (*b*) contain the following:—

	Minimum	Maximum
Wheat by-products	10	35
Maize	20	25
Dried potato products	—	15
Barley	10	15
Oats	—	20
Wheat	—	20
Low protein oilseed cake	—	5
Any animal protein rich substances of which not less than 5 per cent. by weight of the completed compound shall be fish meal including herring meal	7½	10
Dried-milk products other than dried whey powder	6	7½
Molasses	—	5

(2) The compound shall contain cod-liver oil equivalent to either—
   (*a*) not less than one per cent. of cod-liver oil containing 500 international units of Vitamin A and 50 B.S.I. units of Vitamin D per gramme, or
   (*b*) not less than one half of one per cent. of cod-liver oil containing 800 international units of Vitamin A and 100 B.S.I. units of Vitamin D per gramme.

(3) One-half per cent. unextracted dried yeast may be substituted for each one per cent. of dried-milk products.

(4) " D " flour may be substituted for wheat by-products up to a maximum of 10 per cent. by weight of the completed compound.

(5) The compound shall not contain any—
   (*a*) rye, rye products or rye by-products;
   (*b*) re-conditioned damaged grain;
   (*c*) cottonseed cake or cottonseed meal (decorticated or undecorticated);
   (*d*) rapeseed products or rapeseed by-products;
   (*e*) extracted palm kernel meal or extracted copra meal.

NOTES

1. The following ingredients may be in the form of licensed concentrates:—
Animal protein rich substances;
High protein oilseed cake;
Dried-milk products (except dried whey powder);
Minerals;
Cod-liver oil or cod-liver oil substitutes as prescribed in this Order.

2. Where cod-liver oil is prescribed as an ingredient, substances other than cod-liver oil may be used in its place;
Provided that—
   (*a*) the Vitamin A and Vitamin D contents thereof are not less than those prescribed for cod-liver oil;
   (*b*) such substances are warranted in writing by the maker thereof to be fully effective for poultry in accordance with the Chick Test of the British Standards Institution.

3. Where " D " flour is authorised as an ingredient, flour sweepings and/or sack shakings may be used in its place.

4. The conditions relating to the oil, albuminoid and fibre content found on analysis are subject to the limits of variation specified in the Fertilisers and Feeding Stuffs Regulations, 1932.

PART B.—LIVESTOCK MIXTURES

Column 1	Column 2	Column 3	
Description of Livestock Mixture	Conditions as to the ingredients which the Livestock Mixture may Contain*	Conditions as to proportions of ingredients	
		Percentage by Weight	
		Minimum	Maximum
National Horse Feed Mixture	Any two or more of the following:— Oats, barley, maize, beans, wheat by-products, dried grains, licensed molassed feeding stuffs	—	—
National Horse Chop Mixture No. 1	Oats and crushed oats and beans and kibbled beans (or any one or more of them)	.35	40
	Wheat by-products and dried grains (or any one or more of them) ...	10	15
	Chopped hay	35	50
	Chopped straw	—	15
National Horse Chop Mixture No. 2	Oats and crushed oats and beans and kibbled beans (or any one or more of them)	50	55
	Wheat by-products and dried grains (or any one or more of them) ...	10	20
	Chopped hay	25	35
	Chopped straw	—	10

*No livestock mixture mentioned in the first column of the foregoing table shall contain any ingredient not specified opposite to such livestock mixture in the second column of such table.

Column 1	Column 2	Column 3	
Description of Livestock Mixture	Conditions as to the ingredients which the Livestock Mixture may Contain*	Conditions as to proportions of ingredients	
		Percentage by Weight	
		Minimum	Maximum
National Cereal Mixture	Ground barley, ground wheat, maize meal, maize products, ground oats and ground dredge corn (or any one or more of them)	40	60
	Wheat by-products	—	40
	Low protein oilseed cake	5	15
	Licensed molassed feeding stuffs, dried grains and malt culms (or any one or more of them)	—	15
National Poultry Corn No. 1	Oats and clipped oats (or either of them)	—	50
	Maize	—	25
	Wheat	—	50
	Barley	—	50
	Rye	—	20
National Chick Feed	Cut wheat	40	80
	Fine or coarse maize grits	20	60

*No livestock mixture mentioned in the first column of the foregoing table shall contain any ingredient not specified opposite to such livestock mixture in the second column of such table.

AUTHOR INDEX

(497)

SUBJECT INDEX

Maize—*continued*
corn and cob meal, 132
flaked, 131
good supplements for, 131
varieties and characteristics, 130
Maize by-products, 132
(i) Bran, 132
(ii) Gluten meal, 132
(iii) Gluten feed, 132
(iv) Germ, 132
Maize germ protein, amino-acid composition, 36
Maize gluten protein, amino-acid composition, 36
Maize protein,
amino-acid composition, 36, 131
chemical score, 52
nutritive value, 54
Maize silage, 180
Malt sprouts or culms, 129
Maltase, 9
Maltose (malt sugar), occurrence and properties, 9
Manganese, functions in body, 78
Mangolds, 191, 193
Manioc meal, 232
Mannose, occurrence, 8
Mares, in-foal, feeding of, 385
Markers in feeding trials, 247
Marrow-stem kale, 198
Mashes, for poultry, 433
Mastication, 244
Material balances in nutrition, 246
Meadow,
general description, 151
plant species in, 164
water, 151
Meadow fescue, grass, characteristics, 143
Meadow foxtail, grass, 143
Meadow grass, rough-stalked, characteristics, 143
Meat, suitable for carnivora, 418
Meat " grain ", 27
Meat meal,
amino-acid composition, 37
different grades, 212
feeding to livestock, 215
method of production, 213
nature of, 213
Meat-and-bone meal, nature of, 213
Menhaden meal, 216
Metabolic water, 1
Metabolisable energy,
definition of, 280
factors affecting, 282
of foods, 281
Methane, production in rumen, 16
Methionine, 32, 36, 43
of peas and beans, 210
of sunflower seed, 210
Methionine requirements, species differences in, 44
Mice,
feeding of, 456
growth rates of, 457

Middlings, 126
Milk,
as indicator of protein needs, 256
composition of, 221, 257, 259
influence of specific foods on, 307
production standards for, 310
Milk, dried,
bacterial content, 224
for young stock, 261
nutritive value, 225
production methods, 225
Milk, whole, nutritive value, 220
Milk, skim or separated, 223
Milk ash, 222, 272
Milk composition, factors affecting, 268
Milk curd, in late lactation, 328
Milk energy, 269
Milk fat, 221
effects of excess cod-liver oil, 219
Milk production, dried grass for, 171
Milk protein, 221
amino-acid composition, 37
of different species, 257
Milk sugar, 222
Milk taint,
through cabbages, 198
through roots, 193
Millet, 134
Millet straw, 189
Mine horses, feeding of, 394
Mineral deficiencies in " normal " rations, 82
Mineral intake, of livestock on hay, 167
Mineral licks, for fattening cattle, 342
Mineral matter,
of animal foods, 62, 213, 216
of balanced rations, 82
of cereal grains, 62
of green foods, 197
of roots and tubers, 191
of straws, 187
Mineral requirements,
for growth, 259
for lactation, 272
for livestock, 82
for maintenance, 251
for pregnancy, 266
Minerals,
in rations for livestock, 293
Minerals. *See* Inorganic elements, 60
Mink,
balanced diets for, 422, 429
feeding for growth, 428
feeding routine, 423, 428
maintenance ration for, 424
maintenance standards for, 419
nutritional habits, 418
rations for breeding, 427
requirements for fat, 421
protein, 420
vitamins, 422
suitable foods for, 422, 429
" Mixed meals ", in pig feeding, 404
Moisture, determination of, 11
Molasses, 230
for silage preparation, 176

V.D.

33

Rat,
  feeding and management of, 43, 453
  growth of, 455
  importance of maternal nutrition, 456
  " refection " in, 455

Rations,
  environmental factors and, 316
  exercise and, 319
  factors concerned in framing, 291
  for bacon pigs, 415
  for breeding pigs, 409
  for cattle, average energies of, 284
  for chicks, 443
  for cows, 312
  for dogs, 425, 427
  for fattening cattle, 344
  for fox, 425, 427
  for horses, 393
  for milk production, 312
  for mink, 424, 427
  for poultry, 438, 443, 448
  for rabbits, 401
  for rats, 454
  for sheep, 360, 366, 370
  for young pigs, 412
  specimen, for dairy cows, 314

Red clover, 144
" Refection ", in rats, 455
Regularity, of feeding, need for, 324, 347, 378, 429, 447
Research, need for long range, 456
Reticulum, digestion in, 245
*Reviews cited (a selection):
  Amino-acid requirements, 58 (13)
  Calf feeding, 350 (12, 16)
  Cattle, protein requirements, 277 (20)
  Cows, protein requirements, 278 (42)
  Digestibility of foods, 18 (5)
  Dog, nutritional requirements, 118 (52)
  Dried grass and silage, 157 (9)
  Dynamics of body constituents, 29 (4)
  Efficiency of food conversion, 468 (2)
  Energy value of foods, 289 (10)
  Folic acid, 119 (96)
  Laboratory animals, needs of, 459 (2, 3, 4, 5)
  Microflora in ruminants, 18 (19)
  Mineral deficiencies and excesses, 83 (41)
  Nutritional deficiencies of livestock, 278 (35)
  Nutritive values of proteins, 58 (1)
  Pigs, feeding standards for, 119 (87)
  Poultry, feeding of, 278 (32), 452 (8)
  Poultry, mineral requirements, 452 (10)

Reviews cited—*continued*
  Rabbit feeding, 403 (6)
  Reproduction, viability of young, and diet, 459 (2)
  Ruminant digestion, 18 (19)
  Vitamin A needs of farm mammals, 278 (25)
  Water requirements of livestock, 6 (4)

Rhamnose, 8
Rhodopsin, 92
Ribgrass, 145
Riboflavin,
  carbohydrate metabolism and, 107
  chemistry of, 107
  dietary sources, 108
  species differences in needs for, 108
Rice, general characteristics, 133
Rice by-products, (i) bran, (ii) polishings, (iii) slump, 133
Rice protein, amino-acid composition, 36
Rice straw, 189
Rickets, 69
Rickets in dogs and foxes, 421
Rock phosphate, fluorine in, 80
Rodents, type of milk secreted by, 257, 272
Roots and tubers, comparative properties, 191
  for calves, 326, 332
  for cows, 308, 314
  for fattening cattle, 341
  for horses, 381, 387
  for sheep, 355, 359, 362, 364, 366, 368, 371
" Roup ", nutritional, 97
Rubner's Surface Law, 384. *See* Brody's Equation.
Rumen,
  food capacity of, 293
  functions of, 245
Rumen development, 330, 332, 358
Ruminants, anatomy and physiology of, 244
Ruminants. *See also* Cattle, Sheep and Goats.
Rutabaga, 193
Rye, 134
Rye-grasses, characteristics, 142
Rye protein, amino-acid composition, 36
Rye straw, 189

S

Safflower seed, 209
Sago pith meal, 232
Salt,
  addition to cattle rations, 73
  permitted content of foods, 73

* Extremely useful sources of additional reviews are " Nutrition Abstracts and Reviews " (Commonwealth Bureau of Animal Nutrition, Rowett Research Institute, Aberdeenshire, Scotland), the publications of the Ministry of Agriculture (H.M. Stationery Office), and the excellent " Yearbooks " of the United States Department of Agriculture (Superintendent of Documents, Washington, D.C., U.S.A.).

N.B.—Both the nature of the food and the circumstances in which it is fed require very careful consideration before any conclusions as to toxicity may be drawn.

PLATE 1

DIGESTIVE SYSTEMS OF SOME DOMESTIC ANIMALS

COW

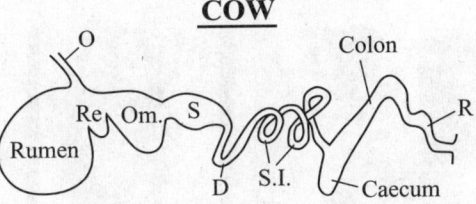

HORSE

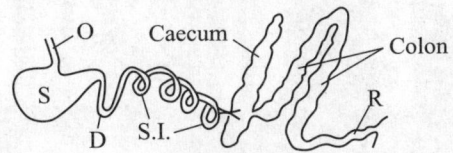

RABBIT

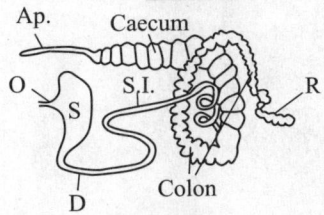

PIG

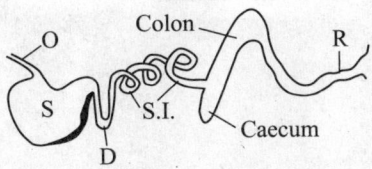

HEN (*Gallus*)

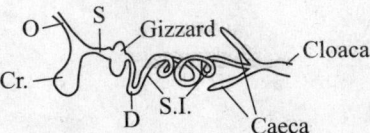

O=oesophagus; Re=reticulum; Om=omasum; S=true stomach; D=duodenum;
S.I.=small intestine; R=rectum; Ap=Vermiform appendix; Cr = crop.

OWEN (1946)   Proc. Nutrition Soc., 5, 186.

(*By courtesy of the author and the Nutrition Society*)

PLATE 2

MECHANICAL AND MICROBIAL AGENCIES
IN RUMINANT DIGESTION

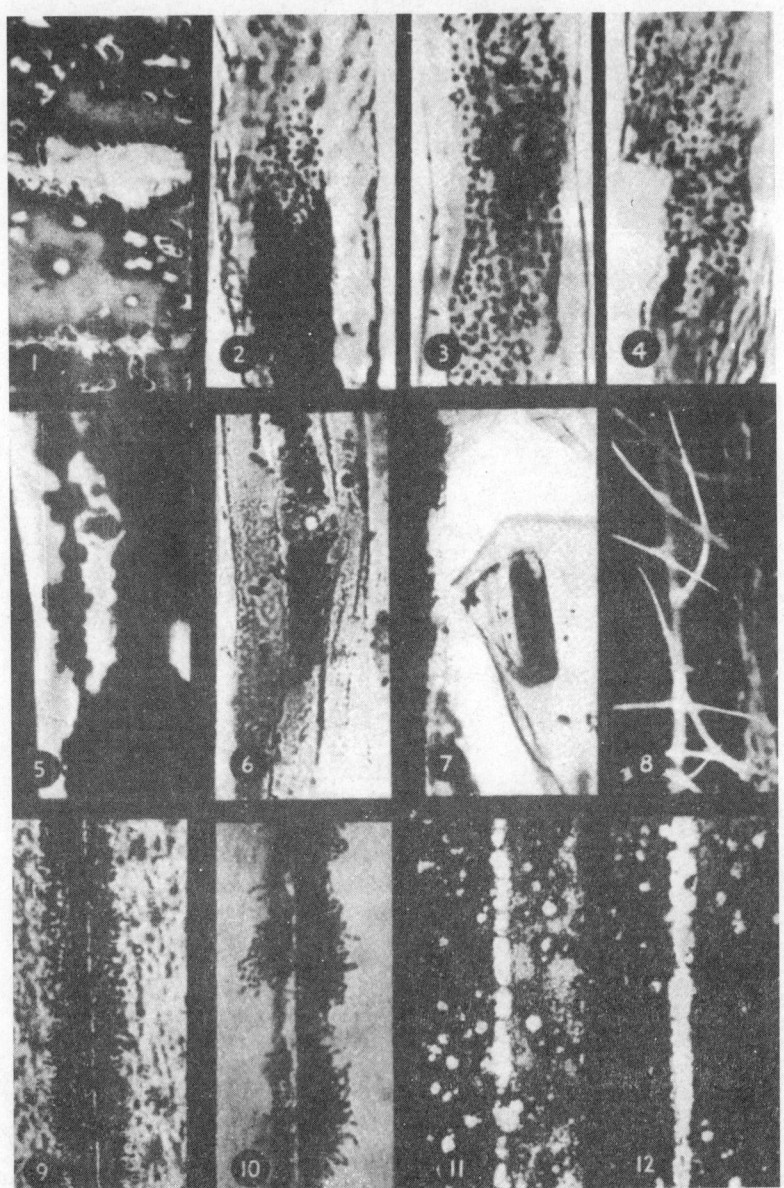

BAKER, HARRISS (1947)

Nutrition Abs. Rev., *17*, 3

(By courtesy of the author and the Imperial Bureau of Animal Nutrition)

The photomicrographs of Plate 2 show the breakdown of plant materials and of pure cellulose by microbial action.

DIGESTION *IN VIVO* AND *IN VITRO*.

1. Surface view of epidermal cells of grass blade taken from rumen of slaughtered sheep. Vibrios and small, large and giant iodophile coccoids within enzymic cavities.

× 800 (approx.)

2. Filter paper (cellulose) after 48 hours in rumen of fistula sheep. Small coccoids within lumen of disintegrating fibre.

× 1000 (approx.)

3. Filter paper after 48 hours incubation *in vitro* at 39° C. in ruminal filtrate inoculated with fresh rumen contents.

× 1000 (approx.)

4. Filter paper after 48 hours incubation *in vitro* at 39° C. in Vartiovaara's medium inoculated from sub-culture of rumen micro-organisms in same medium.

× 1000 (approx.)

5. Surface view of epidermal cells of blade of Timothy grass after 48 hours in rumen of fistula sheep, polarised light under crossed nicols, showing loss of birefrigence in the enzymic cavities.

× 800 (approx.)

6. Same preparation, nicols uncrossed, showing large iodophile micro-organisms *in situ*.

INDIGESTIBLE PORTIONS OF PLANT MATERIALS.

7. Surface view of epidermis of grass in late phase of disintegration, from rumen of slaughtered sheep, showing undigested cutinised residue comprising guard cell and cuticle.

× 500 (approx.)

8. Undigested residue of blade of Yorkshire Fog after 48 hours in rumen of fistula sheep, showing resistance of epidermal hairs and sclerenchyma. Photographed in low frequency ultra-violet light.

× 100 (approx.)

MICROBIAL ACTION ALONG LINES OF WEAKNESS.

The interesting feature of these photographs is that they show how mechanical disrupture of plant materials as in mastication, may facilitate microbial action.

9. Surface of scored cellophane after 48 hours in rumen of fistula sheep, showing preferential growth of micro-organisms along scratch.

× 100 (approx.)

10. Similar cellophane preparation showing individual colonies of micro-organisms.

× 500 (approx.)

11. Surface of scored cellophane. Congo red preparation showing preferential decomposition of cellulose along scratch. The white patches are enzymic cavities.

× 100 (approx.)

12 Similar preparation. Later phase showing complete fusion of enzymic cavities along scratch.

PLATE 3

INFLUENCE OF VITAMIN D ON BONE CALCIFICATION

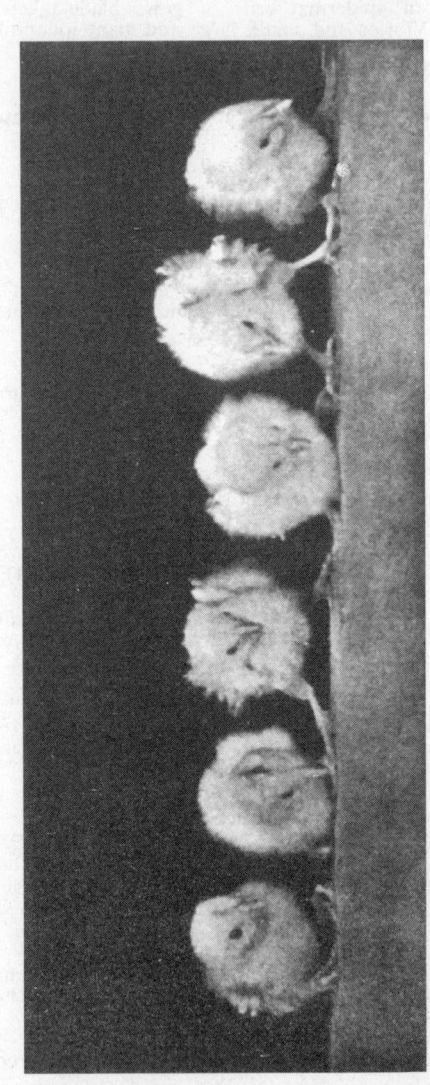

Rachitic chicks at 3 weeks old.

J. Agric. Sci., *31*, 161.

WRIGHT (1941)

(*By courtesy of the author and the Cambridge University Press*)

PLATE 4

INFLUENCE OF VITAMIN D ON BONE CALCIFICATION

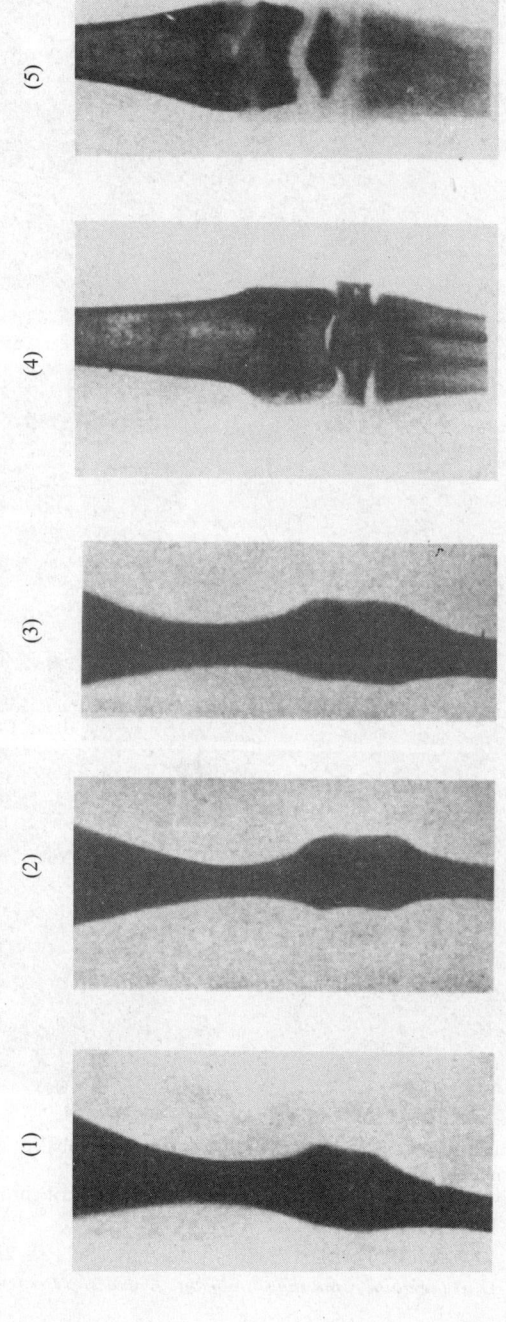

(1) Normal hock-joint at 3 weeks.
(2) and (3) Hock-joints from rachitic birds at 3 weeks.
(4) Normal calcification at 15 weeks old.
(5) Defective calcification at 15 weeks old.

WRIGHT (1941)

J. Agric. Sci., 31, 161.

(By courtesy of the author and the Cambridge University Press)

PLATE 5

COBALT AND COPPER DEFICIENCIES IN SHEEP

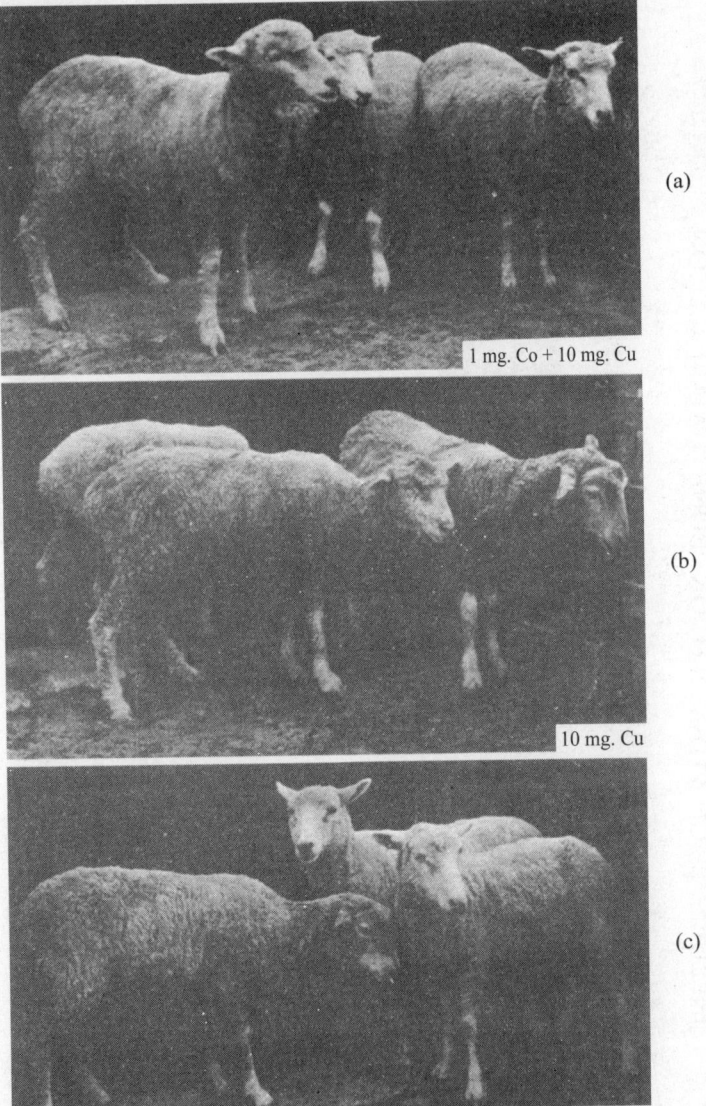

(a)

1 mg. Co + 10 mg. Cu

(b)

10 mg. Cu

(c)

1 mg. Co

(a) Normal, healthy alert sheep, receiving both copper and cobalt.
(b) Listless, rheumy animals receiving copper only.
(c) Sheep, with rather open fleeces, showing early symptoms of chronic copper deficiency.

MARSTON, LEE, McDONALD (1948)   J. Agric. Sci., *38*, 222.

(By courtesy of the author and the Cambridge University Press)

PLATE 6

THE EFFECT OF COPPER DEFICIENCY ON MERINO WOOL

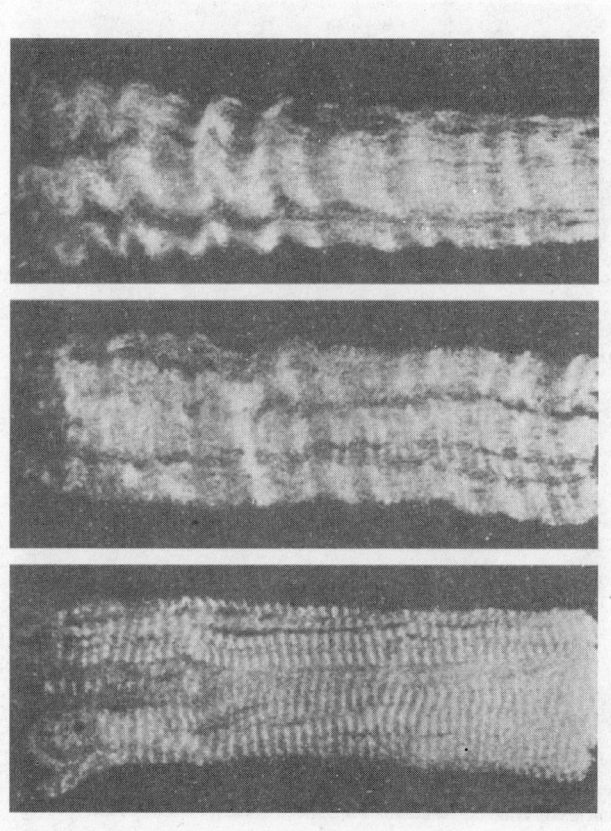

Nov. 1941   Nov. 1942   Nov. 1943

Deterioration of wool quality after sheep had been confined to copper deficient terrain.

MARSTON, LEE (1948)

J. Agric. Sci., 38, 229.

(By courtesy of the author and the Cambridge University Press)

PLATE 7

354

VITAMIN A DEFICIENCY IN THE PIG

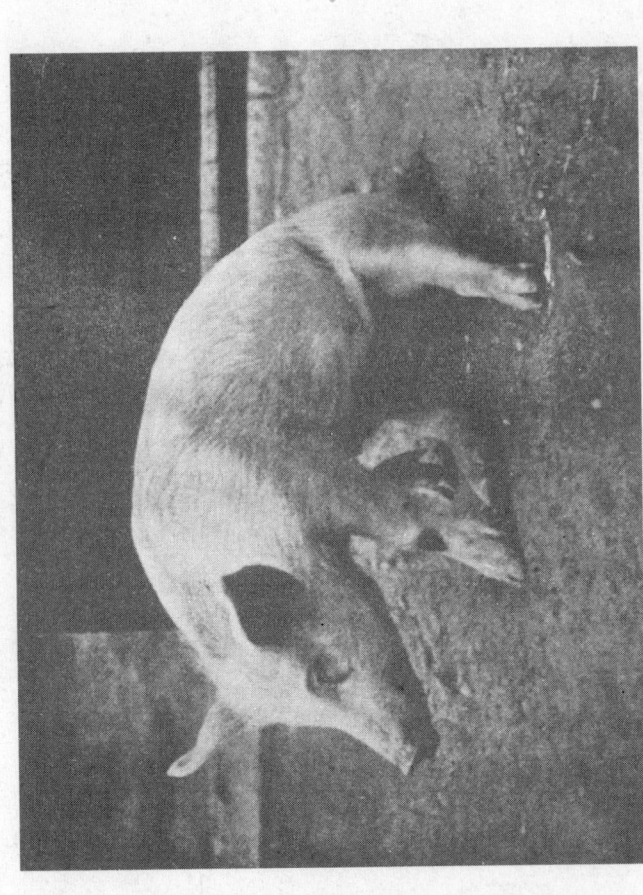

Pig, 267 days old, after being maintained on vitamin A-deficient diet since it commenced to eat. The pig was unable to move without support, vision had become defective and growth was much below normal.

FOOT, HENRY, KON & MACKINTOSH (1939)

J. Agric. Sci., 29, 142.

(By courtesy of the author and the Cambridge University Press)